Essentials of Gastroenterology

Essentials of Gastroenterology

Editor: Cyrus Holt

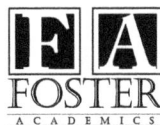

FOSTER
ACADEMICS

www.fosteracademics.com

www.fosteracademics.com

FA
FOSTER
ACADEMICS

Cataloging-in-Publication Data

Essentials of gastroenterology / edited by Cyrus Holt.
    p. cm.
Includes bibliographical references and index.
ISBN 978-1-63242-656-7
1. Gastroenterology. 2. Digestive organs--Diseases. 3. Internal medicine. I. Holt, Cyrus.
RC801 .E87 2019
616.3--dc23

Foster Academics,
118-35 Queens Blvd., Suite 400,
Forest Hills, NY 11375, USA

ISBN 978-1-63242-656-7 (Hardback)

Contents

Preface

Gastroenterology is a branch of medicine. Its area of focus is the functioning of the digestive system and its disorders. Hepatology and proctology are two important sub-fields of gastroenterology. Hepatology is a branch concerned with diseases related to the liver, bile ducts, gallbladder and pancreas, whereas, proctology is a branch that studies the disorders related to the rectum, colon and anus. Doctors who specialize in the field of gastroenterology are known as gastroenterologists. Some of the diagnostic and therapeutic procedures they perform include endoscopy, endoscopic ultrasound, endoscopic retrograde cholangiopancreatography and colonoscopy. The objective of this book is to give a general view of the different aspects of gastroenterology. It is a valuable compilation of topics, ranging from the basic to the most complex advancements in this field. Students, researchers, doctors and all associated with gastroenterology will benefit alike from this book.

The information shared in this book is based on empirical researches made by veterans in this field of study. The elaborative information provided in this book will help the readers further their scope of knowledge leading to advancements in this field.

Finally, I would like to thank my fellow researchers who gave constructive feedback and my family members who supported me at every step of my research.

Editor

Sex and ethnic/racial-specific risk factors for gallbladder disease

Jane C. Figueiredo[1,2*], Christopher Haiman[1,3], Jacqueline Porcel[3], James Buxbaum[4], Daniel Stram[1], Neal Tambe[1], Wendy Cozen[1,3,5], Lynne Wilkens[6], Loic Le Marchand[6] and Veronica Wendy Setiawan[1,3]

Abstract

Background: Gallbladder disease (GBD) is a highly prevalent condition; however, little is known about potential differences in risk factors by sex and ethnicity/race. Our aim was to evaluate dietary, reproductive and obesity-related factors and GBD in multiethnic populations.

Methods: We performed a prospective analysis from the Multiethnic Cohort study who self-identified as non-Hispanic White ($n = 32{,}103$), African American ($n = 30{,}209$), Japanese ($n = 35{,}987$), Native Hawaiian ($n = 6942$) and Latino ($n = 39{,}168$). GBD cases were identified using Medicare and California hospital discharge files (1993–2012) and self-completed questionnaires. We used exposure information on the baseline questionnaire to identify exposures of interest. Associations were estimated by hazard ratios and 95% confidence intervals using Cox models adjusted for confounders.

Result: After a median 10.7 years of follow-up, there were 13,437 GBD cases. BMI over 25 kg/m^2, diabetes, past and current smoking, red meat consumption, saturated fat and cholesterol were significant risk factors across ethnic/racial populations (p-trends < 0.01). Protective factors included vigorous physical activity, alcohol use, fruits, vegetables and foods rich in dietary fiber (p-trends < 0.01). Carbohydrates were inversely associated with GBD risk only among women and Latinos born in South America/Mexico (p-trend < 0.003). Parity was a significant risk factor among women; post-menopausal hormones use was only associated with an increased risk among White women (estrogen-only: HR = 1.24; 95% CI = 1.07–1.43 and estrogen + progesterone: HR = 1.23; 95% CI = 1.06–1.42).

Conclusion: Overall, dietary, reproductive and obesity-related factors are strong risk factors for GBD affecting men and women of different ethnicities/races; however some risk factors appear stronger in women and certain ethnic groups.

Keywords: Gallbladder, Stones, Cholecystectomy, Ethnicity/race

Background

Gallbladder disease (GBD) is a highly prevalent condition affecting up to 15% of the adult U.S. population and is a leading cause of hospital admissions [1]. In developed countries, GBD occurs largely as a result of formation of cholesterol gallstones. While most gallstones are clinically silent, 20% of people harboring stones experience biliary symptoms that at some point require surgical removal of the gallbladder [2]. Over 700,000 cholecystectomies are performed annually in the U.S. at a cost of approximately $6.5 billion [3].

The basis for GBD is multifactorial including infections, genetic susceptibility and modifiable lifestyle factors. Of particular note is the significant difference in rates of GBD by ethnicity/race and geography. The prevalence is highest among Hispanic populations of Central and South American and in individuals with Native American ancestry [4]. In the U.S., the prevalence of GBD is also notably higher in Hispanics compared to any other ethnic/racial group [5]. Genetic factors in part explain some of the observed racial differences in incidence; large population-based twin studies have estimated that genetic effects account for 25% (95% CI = 9–40%) [6]. Other factors may explain a larger fraction of the attributable risk associated with

* Correspondence: jane.figueiredo@cshs.org
[1]Department of Preventive Medicine, Keck School of Medicine of University of Southern California, Los Angeles, California, USA
[2]Samuel Oschin Comprehensive Cancer Institute, Cedars-Sinai Medical Center, Los Angeles, California, USA
Full list of author information is available at the end of the article

GBD, including lifestyle factors related to obesity and diet.

Diet constitutes a major source of cholesterol and several factors directly related to diet including high caloric intake and low dietary fiber intake, have been identified as risk factors for gallstone formation in both population-based studies and experimental animal models [7]. Although there exist inconsistencies across studies, diets high in vegetables, fruits and total fiber have been shown to reduce risk of GBD, and diets high in animal protein, carbohydrates and cholesterol increase risk [8–10]. Obesity, particularly abdominal or centripetal obesity, has also been observed as a risk factor for gallstone disease in some studies in the U.S. [11], Europe [12] and China [13]; other studies have observed no association in Mexicans [14] and Japanese [15] populations. Lifestyle behaviors that help maintain body weight including increased physical activity appear to lower risk in some [13, 16–18], but not all studies [19, 20]. Other behaviors including smoking and alcohol use have also been inconsistently associated with GBD risk [21–26], and may depend on patient characteristics including sex, ethnicity/race and country.

Several studies have documented a disproportionate number of women diagnosed with GBD compared to men. Overall, women are almost twice as likely as men to form gallstones, undergo cholecystectomy and to be diagnosed with gallbladder cancer [3], but these sex differences tends to narrow with increasing age [27]. The sex disparity has been attributed to hormonal factors, in particular estrogen. Several observational studies in non-Hispanic Whites have observed a modest increased risk of GBD associated with use of oral contraceptives [28] and post-menopausal hormones [29, 30]. Overall, parity appears to be the most consistent reproductive risk factor and has been observed in studies in the U.S. [31, 32].

In this study, we examined the association between dietary, reproductive and obesity-related factors and GBD by sex and ethnicity/race: African Americans, Japanese Americans, Native Hawaiians, Latinos and Whites, in the Multiethnic Cohort (MEC) study.

Methods
Study population
The MEC is an ongoing population-based prospective cohort study with over 215,000 men and women from Hawaii and California assembled between 1993 and 1996. The details of the study design and baseline characteristics have been published [33]. Briefly, the cohort is comprised predominantly of African Americans, Native Hawaiians, Japanese Americans, Latinos, and Whites (aged 45–75 years). The baseline mailed questionnaire assessed diet, lifestyle, anthropometrics, family and personal medical history, and for women menstrual,

reproductive history and exogenous hormone use. The MEC participants older than 65 years were linked to Centers for Medicare Services (CMS) claims (1999–2012) using Social Security number, sex, and date of birth, and 93% of these participants were successfully linked [34]. California participants were also linked to the Office of Statewide Health Planning and Development Hospital Discharge Data (1993–2012).

For this study, we excluded participants ($N = 22,824$) who were not from the five major ethnic groups or who had missing baseline information on the established GBD risk factors and important covariates (i.e. smoking status, body mass index, diabetes, alcohol intake, and education level). Participants with a diagnosis of gallbladder cancer identified via tumor registries ($N = 8$) or GBD identified via baseline questionnaire or the California hospital discharge data ($N = 1426$) before cohort entry were excluded. Hawaii participants who were not Medicare members (N = 14,035) or who were not fee-for-service (FFS) members were excluded ($N = 28,438$), as we had no opportunity to discover a GBD diagnosis in this group. A total of 144,409 eligible participants were available for analysis.

GBD case identification
We considered individuals with gallstones [International Classification of Diseases, 9th Revision (ICD-9), code 574.x], cholelithiasis (575.x) or those who had undergone a cholecystectomy (procedure codes 51.2× and CPT codes 47,480, 47,490, 47,562 47,563, 47,564, 47,600, 47,605, 47,610, 47,612, 47,620, 56,340, 56,341, 56,342) as cases with GBD. Cases were identified from one or more claims in the MedPAR (hospitalization) or the CHDD or two or more claims if they were from outpatient files. We identified 13,513 GBD cases through December 31, 2012; 76 cases were excluded because we could not identify eligible non-cases for the risk set.

Exposure assessment
Data on demographic factors and known/potential risk factors for GBD including anthropometry, alcohol intake, smoking history, physician-diagnosed type 2 diabetes, physical activity, and dietary factors were obtained from the MEC baseline questionnaire (available in Additional file 1). Body mass index (BMI) was calculated as weight in kg divided by height in m^2 and categorized as <25, 25- < 30, and ≥30 kg/m^2. Vigorous activity (hours/day) were categorized using quartile distributions in the cohort. Alcohol intake was categorized as non-drinkers, < 24, 24- ≤ 48, and > 48 g ethanol/day. Smoking status was categorized as never, past, and current, and for past and current smoking, they were further stratified by < 20 and ≥ 20 pack years. Dietary factors and nutrients (e.g. red meat, fruits, vegetables,

fiber, saturated fat, cholesterol, and carbohydrate, etc.) were categorized using overall quartile distributions in the cohort. The reference period for the dietary factors was the past year.

Statistical analysis

We used the date of the first GBD claim as the event date. As the time of diagnosis was not measured precisely, but was based on claim date, we used a Cox proportional hazards model for interval data based on a logistic model with a complementary log-log link. For each case, we constructed the set of at-risk individuals (alive and without a GBD diagnosis at the date of index case's diagnosis) matched on ethnicity, sex, exact birth year, study area, and if a case was identified via Medicare, length of Medicare coverage (±1 year). The associations between risk factors and GBD were estimated by hazard ratio (HR) and its 95% confidence interval (CI) adjusted for education, BMI, history of diabetes, smoking status and pack-years, and alcohol intake. Further adjustment for caloric intake was done for the diet analysis. Tests for trend were performed by entering the ordinal values representing categories of exposures as continuous variables in the models. Statistical analyses were performed with SAS 9.3 software (SAS Institute, Inc., Cary, NC). All p-values were two sided.

Results

After a mean 10.7 years of follow-up (SD = 5.0), there were 13,437 incident cases of GBD among the 144,409 at-risk cohort participants (Table 1). Overall the mean age at diagnosis was 73.5 (range = 45.3–94.8) years. The majority of cases of GBD were reports of gallstone only (40.2%) and 49.2% of all cases had a cholecystectomy. GBD cases included more women (57.9%) than men (42.1%). The cases' ethnicity breakdown was 35.2% Latinos, 23.3% Japanese, 19.4% whites, 18.4% African Americans, and 3.8% Native Hawaiians. The characteristics and distributions of selected risk factors by ethnicity/race are shown in Additional file 2: Table S1.

Both overweight and obese men and women were at significantly higher risk compared to those with a BMI under 25 kg/m² (p-trends < 0.0001, Table 2) with no differences by ethnicity/race (Table 3). Concomitant and past diabetes was associated with GBD risk in men (HR = 1.44; 95% CI = 1.34–1.55) and women (HR = 1.46; 95% CI = 1.37–1.56). Diabetes was also consistently associated with a higher risk of GBD in all ethnic/racial groups (p-values ≤ 0.0257). Past and current smoking were also significantly associated with risk of GBD among men and women (HR range = 1.09–1.37; with increasing RRs with increasing pack years; p-trends < 0.0001). By ethnicity/race, current smoking (> 20 pack-years) was associated with a

Table 1 Characteristics of study participants in the Multiethnic Cohort

	Total N = 144,409		GBD cases N = 13,437	
	N	%	N	%
Age at GBD occurrence, years				
Mean (range)			73.5 (45.3–94.8)	
Age at cohort entry, years				
< 50	19,307	13.4	758	5.6
50–54	22,658	15.7	1483	11.0
55–59	25,808	17.9	2542	18.9
60–64	26,559	18.4	2992	22.3
65–69	25,739	17.8	3053	22.7
≥ 70	24,338	16.9	2609	19.4
Gender				
Men	64,901	44.9	5658	42.1
Women	79,508	55.1	7779	57.9
Race/ethnicity				
White	32,103	22.2	2600	19.4
African American	30,209	20.9	2469	18.4
Native Hawaiian	6942	4.8	511	3.8
Japanese American	35,987	24.9	3133	23.3
Latino – US born	20,405	14.1	2398	17.9
Latino – Mexico/South America born	18,763	13.0	2326	17.3
Area				
Hawaii	51,579	35.7	4100	30.5
California	92,830	64.3	9337	69.5
Type				
Gallstones only			5395	40.2
Cholecystitis only			927	6.9
Cholecystectomy only			123	0.9
Gallstones and Cholecystitis			507	3.8
Gallstones and Cholecystectomy			3882	28.9
Cholecystitis and Cholecystectomy			505	3.8
Gallstones, Cholecystitis, and Cholecystectomy			2098	15.6
Year of diagnosis[a,b]				
1993–1997			1352	10.1
1998–2002			3362	25.0
2003–2007			4243	31.6
2008–2012			4480	33.3

[a]Gallbladder disease included gallstone (574.XX), cholecystitis (575.XX), and cholecystectomy (procedure codes 51.2X and CPT codes 47,480, 47,490, 47,562 47,563, 47,564, 47,600, 47,605, 47,610, 47,612, 47,620, 56,340, 56,341, 56,342), whichever came first
[b]Cases diagnosed before 1999 were identified from CHDD; between 1999 and 2012 were from both CHDD and Medicare

Table 2 Associations between modifiable risk factors and GBD risk by sex

Risk Factors	Men		Women	
	No. Cases	HR[a](95% CI)	No. Cases	HR[a](95% CI)
BMI (kg/m^2)				
< 25	1577	1.00 (ref.)	2463	1.00 (ref.)
25 - < 30	2612	1.23 (1.15–1.31)	2444	1.33 (1.25–1.41)
≥ 30	1076	1.55 (1.43–1.69)	2213	1.74 (1.63–1.85)
P trend		< .0001		< .0001
Diabetes				
No	4360	1.00 (ref.)	5968	1.00 (ref.)
Yes	905	1.44 (1.34–1.55)	1152	1.46 (1.37–1.56)
Smoking (pack-years)				
Never	1537	1.00 (ref.)	4003	1.00 (ref.)
Past, < 20	2013	1.09 (1.01–1.16)	1740	1.10 (1.04–1.16)
Past, ≥ 20	888	1.16 (1.07–1.27)	418	1.30 (1.17–1.44)
Current, < 20	411	1.16 (1.04–1.30)	582	1.17 (1.08–1.28)
Current, ≥ 20	416	1.22 (1.09–1.37)	377	1.37 (1.23–1.53)
P trend		< .0001		< .0001
Alcohol intake (ethanol g/day)				
0	2185	1.00 (ref.)	4755	1.00 (ref.)
< 24	2256	0.92 (0.86–0.97)	2083	0.86 (0.82–0.91)
24- ≤ 48	501	0.85 (0.77–0.94)	190	0.80 (0.69–0.93)
> 48	323	0.86 (0.76–0.97)	92	0.92 (0.74–1.14)
P trend		0.0001		< .0001
Vigorous Activity (hrs/day)				
0	2063	1.00 (ref.)	4567	1.00 (ref.)
> 0- ≤ 0.21	892	0.89 (0.82–0.96)	1078	0.90 (0.84–0.97)
> 0.21- ≤ 0.46	831	0.86 (0.79–0.94)	740	0.95 (0.87–1.03)
> 0.46	1479	0.80 (0.74–0.86)	735	0.90 (0.83–0.98)
P trend		< .0001		0.0041
Parity[b]				
0 children			771	1.00 (ref.)
1 child			746	1.09 (0.98–1.20)
2–3 children			2906	1.05 (0.97–1.14)
≥ 4 children			2899	1.14 (1.05–1.23)
P trend				0.0036
Age at First Live Birth (years)[b]				
No children			771	1.00 (ref.)
≤ 20			2505	1.10 (1.01–1.20)
21–30			3613	1.07 (0.99–1.15)
> 30			433	1.05 (0.94–1.19)
P trend				0.5200
Ever Used Birth Control[b]				
No			4714	1.00 (ref.)
Yes			2608	1.05 (0.99–1.11)

Table 2 Associations between modifiable risk factors and GBD risk by sex *(Continued)*

Risk Factors	Men		Women	
	No. Cases	HR[a](95% CI)	No. Cases	HR[a](95% CI)
Menopausal Hormone Use[b]				
Never users			3383	1.00 (ref.)
Past users			1442	0.97 (0.91–1.04)
Current estrogen-only			1113	1.09 (1.02–1.17)
Current estrogen + progesterone			1099	1.06 (0.99–1.14)

[a]HR stratified by set number (defined by matching factors: birth year, sex, ethnicity, study area, duration of Medicare enrollment—for cases identified from Medicare) and adjusted for smoking-pack years (never, past < 20, past ≥ 20, current < 20, current ≥ 20), alcohol intake (0, < 24, 24- ≤ 48, > 48 ethanol g/day), body mass index (< 25, 25- < 30, 30+ kg/m^2), diabetes (no/yes), and education (≤ High School, some college, ≥college graduate). Menopausal hormone use limited to postmenopausal women
[b]Females only

significant increased risk in Whites, African Americans and Japanese Americans and US-born Latinos (p-trends ≤ 0.0055). There was a non-significant increased risk between past or current smoking and GBD among Native Hawaiians; and only past smoking > 20 pack-years were significantly associated with GBD in Mexican/SA-born Latinos (HR = 1.38; 1.12–1.69). Daily consumption of alcohol significantly reduced the risk of GBD among men and women (p-trends ≤ 0.0001). Vigorous physical activity was also inversely associated with GBD risk in all categories for men and women compared to no activity (p-trends ≤ 0.004). The highest level of vigorous activity was associated with a reduced the risk of GBD among all groups; the estimates for the trend were non-significant in Native Hawaiians, Japanese and US-born Latinos, but in the same direction.

Among women, selected reproductive factors were evaluated as risk factors for GBD (Table 2). The risk associated with giving birth to 4 or more children was 14% higher compared to nulliparity (HR = 1.14; 95% CI = 1.05–1.23, p-trend = 0.0036). Women who reported having their first child prior to age 20 were at higher risk of GBD (HR = 1.10; 95% CI = 1.01–1.20) compared to those who never had children. Ever use of oral contraceptives was not associated with GBD; age at first use and duration of use did not modify this association (data not shown). Current use of estrogen-only menopausal hormones was also associated with GBD risk (HR = 1.09; 95% CI: 1.02–1.17). Post-menopausal estrogen and progesterone use was only marginally significant (HR = 1.06; 95% CI = 0.99–1.14). By ethnicity/race, these associations were limited to White women (HR = 1.24; 95% CI = 1.07–1.43 and HR = 1.23; 95% CI = 1.06–1.42, respectively, Table 3).

Significant trend in reducing risk was observed for increasing intake of vegetables, fruits and fiber-rich foods among men and women (p-trends < 0.0001, Table 4). Among women, increasing quartiles of carbohydrates were inversely associated with GBD risk (HR quartile 4 vs. quartile 1 = 0.86; 95% CI = 0.80–0.93, *p*-trend < 0.0001);

no association was observed in men. Conversely, significant increased risk of GBD was observed for increasing amount of red meat, and foods rich in saturated fat and cholesterol (p-trends < 0.0001). We observed consistently significant estimates of risk with GBD among Whites, African-Americans and Latinos for dietary fiber, vegetables, fruits, red meat, saturated fat and cholesterol (Table 5). Carbohydrates were not associated with GBD risk, except for Latinos from Mexico/South America (HR quartile 4 vs. quartile 1 = 0.82; 9%CI = 0.71–0.93, p-trend = 0.0028). Among Native Hawaiians and Japanese Americans we observed no statistically significant findings, except for a decreased risk of GBD with dietary fiber (p-trend = 0.015) and increased risk associated with red meat intake (p-trend = 0.0024) and saturated fat (p-trend = 0.045) among Japanese Americans.

In a sensitivity analysis excluding cases who had a cholecystectomy without a report of gallstone or chole-cystitis, we observed similar results (data not shown).

Discussion

These findings from the large population-based MEC, suggest that several lifestyle factors increase the risk of GBD in both men and women across different ethnic/racial groups. Our observations are consistent with previous observational studies with much smaller sample sizes, provide better estimation of risk associated with various factors, and importantly compare risks across understudied minorities in the U.S. Results from the Third National Health and Nutrition Examination Survey study was limited to three ethnic/racial populations and selected lifestyle factors over a shorter duration of follow-up and did not report on dietary factors [35]. Here we obtained stronger evidence for the role of dietary factors in GBD across all ethnic/racial groups, except Native Hawaiians. In addition, we confirm known associations between obesity, diabetes, physical activity, smoking and parity across ethnic/racial groups. We did not observe appreciable differences in the associations by sex or ethnicity/race, except for an

Table 3 Association between modifiable risk factors and GBD (HR[a] and 95% CI) by race/ethnicity

	NH-White N = 2600	African American N = 2469	Native Hawaiian N = 511	Japanese American N = 3133	Latino US born N = 2398	Latino Mexico/SA born N = 2326
BMI (kg/m²)						
< 25	1.00 (ref.)	1.00 (ref.)	1.00 (ref.)	1.00 (ref.)	1.00 (ref.)	1.00 (ref.)
25 - < 30	1.30 (1.19–1.43)	1.21 (1.08–1.36)	1.27 (0.99–1.63)	1.37 (1.26–1.48)	1.20 (1.08–1.34)	1.29 (1.15–1.44)
≥ 30	1.68 (1.50–1.87)	1.56 (1.39–1.75)	1.62 (1.26–2.10)	1.73 (1.51–1.99)	1.56 (1.39–1.75)	1.74 (1.54–1.97)
P trend	<.0001	<.0001	0.0002	<.0001	<.0001	<.0001
Diabetes						
No	1.00 (ref.)	1.00 (ref.)	1.00 (ref.)	1.00 (ref.)	1.00 (ref.)	1.00 (ref.)
Yes	1.35 (1.16–1.57)	1.58 (1.43–1.76)	1.33 (1.04–1.72)	1.27 (1.14–1.42)	1.57 (1.41–1.74)	1.47 (1.31–1.64)
Smoking (pack-years)						
Never	1.00 (ref.)	1.00 (ref.)	1.00 (ref.)	1.00 (ref.)	1.00 (ref.)	1.00 (ref.)
Past, < 20	1.03 (0.93–1.14)	1.17 (1.06–1.29)	1.00 (0.80–1.25)	1.11 (1.02–1.22)	1.12 (1.01–1.23)	1.07 (0.96–1.19)
Past, ≥ 20	1.10 (0.97–1.24)	1.32 (1.13–1.55)	0.93 (0.68–1.28)	1.34 (1.19–1.51)	1.09 (0.91–1.31)	1.38 (1.11–1.71)
Current, <20	1.33 (1.11–1.59)	1.26 (1.10–1.44)	1.06 (0.75–1.51)	1.05 (0.87–1.27)	1.10 (0.94–1.29)	1.11 (0.95–1.30)
Current, ≥ 20	1.30 (1.12–1.50)	1.50 (1.27–1.77)	0.87 (0.61–1.24)	1.3 (1.1–1.54)	1.38 (1.12–1.69)	0.90 (0.66–1.21)
P trend	<.0001	<.0001	0.5831	<.0001	0.0055	0.1849
Alcohol intake (ethanol g/day)						
0	1.00 (ref.)	1.00 (ref.)	1.00 (ref.)	1.00 (ref.)	1.00 (ref.)	1.00 (ref.)
< 24	0.86 (0.78–0.94)	0.89 (0.81–0.98)	0.94 (0.76–1.16)	0.93 (0.86–1.01)	0.89 (0.81–0.98)	0.84 (0.76–0.93)
24-≤ 48	0.82 (0.71–0.95)	0.94 (0.76–1.16)	1.05 (0.71–1.56)	0.83 (0.7–0.99)	0.77 (0.63–0.94)	0.74 (0.57–0.94)
> 48	0.83 (0.69–1.00)	1.16 (0.93–1.46)	0.77 (0.45–1.32)	0.70 (0.52–0.93)	0.82 (0.65–1.03)	0.87 (0.65–1.16)
P trend	0.0011	0.5926	0.4816	0.0016	0.0016	0.0008
Vigorous activity (hrs/day)						
0	1.00 (ref.)	1.00 (ref.)	1.00 (ref.)	1.00 (ref.)	1.00 (ref.)	1.00 (ref.)
> 0- ≤ 0.21	0.91 (0.81–1.03)	0.96 (0.85–1.07)	1.20 (0.91–1.59)	0.91 (0.82–1.01)	0.87 (0.77–0.99)	0.79 (0.69–0.91)
> 0.21- ≤ 0.46	0.88 (0.77–1.00)	0.80 (0.69–0.93)	1.10 (0.83–1.46)	1.05 (0.94–1.18)	0.94 (0.82–1.07)	0.79 (0.68–0.92)
> 0.46	0.79 (0.71–0.89)	0.68 (0.59–0.80)	0.96 (0.75–1.24)	0.92 (0.82–1.03)	0.97 (0.86–1.09)	0.80 (0.71–0.91)
P trend	<.0001	<.0001	0.7369	0.3474	0.4939	0.0001
Parity[b]						
0 children	1.00 (ref.)	1.00 (ref.)	1.00 (ref.)	1.00 (ref.)	1.00 (ref.)	1.00 (ref.)
1 child	1.12 (0.91–1.37)	1.13 (0.94–1.35)	1.26 (0.61–2.60)	1.04 (0.84–1.29)	1.19 (0.88–1.62)	0.89 (0.66–1.20)
2–3 children	1.11 (0.95–1.31)	1.01 (0.86–1.19)	0.97 (0.55–1.72)	1.14 (0.97–1.34)	1.00 (0.79–1.27)	0.89 (0.70–1.12)
≥ 4 children	1.09 (0.91–1.29)	1.12 (0.95–1.32)	1.14 (0.65–1.99)	1.14 (0.94–1.37)	1.15 (0.92–1.45)	1.08 (0.87–1.33)
P trend	0.4436	0.3186	0.6047	0.0987	0.1931	0.0851
Age at first live birth (years)[b]						
No children	1.00 (ref.)	1.00 (ref.)	1.00 (ref.)	1.00 (ref.)	1.00 (ref.)	1.00 (ref.)
≤ 20	1.20 (1.00–1.44)	1.04 (0.89–1.22)	1.19 (0.68–2.10)	1.09 (0.86–1.38)	1.10 (0.87–1.39)	0.99 (0.79–1.23)
21–30	1.07 (0.91–1.25)	1.06 (0.90–1.24)	0.94 (0.54–1.65)	1.15 (0.98–1.34)	1.07 (0.85–1.34)	0.99 (0.80–1.23)
> 30	0.98 (0.76–1.27)	1.14 (0.87–1.50)	1.03 (0.40–2.67)	1.11 (0.89–1.38)	1.10 (0.76–1.60)	0.97 (0.72–1.30)
P trend	0.6757	0.3744	0.2289	0.1600	0.8651	0.9194
Ever used birth control[b]						
No	1.00 (ref.)	1.00 (ref.)	1.00 (ref.)	1.00 (ref.)	1.00 (ref.)	1.00 (ref.)
Yes	1.11 (0.98–1.25)	1.01 (0.89–1.13)	0.80 (0.59–1.08)	1.10 (0.96–1.25)	1.02 (0.89–1.17)	1.06 (0.92–1.21)

Table 3 Association between modifiable risk factors and GBD (HR[a] and 95% CI) by race/ethnicity *(Continued)*

	NH-White N = 2600	African American N = 2469	Native Hawaiian N = 511	Japanese American N = 3133	Latino US born N = 2398	Latino Mexico/SA born N = 2326
Menopausal Hormone Use[b]						
Never users	1.00 (ref.)	1.00 (ref.)	1.00 (ref.)	1.00 (ref.)	1.00 (ref.)	1.00 (ref.)
Past users	0.94 (0.81–1.10)	0.95 (0.84–1.08)	0.90 (0.63–1.28)	1.03 (0.88–1.20)	1.09 (0.93–1.27)	0.89 (0.75–1.04)
Current estrogen only	1.24 (1.07–1.43)	1.14 (0.98–1.34)	0.83 (0.55–1.24)	1.06 (0.92–1.23)	0.94 (0.79–1.13)	1.14 (0.92–1.40)
Current estrogen + progesterone	1.23 (1.06–1.42)	1.14 (0.93–1.39)	0.85 (0.57–1.27)	0.97 (0.84–1.11)	1.07 (0.88–1.28)	0.96 (0.76–1.21)

[a]HR stratified by set number (defined by matching factors: birth year, ethnicity, study area, duration of Medicare enrollment—for cases identified from Medicare) and adjusted for smoking-pack years (never, past <20, past ≥20, current <20, current ≥20), alcohol intake (0, <24, 24- ≤ 48, >48 ethanol g/day), body mass index (<25, 25- < 30, 30+ kg/m2), diabetes (no/yes), and education (≤ High School, some college, ≥college graduate)
[b]Females only

increased risk of post-menopausal hormone use in White women.

Cholesterol hypersaturation of the bile and cholesterol nucleation leading to dysmotility have been implicated in the pathogenesis of GBD [36]. These observations have led to intense investigation of the roles of specific dietary components in gallbladder physiology and gallstone formation. Although results have not been entirely consistent across studies likely due to methodological differences, the overall body of evidence supports the hypothesis that a diet characterized by high caloric intake, refined carbohydrates, animal protein and cholesterol and low in vegetables and dietary fiber increase risk of GBD [8–10]. Early ecological studies noted an increased prevalence of GBD associated with diets characterized by higher intake of fat and refined carbohydrate and lower dietary fiber in the U.S. and Japan [37, 38]. In the Nurses' Health Study of primarily non-Hispanic women, fruit and vegetable consumption were significantly inversely associated with risk of cholecystectomy [39]. Data in other ethnic/racial group are limited; a study from the Third National Health and Nutrition Examination Survey among Mexican Americans investigated dietary patterns and risk of GBD finding distinct differences by sex but no significant associations with GBD risk [40].

Obesity and associated co-morbidities, strongly linked with poor diet and positive energy balance, have also been recognized as important risk factors for GBD. In the Nurses' Health Study among largely non-Hispanic White women, obese participants (BMI ≥ 30 kg/m^2) had a 2-fold excess risk and extremely obese women (BMI ≥ 45 kg/m^2) had a 7-fold increased risk of symptomatic gallstones compared to women with a BMI < 24 kg/m^2 [41]. While studies in China [13], Mexico [14] and Japan [15] have reported variable results, although the overall summary estimates have suggested an increased risk associated with obesity. We also observed a strong association between type II diabetes and GBD risk across ethnic/racial

populations. In agreement, the Strong Heart Study also reported that diabetes was associated with GBD in women; however their analysis did not confirm the association among men [35]. In agreement with our results, low physical activity, high body-mass-index and diabetes were found to increase GBD risk in most [13, 16–18, 42], but not all studies [19, 20].

Smoking is a known risk factor for diseases in several organs, including those not directly exposed to inhaled smoke, including the gastrointestinal tract. In the gallbladder, smoking is suspected to lead to disruption in emptying, which is thought to be associated with gallstone formation. Both bile stasis and disrupted gallbladder motility are important factors for gallstone formation. Several studies have investigated the association between smoking and GBD with inconsistent results; among Japanese men and women some studies [21, 22], but not all [23, 24] have observed an increased risk associated with active smoking; similar inconsistencies have been observed among Europeans [25, 26]. In terms of alcohol use, most previous studies in the U.S., Europe and Japan have found an inverse association between alcohol intake and GBD [15, 21, 22, 43–45]. Moderate alcohol intake may protect against gallstone development through its association with reduced biliary cholesterol saturation and higher serum HDL [46]. Overall our results across a large sample size of diverse populations provide confirmatory evidence of the increased risk associated with smoking and decreased risk associated with alcohol use.

Sex disparities in the incidence of several diseases have been reported. For GBD, the rates reported are 1.5–3-times higher in women compared to men [47]. Possible explanations for these discrepancies may be due to sex hormones and potentially other differences in dietary patterns and tobacco and alcohol exposures or other lifestyle-related behaviors. Overall, in agreement with our study, pregnancy has been found to be the most consistent risk factor for GBD in previous studies [48], in particular among overweight or obese women [49].

Table 4 Associations between selected dietary factors and GBD by sex

	Men		Women	
	No. Cases	HR[a](95% CI)	No. Cases	HR[a](95% CI)
Dietary Fiber (g/1000 kcal/day)				
≤ 9.0	1723	1.00 (ref.)	1409	1.00 (ref.)
> 9.0 – ≤ 11.6	1587	1.00 (0.93–1.08)	1912	0.96 (0.90–1.04)
> 11.6 – ≤ 14.8	1300	0.91 (0.84–0.98)	2142	0.88 (0.81–0.94)
> 14.8	1048	0.80 (0.74–0.88)	2316	0.81 (0.75–0.87)
P trend		< .0001		< .0001
Total Vegetables (g/1000 kcal/day)				
≤ 109.3	1744	1.00 (ref.)	1569	1.00 (ref.)
> 109.3 – ≤ 150.1	1582	1.00 (0.93–1.07)	1788	0.96 (0.89–1.03)
> 150.1 – ≤ 202.6	1298	0.89 (0.82–0.96)	2084	0.96 (0.89–1.02)
> 202.6	1034	0.85 (0.78–0.92)	2338	0.89 (0.83–0.95)
P trend		< .0001		0.0007
Total Fruits (g/1000 kcal/day)				
≤ 78.9	1741	1.00 (ref.)	1591	1.00 (ref.)
> 78.9 – ≤ 145.9	1558	0.93 (0.87–1.00)	1723	0.91 (0.84–0.97)
> 145.9 – ≤ 239.8	1307	0.89 (0.82–0.96)	2128	0.93 (0.87–1.00)
> 239.8	1052	0.93 (0.85–1.01)	2337	0.85 (0.80–0.91)
P trend		0.0216		<.0001
Red Meat (g/1000 kcal/day)				
≤ 14.3	1022	1.00 (ref.)	2087	1.00 (ref.)
> 14.3 – ≤ 24.4	1305	1.07 (0.98–1.17)	2057	1.08 (1.01–1.15)
> 24.4 – ≤ 36.1	1528	1.08 (0.99–1.17)	1860	1.13 (1.06–1.21)
> 36.1	1803	1.13 (1.04–1.23)	1775	1.23 (1.15–1.31)
P trend		0.0055		<.0001
% Calories from Saturated Fat				
≤ 7.1	1269	1.00 (ref.)	1878	1.00 (ref.)
> 7.1 – ≤ 8.9	1433	1.12 (1.04–1.21)	1875	1.02 (0.96–1.10)
> 8.9 – ≤ 10.8	1423	1.09 (1.00–1.18)	1962	1.11 (1.04–1.19)
> 10.8	1533	1.14 (1.04–1.24)	2064	1.20 (1.12–1.29)
P trend		0.0134		< .0001
Cholesterol (mg/1000 kcal/day)				
≤ 77.8	1241	1.00 (ref.)	1925	1.00 (ref.)
> 77.8 – ≤ 101.7	1383	1.06 (0.98–1.15)	1937	1.06 (0.99–1.13)
> 101.7 – ≤ 128.7	1456	1.08 (1.00–1.17)	1966	1.14 (1.06–1.22)
> 128.7	1578	1.06 (0.98–1.15)	1951	1.22 (1.14–1.31)
P trend		0.1823		< .0001
% Calories from Carbohydrate				
≤ 46.1	1619	1.00 (ref.)	1676	1.00 (ref.)
> 46.1 – ≤ 52.1	1494	1.00 (0.93–1.08)	1907	0.94 (0.88–1.01)
> 52.1 – ≤ 58.2	1327	0.98 (0.90–1.06)	2083	0.91 (0.85–0.97)
> 58.2	1218	0.99 (0.91–1.09)	2113	0.86 (0.80–0.93)
P trend		0.7258		< .0001

[a]HR stratified by set number (defined by matching factors: birth year, sex, ethnicity, study area, duration of Medicare enrollment) and adjusted for smoking-pack years (never, past <20, past ≥20, current <20, current ≥20), alcohol intake (0, <24, 24- ≤ 48, >48 ethanol g/day), body mass index (<25, 25- < 30, 30+ kg/m2), diabetes (no/yes), calories, and education (≤ High School, some college, ≥college graduate)

Table 5 Associations between selected dietary factors and GBD (HR[a] and 95% CI) by race/ethnicity

	NH-White N = 2600	African American N = 2469	Native Hawaiian N = 511	Japanese American N = 3133	Latino US born N = 2398	Latino Mexico/SA born N = 2326
Dietary Fiber (g/1000 kcal/day)						
≤ 9.0	1.00 (ref.)	1.00 (ref.)	1.00 (ref.)	1.00 (ref.)	1.00 (ref.)	1.00 (ref.)
> 9.0 – ≤ 11.6	0.91 (0.82–1.03)	0.90 (0.80–1.01)	0.84 (0.66–1.07)	1.04 (0.94–1.14)	1.11 (0.97–1.27)	0.98 (0.83–1.16)
> 11.6 – ≤ 14.8	0.92 (0.82–1.03)	0.82 (0.73–0.93)	0.79 (0.60–1.03)	0.99 (0.89–1.10)	0.94 (0.82–1.08)	0.80 (0.68–0.94)
> 14.8	0.75 (0.66–0.85)	0.78 (0.68–0.88)	0.83 (0.62–1.12)	0.85 (0.76–0.96)	0.89 (0.77–1.02)	0.78 (0.67–0.91)
P trend	< .0001	< .0001	0.1166	0.0146	0.0033	< .0001
Total Vegetables (g/1000 kcal/day)						
≤ 109.3	1.00 (ref.)	1.00 (ref.)	1.00 (ref.)	1.00 (ref.)	1.00 (ref.)	1.00 (ref.)
> 109.3 – ≤ 150.1	1.03 (0.92–1.15)	0.99 (0.89–1.10)	0.91 (0.70–1.18)	1.02 (0.92–1.13)	0.89 (0.79–1.00)	0.94 (0.82–1.09)
> 150.1 – ≤ 202.6	0.91 (0.81–1.02)	0.88 (0.78–0.99)	1.02 (0.78–1.33)	0.98 (0.88–1.09)	0.91 (0.81–1.03)	0.92 (0.80–1.05)
> 202.6	0.86 (0.76–0.97)	0.88 (0.78–0.99)	0.94 (0.71–1.23)	0.93 (0.83–1.04)	0.83 (0.74–0.94)	0.85 (0.74–0.97)
P trend	0.0024	0.0094	0.8386	0.1317	0.0079	0.0085
Total Fruits (g/1000 kcal/day)						
≤ 78.9	1.00 (ref.)	1.00 (ref.)	1.00 (ref.)	1.00 (ref.)	1.00 (ref.)	1.00 (ref.)
> 78.9 – ≤ 145.9	0.85 (0.76–0.95)	0.83 (0.74–0.94)	1.03 (0.80–1.33)	0.93 (0.84–1.04)	1.08 (0.96–1.21)	0.89 (0.78–1.00)
> 145.9 – ≤ 239.8	0.81 (0.72–0.91)	0.92 (0.82–1.04)	0.96 (0.73–1.26)	0.94 (0.85–1.05)	1.02 (0.90–1.15)	0.90 (0.79–1.02)
> 239.8	0.85 (0.76–0.96)	0.83 (0.74–0.94)	0.76 (0.57–1.02)	0.93 (0.84–1.04)	1.02 (0.90–1.16)	0.78 (0.69–0.88)
P trend	0.0076	0.0245	0.0586	0.3021	0.9962	0.0002
Red Meat (g/1000 kcal/day)						
≤ 14.3	1.00 (ref.)	1.00 (ref.)	1.00 (ref.)	1.00 (ref.)	1.00 (ref.)	1.00 (ref.)
> 14.3 – ≤ 24.4	1.06 (0.95–1.18)	1.12 (1.00–1.27)	0.88 (0.66–1.18)	1.06 (0.96–1.18)	1.08 (0.94–1.23)	1.10 (0.97–1.25)
> 24.4 – ≤ 36.1	1.18 (1.06–1.32)	1.08 (0.95–1.22)	0.91 (0.69–1.22)	1.15 (1.04–1.27)	1.06 (0.93–1.21)	1.09 (0.96–1.24)
> 36.1	1.13 (1.00–1.28)	1.32 (1.17–1.49)	1.20 (0.91–1.58)	1.16 (1.04–1.30)	1.15 (1.01–1.30)	1.13 (1.00–1.28)
P trend	0.0100	< .0001	0.1033	0.0024	0.0545	0.0934
% Calories from Saturated Fat						
≤ 7.1	1.00 (ref.)	1.00 (ref.)	1.00 (ref.)	1.00 (ref.)	1.00 (ref.)	1.00 (ref.)
> 7.1 – ≤ 8.9	1.02 (0.91–1.15)	1.03 (0.90–1.18)	1.16 (0.91–1.49)	1.07 (0.98–1.17)	1.11 (0.95–1.29)	1.08 (0.94–1.25)
> 8.9 – ≤ 10.8	1.07 (0.95–1.20)	1.08 (0.95–1.23)	1.01 (0.77–1.32)	1.11 (1.00–1.23)	1.18 (1.02–1.36)	1.14 (0.99–1.30)
> 10.8	1.13 (1.00–1.27)	1.18 (1.04–1.35)	1.06 (0.78–1.42)	1.09 (0.93–1.27)	1.20 (1.04–1.39)	1.27 (1.11–1.46)
P trend	0.0361	0.0039	0.9779	0.0452	0.0104	0.0003
Cholesterol (mg/1000 kcal/day)						
≤ 77.8	1.00 (ref.)	1.00 (ref.)	1.00 (ref.)	1.00 (ref.)	1.00 (ref.)	1.00 (ref.)
> 77.8 – ≤ 101.7	1.05 (0.94–1.18)	1.09 (0.95–1.26)	0.94 (0.72–1.23)	1.09 (1.00–1.19)	1.09 (0.96–1.25)	1.04 (0.91–1.18)
> 101.7 – ≤ 128.7	1.08 (0.97–1.21)	1.19 (1.04–1.36)	1.15 (0.88–1.50)	1.03 (0.93–1.14)	1.24 (1.10–1.41)	1.08 (0.96–1.23)
> 128.7	1.18 (1.05–1.33)	1.20 (1.05–1.36)	1.30 (0.99–1.70)	1.10 (0.98–1.23)	1.16 (1.02–1.32)	1.14 (1.01–1.30)
P trend	0.0069	0.0043	0.0252	0.1768	0.0115	0.0271
% Calories from Carbohydrate						
≤ 46.1	1.00 (ref.)	1.00 (ref.)	1.00 (ref.)	1.00 (ref.)	1.00 (ref.)	1.00 (ref.)
> 46.1 – ≤ 52.1	0.99 (0.88–1.10)	0.89 (0.80–0.99)	0.89 (0.66–1.20)	1.03 (0.89–1.19)	1.12 (1.00–1.25)	0.88 (0.78–1.00)
> 52.1 – ≤ 58.2	0.94 (0.84–1.06)	0.92 (0.82–1.03)	0.92 (0.69–1.24)	1.00 (0.86–1.15)	1.01 (0.90–1.15)	0.84 (0.74–0.96)
> 58.2	0.90 (0.80–1.03)	0.89 (0.78–1.01)	0.93 (0.69–1.26)	0.96 (0.83–1.11)	1.01 (0.88–1.16)	0.82 (0.71–0.93)
P trend	0.0891	0.0767	0.8459	0.2587	0.8483	0.0028

[a]HR stratified by matching factors (birth year, ethnicity, study area, duration of Medicare enrollment) and adjusted for smoking-pack years (never, past < 20, past ≥ 20, current < 20, current ≥ 20), alcohol intake (0, < 24, 24-≤ 48, > 48 ethanol g/day), body mass index (< 25, 25-< 30, 30+ kg/m2), diabetes (no/yes), calories, and education (≤ High School, some college, ≥ college graduate

Pregnancy is a critical time period of increased risk of insulin resistance (gestational diabetes) [50] as well as biliary sludge, a suspected to be a potential precursor to gallstones. Biliary sludge, a mixture of cholesterol and calcium bilirubinate crystals in bile, develops in up to 30% of women [31] and likely represents a precursor of gallstones [51]. We observed the highest risk of GBD among women who reported having a child before age 20. No other reproductive variables were significant in our study, except for postmenopausal use among White women only. A previous meta-analysis found highly inconsistent results across studies for oral contraceptives; the summary estimate was RR = 1.36 (95% CI = 1.15–1.62) [28]. Secondary analysis of randomized clinical trials of post-menopausal hormones among largely non-Hispanic Whites have observed significantly elevated risk of GBD among women randomized to the treatment arm compared to placebo; in the Heart and Estrogen/progestin Replacement Study, RR (estrogen + progestin) =1.38 (95% CI, 1.00–1.92) [29] and the Women's Health Initiative, RR (estrogen-only) = 1.67 (95% CI = 1.35–2.06) and RR (estrogen + progestin) = 1.59 (95% CI = 1.28–1.97) [30].

Our study has several strengths and some limitations. To date no other study has been able to compare risk estimates across sex and ethnicity/race in a single study with uniform data collection on risk factors collected up to 19 years prior to diagnosis. In addition, the MEC has been shown to be representative of the populations represented in the cohort [33], and thus our results are broadly generalizable to U.S. populations. We also excluded subjects with GBD at baseline to investigate prospectively risk factors for incident GBD. One limitation is that our analysis is based on exposure data collected from self-reported questionnaires; however measurement error is likely to be non-differential. Furthermore, we defined GBD as any occurrence of gallstones, cholelithiasis and cholecystectomy from claim records. The validity of the algorithm to accurately define cases has not been evaluated in the MEC; however, in our own sensitivity analysis comparing results obtained with our broad definition of GBD with those obtained using claims of cholecystectomy alone, we did not observe significant differences in the results.

Conclusion

Our study represents the first prospective analysis from multiethnic US populations with varying exposure levels across men and women by ethnicity/race and risk for GBD. Our results strongly support a substantial role of several lifestyle factors in the development of GBD across diverse populations.

Abbreviations
BMI: Body Mass Index; CI: Confidence interval; GBD: Gallbladder disease; HR: Hazard ratio; MEC: Multiethnic cohort study

Acknowledgements
We thank the MEC participants for their participation and commitment. We would also like to especially acknowledge Dr. Brian E. Henderson, who passed away before this paper was submitted. Without his mentorship and tremendous efforts in co-founding the MEC, this work would not have been possible.

Funding
The MEC is supported by NCI UM1 CA164973 which had no role in the study design, recruitment, data collection, analysis and interpretation of data and in writing the manuscript.

Authors' contributions
JCF, JP and VWS were involved in the study concept and design, analysis and interpretation of data, drafting the manuscript, statistical analysis and critical revision of the manuscript for important intellectual content. LLM and CH were involved in acquisition of data; analysis and interpretation of data; drafting of the manuscript and obtained funding. DS and LW were involved in the statistical analysis, interpretation of the data and drafting of the manuscript. NT, WC and JB were involved in the interpretation of data, drafting the manuscript, and critical revision of the manuscript for important intellectual content. All authors have read and approved the final version of this manuscript.

Competing interests
All authors disclose that there are no competing interests.

Author details
[1]Department of Preventive Medicine, Keck School of Medicine of University of Southern California, Los Angeles, California, USA. [2]Samuel Oschin Comprehensive Cancer Institute, Cedars-Sinai Medical Center, Los Angeles, California, USA. [3]Norris Comprehensive Cancer Center, Keck School of Medicine of University of Southern California, Los Angeles, California, USA. [4]Department of Medicine, Keck School of Medicine, University of Southern California, Los Angeles, California, USA. [5]Department of Pathology, Keck School of Medicine, University of Southern California, Los Angeles, California, USA. [6]Epidemiology Program, University of Hawaii Cancer Center, Honolulu, Hawaii, USA.

References
1. Stinton LM, Myers RP, Shaffer EA. Epidemiology of gallstones. Gastroenterol Clin N Am. 2010;39(2):157–69. vii
2. Ransohoff DF, Gracie WA, Wolfenson LB, Neuhauser D. Prophylactic cholecystectomy or expectant management for silent gallstones. A decision analysis to assess survival. Ann Intern Med. 1983;99(2):199–204.
3. Shaffer EA. Gallstone disease: epidemiology of gallbladder stone disease. Best Pract Res Clin Gastroenterol. 2006;20(6):981–96.
4. Miquel JF, Covarrubias C, Villaroel L, Mingrone G, Greco AV, Puglielli L, Carvallo P, Marshall G, Del Pino G, Nervi F. Genetic epidemiology of cholesterol cholelithiasis among Chilean Hispanics, Amerindians, and Maoris. Gastroenterol. 1998;115(4):937–46.
5. Maurer KR, Everhart JE, Ezzati TM, Johannes RS, Knowler WC, Larson DL, Sanders R, Shawker TH, Roth HP. Prevalence of gallstone disease in Hispanic populations in the United States. Gastroenterol. 1989;96(2 Pt 1):487–92.
6. Katsika D, Grjibovski A, Einarsson C, Lammert F, Lichtenstein P, Marschall HU. Genetic and environmental influences on symptomatic gallstone disease: a Swedish study of 43,141 twin pairs. Hepatol. 2005;41(5):1138 43.

7. Cuevas A, Miquel JF, Reyes MS, Zanlungo S, Nervi F. Diet as a risk factor for cholesterol gallstone disease. J Am Coll Nutr. 2004;23(3):187–96.

8. Moerman CJ, Bueno de Mesquita HB, Smeets FW, Runia S. lifestyle factors including diet and cancer of the gallbladder and bile duct: a population-based case-control study in The Netherlands. Eur J Cancer Prev. 1997;6(2):139–42.

9. Pandey M, Shukla VK. Diet and gallbladder cancer: a case-control study. Eur J Cancer Prev. 2002;11(4):365–8.

10. Mendez-Sanchez N, Zamora-Valdes D, Chavez-Tapia NC, Uribe M. Role of diet in cholesterol gallstone formation. Clin Chim Acta. 2007;376(1–2):1–8.

11. Ruhl CE, Everhart JE. Relationship of serum leptin concentration and other measures of adiposity with gallbladder disease. Hepatology. 2001;34(5):877–83.

12. Heaton KW, Emmett PM, Symes CL, Braddon FE. An explanation for gallstones in normal-weight women: slow intestinal transit. Lancet. 1993; 341(8836):8–10.

13. Hou L, Shu XO, Gao YT, Ji BT, Weiss JM, Yang G, Li HL, Blair A, Zheng W, Chow WH. Anthropometric measurements, physical activity, and the risk of symptomatic gallstone disease in Chinese women. Ann Epidemiol. 2009; 19(5):344–50.

14. Gonzalez Villalpando C, Rivera Martinez D, Arredondo Perez B, Martinez Diaz S, Gonzalez Villalpando ME, Haffner SM, Stern MP. High prevalence of cholelithiasis in a low income Mexican population: an ultrasonographic survey. Arch Med Res. 1997;28(4):543–7.

15. Kono S, Shinchi K, Todoroki I, Honjo S, Sakurai Y, Wakabayashi K, Imanishi K, Nishikawa H, Ogawa S, Katsurada M. Gallstone disease among Japanese men in relation to obesity, glucose intolerance, exercise, alcohol use, and smoking. Scand J Gastroenterol. 1995;30(4):372–6.

16. Leitzmann MF, Rimm EB, Willett WC, Spiegelman D, Grodstein F, Stampfer MJ, Colditz GA, Giovannucci E. Recreational physical activity and the risk of cholecystectomy in women. N Engl J Med. 1999;341(11):777–84.

17. Chuang CZ, Martin LF, LeGardeur BY, Lopez A. Physical activity, biliary lipids, and gallstones in obese subjects. Am J Gastroenterol. 2001;96(6):1860–5.

18. Storti KL, Brach JS, FitzGerald SJ, Zmuda JM, Cauley JA, Kriska AM. Physical activity and decreased risk of clinical gallstone disease among post-menopausal women. Prev Med. 2005;41(3–4):772–7.

19. Basso L, McCollum PT, Darling MR, Tocchi A, Tanner WA. A descriptive study of pregnant women with gallstones. Relation to dietary and social habits, education, physical activity, height, and weight. Eur J Epidemiol. 1992;8(5): 629–33.

20. Jorgensen T, Kay L, Schultz-Larsen K. The epidemiology of gallstones in a 70-year-old Danish population. Scand J Gastroenterol. 1990;25(4):335–40.

21. Kato I, Nomura A, Stemmermann GN, Chyou PH. Prospective study of clinical gallbladder disease and its association with obesity, physical activity, and other factors. Dig Dis Sci. 1992;37(5):784–90.

22. Kono S, Shinchi K, Ikeda N, Yanai F, Imanishi K. Prevalence of gallstone disease in relation to smoking, alcohol use, obesity, and glucose tolerance: a study of self-defense officials in Japan. Am J Epidemiol. 1992;136(5):787–94.

23. Kono S, Eguchi H, Honjo S, Todoroki I, Oda T, Shinchi K, Ogawa S, Nakagawa K. Cigarette smoking, alcohol use, and gallstone risk in Japanese men. Digestion. 2002;65(3):177–83.

24. Okamoto M, Yamagata Z, Takeda Y, Yoda Y, Kobayashi K, Fujino MA. The relationship between gallbladder disease and smoking and drinking habits in middle-aged Japanese. J Gastroenterol. 2002;37(6):455–62.

25. Murray FE, Logan RF, Hannaford PC, Kay CR. Cigarette smoking and parity as risk factors for the development of symptomatic gall bladder disease in women: results of the Royal College of general Practitioners' oral contraceptive study. Gut. 1994;35(1):107–11.

26. Attili AF, Scafato E, Marchioli R, Marfisi RM, Festi D. Diet and gallstones in Italy: the cross-sectional MICOL results. Hepatology. 1998;27(6):1492–8.

27. Shaffer EA. Epidemiology and risk factors for gallstone disease: has the paradigm changed in the 21st century? Current Gastroenterol Rep. 2005; 7(2):132–40.

28. Thijs C, Knipschild P. Oral contraceptives and the risk of gallbladder disease: a meta-analysis. Am J Public Health. 1993;83(8):1113–20.

29. Hulley S, Grady D, Bush T, Furberg C, Herrington D, Riggs B, Vittinghoff E. Randomized trial of estrogen plus progestin for secondary prevention of coronary heart disease in postmenopausal women. Heart and estrogen/progestin replacement study (HERS) research group. JAMA. 1998;280(7):605–13.

30. Cirillo DJ, Wallace RB, Rodabough RJ, Greenland P, LaCroix AZ, Limacher MC, Larson JC. Effect of estrogen therapy on gallbladder disease. JAMA. 2005; 293(3):330–9.

31. Maringhini A, Ciambra M, Baccelliere P, Raimondo M, Orlando A, Tine F, Grasso R, Randazzo MA, Barresi L, Gullo D, et al. Biliary sludge and gallstones in pregnancy: incidence, risk factors, and natural history. Ann Intern Med. 1993;119(2):116–20.

32. Valdivieso V, Covarrubias C, Siegel F, Cruz F. Pregnancy and cholelithiasis: pathogenesis and natural course of gallstones diagnosed in early puerperium. Hepatology. 1993;17(1):1–4.

33. Kolonel LN, Henderson BE, Hankin JH, Nomura AM, Wilkens LR, Pike MC, Stram DO, Monroe KR, Earle ME, Nagamine FS. A multiethnic cohort in Hawaii and Los Angeles: baseline characteristics. Am J Epidemiol. 2000; 151(4):346–57.

34. Setiawan VW, Virnig BA, Porcel J, Henderson BE, Le Marchand L, Wilkens LR, Monroe KR. Linking data from the multiethnic cohort study to Medicare data: linkage results and application to chronic disease research. Am J Epidemiol. 2015;

35. Everhart JE, Khare M, Hill M, Maurer KR. Prevalence and ethnic differences in gallbladder disease in the United States. Gastroenterol. 1999;117(3):632–9.

36. Mendez-Sanchez N, Cardenas-Vazquez R, Ponciano-Rodriguez G, Uribe M. Pathophysiology of cholesterol gallstone disease. Arch Med Res. 1996;27(4): 433–41.

37. Heaton KW. The epidemiology of gallstones and suggested aetiology. Clin Gastroenterol. 1973;2(1):67–83.

38. Nakayama F, Miyake H. Changing state of gallstone disease in Japan. Composition of the stones and treatment of the condition. Am J Surg. 1970;120(6):794–9.

39. Tsai CJ, Leitzmann MF, Willett WC, Giovannucci EL. Fruit and vegetable consumption and risk of cholecystectomy in women. The Am J Med. 2006; 119(9):760–7.

40. Tseng M, DeVellis RF, Maurer KR, Khare M, Kohlmeier L, Everhart JE, Sandler RS. Food intake patterns and gallbladder disease in Mexican Americans. Public Health Nutr. 2000;3(2):233–43.

41. Stampfer MJ, Maclure KM, Colditz GA, Manson JE, Willett WC. Risk of symptomatic gallstones in women with severe obesity. Am J Clin Nutr. 1992;55(3):652–8.

42. Leitzmann MF, Giovannucci EL, Rimm EB, Stampfer MJ, Spiegelman D, Wing AL, Willett WC. The relation of physical activity to risk for symptomatic gallstone disease in men. Ann Intern Med. 1998;128(6):417–25.

43. Maclure KM, Hayes KC, Colditz GA, Stampfer MJ, Speizer FE, Willett WC. Weight, diet, and the risk of symptomatic gallstones in middle-aged women. N Engl J Med. 1989;321(9):563–9.

44. Friedman GD, Kannel WB, Dawber TR. The epidemiology of gallbladder disease: observations in the Framingham study. J Chron Dis. 1966;19(3):273–92.

45. La Vecchia C, Decarli A, Ferraroni M, Negri E. Alcohol drinking and prevalence of self-reported gallstone disease in the 1983 Italian National Health Survey. Epidemiology. 1994;5(5):533–6.

46. Hayes KC, Livingston A, Trautwein EA. Dietary impact on biliary lipids and gallstones. Ann Rev Nutr. 1992;12:299–326.

47. Jorgensen T. Prevalence of gallstones in a Danish population. Am J Epidemiol. 1987;126(5):912–21.

48. Jorgensen T. Gall stones in a Danish population: fertility period, pregnancies, and exogenous female sex hormones. Gut. 1988;29(4):433–9.

49. Ko CW, Beresford SA, Schulte SJ, Matsumoto AM, Lee SP. Incidence, natural history, and risk factors for biliary sludge and stones during pregnancy. Hepatology. 2005;41(2):359–65.

50. Ko CW, Beresford SA, Schulte SJ, Lee SP. Insulin resistance and incident gallbladder disease in pregnancy. Clin Gastroenterol Hepatol. 2008;6(1):76–81.

51. Lee SP, Maher K, Nicholls JF. Origin and fate of biliary sludge. Gastroenterol. 1988;94(1):170–6.

2

Upcoming pharmacological developments in chronic hepatitis B: can we glimpse a cure on the horizon?

Sonia Alonso, Adriana-René Guerra, Lourdes Carreira, Juan-Ángel Ferrer, María-Luisa Gutiérrez and Conrado M. Fernandez-Rodriguez*

Abstract

Background: Hepatitis B virus (HBV) chronic infection affects up to 240 million people in the world and it is a common cause of cirrhosis and hepatocellular carcinoma (HCC). HBV covalently closed circular DNA (cccDNA) plays an essential role in HBV persistence and replication. Current pharmacological treatment with nucleos(t)ide analogues (NA) may suppress HBV replication with little or no impact on cccDNA, hence lifelong treatment is required in the vast majority of patients. Clearances of intrahepatic cccDNA and/or HBsAg are critical endpoints for future antiviral therapy in chronic HBV. Recent promising developments targeting different molecular HBV life cycle steps are being pre-clinically tested or have moved forward in early clinical trials.

Methods: We review the current state of the art of these pharmacological developments, mainly focusing on efficacy and safety results, which are expected to lay the ground for future HBV eradication. An inclusive literature search on new treatments of HBV using the following electronic databases: Pubmed/MEDLINE, AMED, CINAHL and the Cochrane Central Register of Controlled Trials. Full-text manuscripts and abstracts published over the last 12 years, from 2005 to March 2011 were reviewed for relevance and reference lists were crosschecked for additional applicable studies regarding new HBV antiviral treatment.

Results: HBV entry inhibitors, HBV core inhibitors, HBV cccDNA transcripts RNA interference, HBV cell apoptosis inducers, HBV RNA, viral proteins and DNA knock down agents, HBV release inhibitors, anti-sense nucleosides, exogenous interferon stimulation, interferon response stimulation and HBV therapeutic vaccines were reviewed.

Conclusion: This review will provide readers with an updated vision of current and foreseeable therapeutic developments in chronic hepatitis B.

Keywords: Hepatitis B virus clearance, Latest pharmacological developments, HBV cccDNA, HBV functional cure, HBV eradication

Background

The percentage of the world's population chronically infected with the Hepatitis B virus is approximately 5%. This infection is the main cause of chronic liver disease and hepatocellular carcinoma (HCC) globally. From 1990 to 2005 there has been a global decrease in HBV chronic infection prevalence due to expanded vaccination [1]. However, this condition is still a leading cause of global mortality and its overall burden and relative rank of mortality and disability rose between 1990 and 2013 [2]. Although there is important geographic variation with 75% of the infected population living in China and the highest prevalence occurring in central sub-Saharan Africa [1], HBV represents an important global public health issue with a considerable burden to almost all health systems [3–5]. Whilst universal vaccination might provide a key step forward in the HBV global eradication horizon, current therapies only confer clinical control through antiviral activity with few patients achieving HBsAg loss [6], a functional cure not equivalent to viral eradication. In the era of direct antiviral

* Correspondence: cfernandez@fhalcorcon.es
Unit of Gastroenterology, Hospital Universitario Fundación Alcorcón, Av. Budapest-1, 28922 Alcorcon, Madrid, Spain

agents (DAAs), more than 95% of hepatitis C virus (HCV) patients achieve viral eradication, which contrasts with the therapeutic outcome in HBV chronic infection. HBV therapeutic guidelines recommend treatment to prevent liver disease progression, decompensation of cirrhosis and HCC development [7, 8]. The current standard of care includes administration of nucleos(t)ide analogues (NAs) and peginterferon. Cure of HBV infection is uncommon, influenced by the tenacity of covalently closed circular DNA (cccDNA) in the hepatocytes nuclei. Interferon-based therapies are usually recommended for 48 weeks and may provide more benefit in HBeAg positive patients with low viremia, elevated ALT and HBV genotype-A [9, 10] however, the benefit in terms of HBV clearance is still low. NAs (Entecavir and Tenofovir), inhibit the HBV polymerase activity and thus viral replication, but with no major impact on cccDNA which is used to transcribe viral RNAs. Consequently, NAs do not prevent the expression of HBV genes from cccDNA or the production of sub-viral particles. Long-term NAs administration achieves HBV eradication in only 5–8% of cases [6, 11]. Hence, the vast majority of patients require lifelong treatment and rebounding of viral replication frequently follows drug cessation. Furthermore, HCC risk is reduced but not eliminated, even after long-term effective viral suppression [12]. On the long-term, sustained virological response (SVR) or functional cure occurs in less than 10% of patients [13, 14]. Hence, new therapies to eliminate HBV are needed. Research developments in HBV molecular virology have resulted in relevant advances in discerning potential therapeutic targets. This review outlines recent pre-clinical and early clinical drug developments aimed at HBV clearance including HBV entry inhibitors, 2nd generation Core inhibitors, TLR (*toll-like receptor*) agonists, anti-sense nucleotides and cccDNA targeting agents.

HBV Life cycle

The viral entry to hepatocytes starts with a reversible attachment to the low affinity host cell surface heparansulfate proteoglycans. This is continued with a more specific attachment of the receptor-binding region of pre-S1 to the extracellular loops of the hepatocyte specific receptor sodium taurocholate co-transporting polypeptide (NTCP), a multiple transmembrane transporter [15]. NTCP discovery has been a significant breakthrough in the field of HBV molecular biology as it has allowed the development of reliable HBV cell cultures to explore both the HBV and HDV life cycle as well as in vitro drug testing. The binding of the pre-S1 region to NTCP elicits endocytosis before the HBV nucleocapsid transfers to the cell nucleus [16]. However, key steps in replication such as viral particle and cell membrane fusion,

uncoating, and transference of HBV relaxed circular DNA (rcDNA) to the nucleus, are still incompletely understood. Once in the nucleus, rcDNA is transformed into covalently closed circular DNA (cccDNA), which acts as the template for the transcription of all viral mRNAs and pregenomic RNA (pgRNA). The pgRNA is encapsidated with the P protein. Once in the nucleocapsid, the pgRNA is reverse transcribed into negative-strand DNA. From the negative-strand DNA, the rcDNA is produced by plus-strand synthesis and the nucleocapsids are then either re-imported to the nucleus for cccDNA amplification or else enveloped and released via the endoplasmic reticulum (ER). Inhibition of these stages is an important target of drugs under development [17]. Epigenetic modifications such as histone acetylations and methylations and the HBx protein regulate the transcriptional activity of cccDNA [18].

Furthermore, there are viral and host factors involved in the synthesis, stability and transcriptional regulation of cccDNA synthesis. One of them has recently been discovered as the tyrosyl-DNA phosphodiesterase 2 (TDP2) which is involved in the first step of cccDNA formation and offers a potential target for the development of drugs directed at HBV eradication [19]. In addition, an inactivation of cccDNA transcription by hyperchromatination, has been pointed to as another potential tool to achieve functional cure ("locking" cccDNA) (Fig. 1).

Current therapies

Current standard of care includes peginterferon alfa2a, and NAs (tenofovir and entecavir) as first line therapies to suppress HBV viral replication, which is followed by a biochemical response and improvement in liver histology [20, 21].

Peginterferon α has antiviral, anti-proliferative, and immunomodulatory effects. In hepatitis B e antigen (HBeAg)-positive patients, 1-year peginterferon monotherapy leads to HBeAg and HBsAg seroconversion in 29–32% and 3–5% at 6 months of follow-up, respectively [9]. ALT normalization and sustained viral suppression of HBV (DNA < 400 copies/ml) is achieved in about 15% of HBeAg negative patients [10].

Importantly, peginterferon-α treatment allows finite treatment duration with a 4% of HBsAg loss reported at 6 months off-therapy, which progressively increased to 11% after 4 years of follow-up [9, 10]. However, its long-term use is limited by the side effects.

Although both entecavir (ETV) and tenofovir (TDF) are potent nucleos(t)ide HBV polymerase inhibitors with a high genetic barrier to drug resistance, they do not affect the transcriptional activity of cccDNA and lifelong treatment to achieve a significant reduction of the cccDNA pool would be required. They also have a

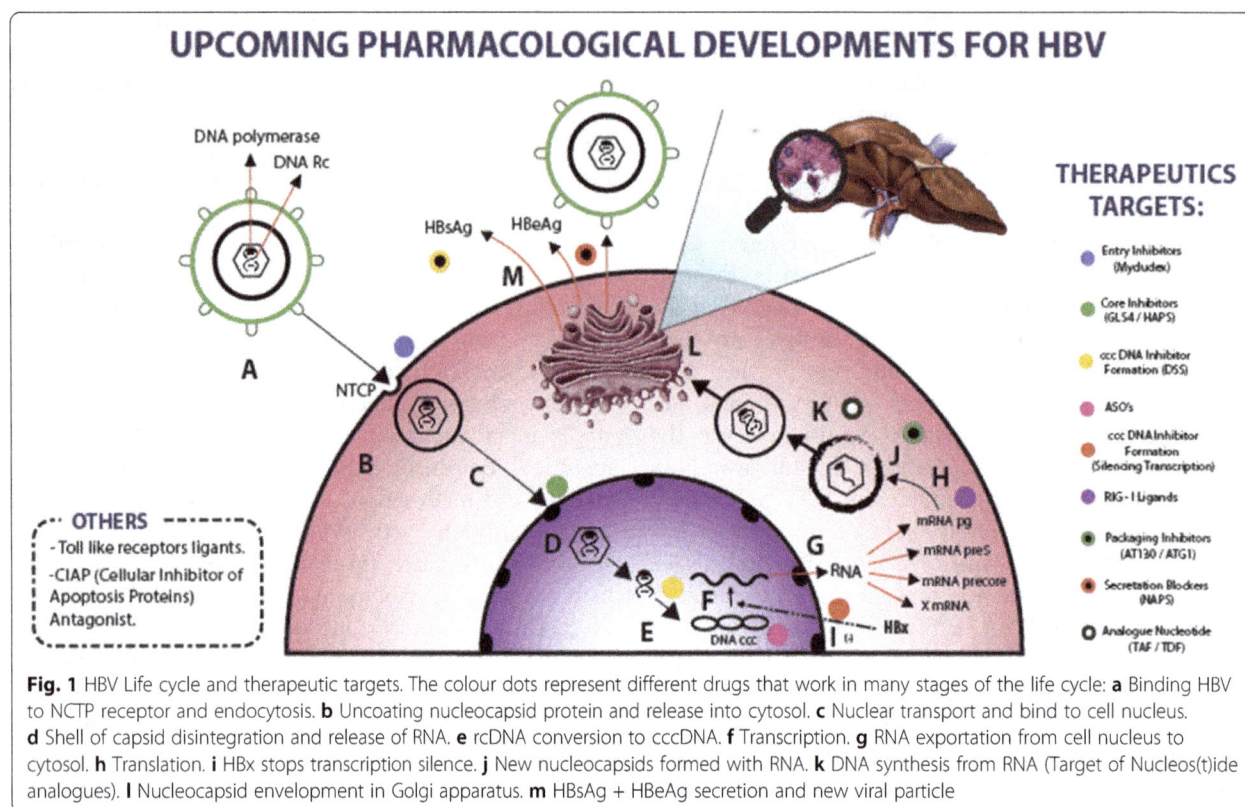

Fig. 1 HBV Life cycle and therapeutic targets. The colour dots represent different drugs that work in many stages of the life cycle: **a** Binding HBV to NCTP receptor and endocytosis. **b** Uncoating nucleocapsid protein and release into cytosol. **c** Nuclear transport and bind to cell nucleus. **d** Shell of capsid disintegration and release of RNA. **e** rcDNA conversion to cccDNA. **f** Transcription. **g** RNA exportation from cell nucleus to cytosol. **h** Translation. **i** HBx stops transcription silence. **j** New nucleocapsids formed with RNA. **k** DNA synthesis from RNA (Target of Nucleos(t)ide analogues). **l** Nucleocapsid envelopment in Golgi apparatus. **m** HBsAg + HBeAg secretion and new viral particle

modest effect on the HBsAg level as well as poor immunological control [22]. Nevertheless, either HBe Ag-positive or negative treatment-*naïve* patients achieve more than 90% rate of HBV undetectability after long-term treatment with ETV [14] and TDF [13]. On the other hand, HBeAg seroconversion occurred in 21% of patients after 1-year of ETV and TDF therapy [14, 23], and more importantly, HBsAg loss was achieved in 11.8% of HBeAg-positive patients after 7 years of TDF treatment. 5-year cumulative probability of genotype resistance in patients treated with ETV was 1,2% [24] and resistance to TDF has not been reported after 7 years of treatment [13].

This maintained viral suppression is associated with improvement in necro-inflammation and fibrosis scores in most patients [20] and to a reduction in HCC risk in patients receiving ETV compared to untreated historical controls in an Asian [25] but not in a Caucasian population [26]. Although resistance rates are so far extremely low in the case of ETV and not yet described with TDF, concerns about long-term resistance and safety remain as critical unmet needs.

Long-term, perhaps indefinite, NA therapy is normally administered to HBeAg-negative patients. Recent evidence from a Greek study suggests that long-term (≥ 4-year) ETV/TDF therapy may be safely discontinued in noncirrhotic HBeAg negative patients, particularly with mild to moderate fibrosis, although retreatment rates were 0%, 15%, 18%, 24%, 26% at 1, 2, 3, 6, 9 months after ETV/TDF cessation [27].

Combination therapy with IFNα and NAs, add-on or switch may have a synergistic effect by combining antiviral and immunomodulatory mechanisms. Although TDF and peginterferon-alfa2a combination resulted in an increased rate of HBsAg loss than either therapy alone, this rate (9.1%) still remains low [23]. Whilst add-on ETV to peginterferon treatment in HBeAg positive patients failed to show significant benefit [28], switch to peginterferon in HBeAg positive patients on ETV achieved higher HBeAg seroconversion and 8.5% of HBsAg loss. Predictors of response included an early-on decline of HBsAg or baseline levels of < 1500 IU/ml [29]. Recently a multicentre randomised trial comparing add-on or switch to peginterferon alpha 2b for 48 weeks in HBeAg patients on NA therapy, compared to continuing NA, showed that HBeAg loss or decrease in HBsAg levels >1 log at week 72 was significantly higher in the add-on but not the switch arm, compared to the controls. This suggests that compared to the other two options, add-on therapy is a superior strategy [30]. A recent randomized controlled open trial evaluated the efficacy and safety of addition of a 48 week course of peginterferon in HBeAg-negative chronic hepatitis B patients on NA therapy with undetectable HBV DNA for a least 1 year. Addition of Peginterferon to NAs therapy in 92 patients was poorly tolerated with no differences in HBsAg clearance, when compared to 93 patients who continued NA therapy alone (difference 4,6% [95% CI -2·6 to 12·5]; $p = 0·15$) [31]. To date, combination treatment strategies are not recommended and require further assessment of efficacy and safety. Therefore, new therapies to eliminate intrahepatic cccDNA are prompted for patients with an increased risk of developing cirrhosis and HCC.

New NAs

Tenofovir alafenamide (TAF) is a second-generation prodrug of tenofovir and is mainly metabolized intracellularly to tenofovir diphosphate showing lower levels of tenofovir in plasma than TDF [32]. Recently two phase III studies, showed non-inferior efficacy of 25 mg of TAF to TDF on virological suppression at week 48 in HBeAg positive and negative patients. Patients who received TAF had less changes in bone and renal parameters due to the absence of renal organic anion transporters, OAT1 and OAT3-dependent cytotoxicity [33, 34].

Besifovir (LB80380) is a novel guanosine analogue with potent anti-HBV activity and works even against viruses resistant to approved NAs [35]. In a multicenter randomised trial, besifovir showed similar rates of virological response and HBeAg seroconversion compared to entecavir [36]. Although both TAF and besifovir might represent important advances, they do not clear intrahepatic cccDNA, and thus do not achieve a cure for HBV infection alone.

Novel developments and potential therapeutic approaches

Extensive research on HBV life cycle and virus-host interactions has shed light on potential viral and host targets that are accountable for persistent HBV infection (Table 1).

HBV attachment inhibitors

The basis of HBV entry inhibitors is the disruption of viral propagation that potentially could prevent post-exposure infection in some situations, such as after liver transplantation and in neonates of infected mothers. Moreover, addition of entry inhibitors to other antivirals could allow the inhibition of de novo infection of *naïve* hepatocytes and elimination of infected hepatocytes through induced immunomodulation while allowing the

Table 1 Novel agents against HBV and phase of development

Mode of action	Target	Drug	Clinical phase
Direct acting antivirals			
Polymerase inhibition	HBV polymerase	Tenofovir alafenamide	Phase 3
		Besifovir	Phase 3
Entry inhibition	NTCP	Myrcludex-B	Phase 2a
Core inhibitors	Nucleocapsid assembly	NVR 3–778	Phase 2
		AT-61, AT130, Bay 41–4109	Preclinical
Cleavage of DNA	ccc-DNA	ZFNs,TALENs,CRISPR/Cas	Preclinical
Inhibition of ccc-DNA formation		CCC-0975 and CCC-0346	Preclinical
Non-cytolitic cccDNA degradation by inducing APOBEC3A and APOBEC3B		Lymphotoxin-b receptor agonist	Preclinical
Apoptosis induction by inhibiting cIAPs	cIAPs	Birinapant	Phase 1
Knock down HBV RNA, viral proteins and HBV DNA	HBV RNA	ARC-520, ARC-521	Phase 2
Block release of HBsAg		REP-2139	Phase 2
Antisense nucleotides	Target RNA	ASOs	Preclinical
Host targeting agents			
Exogenous interferon stimulation	Innate immunity TLR7	Toll-like receptor (TLR) agonist (GS-9620)	Phase 2
Stimulate IFN response	Innate immunity RIG-I	SB 9200	Phase 2
Therapeutic vaccination	Adaptive immunity	GS-4774 (Tarmogen)	Phase 2b
		ABX203	Phase 2b

APOBEC apolipoprotein B mRNA editing enzyme, catalytic polypeptide 3A and 3B, *ASO* antisense nucleotides, *cccDNA* covalently closed circular DNA, *CIAPs* Cellular inhibitor of apoptosis proteins, *CRISPR/Cas* clustered regulatory interspaced short palindromic repeats (CRISPR) and CRISPR associated (Cas) systems, *NTCP* sodium taurocholate co-transporting polypeptide, *RIG-I* Retinoic acid-inducible gene, *TALENs* transcription activator-like effector nucleases, *ZFNs* zinc-finger nucleases

development of uninfected hepatocytes, thereby "clearing" the liver from HBV [37]. As previously commented, NTCP has been identified as a specific binding receptor of the pre-S1 domain of the HBV envelope protein for HBV entry into the host cell [15], therefore, is a potential therapeutic target.

Myrcludex-B, is a synthetic lipopeptide coming from the pre-S1 domain of the HBV envelope protein, which targets NTCP and inhibits HBV entry by competing for the NTCP receptor [37, 38]. This compound was well tolerated at the highest intravenous dose of 20 mg in 36 healthy volunteers [39]. In immunodeficient humanized mice (human liver chimeric uPA/SCID mice) infected with HBV, the serum viral load and HBsAg levels were reduced, showing its effect on the inhibition of amplification of intrahepatic cccDNA and preventing intrahepatic viral spreading [40]. In 2012, Phase I clinical trials in HBV patients were completed [38]. In a phase IIa clinical study, 75% of patients achieved > 1 log decrease in serum HBV DNA with once daily subcutaneous Myrcludex B. Higher doses were related to a clinically non-significant raise in serum bile acid levels [41]. Among patients with hepatitis D virus (HDV) coinfection, monotherapy with Myrcludex B showed a significant reduction on HDV RNA serum levels and ALT normalization. When added to peginterferon-alfa2a a synergistic antiviral effect on HDV RNA and HBV DNA was observed [42].. This pilot study was a sub-study of a phase Ib/IIa randomized, open-label clinical trial which compared daily myrcludex B vs. entecavir administration in patients with CHB. A liposomal formulation of Myrcludex B allows oral administration and long-term storage [43].

Combination regimens of Myrcludex B with immunomodulator or antiviral agents may improve efficacy and further clarify safety concerns. The combination of NAs and entry inhibitors might accelerate the elimination of infected cells preventing reformation of cccDNA after removal of NAs and induction of relapse and subsequently viral clearance.

Heparan Sulfate and Glypican 5 [44] are other NTCP co-receptors, but their role as HBV entry inhibitors has not yet been evaluated.

Polyethylenimines (PEI) are polymers that block the interaction between viruses and proteoglycans on the cell membrane, thus preventing viral entry. This polymer reduced the production of HBsAg and core-associated HBV DNA by 80% and more than 60%, respectively, when equated to the control in HepG2-hNTCP cells [45].

Core inhibitors

Pregenomic RNA encapsidation is vital for the subsequent HBV-DNA synthesis. Core inhibitors may additionally inhibit capsid disassembly at the nuclear pore and affect occupancy of cccDNA in the nucleus. The hetero-aryl-dihydropyrimidines (HAPs) are potent inhibitors of capsid assembly with the construction of aberrant core particles. BAY 41-4109 is one of these compounds that has been tested in different HBV models [46, 47] and achieved a rapid reduction in HVB DNA replication, but a rapid rebound after the end of the treatment in an animal model [48]. GLS4 is another member of the HAP family with in vitro *activity* inhibiting HBV replication of adefovir resistant strains [49] and entered early clinical development in China. GLS4JHS and Ritonavir have been shown as a safe combination and revealed a significant and rapid reduction in HBV-DNA and HBsAg levels in patients with chronic HBV infection [50]. Recently, third-generation 4-H HAPs have shown improved anti-HBV activity in vitro and in vivo and better drug-like properties compared to the first- and second-generations. They have been subsequently selected for further development as oral anti-HBV infection agents [51].

Both phenyl-propenamide AT-61 and AT-130 affect HBV-RNA packaging and formation of capsids [52], but must be proven in clinical trials.

Compounds with more advanced research are sulphamoyl-benzamide derivatives, which inhibit the encapsidation of viral pregenomic RNA into nucleocapsids and block the secretion of virions and particles containing RNA. A prototype of these core inhibitors, NVR 3–778, has shown superiority over peginterferon in the humanized uPA/SCID mouse model [53] and showed a good safety profile in a phase Ia trial in healthy adult volunteers [54]. Different doses of NVR 3–778 were well tolerated in a phase Ib clinical trial enrolling 36 HBeAg positive chronic hepatitis B patients. Significant HBV-DNA decline was observed only with the higher 1200 mg (600 mg b.i.d.) dose [55]. Currently, NVR 3–778 in combination with peginterferon, as well as with nucleoside analogs, is being explored. In a four week interim analysis, NVR 3–778 (400 and 600 mg) plus peginterferon was associated with reduction of both HBV DNA (1.97 log DNA-HBV for peginterferon and NVR 3–778 combination) and HBeAg, but not to HBsAg reduction, which is likely due to the short treatment duration [56, 57].

When AB-423, which is a novel antiviral agent, is combined with nucleoside or RNAi agents in vitro it has shown a potent inhibition of HBV replication.. Its high potential is sustained by inhibition of pgRNA encapsidation and the formation of cccDNA. Evaluation of AB-423 for advancement into clinical development is underway. [58].

Core Protein Assembly Modifiers (CPAMs) are compounds that target core protein. A recent study comparing a series of CPAMs with entecavir has shown their capacity in suppressing both HBV replication and formation of cccDNA. They can inhibit new rcDNA synthesis by interfering with pgRNA encapsidation and suppressing HBV DNA replication. Reductions in HBeAg, HBsAg and pgRNA levels in cell cultures prove its ability to block HBV de novo infection [59], unlike ETV.

cccDNA inhibitors

As commented, the cccDNA mini-chromosome is a key intermediate in the HBV life cycle, is responsible for HBV infection persistence and resides in the nucleus of infected cells (Fig. 1). There are several options for cccDNA targeting: inhibition of its formation, silencing its transcription or eliminating already existing cccDNA.

Another challenge is the lack of standardized assays for specific cccDNA quantification in cells and tissues, for the discrimination between rcDNA and cccDNA pools and markers of cccDNA activity to assess efficacy of treatments.

a) Inhibition of cccDNA formation: di-substituted sulfonamide (DSS) termed CCC-0975 and CCC-0346 has proven its capacity to interfere with the conversion of rcDNA into cccDNA in cell culture [60]. As cccDNA has a long life, these compounds would have a role during the first phase of infection or high hepatocyte turnover [61].

b) Silencing cccDNA transcription: cccDNA transcription and HBV gene expression are controlled by the regulation of HBV chromatin and cccDNA-bound histone post-translational modifications (PTMs) [62]. The ability of Peginterferon to inhibit cccDNA transcription relies on the reduction of cccDNA-bound histones acetylation [63]. HBx may represent a target for direct-acting antivirals as it appears necessary to block cellular factors that inhibit cccDNA transcription [64]. Some recent work has defined the role of the HBx protein interacting with "structural maintenance of chromosome" Smc complex Smc5/6, which inhibits extrachromosomal DNA transcription. HBx relieves the inhibition of HBV gene expression by destroying this Smc5/6 complex [65, 66]. Another study determined that the Smc5/6 complex limits hepatitis B virus transcription when confined to ND10 (Nuclear Domain 10) in human hepatocytes and that this association is important for transcriptional silencing of cccDNA in the absence of HBx [67]. Induction of PTMs on cccDNA bound histones by small compounds [68] can reduce cccDNA transcription and therefore inhibit viral replication, opening the possibility for an epigenetic silencing of cccDNA as a new approach. Although it must be confirmed *in vivo*, this strategy could achieve a functional cure.

c) Elimination of cccDNA: Non-cytolytic elimination ('curing'), or destruction of all cells harbouring cccDNA by T cells ('killing') and replacement by non-infected cells are the two ways for cccDNA clearance from hepatocytes [69]. Cytokines and downstream effectors play an important role, which is not yet completely known. In this way, the results of a recent study showed T-cells derived IFNγ and TNF-α to decrease levels of HBV cccDNA in hepatocytes by inducing deamination and subsequent cccDNA decay in vitro [70]. Lymphotoxin-b receptor agonists activate apolipoprotein B mRNA editing enzyme, catalytic polypeptide 3A and 3B (APOBEC3A and APOBEC3B) cytidine deaminases in HBV infected cells, inducing non-cytolytic cccDNA degradation [61]. Nevertheless, a fraction of cccDNA may persist refractory to immune-mediated clearance and degradation. New tools for targeting and cleaving cccDNA have been explored in cell models, such as zinc-finger nucleases (ZFNs), transcription activator-like endonucleases (TALENs) or the RNA-guided clustered regularly interspaced short palindromic repeats (CRISPR)/Cas system. ZFNs target sequences within the HBV polymerase, core and X genes, and break the DNA double strand with imprecise repair that leads to mutation which inactivates HBV genes. In a recent study [71], delivery of 3 HBV specific ZFNs, using self-complementary adeno-associated virus vectors, achieved total inhibition of HBV DNA replication and manufacture of infectious HBV virions in HepAD38 cells. In vivo murine hydrodynamic injection model of HBV replication with TALEN led to a targeted mutation in approximately 35% of cccDNA molecules without evidence of toxicity [72]. Finally, a recent study showed that over 90% of HBV DNA was cleaved in by Cas9 [73]. Despite their potential, it is necessary to elucidate efficacy of these compounds in animal models of chronic HBV infection prior to clinical development and to assess aspects related with off-target effects affecting the host genome.

Apoptosis inductors: SMAC mimetic drugs

Cellular inhibitor of apoptosis proteins (cIAPs) prevent TNF-mediated killing/death of infected cells, thus impairing the clearance of HBV infection [74]. Drug inhibitors of cIAPs are also known as Smac (second mitocondria-derived activator of caspase) mimetics, because they mimic the action of the endogenous protein Smac/Diablo that antagonizes cIAP function. Recent studies have shown that birinapant and other Smac mimetics produced a rapid decrease in serum HBV-DNA and HBV surface antigen and promoted the removal of hepatocytes containing HBV core antigen in an immunocompetent mouse model of chronic HBV infection. Liver enzymes were transiently elevated showing non-significant liver damage related to the action of birinapant. The effect of birinapant and ETV in combination was higher than either drug alone in promoting clearance of serum HBV DNA with no overt evidence of toxicity [75]. In 2015, a phase II study of birinapant for the treatment of HBV was initiated.

Inhibition of HBV gene expression

As collapse and dysfunction of HBV-specific T-cell immunity in chronic hepatitis B might be related to the presence of increased levels of viral load, a reduction or disruption of HBV gene expression may be a potential tool to achieve immune restoration [62].

a) *Secretion pathways*: Nucleic Acid Polymers (NAPs), blocked the release of HBsAg. REP9-AC (REP 2055), a 40-nucleotide DNA polymer, led to rapid clearance of serum HBsAg and anti-HBs appearance [76]. REP-2139, a modified compound with no inflammatory effect showed a synergistic antiviral effect when peginterferon was added-on after HBsAg clearance and also in combination with peginterferon in patients with HBeAg positive chronic HBV infection [77].. In both studies NAP monotherapy for 40 weeks, resulted in 2–7 log reductions of serum HBsAg, 3–9 log reductions in serum HBV DNA and development of serum anti-HBsAg antibodies. In the randomized, controlled trial REP 401 protocol (NCT02565719), triple antiviral therapy with NAPs, peginterferon and TDF in Caucasian patients with HBeAg negative chronic HBV are currently being evaluated. Efficacy and tolerability of REP 2139 and REP 2165 in combination with peg-IFN and TDF have been proven in 34 patients with HBeAg negative chronic HBV infection. 9/9 patients receiving REP 2139 and 7/9 patients receiving REP 2165 achieved >1 log reduction in serum HBsAg [78]. Larger controlled studies are needed to confirm whether immune restoration occurs after NAPs induced HBsAg clearance.

b) *RNA interference:* In gene expression disruption RNA interference is one of the most widely used approaches. As mentioned above, high levels of viral antigens such as HBsAg might alter HBV-specific T-cell immunity in chronic hepatitis B. Thus, it is conceivable that reduction of HBV gene expression might lead to immune restoration. ARC-520 is a combination of a hepatocyte-targeted, N-acetyl-galactosamine conjugated Melittin-like peptide with a liver-tropic cholesterol-conjugated small interfering RNA (siRNA). It is directed against conserved HBV RNA sequences that require intravenous administration to effectively knock down HBV-RNA, HBsAg and DNA levels in chimpanzees. Of note,

ALT flares were observed reflecting immune reconstitution [79, 80]. Data from a phase IIa clinical trial confirm tolerability and efficacy of ARC-520 showing significant, dose-dependent reduction in HBsAg for up to 57 days in CHB patients [81, 82]. The beneficial effect of multi-dose treatment with ARC-520 in chimps previously treated with NAs may lead to the effective knockdown of target genes with no development of drug resistance by triggering two sites [83]. Furthermore, a recent study has shown that ARC-520 (siRNA) and entecavir led to quick HBV-DNA suppression in all HBeAg positive patients achieving up to 5.5 log reductions of HBV-DNA. This also occurred in all HBeAg negative treatment naïve patients achieving decreases up to below the limit of quantitation. After a single dose was administered to HBV patients, ARC-520 inhibited HBV cccDNA-derived mRNA, as up to a 2-log viral protein reduction was observed [84].

A preclinical study, using cell culture models, found that in HepBHAe82 cells, the capsid inhibitor AB-423 in combination with a second-generation siRNA agent, ARB-1740, displayed synergistic activity against HBV relaxed circular DNA. Their activity also led to an important decline in HBV DNA, whilst maintaining the serum HBsAg inhibition mediated by ARB-1740 and the HBeAg level when added to Peginterferon or entecavir during a 28 day period [85]. ARB-1467 contains three double-stranded siRNAs, which target three different sites in the viral genome to realize post-transcriptional gene suppression of HBV proteins. These proteins are generated from both cccDNA and integrated DNA, including the surface antigen (HBsAg). The safety and efficacy of ARB-1467 was evaluated in a recent study over a period of 12 weeks in 24 subjects and showed declines in HBsAg levels with single and multiple doses [86]. BB-103 is a recombinant AAV8 vector which is designed to treat chronic HBV infection using RNAi, and targets three sequences in the Core, S-antigen and X protein regions on the HBV viral RNA. When combining a single dose of this compound with Peginterferon or entecavir in a mouse model, HBV DNA was reduced nearly 4 log while also achieving a 2 log drop in HBsAg [87].

Recently, a biodegradable nanoparticle, which can deliver HBV-targeting unlocked nucleomonomer agent (UNA) oligomers successfully to hepatocytes, has been proven to show an excellent tolerability. A combination of three UNA oligomers with capacity to target all viral transcripts and cover all HBV genotypes has shown potent activity against HBV in HBV-infected human hepatocytes and in two mouse models of HBV infection [88].

Cyclophilin inhibitors

Cyclophilins are cytoplasmic proteins used by several viruses for replication. Alisporivir, which was developed for the treatment of HCV, is a cyclophilin A inhibitor that has recently been shown to have an effect in reducing the replication of HBV DNA and HBsAg production and secretion and these effects were potentiated with telbivudine addition in a preclinical study [89].

Inmunological approaches

a) Innate immune ligands

-*Toll-like Receptor (TLR) ligands:* The toll-like receptor family is an important regulator of innate and adaptive immune response through the recognition of foreign pathogens, which triggers the expression of genes involved in cytokines and antigen specific adaptive immunity. In mice models, HBV can be suppressed by TLR induced antiviral activity [90]. A TLR subfamily composed of TLR3, 7/8 and TLR9 recognize endosomal viral nucleic acids and induce a type-1 interferon response.

Short-term oral administration of the TLR7 agonist GS-9620 in chimpanzees, achieved reduction in serum and liver HBV-DNA and in HBsAg and HBeAg [91].GS-9620 stimulated the creation of interferon-alpha and other cytokines and chemokines, and activated interferon-stimulated genes and natural killer cells. A short course of oral GS-9620 in a phase Ib clinical trial did not show changes in HBsAg or HBV DNA levels although it was proven to be safe and well tolerated [92]. It is unknown whether longer therapy duration will improve this response. Results from a phase II study comparing GS-9620 during 4, 8 and 12 weeks in patients with viral suppression receiving tenofovir, did not show a decline of HBsAg levels [93]. As part of the SG-US-283-1059 study, 28 HBeAg negative with genotype D HBV infected patients in treatment with NUCs were randomized to receive either placebo or one of three different GS-9620 doses (1,2 and 4 mg, weekly for 12 weeks). All in vitro analyzed HBV-specific T cell responses were significantly stronger in virally-suppressed patients at baseline, mainly IFN-γ production and CD4 responses. When adding GS-9620 to NUC, production of IL-2 and CD8 responses are enhanced, as with the overall NK cell function, but changes in T cell/NK cell function and HBsAg decline were not correlated. The role of GS-9620 associated to other anti-HBV therapy might be investigated in different clinical settings [94].

-*STING agonists:* 5,6-dimethylxanthenone-4-acetic acid (DMXAA) is an agonist of the mouse stimulator of interferon genes (STING), and has been found to suppress HBV replication in mouse hepatocytes by inducing a robust cytokine response in macrophages followed by reducing the amount of cytoplasmic viral nucleocapsids. The STING agonist induced a cytokine response mainly by type I interferons, which is unlike the TLR agonists that induced a predominant inflammatory cytokine/chemokine response. [95].

-*RIG-I ligands:* Retinoic acid-inducible gene (RIG-I)-like RNA helicases (RLHs) recognize RNA in the cytoplasm and induce an IFN response as well as interfere with the interaction of the HBV polymerase with pgRNA to suppress viral replication. The active SB-9000, an oral dinucleotide prodrug, isomer products bind to RIG-I and NOD2 to stimulate an interferon response. Pretreatment with SB 9200 to induce a host immune response followed by ETV in woodchucks was found to have a significant reduction in viral DNA, RNA, and antigens compared to viral reduction with ETV followed by immune modulation. A Phase II clinical trial of SB 9200 alone and in combination with a nucleoside to treat chronic HBV is therefore planned [96].

b) Therapeutic vaccines

The basis for therapeutic vaccination is the achievement of breaking T cell tolerance to HBV proteins (HBsAg, HBcAg) and stimulation of HBV-specific T cell immunity in patients with chronic HBV infection. GS-4774 elicits an HBV-specific T-cell response through a heat-inactivated yeast-based therapeutic T-cell vaccine expressing a recombinant protein containing HBV core, surface, and X proteins. Recently, data from a 2phase IIb clinical trial have been published. 178 patients with non-cirrhotic chronic HBV infection with viral suppression by NUC therapy were randomized to continue antiviral therapy alone or receive NUC plus GS-4774 subcutaneously every 4 weeks. There were no significant differences between groups in mean HBsAg decreases from baseline to week 24 or 48 and no patient experienced loss of serum HBsAg [97]. The vaccine was safe and well tolerated in spite of poor clinical benefit. The investigators speculate with the possibility of better results in patients with shorter duration of infection.

Recent results from a randomized phase II study assessing the GS-4774 vaccine + TDF in 195 patients with chronic HBV who were not on antivirals evidenced modest reductions in HBsAg in the GS-4774 + TDF group when compared to the TDF group alone through week 48 and no patients lost HBsAg [93, 98].

A phase IIb study is currently evaluating the efficacy of a therapeutic vaccine composed of HBsAg and HBcAg recombinant proteins (ABX203) in HBeAg-negative patients after cessation of NA therapy [62].

In a recent preclinical mice model, reducing viral antigens with an adeno-associated virus targeting HBV transcripts via RNAi, prior to vaccination with a protein prime/modified vaccinia virus Ankara (MVA), induced higher HBs and HBc specific CD8 T-cell responses. This is due to the high levels of viral antigens promoting HBV tolerance [99].

Transfer of T-cells engineered to express a HBV specific T-cell receptor may reconstitute the immune response against HBV and reduced serological and intrahepatic viral loads in human liver chimeric mice [100].

Anti-sense nucleotides (ASOs)

ASOs are small single-stranded nucleic acids (8–50 nucleotides) which are complementary to their target RNA, and bind via base pairing, leading to the degradation of the specific target RNA. This is followed by reduction of HBV antigenemia with limited off-target effects [101]. Recently, in vitro and in vivo antiviral effects of first generation ASOs against HBV have been described [102, 103], but toxicity has limited their use in vivo. Second generation ASOs have provided improved potency, stability, specificity and safety [102]. A lead ASO identified in vitro, efficiently reduced HBV gene expression, replication, viremia and antigenemia in HBV transgenic mice. HBsAg decreased 2-logs in a week after a single ASO injection, as well as combined with ETV, while the NUC alone did not. Also, cccDNA-driven HBV gene expression is ASO sensitive in HBV infected cells *in vitro* [104]. Advantages of ASOs

compared to siRNA compounds, such as ARC-520 [84], may consist in specific formulation required for the siRNA and the need of intravenous administration due to instability and delivery limitations of siRNA compounds.

Ribonuclease H inhibitors

The HBV ribonuclease H (RNaseH) has been recently evaluated as a drug target as it is essential for viral replication, since HBV is a DNA virus that replicates by reverse transcription via an RNA intermediate. N-hydroxyisoquinolinedione (HID), 3-hydroxypyrimidine-2,4-diones and α-hydroxytropolone compounds have confirmed its activity against viral replication by inhibiting RNaseH [105].

Conclusions

Recent developments of new highly effective antiviral therapy against HCV infection have fueled the research for a cure of chronic HBV infection or HBsAg loss. Intranuclear cccDNA and HBV-DNA integration remain as critical barriers for HBV cure. Albeit, new preclinical and early-clinical development show promising proof of concept results, although most of the trials, even the more advanced, ones did not set HBsAg loss as a principal endpoint. Furthermore, which biomarkers are necessary to accurately assess sterilizing cure remains unclear. Thus, we are currently quite far from foreseeing which

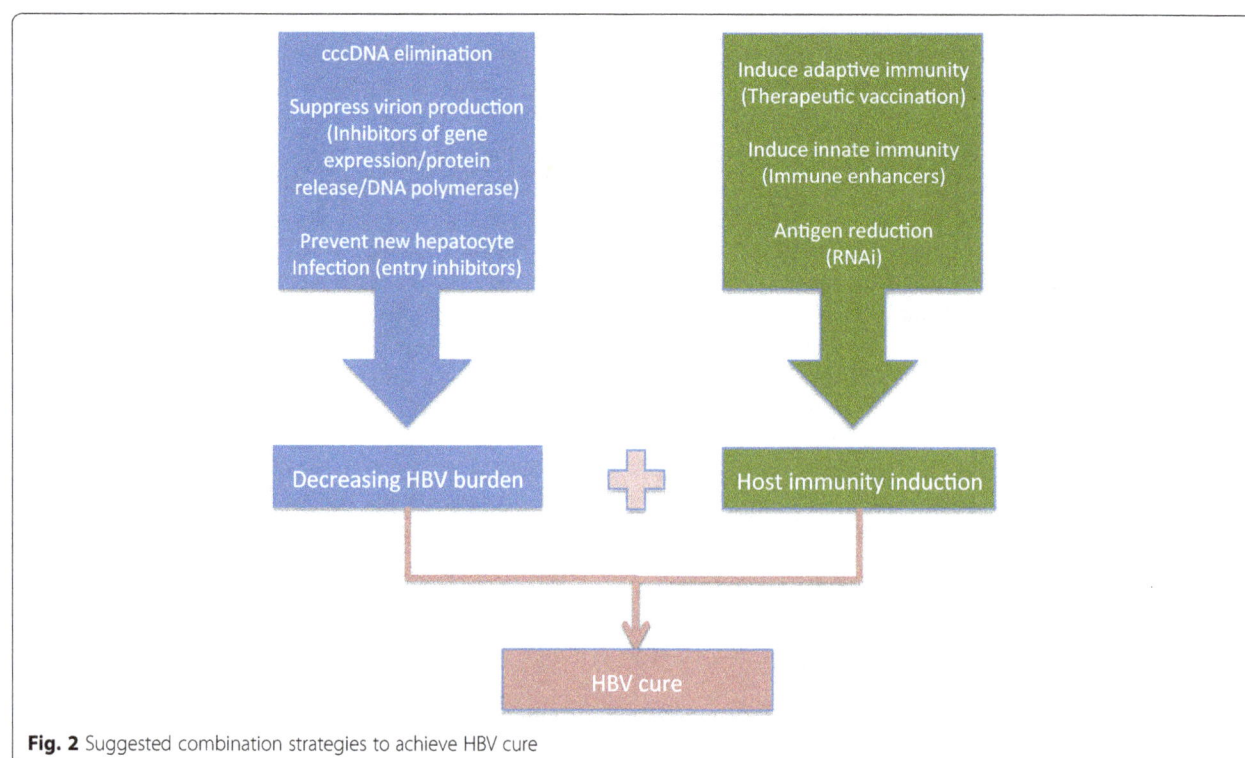

Fig. 2 Suggested combination strategies to achieve HBV cure

drugs or which combinations will eventually succeed in eliminating cccDNA. It is likely that combining agents directed at different specific steps in the viral life-cycle, including cccDNA targets, with those aimed at activating and restoring host anti-viral immunity will be needed to overcome HBV chronic infection. These therapeutic strategies are expected to be tested and enter clinical assessment in the next few years (Fig. 2). Additional concerns about safety of host targeting drugs remain to be elucidated. In this sense, a non-cytolytic purging of cccDNA containing hepatocytes stands out as the preferred approach.

Although we still seem to be a long way from definitely curing HBV infection, combining efforts of basic, translational, clinical research and awareness of regulatory agencies of the need for early combination trials, will hopefully pave the way to the cure of HBV infection in the next two decades.

Abbreviations
ALT: Alanine Aminotransferase; cccDNA: Covalently circular closed DNA; cccDNA: HBV covalently closed circular DNA; DAAs: Direct Antiviral Agents; DMXAA: 5,6-dimethylxanthenone-4-acetic acid; ER: Endoplasmic reticulum; ETV: Entecavir; HBeAg: Hepatitis B e Antigen; HBsAg: Hepatitis B surface Antigen; HBV: Hepatitis B virus; HCC: Hepatocellular carcinoma; HCV: Hepatitis C virus; NAs: Nucleos(t)ide analogues (NAs); NTCP: Sodium taurocholate co-transporting polypeptide; OAT: Organic anion transporters; pgRNA: Pregenomic RNA; rcDNA: Relaxed circular DNA; SMAC: second mitochondrial-derived activator of caspases; STING: stimulator of interferon genes; SVR: Sustained virological response; TAF: Tenofovir alafenamide; TDF: Tenofovir fumarate; TDP2: Tyrosyl-DNA phosphodiesterase 2; TLR: Toll-like receptor; UNA: Unlocked nucleomonomer agent

Acknowledgements
Authors acknowledge Christian Correa for graphic design and Elena Stalling for editorial assistance.

Funding
None.

Authors' contributions
All authors equally contributed to bibliographic search, redaction, review and graphic design contained in the manuscript. All authors read and approved the final manuscript.

Competing interests
The authors declare that they have no competing interests.

References
1. Ott JJ, Stevens GA, Groeger J, Wiersma ST. Global epidemiology of hepatitis B virus infection: new estimates of age-specific HBsAg seroprevalence and endemicity. Vaccine. 2012;30:2212–9.
2. Stanaway JD, Flaxman AD, Naghavi M, Fitzmaurice C, Vos T, Abubakar I, et al. The global burden of viral hepatitis from 1990 to 2013: findings from the global burden of disease study 2013. Lancet. 2016;388:1081–8.
3. Lok AS. Chronic hepatitis B. N Engl J Med. 2002;346:1682–3.
4. El-Serag HB. Hepatocellular carcinoma. N Engl J Med. 2011;365:1118–27.
5. Ganem D, Prince AM. Hepatitis B virus infection–natural history and clinical consequences. N Engl J Med. 2004;350:1118–29.
6. Heathcote EJ, Marcellin P, Buti M, Gane E, De Man RA, Krastev Z, et al. Three-year efficacy and safety of tenofovir disoproxil fumarate treatment for chronic hepatitis B. Gastroenterology. 2011;140:132–43.
7. European Association For The Study Of The Liver. EASL clinical practice guidelines: management of chronic hepatitis B virus infection. J Hepatol. 2012;57:167–85.
8. Lok AS, McMahon BJ. Chronic hepatitis B: update 2009. Hepatology. 2009;50:661–2.
9. Janssen HL, van Zonneveld M, Senturk H, Zeuzem S, Akarca US, Cakaloglu Y, et al. Pegylated interferon alfa-2b alone or in combination with lamivudine for HBeAg-positive chronic hepatitis B: a randomised trial. Lancet. 2005;365:123–9.
10. Marcellin P, Lau GK, Bonino F, Farci P, Hadziyannis S, Jin R, et al. Peginterferon alfa-2a alone, lamivudine alone, and the two in combination in patients with HBeAg-negative chronic hepatitis B. N Engl J Med. 2004; 351:1206–17.
11. Marcellin P, Heathcote EJ, Buti M, Gane E, de Man RA, Krastev Z, et al. Tenofovir disoproxil fumarate versus adefovir dipivoxil for chronic hepatitis B. N Engl J Med. 2008;359:2442–55.
12. Lai CL, Yuen MF. Prevention of hepatitis B virus-related hepatocellular carcinoma with antiviral therapy. Hepatology. 2013;57:399–408.
13. Buti M, Tsai N, Petersen J, Flisiak R, Gurel S, Krastev Z, et al. Seven-year efficacy and safety of treatment with tenofovir disoproxil fumarate for chronic hepatitis B virus infection. Dig Dis Sci. 2015;60:1457–64.
14. Chang TT, Lai CL, Kew Yoon S, Lee SS, Coelho HS, Carrilho FJ, et al. Entecavir treatment for up to 5 years in patients with hepatitis B e antigen-positive chronic hepatitis B. Hepatology. 2010;51:422–30.
15. Yan H, Zhong G, Xu G, He W, Jing Z, Gao Z, et al. Sodium taurocholate cotransporting polypeptide is a functional receptor for human hepatitis B and D virus. elife. 2012;1:e00049.
16. Li W, Urban S. Entry of hepatitis B and hepatitis D virus into hepatocytes: basic insights and clinical implications. J Hepatol. 2016;64:S32–40.
17. Nassal M. Hepatitis B viruses: reverse transcription a different way. Virus Res. 2008;134:235–49.
18. Belloni L, Pollicino T, De Nicola F, Guerrieri F, Raffa G, Fanciulli M, et al. Nuclear HBx binds the HBV minichromosome and modifies the epigenetic regulation of cccDNA function. Proc Natl Acad Sci U S A. 2009;106:19975–9.
19. Koniger C, Wingert I, Marsmann M, Rosler C, Beck J, Nassal M. Involvement of the host DNA-repair enzyme TDP2 in formation of the covalently closed circular DNA persistence reservoir of hepatitis B viruses. Proc Natl Acad Sci U S A. 2014;111:E4244–53.
20. Marcellin P, Gane E, Buti M, Afdhal N, Sievert W, Jacobson IM, et al. Regression of cirrhosis during treatment with tenofovir disoproxil fumarate for chronic hepatitis B: a 5-year open-label follow-up study. Lancet. 2013; 381:468–75.
21. Wong GL, Chan HL, Mak CW, Lee SK, Ip ZM, Lam AT, et al. Entecavir treatment reduces hepatic events and deaths in chronic hepatitis B patients with liver cirrhosis. Hepatology. 2013;58:1537–47.
22. Werle-Lapostolle B, Bowden S, Locarnini S, Wursthorn K, Petersen J, Lau G, et al. Persistence of cccDNA during the natural history of chronic hepatitis B and decline during adefovir dipivoxil therapy. Gastroenterology. 2004;126:1750–8.
23. Marcellin P, Ahn SH, Ma X, Caruntu FA, Tak WY, Elkashab M, et al. Combination of Tenofovir Disoproxil Fumarate and Peginterferon alpha-2a increases loss of hepatitis B surface antigen in patients with chronic hepatitis B. Gastroenterology. 2016;150:134–44. e10
24. Tenney DJ, Rose RE, Baldick CJ, Pokornowski KA, Eggers BJ, Fang J, et al. Long-term monitoring shows hepatitis B virus resistance to entecavir in nucleoside-naive patients is rare through 5 years of therapy. Hepatology. 2009;49:1503–14.

25. Wu CY, Lin JT, Ho HJ, Su CW, Lee TY, Wang SY, et al. Association of nucleos(t)ide analogue therapy with reduced risk of hepatocellular carcinoma in patients with chronic hepatitis B: a nationwide cohort study. Gastroenterology. 2014;147:143–51. e5

26. Papatheodoridis GV, Chan HL, Hansen BE, Janssen HL, Lampertico P. Risk of hepatocellular carcinoma in chronic hepatitis B: assessment and modification with current antiviral therapy. J Hepatol. 2015;62:956–67.

27. Papatheodoridis G, Rigopoulou E, Papatheodoridi M, Zachou K, Xourafas V, Gatselis N, et al. DARING-B: discontinuation of effective entecavir or tenofovir therapy in non-cirrhotic HBeAg-negative chronic hepatitis B patients: a prospective greek study. J Hepatol. 2017;66:S26.

28. Xie Q, Zhou H, Bai X, Wu S, Chen JJ, Sheng J, et al. A randomized, open-label clinical study of combined pegylated interferon Alfa-2a (40KD) and entecavir treatment for hepatitis B "e" antigen-positive chronic hepatitis B. Clin Infect Dis. 2014;59:1714–23.

29. Ning Q, Han M, Sun Y, Jiang J, Tan D, Hou J, et al. Switching from entecavir to PegIFN alfa-2a in patients with HBeAg-positive chronic hepatitis B: a randomised open-label trial (OSST trial). J Hepatol. 2014;61:777–84.

30. Lim SG, Yang WL, Ngu J, Tan J, Ahmed T, Dan YY, et al. Switch or add-on peginterferon for chronic hepatitis B patients already on nucleos(t)ide analogue therapy (SWAP study): provisional analysis – add-on therapy superior. J Hepatol. 2017;66:S60.

31. Bourliere M, Rabiega P, Ganne-Carrie N, Serfaty L, Marcellin P, Barthe Y, et al. Effect on HBs antigen clearance of addition of pegylated interferon alfa-2a to nucleos(t)ide analogue therapy versus nucleos(t)ide analogue therapy alone in patients with HBe antigen-negative chronic hepatitis B and sustained undetectable plasma hepatitis B virus DNA: a randomised, controlled, open-label trial. Lancet Gastroenterol Hepatol. 2017;2:177–88.

32. Murakami E, Wang T, Park Y, Hao J, Lepist EI, Babusis D, et al. Implications of efficient hepatic delivery by tenofovir alafenamide (GS-7340) for hepatitis B virus therapy. Antimicrob Agents Chemother. 2015;59:3563–9.

33. Chan HLY, Fung S, Seto WK, et al. A phase 3 study of tenofovir alafenamide compared with tenofovir disoproxil fumarate in patients with HBeAg positive chronic HBV: week 48 efficacy and safety results. J Hepatol. 2016;64:S161.

34. Buti M, Gane E, Seto WK, et al. A phase 3 study of tenofovir alafenamide compared with tenofovir disoproxil fumarate in patients with HBeAg negative, chronic hepatitis B: week 48 efficacy and safety results. J Hepatol. 2016;64:S135.

35. Lai CL, Ahn SH, Lee KS, Um SH, Cho M, Yoon SK, et al. Phase IIb multicentred randomised trial of besifovir (LB80380) versus entecavir in Asian patients with chronic hepatitis B. Gut. 2014;63:996–1004.

36. Yuen MF, Ahn SH, Lee KS, Um SH, Cho M, Yoon SK, et al. Two-year treatment outcome of chronic hepatitis B infection treated with besifovir vs. entecavir: results from a multicentre study. J Hepatol. 2015;62:526–32.

37. Urban S, Bartenschlager R, Kubitz R, Zoulim F. Strategies to inhibit entry of HBV and HDV into hepatocytes. Gastroenterology. 2014;147:48–64.

38. Volz T, Allweiss L, Ben MBarek M, Warlich M, Lohse AW, Pollok JM, et al. The entry inhibitor Myrcludex-B efficiently blocks intrahepatic virus spreading in humanized mice previously infected with hepatitis B virus. J Hepatol. 2013; 58:861–7.

39. Blank A, Markert C, Hohmann N, Carls A, Mikus G, Lehr T, et al. First-in-human application of the novel hepatitis B and hepatitis D virus entry inhibitor Myrcludex B. J Hepatol. 2016;65(3):483–9.

40. Petersen J, Dandri M, Mier W, Lutgehetmann M, Volz T, von Weizsacker F, et al. Prevention of hepatitis B virus infection in vivo by entry inhibitors derived from the large envelope protein. Nat Biotechnol. 2008;26:335–41.

41. Bogomolov P, Voronkova N, Allweiss L, Dandri M, Schwab M, Lempp FA, et al. A proof-of-concept phase 2a clinical trial with HBV/HDV entry inhibitor Myrcludex B. Hepatology. 2014;60:1279A–80A.

42. Bogomolov P, Alexandrov A, Voronkova N, Macievich M, Kokina K, Petrachenkova M, et al. Treatment of chronic hepatitis D with the entry inhibitor myrcludex B: first results of a phase Ib/IIa study. J Hepatol. 2016; 65(3):490–8.

43. Uhl P, Helm F, Hofhaus G, Brings S, Kaufman C, Leotta K, et al. A liposomal formulation for the oral application of the investigational hepatitis B drug Myrcludex B. Eur J Pharm Biopharm. 2016;103:159–66.

44. Verrier ER, Colpitts CC, Bach C, Heydmann L, Weiss A, Renaud M, et al. A targeted functional RNA interference screen uncovers glypican 5 as an entry factor for hepatitis B and D viruses. Hepatology. 2016;63:35–48.

45. Lee GH, Aung MM, Yang C, Hedrick JL, Lim SG, Yang YY, et al. Polyethylenimines (PEI) polymer functionalized with L-mannose moieties

inhibits hepatitis B virus (HBV) entry into HepG2-hNTCP cells with negligible cellular toxicity. Hepatology. 2017;64:938A.

46. Deres K, Schroder CH, Paessens A, Goldmann S, Hacker HJ, Weber O, et al. Inhibition of hepatitis B virus replication by drug-induced depletion of nucleocapsids. Science. 2003;299:893–6.

47. Stray SJ, Bourne CR, Punna S, Lewis WG, Finn MG, Zlotnick A. A heteroaryldihydropyrimidine activates and can misdirect hepatitis B virus capsid assembly. Proc Natl Acad Sci U S A. 2005;102:8138–43.

48. Brezillon N, Brunelle MN, Massinet H, Giang E, Lamant C, DaSilva L, et al. Antiviral activity of bay 41-4109 on hepatitis B virus in humanized alb-uPA/SCID mice. PLoS One. 2011;6:e25096.

49. Wang XY, Wei ZM, Wu GY, Wang JH, Zhang YJ, Li J, et al. In vitro inhibition of HBV replication by a novel compound, GLS4, and its efficacy against adefovir-dipivoxil-resistant HBV mutations. Antivir Ther. 2012;17:793–803.

50. Ding Y, Zhang H, Niu J, Chen H, Liu C, Li X, Wang F. Multiple dose study of GLS4JHS, interfering with the assembly of hepatitis B virus core particles, in patients infected with hepatitis B virus. J Hepatol. 2017;66:S27.

51. Qiu Z, Lin X, Zhang W, Zhou M, Guo L, Kocer B, et al. Discovery and pre-clinical characterization of third-generation 4-H Heteroaryldihydropyrimidine (HAP) analogues as hepatitis B virus (HBV) Capsid inhibitors. J Med Chem. 2017;60:3352–71.

52. Feld JJ, Colledge D, Sozzi V, Edwards R, Littlejohn M, Locarnini SA. The phenylpropenamide derivative AT-130 blocks HBV replication at the level of viral RNA packaging. Antivir Res. 2007;76:168–77.

53. Klumpp K, Shimada T, Allweiss L, Volz T, Luetgehetman M, Flores O, et al. High antiviral activity of the HBV core inhibitor NVR 3-778 in the humanized uPA/SCID mouse model. J Hepatol. 2015;62:S214.

54. Gane EJ, Schwabe S, Walker K, Flores L, Hartman GD, Klumpp K, et al. Phase 1a safety and pharmacokinetics of NVR 3-778, a potential first-in-class HBV Core inhibitor. Hepatology. 2014;60:1279A.

55. Yuen MF, Kim DJ, Weilert F, Chan HLY, Lalezari JP, Hwang SG, et al. NVR 3-778, a first in class core inhibitor, alone and in combination with PEG-interferon (PEGIFN), in treatment naïve HBeAg-positive patients: early reductions in HBV DNA and HBeAg. J Hepatol. 2016;64:S208.

56. Yuen MF, Kim DL, Weilert F, Chan HL, Jacob P, Lalezari JP, et al. Phase 1b efficacy and safety of NVR 3-778, a first-in- class HBV Core inhibitor, in HBeAg-positive patients with chronic HBV infection. Hepatology. 2015; 62(S1):1385A.

57. Yuen MF, Kim DJ, Weilert F, HLY C, Lalezari JP, Hwang SG, Nguyen T, Liaw S, Brown N, et al. NVR 3-778, a first-in-class HBV core inhibitor, alone and in combination with PEG-interferon (PEGIFN), in treatment-naive HBeAg positive patients: early reductions in HBV DNA and HBeAg. J Hepatol. 2016; 64:S210.

58. Mani N, Cole AG, Ardzinsk A, Cai D, Cuconati A, Dorsey BD, Guo H, et al. The HBV capsid inhibitor AB-423 exhibits a dual mode of action and displays additive/synergistic effects in in vitro combination studies. Hepatology. 2016;64:123A.

59. Huang Q, Zong Y, Mercier A, Kumar R, Mahon C, Zhou Y, Li PC, Guo L, et al. Blockage of HBV virus replication and inhibition of cccDNA establishment by Core protein Allosteric modifiers (CpAMs). Hepatology. 2016;64:937A.

60. Cai D, Mills C, Yu W, Yan R, Aldrich CE, Saputelli JR, et al. Identification of disubstituted sulfonamide compounds as specific inhibitors of hepatitis B virus covalently closed circular DNA formation. Antimicrob Agents Chemother. 2012;56:4277–88.

61. Lucifora J, Protzer U. Attacking hepatitis B virus cccDNA - the holy grail to hepatitis B cure. J Hepatol. 2016;64:S41–8.

62. Petersen J, Thompson AJ, Levrero M. Aiming for cure in HBV and HDV infection. J Hepatol. 2016;65(4):835–48.

63. Belloni L, Allweiss L, Guerrieri F, Pediconi N, Volz T, Pollicino T, et al. IFN-alpha inhibits HBV transcription and replication in cell culture and in humanized mice by targeting the epigenetic regulation of the nuclear cccDNA minichromosome. J Clin Invest. 2012;122:529–37.

64. Lucifora J, Arzberger S, Durantel D, Belloni L, Strubin M, Levrero M, et al. Hepatitis B virus X protein is essential to initiate and maintain virus replication after infection. J Hepatol. 2011;55:996–1003.

65. Decorsiere A, Mueller H, van Breugel PC, Abdul F, Gerossier L, Beran RK, et al. Hepatitis B virus X protein identifies the Smc5/6 complex as a host restriction factor. Nature. 2016;531:386–9.

66. Murphy CM, Xu Y, Li F, Nio K, Reszka-Blanco N, Li X, et al. Hepatitis B virus X protein promotes degradation of SMC5/6 to enhance HBV replication. Cell Rep. 2016;16:2846–54.

67. Livingston CM, Beran RK, Ramakrishnan D, Strubin M, Delaney WE, Fletcher SP. The Smc5/6 complex restricts hepatitis B virus transcription when localized to ND10. Hepatology. 2016;64:7A.

68. Tropberger P, Mercier A, Robinson M, Zhong W, Ganem DE, Holdorf M. Mapping of histone modifications in episomal HBV cccDNA uncovers an unusual chromatin organization amenable to epigenetic manipulation. Proc Natl Acad Sci U S A. 2015;112:E5715–24.

69. Nassal M. HBV cccDNA: viral persistence reservoir and key obstacle for a cure of chronic hepatitis B. Gut. 2015;64:1972–84.

70. Xia Y, Stadler D, Lucifora J, Reisinger F, Webb D, Hosel M, et al. Interferon-gamma and tumor necrosis factor-alpha produced by T cells reduce the HBV persistence form, cccDNA, without cytolysis. Gastroenterology. 2016;150:194–205.

71. Weber ND, Stone D, Sedlak RH, De Silva Feelixge HS, Roychoudhury P, Schiffer JT, et al. AAV-mediated delivery of zinc finger nucleases targeting hepatitis B virus inhibits active replication. PLoS One. 2014;9:e97579.

72. Bloom K, Ely A, Mussolino C, Cathomen T, Arbuthnot P. Inactivation of hepatitis B virus replication in cultured cells and in vivo with engineered transcription activator-like effector nucleases. Mol Ther. 2013;21:1889–97.

73. Seeger C, Sohn JA. Complete Spectrum of CRISPR/Cas9-induced mutations on HBV cccDNA. Mol Ther. 2016;24(7):1258–66.

74. Ebert G, Preston S, Allison C, Cooney J, Toe JG, Stutz MD, et al. Cellular inhibitor of apoptosis proteins prevent clearance of hepatitis B virus. Proc Natl Acad Sci U S A. 2015;112:5797–802.

75. Ebert G, Allison C, Preston S, Cooney J, Toe JG, Stutz MD, et al. Eliminating hepatitis B by antagonizing cellular inhibitors of apoptosis. Proc Natl Acad Sci U S A. 2015;112:5803–8.

76. Mahtab MA, Bazinet M, Patient R, Roingeard P, Vaillant A. Nucleic acid polymers REP 9 AC/REP 9 AC' elicit sustained immunologic control of chronic HBV infection. Glob Antiviral J. 2011;7:64A.

77. Al-Mahtab M, Bazinet M, Vaillant A. Safety and efficacy of nucleic acid polymers in Monotherapy and combined with immunotherapy in treatment-naive Bangladeshi patients with HBeAg+ chronic hepatitis B infection. PLoS One. 2016;11:e0156667.

78. Bazinet M, Pantea V, Placinta G, Moscalu I, Cebotarescu V, Cojuhari L, Jimbei P, et al. Update on safety and efficacy in the REP 401 protocol: REP 2139-Mgor REP 2165-mg used in combination with tenofovir disoproxil fumarate and pegylated interferon alpha-2a in treatment naïve caucasian patients with chronic HBeAg negative HBV infection. J Hepatol. 2017;66:S256.

79. Lanford R, Wooddell Cl, Chavez D, Oropeza C, Chu Q, Hamilton HL, et al. ARC-520 RNAi therapeutic reduces HBV DNA, s and e antigen in a chimpanzee with a very high viral titer. Hepatology. 2013;58:707A.

80. Sebestyen MG, Wong SC, Trubetskoy V, Lewis DL, Wooddell Cl. Targeted in vivo delivery of siRNA and an endosome-releasing agent to hepatocytes. Methods Mol Biol. 2015;1218:163–86.

81. Man-Fung Yuen MF, HLY C, Given BD, Hamilton J, Schluep T, Lewis DL, et al. Phase II, dose-ranging study of ARC-520, a siRNA-based therapeutic, in patients with chronic hepatitis B virus infection. Hepatology. 2014;60:LB21.

82. Gish RG, Yuen MF, Chan HL, Given BD, Lai CL, Locarnini SA, et al. Synthetic RNAi triggers and their use in chronic hepatitis B therapies with curative intent. Antivir Res. 2015;121:97–108.

83. Xu D, Chavez D, Guerra B, Littlejohn M, Peterson R, Locarnini S, Gish R, et al. Tratment of chronically HBV-infected chimpanzees with RNA interference therapeutic ARC-520 led to potent reduction of viral mRNA, DNA and proteins without observed drug resistance. J Hepatol. 2016;64:S398.

84. Yuen MF, Chan HL, Liu K, Given BD, Schluep T, Hamilton J, Lai C-L, Locarnini SA, et al. Differential reductions in viral antigens expressed from ccDNA integrated DNA in treatment naive HBeAg positive and negative patients with chronic HBV after RNA interference therapy with ARC-520. J Hepatol. 2016;64:S390.

85. Lee AC, Dhillon AP, Reid SP, Thi EP, Phelps JR, McClintock M, Li AH, et al. Exploring combination therapy for curing HBV: preclinical studies with Capsid inhibitor AB-423 and a siRNA agent, ARB-1740. Hepatology. 2016;64:122A.

86. Streinu-Cercel A, Gane E, Cheng W, Sievert W, Roberts S, Ahn SH, Kim YJ, et al. A phase 2a study evaluating the multi-dose activity of ARB-1467 in HBeAg positive and negative virally suppressed subjects with hepatitis B. J Hepatol. 2017;66:S688.

87. Mao T, Zhang K, Kloth C, Roelvink P, Suhy D. Superior suppression of hepatitis B virus DNA and antigen levels in a chimeric mouse model when BB-103, a DNA-directed RNA interference agent, is coupled with standard of care drugs. J Hepatol. 2017;66:S260.

88. Esau C, Linphong P, Tachikawa K, McSwiggen J, Taylor W, Figa PK, et al. LUNAR™-HBV, a UNA oligomer combination for the treatment of chronic hepatitis B virus infection. Hepatology. 2016;64:912A.

89. Phillips S, Chokshi S, Chatterji U, Riva A, Bobardt M, Williams R, et al. Alisporivir inhibition of hepatocyte cyclophilins reduces HBV replication and hepatitis B surface antigen production. Gastroenterology. 2015;148:403–14. e7

90. Wu J, Meng Z, Jiang M, Pei R, Trippler M, Broering R, et al. Hepatitis B virus suppresses toll-like receptor-mediated innate immune responses in murine parenchymal and nonparenchymal liver cells. Hepatology. 2009;49:1132–40.

91. Lanford RE, Guerra B, Chavez D, Giavedoni L, Hodara VL, Brasky KM, et al. GS-9620, an oral agonist of toll-like receptor-7, induces prolonged suppression of hepatitis B virus in chronically infected chimpanzees. Gastroenterology. 2013;144:1508–17. 1517.e1-10

92. Gane EJ, Lim YS, Gordon SC, Visvanathan K, Sicard E, Fedorak RN, et al. The oral toll-like receptor-7 agonist GS-9620 in patients with chronic hepatitis B virus infection. J Hepatol. 2015;63:320–8.

93. Janssen HL, Brunetto MR, Kim YJ, Ferrari C, Massetto B, Nguyen AH, Gaggar A, et al. Safety and efficacy of GS-9620 in virally-suppressed patients with chronic hepatitis B. Hepatology. 2016;64:913A.

94. Boni C, Vecchi A, Rossi M, Laccabue D, Giuberti TG, Alfieri A, Lampertico P, et al. TLR-7 agonist GS-9620 can improve HBV-specific T cell and NK cell responses in nucleos(t)ide suppressed patients with chronic hepatitis B. Hepatology. 2016;64:7A.

95. Guo F, Tang L, Shu S, Sehgal M, Sheraz M, Liu B, et al. Activation of STING in hepatocytes suppresses the replication of hepatitis B virus. Antimicrob Agents Chemother. 2017. PMID 28717041. doi: 10.1128/AAC.00771-17.

96. Korolowicz K, Balarezo M, Iyer R, Padmanabhan S, Cleary D, Gimi R, Sheri A, Suresh M, et al. Antiviral efficacy and host immune response induction with SB 9200, an oral prodrug of the dinucleotide SB 9000, in combination with entecavir in the woodchuck model of chronic hepatitis B. J Hepatol. 2016; 64:S602.

97. Lok AS, Pan CQ, Han SB, Trinh HN, Fessel WJ, Rodell T, et al. Randomized phase II study of GS-4774 as a therapeutic vaccine in virally suppressed patients with chronic hepatitis B. J Hepatol. 2016;65(3):509–16.

98. Janssen HL, Yoon SK, Yoshida EM, Trinh HN, Rodell TC, Nguyen AH, Caggar A, et al. Safety and efficacy of GS-4774 in combination with TDF in patients with chronic hepatitis B not on antiviral medication. Hepatology. 2016;64:122A.

99. Michler T, Kosinska A, Jäger C, Röder N, Grimm D, Heikenwälder M, et al. RNA interference mediated suppression of HBV transcripts restores HBV-specific immunity and enhances the efficacy of therapeutic vaccination. J Hepatol. 2016;64:S133.

100. Kah J, Koh S, Volz T, Allweiss L, Lohse A, Lütgehetmann M, et al. Immunotherapy using T cells redirected against HBV results in reduced viral loads and enhanced immune responses in humanized mice. J Hepatol. 2016;64:S151.

101. Bennett CF, Swayze EE. RNA targeting therapeutics: molecular mechanisms of antisense oligonucleotides as a therapeutic platform. Annu Rev Pharmacol Toxicol. 2010;50:259–93.

102. Zheng SJ, Zhong S, Zhang JJ, Chen F, Ren H, Deng CL. Distribution and anti-HBV effects of antisense oligodeoxynucleotides conjugated to galactosylated poly-L-lysine. World J Gastroenterol. 2003;9:1251–5.

103. Ding X, Yang J, Wang S. Antisense oligonucleotides targeting abhydrolase domain containing 2 block human hepatitis B virus propagation. Oligonucleotides. 2011;21:77–84.

104. Billioud G, Kruse RL, Carrillo M, Whitten-Bauer C, Gao D, Kim A, et al. In vivo reduction of hepatitis B virus antigenemia and viremia by antisense oligonucleotides. J Hepatol. 2016;64:781–9.

105. Lomonosova E, Daw J, Garimallaprabhakaran AK, Agyemang NB, Ashani Y, Murelli RP, et al. Efficacy and cytotoxicity in cell culture of novel alpha-hydroxytropolone inhibitors of hepatitis B virus ribonuclease H. Antivir Res. 2017;144:164–72.

3

Time-varying serum gradient of hepatitis B surface antigen predicts risk of relapses after off-NA therapy

Nai-Hsuan Chien[1,2,12], Yen-Tsung Huang[3], Chun-Ying Wu[4,5], Chi-Yang Chang[2,6,10], Ming-Shiang Wu[7], Jia-Horng Kao[7,8], Lein-Ray Mo[9], Chi-Ming Tai[10], Chih-Wen Lin[10], Tzeng-Huey Yang[11], Jaw-Town Lin[2,6,10] and Yao-Chun Hsu[2,6,10,13*]

Abstract

Background: The serum gradient of hepatitis B surface antigen (HBsAg) varies over time after cessation of nucleos(t)ide analog (NA) treatment in patients with chronic hepatitis B (CHB). The association between the time-varying HBsAg serum gradient and risk of relapse has not been elucidated.

Methods: This multicenter cohort study prospectively enrolled CHB patients who discontinued 3 year-NA treatment. Eligible patients were serologically negative for HBeAg and viral DNA at NA cessation. The participants (n = 140) were followed every 3 months through HBsAg quantification. Virological and clinical relapses were defined as viral DNA levels >2000 IU/mL and alanine aminotransferase (ALT) levels >80 U/mL, respectively. The association of time-varying HBsAg levels with relapses was assessed through a time-dependent Cox analysis.

Results: During a median follow-up of 19.9 (interquartile range [IQR], 10.6–25.3) months, virological and clinical relapses occurred in 94 and 49 patients, with a 2-year cumulative incidence of 79.2% (95% confidence interval [CI], 70.9%–86.4%) and 42.9% (95% CI, 34.1%–52.8%), respectively. The serum level of HBsAg was associated with virological ($P < 0.001$) and clinical ($P = 0.01$) relapses in a dose–response manner, with adjusted hazard ratios of 2.10 (95% CI, 1.45–3.04) and 2.32 (95% CI, 1.28–4.21). Among the patients (n = 19) whose HBsAg levels ever dropped below 10 IU/mL, only one and three patients subsequently developed clinical and virological relapses.

Conclusion: The serum gradient of HBsAg measured throughout the off-therapy observation is associated with the subsequent occurrence of virological and clinical relapses in CHB patients who discontinue NA treatment.

Keywords: Chronic hepatitis B, Nucleos(t)ide analogs, Hepatitis B surface antigen quantification, Time-dependent Cox proportion hazards model

Background

Chronic infection with hepatitis B virus (HBV) is the leading cause of liver-related morbidity and mortality worldwide, particularly in Asian countries [1]. Management of patients with chronic hepatitis B (CHB) has reached an era of anti-viral therapy, with approved regimens consisting of interferon alpha and nucleos(t)ide analogs (NAs) [2–5]. Through the effective inhibition of viral replication, NAs not only ameliorate viremia and reduce hepatic inflammation, but also may prevent and even reverse liver fibrosis [6–8]. A large body of evidence corroborates the effectiveness of NAs in improving clinical outcomes [9, 10]. However, off-therapy durability after discontinuation of NA treatment is typically unsustainable [11–19].

Because of high off-therapy relapse rates, major international guidelines currently recommend an indefinite prolongation of NA therapy, possibly until loss of hepatitis B surface antigen (HBsAg) with or without appearance of accompanying antibodies [12]. However, this strategy entails life-long treatment for most treated patients [13] and is not affordable in regions with

* Correspondence: gatsbyhsu@yahoo.com.tw; holdenhsu@gmail.com
[2]School of Medicine, Fu Jen Catholic University, New Taipei, Taiwan
[6]Division of Gastroenterology, Fu-Jen Catholic University Hospital, New Taipei, Taiwan
Full list of author information is available at the end of the article

resource-constrained health care systems, where, ironically, CHB is most prevalent [14]. Therefore, it is important to find out some factors to predict the risk of off-therapy relapse. Recently, intense research has been carried out to clarify predictors of off-therapy relapse and identify patients who maintain remission without resuming medication [17–22].

In response to the challenges associated with the safe discontinuation of NAs, we prospectively followed a multicenter cohort who discontinued NAs after a minimum of 3 years on therapy. We observed that the serum gradient of HBsAg observed at the end of treatment (EOT), in addition to serum alanine aminotransferase (ALT) levels and age, stratified the risks of both virological and clinical relapses [20]. After the cessation of NA therapy, the level of HBsAg may change over time, but its clinical implication has not been elucidated. Therefore, we conducted this study to explore the association between relapse risks and time-varying serum gradients of HBsAg measured during an off-therapy follow-up.

Methods

Design and setting

This prospective cohort study was conducted in three different regional teaching hospitals (E-Da Hospital, Kaohsiung, Lotung Poh-Ai Hospital, Yilan, and National Taiwan University Hospital Yun-Lin Branch, Yunlin) in Taiwan. Institutional review boards approved the study protocol (EMRP100–049) in all hospitals for patient recruitment and database establishment. Data analysis specifically for this study was also approved (EMRP-104-082). Written informed consent was obtained from all participants prior to their enrollment.

Study participants

We consecutively screened adult patients with CHB who were going to discontinue NA therapy between July 1, 2011 and April 1, 2015, and we evaluated their eligibility. Patients were included if they had been diagnosed with CHB for at least 6 months prior to NA treatment, continuously received any NA (lamivudine, adefovir, telbivudine, entecavir, or tenofovir) for at least 3 years, were serologically negative for HBeAg, and showed undetectable levels of HBV DNA at the end of NA therapy. Patients were excluded in the presence of coinfection with human immunodeficiency virus or hepatitis C virus, any malignancy, liver cirrhosis, hepatic encephalopathy, variceal hemorrhage, organ transplantation, previous use of interferon alpha for 1 month or longer, and concurrent use of cytotoxic or immunosuppressive medication. The diagnosis of liver cirrhosis was based on pathological proof or clinical criteria that included splenomegaly or esophagogastric varices in addition to typical sonographic features.

Patients had to discontinue NAs because of the national health insurance policy. Details of the reimbursement regulations have been previously reported.[10] In brief, the therapeutic duration was principally restricted to 3 years among general patients without cirrhosis. Those who experienced HBeAg seroconversion on therapy were entitled to treatment consolidation for an additional 1 year.

Follow-up after cessation of NAs

Pertinent demographic, biochemical, serological, and virological data were collected at enrollment. After discontinuation of NAs, patients were monitored at a close interval of 3 months. The patients underwent physical checkup and laboratory measurement at each follow-up visit. They also underwent abdominal sonography along with serum alpha-fetoprotein estimation tests every 6 months for the surveillance of liver cancer.

Standardized quantification of serum HBsAg and viral DNA was carried out in the Taipei Pathology Institutes (Taipei, Taiwan). Serum HBsAg levels were measured through an automated immunoassay (Abbott Architect i2000, Abbott Park, IL, USA). Samples with HBsAg levels exceeding the upper limit of automatic detection (250 IU/mL) were manually diluted before quantification. Serum HBV DNA was quantified through a commercialized polymerase chain reaction method (COBAS TaqMan HBV Test, version 2.0, Roche Molecular Systems, Inc., Branchburg, NJ, USA) with a detection range of $20–1.7 \times 10^8$ IU/mL.

Definitions of virological and clinical relapses

Virological relapse was defined as the reappearance of >2000 IU/mL HBV DNA in serum. Clinical relapse was defined as an episode of elevated ALT (>80 IU/mL, >2 times the normal conventional upper limit) and >2000 IU/mL HBV DNA. Patients did not resume antiviral therapy until clinical hepatitis persisted for 3 months or longer, unless a risk of hepatic decompensation (serum bilirubin >2 mg/dL or prothrombin time prolonged >3 s) was observed.

Data analyses and statistical methods

Continuous and categorical variables were summarized using the median and interquartile range (IQR) and proportion with exact numbers, respectively. The incidence rates of virological and clinical relapses were estimated using the Kaplan–Meier method. In a multivariate-adjusted Cox proportional hazards model for off-therapy relapses, the serum level of HBsAg was a time-varying variable that denoted each measurement after NA cessation. The dose–response relationship for the association between HBsAg levels and off-therapy relapses was illustrated by penalized splines in the Cox model. The results were reported as hazard ratios along with 95% confidence intervals

(CIs). Data were analyzed using commercial software (Stata, version 13.0; Stata Corp, College Station, TX, USA). All statistical analyses were two-sided with significance set at $P < 0.05$.

Results

Baseline characteristics of the participants

We monitored a total of 140 patients who discontinued NA therapy after a minimum of 3 years (median, 36.6; IQR, 36.4–37.0 months) between July 1, 2011 and April 1, 2015 (Fig. 1). They were followed for a median of 19.9 (IQR, 10.6–25.3) months following the cessation of NA therapy. The mean time interval between initial HBsAg level and last HBsAg level is 19.15 ± 11 months. Table 1 presents a summary of the characteristics of this study population, which was predominantly male (77.9%, $n = 109$) with a median age of 49.1 (IQR, 39.2–57.5) years. Prior to antiviral treatment, 39 patients were initially HBeAg-positive. They were all serologically negative for HBeAg after treatment and had been consolidated for at least 1 year (median, 18.2; IQR, 12.2–25.4 months) following HBeAg loss. The median levels of HBsAg, ALT, and alpha-fetoprotein

Table 1 Characteristics of the study patients

Characteristics	All patients ($N = 140$)
Male gender, n (%)	109 (77.9%)
EOT Age, years	49.1 (39.2, 57.5)
EOT anti-HBe-positive, n (%)	131 (93.6%)
EOT HBsAg, log IU/mL	2.79 (2.13, 3.12)
EOT ALT, U/L	22 (16.5, 34)
EOT AFP, ng/ml	2.7 (1.97, 3.41)
Pretreatment HBeAg-positive, n (%)	39 (27.9%)
Pretreatment anti-HBe-positive, n (%)	100 (71.4%)
Pretreatment viral DNA, log IU/ml	6.21 (4.53, 7.67)
Pretreatment ALT, U/L	154 (95, 451)
On-therapy duration, month	36.6 (36.4, 37.0)
Off-therapy follow-up[a], month	19.9 (10.6, 25.3)
Patients received Entecavir	125 (89.3%)
Patients received Tenofovir,	9 (6.4%)
Patients received Lamivudine or Telbivudine	6 (4.2%)

Notes. [a]patients were followed up until reuse of antiviral therapy; *AFP* alpha-fetoprotein, *ALT* Alanine transaminase, *EOT* end-of-therapy, *HBeAg* hepatitis B e antigen, *HBsAg* hepatitis B surface antigen

were 2.79 (IQR, 2.13–3.12) log IU/mL, 22 (IQR, 16.5–34) U/L, and 2.7 (IQR, 1.97–3.41) ng/mL at the end of treatment, respectively.

Clinical and virological relapses after NA discontinuation

During the off-therapy follow-up, 49 and 94 participants developed clinical and virological relapses, respectively. The cumulative incidence rates of clinical relapses were 28.4% (95% CI, 21.2%–37.5%) and 42.9% (95% CI, 34.1%–52.8%) at 1 and 2 years, respectively, and those of virological relapses were 62.0% (95% CI, 53.5%–70.6%) and 79.2% (95% CI, 70.9%–86.4%) at 1 and 2 years, respectively (Table 2). Seven patients with previous HBeAg positive experienced reoccurrence of HBeAg. Twenty one patients had been treated with NA after relapse. No patient is complicated with hepatic decompensation after secession of NAs therapy in this study.

Dose–response relationship of the time-varying HBsAg level and off-therapy relapses

The penalized splines in the univariate Cox model characterized the dose–response curves between increments

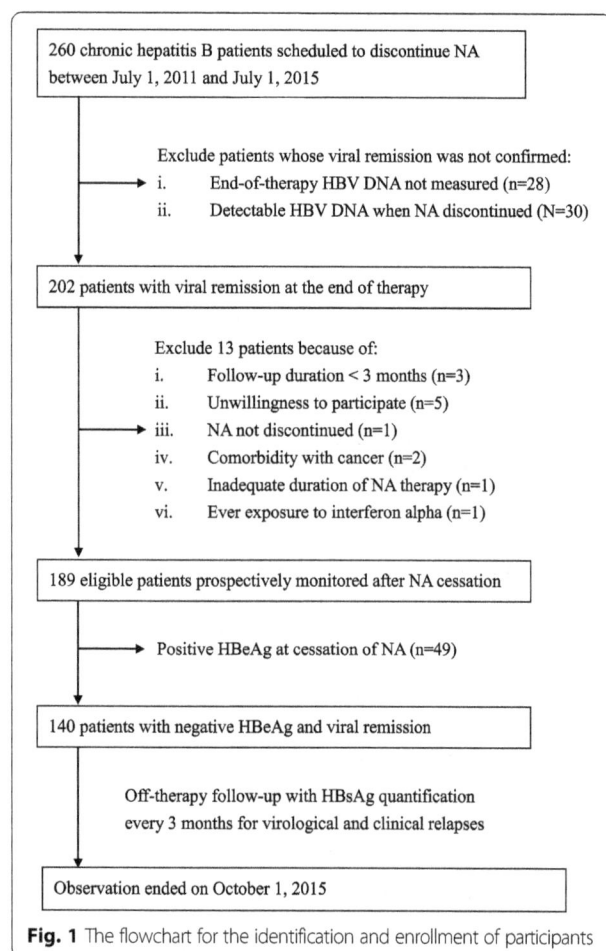

260 chronic hepatitis B patients scheduled to discontinue NA between July 1, 2011 and July 1, 2015

Exclude patients whose viral remission was not confirmed:
i.   End-of-therapy HBV DNA not measured (n=28)
ii. Detectable HBV DNA when NA discontinued (N=30)

202 patients with viral remission at the end of therapy

Exclude 13 patients because of:
i.   Follow-up duration < 3 months (n=3)
ii.   Unwillingness to participate (n=5)
iii. NA not discontinued (n=1)
iv.   Comorbidity with cancer (n=2)
v.   Inadequate duration of NA therapy (n=1)
vi.   Ever exposure to interferon alpha (n=1)

189 eligible patients prospectively monitored after NA cessation

Positive HBeAg at cessation of NA (n=49)

140 patients with negative HBeAg and viral remission

Off-therapy follow-up with HBsAg quantification every 3 months for virological and clinical relapses

Observation ended on October 1, 2015

Fig. 1 The flowchart for the identification and enrollment of participants

Table 2 Clinical and virological relapses after cessation of nucleos(t)ide analogues in patients with negative HBeAg and undetectable viral DNA at the end of treatment

All ($N = 140$)

	First year	Second year
Virological relapse	62.0% (95% CI, 53.5–70.6%)	79.2% (95% CI, 70.9–86.4%)
Clinical relapse	28.4% (95% CI, 21.2–37.5%)	42.9% (95% CI, 34.1–52.8%)

of HBsAg and risks of relapse (Fig. 2). An increase in the serum level of HBsAg following NA cessation was significantly correlated with a higher risk of subsequent virological ($P = 0.00017$) and clinical ($P = 0.012$) relapses. Moreover, no obvious nonlinearity was observed in the dose–response relationship, supporting the use of a linear term in the Cox model to summarize the hazard ratio for one log increase in the HBsAg level.

Multivariate-adjusted analyses for the association between time-varying HBsAg levels and off-therapy relapses

The association between time-varying serum levels of HBsAg and off-therapy relapses was further examined through the multivariate-adjusted Cox proportional hazard analysis, which revealed that HBsAg levels, EOT age, and EOT ALT were significant predictors of both clinical and virological relapses. For virological relapse, the serum level of HBsAg, EOT age, and EOT ALT were associated with adjusted hazard ratios of 2.10 per log IU/mL (95% CI, 1.45–3.04), 1.04 per year (95% CI, 1.02–1.06), and 1.02 per U/L (95% CI, 1.01–1.02), respectively (Table 3). Regarding clinical relapse, the serum level of HBsAg, EOT age, and EOT ALT were associated with adjusted hazard ratios of 2.32 per log IU/mL (95% CI, 1.28–4.21), 1.03 per year (95% CI, 1.00–1.06), and 1.03 per U/L (95% CI, 1.02–1.05), respectively (Table 4). Furthermore, the association of HBsAg levels with outcomes did not vary with time ($P = 0.19$ for virological and 0.71 for clinical relapses), thus satisfying the proportional hazard assumption for the model.

The predictive value of low HBsAg was demonstrated by 19 patients whose respective HBsAg levels ever dropped below 10 IU/mL during the off-therapy follow-up. Among them, only one and three patients subsequently developed clinical and virological relapses,

Table 3 Multivariate Cox porportional hazard model for virological relapse with off-therapy HBsAg level as a time-varying variable

Variables	Adjusted HR	95% CI	P
Time-varying HBsAg level, log IU/mL	2.10	1.45, 3.04	<0.0001
Male sex	1.33	0.58, 3.05	0.49
EOT age, year	1.04	1.02, 1.06	0.0005
EOT ALT, U/L	1.02	1.01, 1.02	<0.0001
EOT AFP, ng/mL	1.06	0.96, 1.16	0.24
EOT anti-HBe-seropositive	0.46	0.16, 1.29	0.14
Pretreatment viral DNA, log IU/mL	1.06	0.90, 1.25	0.52
Pretreatment HBeAg-positive	2.58	0.53, 12.50	0.24
Pretreatment anti-HBe-positive	4.02	0.88, 18.3	0.07

Notes. *AFP* alpha-fetoprotein, *ALT* Alanine transaminase, *CI* confidence interval, *EOT* end-of-therapy, *HBeAg* hepatitis B e antigen, *HBsAg* hepatitis B surface antigen, *HR* hazard ratio

respectively (both $P < 0.0001$), compared with those whose HBsAg levels never fell below10 IU/mL.

Discussion

In our recent study, we demonstrated that the serum gradient of HBsAg measured at the end of treatment, as well as ALT levels and age, stratified the risks of both virological and clinical relapses [20]. The current study further extends the predictive value of HBsAg measurement beyond the time point at NA cessation. We demonstrated that the off-therapy HBsAg level as a time-varying predictor was associated with both clinical and virological relapses in EOT HBeAg-negative patients with CHB. Eextremely low incidence rates of clinical relapse were observed in those whose HBsAg levels fell below 10 IU/mL, indicating the clinical application of HBsAg surveillance in patients attempting NA discontinuation. Therefore, monitoring serum levels of HBsAg

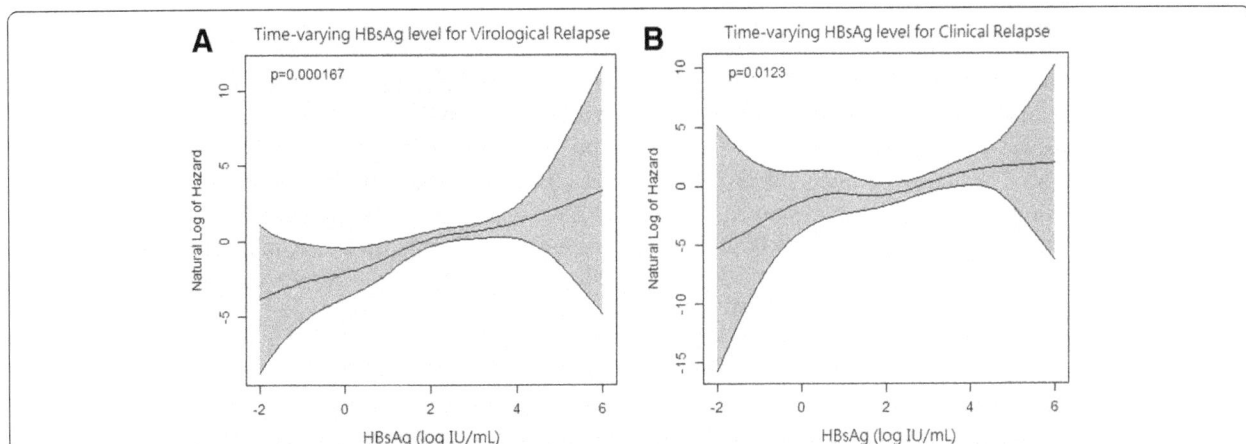

Fig. 2 Dose–response relationship for the association of off-therapy HBsAg levels with virological relapse (**a**) and clinical relapse (**b**). The dose–response curves characterized by penalized splines in the Cox model depict a significantly increasing trend; that is, increases in HBsAg levels are associated with increased risks of virological ($P = 0.00017$) and clinical ($P = 0.012$) relapses.Overall, no obvious nonlinearity was observed in the dose–response relationship, supporting the use of a linear term in the Cox model to summarize the hazard ratio for one log increase of HBsAg level

Table 4 Multivariate Cox porportional hazard model for clinical relapse with off-therapy HBsAg level as a time-varying variable

Variables	Adjusted HR	95% CI	P
Time-varying HBsAg level, log IU/mL	2.32	1.28, 4.21	0.005
Male sex	1.05	0.33, 3.29	0.94
EOT age, year	1.03	1.00, 1.06	0.045
EOT ALT, U/L	1.03	1.02, 1.05	<0.0001
EOT AFP, ng/mL	0.88	0.67, 1.15	0.34
EOT anti-HBe-seropositive	1.27	0.14, 11.60	0.84
Pretreatment viral DNA, log IU/mL	1.03	0.79, 1.36	0.81
Pretreatment HBeAg-positive	0.46	0.66, 3.21	0.43
Pretreatment anti-HBe-positive	0.47	0.70, 3.20	0.44

Notes. *AFP* alpha-fetoprotein, *ALT* Alanine transaminase, *CI* confidence interval, *EOT* end-of-therapy, *HBeAg* hepatitis B e antigen, *HBsAg* hepatitis B surface antigen, *HR* hazard ratio

may guide the selection of patients who can maintain sustained viral suppression.

Inactive carriers have been found to have low HBsAg levels [23–25], with HBsAg levels <1000 U/mL having an 87.9% positive predictive value and 96.7% negative predictive value for patients with HBV DNA <2000 IU/mL. A recent study [21] in Northern Taiwan involving 117 patients receiving entecavir treatment reported that serum HBV DNA levels at 3 and 6 months off-therapy were associated with clinical relapse, and the HBsAg level at 6 months off-therapy had a weak association with clinical relapse. Furthermore, 13.6% of the patients had sustained virological response (undetectable HBV DNA levels at 12 months off -therapy). No clinical relapse was observed during a mean 24.8-month follow-up, suggesting that patients without HBsAg clearance could have sustained clinical and viral remission. However, EOT HBsAg was the only factor associated with sustained virological response (P = 0.009). Another study involving 252 patients in southern Taiwan [26] also showed that the combination of age (<55 years) and EOT HBsAg levels (<150 IU/mL) was associated with a low rate of virologic relapse. The decline level of HBsAg during treatment was higher in patients with HBsAg clearance than in those without HBsAg clearance. However, both studies mainly relied on EOT HBsAg levels to predict outcomes, and the association of HBsAg kinetics and relapse risk was not discussed. Our study is the first to discuss HBsAg as a time-varying factor for durable remission.

Although patients subjected to NA treatment had a favorable response with regard to HBV DNA levels, the observed HBsAg decline in such patients was lower than in those treated with interferon. This is probably due to the mechanism of NA treatment. NA treatment affects the reverse transcription of pregenomic RNA, but it

does not affect covalently closed circular DNA and subgenomic RNA, which have translational activities associated with HBsAg levels [27]. Moreover, serum HBsAg levels reflect active intrahepatic covalently closed circular DNA and have additional value as markers of on-treatment efficacy [28]. However, the NA potentially restores immune responses [29], which possibly results in HBsAg decline. This hypothesis is supported by data that HBsAg decline was strong in patients with higher ALT at the baseline [30] or higher levels of interferon gamma-induced protein 10 at the baseline, which indicates a reasonable level of immune response in such patients. Interferon gamma-induced protein 10 is a chemokine, which is a response to interferon gamma and may reflect the innate immune response against HBV [31]. Our data also show that the serum gradient of HBsAg was associated with the subsequent occurrence of virological and clinical relapses. Especially, the patients, whose HBsAg levels below 10 IU/mL not only at the end of therapy but along the off-therapy follow-up, had very low risk of relapses. Therefore, HBsAg kinetics may be a useful means to monitor NA treatment.

In the current strategies of NA-off follow-up, the HBV DNA and ALT would be monitored routinely and closely. However, elevation of ALT is usually a late event preceded by viral rebound and cannot be regarded as an early predictor. Following abrupt resurgence of viremia, severe acute exacerbation could rapidly ensue and incur the risk of liver failure. Besides, measurement of viral DNA remains costly. Our study showed the HBsAg kinetics has a linear association with relapse risks. Therefore, HBsAg level monitoring, every three months for instance, provides a chance to identify those who may not need frequent viral DNA measurement, and implicates a safe follow-up strategy with less expense.

This study has several strengths. First, we monitored HBsAg levels during the entire follow-up instead of at a single time point. Second, this research was conducted in a real-world setting that reflects "in-field" practice. For external validity, patients were recruited from multiple sites and treatment was not restricted to a single NA. Third, a minimum of 3-year NA therapy enabled most patients to obtain remission status before discontinuing NAs. Finally, stringent monitoring with an interval of 3 months enabled us to observe both virological and clinical relapses closely.

Several limitations were noted in this study. First, because this study prospectively started after NA discontinuation, blood samples prior to the baseline were unavailable. Therefore, we could not ascertain when HBV DNA became undetectable during the treatment by using a standardized protocol. We acknowledge that this is a major limitation because the length of consolidation following remission of viremia has been shown to influence the risk of relapse

[14]. Nonetheless, this limitation is unlikely to bias our finding regarding the dose–response association of time-varying HBsAg with off-therapy relapses. Third, we could not quantify pretreatment HBsAg levels exceeding 250 IU/mL and were thus unable to calculate the exact decline of HBsAg during therapy. Intriguingly, a recent small study in Spain suggested that an on-therapy HBsAg decline of more than 5000 IU/mL might indicate durable remission [32]. Finally, because our study exclusively recruited Asian patients whose viral genotype was either type B or C [33], extrapolation to the Western population requires validation.

Conclusions

In conclusion, this study reveals a dose–response association between time-varying HBsAg and off-therapy relapse following the cessation of NA therapy in patients with CHB. By reporting a negligible risk of subsequent relapse in patients whose HBsAg dropped to a considerably low level (<10 IU/mL), we demonstrate the potential utility of monitoring HBsAg levels in patients with CHB who discontinue NA treatment. These findings may not only implicate a safe strategy to monitor patients who attempt NA cessation but also stimulate further research to elucidate the clinical relevance of HBsAg quantification.

Abbreviations

ALT: Alanine transaminase; CHB: Chronic hepatitis B; CI: Confidence interval; EOT: End of therapy; HBeAg: Hepatitis B envelope antigen; HBsAg: Hepatitis B surface antigen; HBV: Hepatitis B virus; IQR: Interquartile range; NA: Nucleos(t)ide analog

Acknowledgements

The authors are indebted to our colleagues involved in the clinical care of these patients. We also appreciate the efforts by Ms. Ying-Ju Lee, Ms. Hsin-Yi Tsai, and Ms. Tzu-En Tsai.

Grant support

Cathay General Hospital and Fu-Jen University(104-GGH-FJU-11), E-Da Hospital (EDAHP105019), and the Taipei Pathology Institutes (TIP104-2).

Authors' contributions

GUARANTOR OF THE ARTICLE: Y-CH. Concept and design: YCH, Y-TH, and J-TL. Data collection: Y-CH, C-YC, M-SW, T-HY, L-RM, C-MT, and C-WL. Data analysis and interpretation: N-HC, Y-TH, C-YW, Y-CH, and J-HK. Manuscript drafting: N-HC, and Y-CH. Edition and revision of the manuscript: All authors. All authors read and approved the final manuscript.

Competing interests

YCH has received lecture fees from Bristol-Myers Squibb, Roche, and Gilead Sciences. JHK is a consultant for Abbott, Abbvie, Bayer, Boehringer Ingelheim, Bristol-Myers Squibb, Gilead Sciences, GlaxoSmithKline, Johnson & Johnson, Merck Sharp & Dohme, Novartis, and Roche and is on the speaker's bureau for Abbott, Roche, Bayer, Bristol-Myers Squibb, GlaxoSmithKline, and Novartis. JTL has received a research grant from Gilead Sciences in another unrelated study. All other authors have no competing interests to declare.

Author details

[1]Cathay General Hospital, Taipei, Taiwan. [2]School of Medicine, Fu Jen Catholic University, New Taipei, Taiwan. [3]Institute of Statistical Science, Academia Sinica, Taipei, Taiwan. [4]Division of Gastroenterology, Taichung Veterans General Hospital, Taichung, Taiwan. [5]Faculty of Medicine, School of Medicine, National Yang-Ming University, Taipei, Taiwan. [6]Division of Gastroenterology, Fu-Jen Catholic University Hospital, New Taipei, Taiwan. [7]Department of Internal Medicine, National Taiwan University Hospital, Taipei, Taiwan. [8]Graduate Institute of Clinical Medicine, National Taiwan University, Taipei, Taiwan. [9]Department of Internal Medicine, Tainan Municipal Hospital, Tainan, Taiwan. [10]Division of Gastroenterology, E-Da Hospital/I-Shou University, Kaohsiung, Taiwan. [11]Department of Internal Medicine, Lotung Poh-Ai Hospital, Yilan Country, Taiwan. [12]Sijhih Cathay General Hospital, New Taipei, Taiwan. [13]No.510, Zhongzheng Rd., Xinzhuang Dist, New Taipei City 24205, Taiwan.

References

1. Liaw YF, Chu CM. Hepatitis B virus infection. Lancet. 2009;373:582–92.
2. El-Serag HB. Epidemiology of viral hepatitis and hepatocellular carcinoma. Gastroenterology. 2012;142:1264–73.
3. European Association For The Study Of The L. EASL clinical practice guidelines: Management of chronic hepatitis B virus infection. J Hepatol. 2012;57:167–85.
4. Lok AS, McMahon BJ. Chronic hepatitis B: update 2009. Hepatology. 2009;50:661–2.
5. Liaw YF, Kao JH, Piratvisuth T, et al. Asian-Pacific consensus statement on the management of chronic hepatitis B: a 2012 update. Hepatol Int. 2012;6:531–61.
6. Lin CL, Kao JH. Recent advances in the treatment of chronic hepatitis B. Expert Opin Pharmacother. 2011;12:2025–40.
7. Chang TT, Liaw YF, SS W, et al. Long-term entecavir therapy results in the reversal of fibrosis/cirrhosis and continued histological improvement in patients with chronic hepatitis B. Hepatology. 2010;52:886–93.
8. Marcellin P, Gane E, Buti M, et al. Regression of cirrhosis during treatment with tenofovir disoproxil fumarate for chronic hepatitis B: a 5-year open-label follow-up study. Lancet. 2013;381:468–75.
9. CY W, Lin JT, Ho HJ, et al. Association of nucleos(t)ide analogue therapy with reduced risk of hepatocellular carcinoma in patients with chronic hepatitis B: a nationwide cohort study. Gastroenterology. 2014;147:143–51.
10. Chiang CJ, Yang YW, Chen JD, et al. Significant reduction in end-stage liver diseases burden through the national viral hepatitis therapy program in Taiwan. Hepatology. 2015;61:1154–62.
11. Reijnders JG, Perquin MJ, Zhang N, et al. Nucleos(t)ide analogues only induce temporary hepatitis B e antigen seroconversion in most patients with chronic hepatitis B. Gastroenterology. 2010;139:491–8.
12. Chaung KT, Ha NB, Trinh HN, et al. High frequency of recurrent viremia after hepatitis B e antigen seroconversion and consolidation therapy. J Clin Gastroenterol. 2012;46:865–70.
13. Tseng TC, Liu CJ, TH S, et al. Young chronic hepatitis B patients with nucleos(t)ide analogue-induced hepatitis B e antigen seroconversion have a higher risk of HBV reactivation. J Infect Dis. 2012;206:1521–31.

14. Chi H, Hansen BE, Yim C, et al. Reduced risk of relapse after long-term nucleos(t)ide analogue consolidation therapy for chronic hepatitis B. Aliment Pharmacol Ther. 2015;41:867–76.
15. Fung J, Lai CL, Yuen J, et al. Randomized trial of lamivudine versus entecavir in entecavir-treated patients with undetectable hepatitis B virus DNA: outcome at 2 Years. Hepatology. 2011;53:1148–53.
16. Chen CH, SN L, Hung CH, et al. The role of hepatitis B surface antigen quantification in predicting HBsAg loss and HBV relapse after discontinuation of lamivudine treatment. J Hepatol. 2014;61:515–22.
17. Chan HL, Wong GL, Chim AM, et al. Prediction of off-treatment response to lamivudine by serum hepatitis B surface antigen quantification in hepatitis B e antigen-negative patients. Antivir Ther. 2011;16:1249–57.
18. Seto WK, Hui AJ, Wong VW, et al. Treatment cessation of entecavir in Asian patients with hepatitis B e antigen negative chronic hepatitis B: a multicentre prospective study. Gut. 2015;64:667–72.
19. Jeng WJ, Sheen IS, Chen YC, et al. Off-therapy durability of response to entecavir therapy in hepatitis B e antigen-negative chronic hepatitis B patients. Hepatology. 2013;58:1888–96.
20. Hsu YC, Mo LR, Chang CY, et al. Association between serum level of hepatitis B surface antigen at end of entecavir therapy and risk of relapse in E antigen-negative patients. Clin Gastroenterol Hepatol. 2016;14:1490-8.
21. Wang CC, Tseng KC, Hsieh TY, et al. Assessing the durability of Entecavir-treated hepatitis B using quantitative HBsAg. Am J Gastroenterol. 2016;111: 1286-94.
22. Papatheodoridis G, Vlachogiannakos I, Cholongitas E, et al. Discontinuation of oral antivirals in chronic hepatitis B: A systematic review. Hepatology. 2016;63:1481–92.
23. Jaroszewicz J, Calle Serrano B, Wursthorn K, et al. Hepatitis B surface antigen (HBsAg) levels in the natural history of hepatitis B virus (HBV)-infection: a European perspective. J Hepatol. 2010;52:514–22.
24. Martinot-Peignoux M, Lada O, Cardoso AC, et al. Quantitative HBsAg: a new specific marker for the diagnosis of HBsAg inactive carriage. Hepatology. 2010;52:992.
25. Yakut M, Bektas M, Seven G, et al. Characterization of the inactive HBsAg carrier state with 3 year follow-up. J Hepatol. 2011;54:S159.
26. Chen CH, Hung CH, Hu TH, et al. Association between level of hepatitis B surface antigen and relapse after entecavir therapy for chronic hepatitis B virus infection. Clin Gastroenterol Hepatol. 2015;13:1984–92.
27. Manesis EK, Papatheodoridis GV, Tiniakos DG, et al. Hepatitis B surface antigen: relation to hepatitis B replication parameters in HBeAg-negative chronic hepatitis B. J Hepatol. 2011;55:61–8.
28. Chan HL, Wong VW, Tse AM, et al. Serum hepatitis B surface antigen quantitation can reflect hepatitis B virus in the liver and predict treatment response. Clin Gastroenterol Hepatol. 2007;5:1462–8.
29. Boni C, Laccabue D, Lampertico P, et al. Restored function of HBV-specific T Cells after long-term effective therapy with nucleos(t)ide analogues. Gastroenterology. 2012;143:963–73.
30. Zoutendijk R, Hansen BE, van Vuuren AJ, et al. Serum HBsAg decline during long-term potent nucleos(t) ide analogue therapy for chronic hepatitis B and prediction of HBsAg loss. J Infect Dis. 2011;204:415–8.
31. Jaroszewicz J, Ho H, Markova A, et al. Hepatitis B surface antigen (HBsAg) decrease and serum interferon-inducible protein-10 levels as predictive markers for HBsAg loss during treatment with nucleoside/nucleotide analogues. Antivir Ther. 2011;16:915–24.
32. Buti M, Casillas R, Riveiro-Barciela M, Homs M, Tabernero D, Salcedo MT, Rodriguez-Frias F, Esteban R. Tenofovir discontinuation after long-term viral suppression in HBeAg negative chronic hepatitis B. Can HBsAg levels be useful? Clin Virol. 2015;68:61–8.
33. Kao JH, Chen PJ, Lai MY, et al. Hepatitis B genotypes correlate with clinical outcomes in patients with chronic hepatitis B. Gastroenterology. 2000;118:554–9.

4

Multi-disciplinary team for early gastric cancer diagnosis improves the detection rate of early gastric cancer

Lianjun Di[1,2], Huichao Wu[1,2], Rong Zhu[1,2], Youfeng Li[1,2], Xinglong Wu[3], Rui Xie[1,2], Hongping Li[1,2], Haibo Wang[1,2], Hua Zhang[1,2], Hong Xiao[1,2], Hui Chen[4], Hong Zhen[3], Kui Zhao[1,2], Xuefeng Yang[5], Ming Xie[5] and Bigung Tuo[1,2*] (ID)

Abstract

Background: Gastric cancer is a frequent malignant tumor worldwide and its early detection is crucial for curing the disease and enhancing patients' survival rate. This study aimed to assess whether the multi-disciplinary team (MDT) can improve the detection rate of early gastric cancer (EGC).

Methods: The detection rate of EGC at the Digestive Endoscopy Center, Affiliated Hospital, Zunyi Medical College, China between September 2013 and September 2015 was analyzed. MDT for the diagnosis of EGC in the hospital was established in September 2014. The study was divided into 2 time periods: September 1, 2013 to August 31, 2014 (period 1) and September 1, 2014 to September 1, 2015 (period 2).

Results: A total of 60,800 patients' gastroscopies were performed during the two years. 61 of these patients (0.1%) were diagnosed as EGC, accounting for 16.44% (61/371) of total patients with gastric cancer. The EGC detection rate before MDT (period 1) was 0.05% (16/29403), accounting for 9.09% (16/176) of total patients with gastric cancer during this period. In comparison, the EGC detection rate during MDT (period 2) was 0.15% (45/31397), accounting for 23% (45/195) of total patients with gastric cancer during this period ($P < 0.05$). Univariate and multivariate logistic analyses showed that intensive gastroscopy for high risk patients of gastric cancer enhanced the detection rate of EGC in cooperation with Department of Pathology (OR = 10.1, 95% CI 2.39–43.3, $P < 0.05$).

Conclusion: MDT could improve the endoscopic detection rate of EGC.

Keywords: Early gastric cancer, Diagnosis, Intensive gastroscopy, Multi-disciplinary team

Background

Gastric cancer is the fourth frequent malignant tumor and the second leading cause of cancer related death in the world. Every year about 738,000 people die of gastric cancer, and the overall 5-year survival rate is about 20% [1, 2]. The prevalence of gastric cancer has district and gender differences. The incidence of gastric cancer in the North American women is lowest, with average incidence of 3.4 /100000 people, whereas it is highest in Asian men, with average incidence of 26.9/100000, especially in Japan, South Korea, and China [3–9]. Although

the medical advances have reduced gastric cancer mortality, the gastric cancer remains the second leading cause of cancer-related death in Asia [10]. Early gastric cancer (EGC) was first defined by the Japan Gastroscopy Association as an adenocarcinoma limited to the mucosa and submucosa, regardless of lymph node metastasis [11]. Based on this standard, the 5-year survival rate of patients with EGC after surgical treatment has reached 90%, whereas 5-year survival rate of advanced gastric cancer is still less than 30% [12, 13]. Therefore, the early detection of gastric cancer is crucial to enhance survival rate of patients. Japan is the best country in screening EGC work [14]. The National Cancer Center of Japan reported that the ratio of EGC patients in all gastric cancer patients increased from 22% in the 1960s to 75% in the 2000s [15]. China is a high risk area of gastric cancer,

* Correspondence: tuobiguang@aliyun.com
[1]Department of Gastroenterology, Affiliated Hospital, Zunyi Medical College, Zunyi 563003, China
[2]Digestive Endoscopy Center, Affiliated Hospital, Zunyi Medical Colleage, Zunyi, China
Full list of author information is available at the end of the article

with about 400,000 added gastric cancer patients and about 350,000 patients died of this malignant disease each year, and the new and dead patients account for 40% of patients with gastric cancer in the world [16], while the detection rate of EGC in China accounts only for 5% to 20% of total gastric cancer. The low detection rate of EGC in China may be not only related to endoscopist's awareness, experience, ability to identify EGC, and but also related to lack of coordination and cooperation between different departments in the Hospital including Gastroenterology, Pathology, Gastrointestinal Surgery, and Endoscopy Center.

The diagnosis and treatment of gastric cancer should be completed by multi-disciplinary team (MDT) according to Clinical Practice Guidelines of National Comprehensive Cancer Network (NCCN) for gastric cancer in the 2013 version [17]. Improving the detection rate of EGC not only relies on the ability of endoscopist, but also needs multidisciplinary cooperation, especially the cooperation of endoscopist and pathologist. To date, few studies have assessed the association between MDT and the detection rate of EGC. Therefore, in this study, we investigated whether MDT could improve the detection rate of EGC.

Methods

Basic information about the endoscopy center and endoscopists

The Digestive Endoscopy Center of Affiliated Hospital of Zunyi Medical College is one of the largest endoscopy centers in China that meets international standards. Approximately 30,000 gastroscopies were performed annually during the past three years. The endoscopists in the Center are all skilled in endoscopic diagnosis and treatment, and each endoscopist has an experience performing over 3000 gastroscopic examinations.

MDT methods to improve the detection of EGC

MDT for diagnosis and treatment of EGC was established in September 2014, which contains the Departments of Digestive Endoscopy Center, Gastroenterology, Gastrointestinal Surgery, Anesthesiology, and Pathology. The discussion meeting of EGC MDT was held once a month. Digestive Endoscopy Center, Department of Gastroenterology and Department of Pathology were the main members of MDT meeting. The measures of MDT were as follows. First, endoscopists were trained through lectures, watching photos and videos, on-site teaching, and participating discussion meeting for EGC patients in the Center once a week to enhance their awareness and ability to identify EGC. Two senior endoscopists (HuihaoWu and Lianjun Di) made intensive gastroscopies for high-risk patients of gastric cancer (ie, those with atrophic gastritis, gastric ulcer, stomach surgery history, and first-degree relatives of gastric carcinoma patients). During this process,

painless and comfortable gastroscopy was made to facilitate careful examination; mucus decomposing, antifoaming and spasmolytic agents were used to improve the visibility of the gastric mucosa; and standardized gastroscopy photography, white light endoscopy (WLE) indigo carmine staining, narrow band imaging (NBI), and magnifying endoscopy were performed to improve the detection of EGC. Secondly, the Center strengthened the cooperation with Department of Gastroenterology. The gastroenterologists in outpatient service screened high-risk patients of gastric cancer, and then the endoscopist made intensive gastroscopies for the high risk patients. It is most important to use a magnifying endoscopy for intensive gastroscopy. Magnifying endoscopy with narrow-band imaging (M-NBI) can make suspicious lesions more visible. The magnifying endoscopic diagnosis of EGC was determined according to the vessel plus surface (VS) classification system, including an irregular microvascular and/or microsurface pattern together with a clear demarcation line [18]. Thirdly, a regular communication and discussion for the diagnosis of EGC patients between endoscopist and pathologist was made once a week. Fourthly, strengthening cooperation with Department of Gastrointestinal Surgery, all patients with gastric carcinoma who were not suitable for endoscopic submucosal dissection (ESD) were discussed multidisciplinarily within one week to determine the scope and grade of the lesion and operation way. For the patient diagnosed as gastric cancer for many times by endoscopist, but repeated biopsies did not support the diagnosis of gastric cancer, multidisciplinary discussion made a decision whether it needs further surgery. Finally, strengthening cooperation with Department of Anesthesiology, painless endoscopy can eliminate the patient's fear, avoid nausea and vomiting reaction, and slow gastric peristalsis, which is contributive to further intensive gastroscopy for suspicious lesions.

Study design

All gastroscopies performed from September 1, 2013 to September 1, 2015 were reviewed. The study was divided into 2 periods, period 1 (September 1, 2013 to August 31, 2014) and period 2 (September 1, 2014 to September 1, 2015) according to the time of MDT establishment. The endoscopists to undergo endoscopy were same during the two periods. Pathological diagnosis for EGC was performed by gastrointestinal pathologists according to the revised Vienna classification [19]. Mucosal high-grade neoplasia (including high-grade adenoma/dysplasia), noninvasive carcinoma (carcinoma in situ), suspicious for invasive carcinoma, and intramucosal carcinoma were diagnosed as EGC. The diagnosis of EGC before MTD (period 1) was determined by endoscopist according to endoscopic and histological examinations, without collaboration and communication of MDT. The EGC detection

Table 1 The comparison of EGC detection rate before and during MDT

	Before MDT	During MDT	All	P value	χ^2
NG	29,043	31,397	60,800	–	–
EGC/NG(%)	16/29403 (0.05%)	45/31397 (0.15%)	61/60800 (0.1%)	<0.001	11.975
EGC/GC (%)	16/176 (9.09%)	45/195 (23%)	61/371 (16.44%)	<0.001	19.593

NG number of gastroscopies, EGC number of early gastric carcinoma, GC number of total gastric carcinoma

rates before and during MDT were compared. The factors affecting the detection of EGC were analyzed by two endoscopists (HC.W. and LJ.D.). This study was approved by the ethics committee of Zunyi Mecial College, and all patients provided written informed consent for the procedures before endoscopy.

Demographic and clinical characteristics of all patients were evaluated, including age, gender, status (outpatient/inpatient), gastrointestinal symptoms such as abdominal pain and vomiting, past medical history (mainly atrophic gastritis, gastric ulcer), and whether first-degree relatives of gastric carcinoma patients. Endoscopic characteristics to be assessed in the patients with EGC included the site and general morphology of the lesion, surface microstructure, and vascular characteristics.

Statistical analysis

Statistical analysis was processed by using the SPSS PC statistic package. The age with mean ± standard deviation was evaluated using independent samples t test. The Pearson Chi-Square (χ^2) test was applied for the detection rates of EGC between different cooperation departments, sex ratio, and ratio of inpatient and outpatient before and during MDT. The factors affecting the detection of EGC were assessed by univariate and multivariate logistic analyses. Odds ratio (OR) and 95% confidence intervals (CIs) were determined for significant variables found on multivariate analysis. $P < 0.05$ was considered statistically significant.

Results

Rates of EGC detection

From September 1, 2013 to September 1, 2015, the gastroscopies of a total of 60,800 patients were performed in the Digestive Endoscopy Center of Affiliated Hospital of Zunyi Medical College. Among 60,800 patients, 61 patients (0.1%) were diagnosed as EGC, accounting for 16.44% of total 371 diagnosed gastric cancer patients during this period. The EGC detection rate by endoscopists before MDT was 0.05%, accounting for 9.09% of the all diagnosed gastric cancer patients during the period 1. In contrast, the EGC detection rate during MDT was 0.15%, accounting for 23% of the all diagnosed gastric cancer patients during the period 2 (Table 1).

Characteristics of EGC

As shown in Table 2, among the 61 EGCs, 4 were located at the gastric fundus, 3 at the lesser curvature of the gastric corpus, 7 at the greater curvature of the gastric corpus, 4 at the posterior of the gastric corpus, 1 at the anterior of the gastric corpus, 13 at the gastric angle, and 29 at the gastric antrum. 1 was protruding type (0-I), 10 were surface protruding type (0–IIa), 15 were surface depressed type (0–IIc), 2 were flat type (0–IIb), 20 were mixed type (0–IIa + IIc), 2 were mixed type (0–IIc + IIa),

Table 2 Sites and the general morphologic and histologic characteristics of EGCs

	Before MDT	During MDT
Lesion location		
Gastric fundus	0	4
Lesser curvature of gastric corpus	2	1
Greater curvature of gastric corpus	5	2
Posterior of gastric corpus	0	4
Anterior of gastric corpus	0	1
Gastric angle	2	11
Gastric antrum	7	22
Morphological characteristic		
0–I	0	1
0–IIb	0	2
0–IIa	2	8
0–IIc	4	11
0–IIa + IIc	6	14
0-IIc + IIa	0	2
0–III	4	7
Histological characteristic		
Total number of HGIN	9	25
Tub.1and Tub.2.	4	12
Por 1	3	6
Sig	0	2
Depth of tumor invasion		
T1a	13	38
T1b	3	7

Tub.1, well-differentiated adenocarcinoma;Tub.2, moderately-differentiated adenocarcinoma; Por 1, poorly-differentiated adenocarcinoma; Sig, signet-ring cell carcinoma; EGC, early gastric cancer; HGIN, high-grade intraepithelial neoplasias. T1a, Tumor confined to the mucosa (M); T1b, Tumor confined to the submucosa (SM)

and 11 were depressed type (0–III). In general, EGC has various morphological characteristics and the lesion is very subtle. Among the 61 EGCs, images of 24 cases are shown in Fig. 1, including the general morphology of the lesion under the white light imaging (WLI) for these EGCs.

Examples of EGC

Figure 2 shows endoscopic and histopathologic images of 6 typical EGCs, classified as 0–IIa (A), 0–IIb (B), 0–IIc (C), and 0–IIa + IIc (D, E, F) lesions, respectively. Representative endoscopic and histopathologic images of other patients with EGC are shown in Additional file 1 and Additional file 2. Among the 6 EGCs, 4 were located

at the gastric antrum, 2 were located at the gastric corpus and all had typical appearance on M-NBI, including an irregular microvascular and an irregular microsurface pattern with a demarcation line. Pathological examinations of ESD- or surgery-resected specimens showed that there was high-grade intraepithelial neoplasia, signet ring cell carcinoma, or moderately- differentiated adenocarcinoma in these patients.

Impact of MDT on the detection rate of EGC

During September 2013 to September 2015, 60,800 gastroscopies were performed at our center, 2594 patients were underwent biopsies and 620 patients were diagnosed as low-grade intraepithelial neoplasia. Before MDT, from

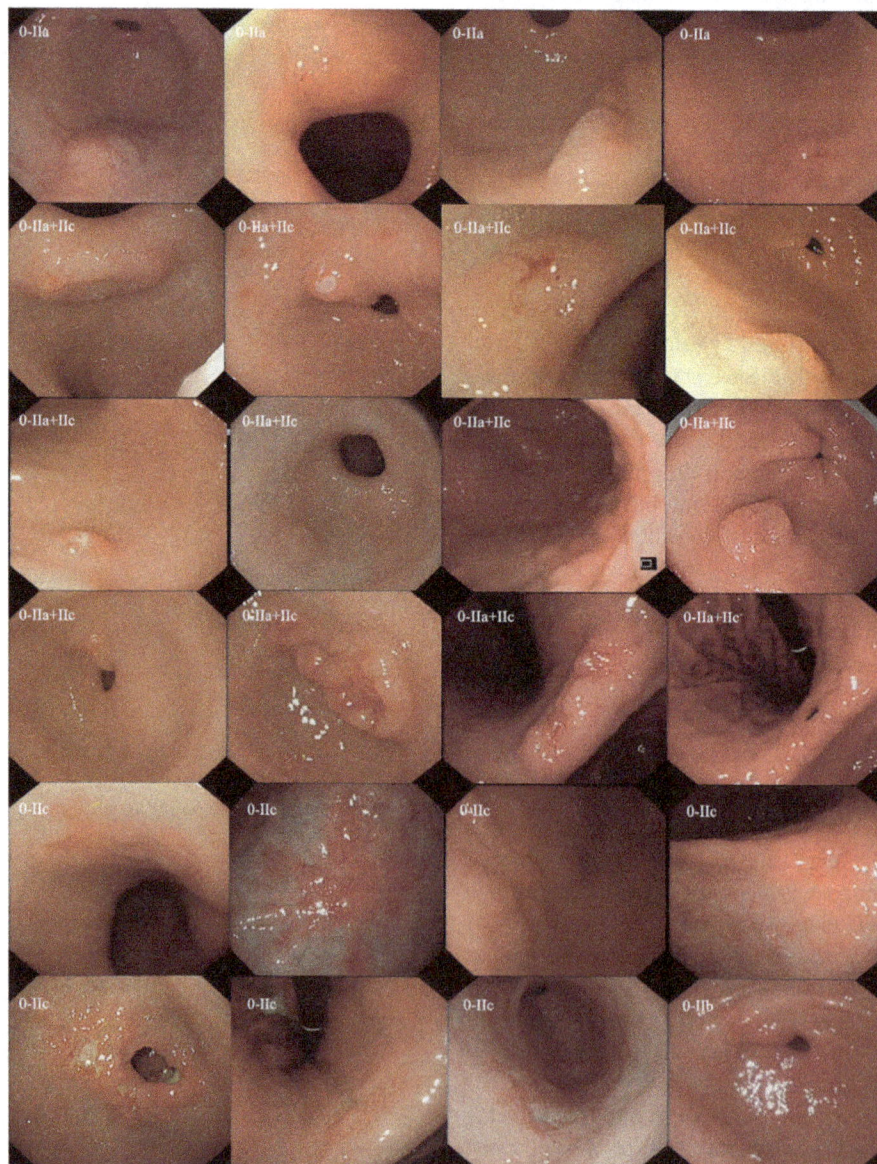

Fig. 1 Representative EGC lesion images under white light imaging

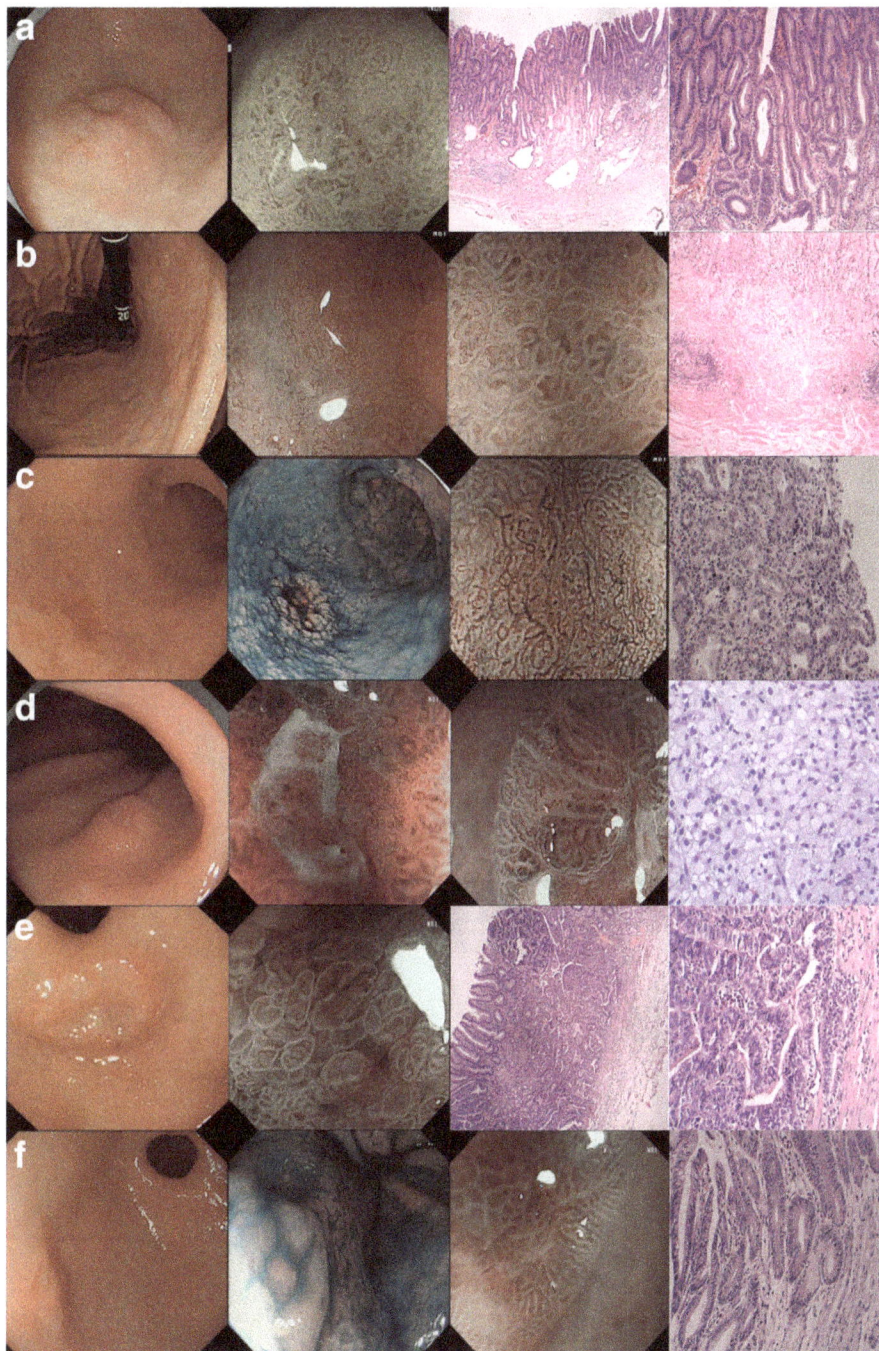

Fig. 2 Typical EGC lesions detected after we underwent intensive endoscopy for high-risk patient of gastric carcinoma. **a** Endoscopic image for 0-IIa in white light imaging and magnifying endoscopy and histopathological image. **b** Endoscopic image for 0-IIb in white light imaging and magnifying endoscopy and histopathological image. **c** Endoscopic image for 0-IIc in white light imaging and indigo carmine staining and magnifying endoscopy and histopathological image. **d** Endoscopic image for 0-IIa + IIc in white light imaging and magnifying endoscopy and histopathological image. **e** Endoscopic image for 0-IIa + IIc in white light imaging and magnifying endoscopy and histopathological image. **f** Endoscopic image for 0-IIa + c in white light imaging and indigo carmine staining and magnifying endoscopy and histopathological image

September 1, 2013 to August 31, 2014, 29,043 gastroscopies were performed, 1152 patients were underwent biopsies, and 253 patients were diagnosed as low-grade intraepithelial neoplasia. 33 patients were suspected EGC under white light imaging (WLI) among 253 patients. After repeatedly biopsies, only 2 patients were diagnosed as EGC. Pathological examination of ESD- or surgery resected specimens showed that 1 was well-differentiated adenocarcinoma and

1 was poorly-differentiated adenocarcinoma. During MDT, from September 1, 2014 to September 1, 2015, 31,397 gastroscopies were performed, 1442 patients were underwent biopsies, and 397 patients were initially diagnosed low-grade intraepithelial neoplasia. 38 patients were suspected EGC under WLI among the 397 patients, and after repeatedly targeted biopsies under M-NBI, 21 patients were diagnosed as high-grade intraepithelial neoplasia and 1 patient was diagnosed as signet ring cell carcinoma among the 38 patients by cooperative consultation with Department of Pathology. Finally, 21 patients with high-grade intraepithelial neoplasia were resected with ESD and 1 patient of signet ring cell carcinoma was treated by surgery. The detection rate of EGC in the low-grade intraepithelial neoplasia was markedly increased from 0.7% to 5.9% before and after cooperation with Department of Pathology (Fig. 3).

Before cooperation with Department of Gastrointestinal Surgery, tissue biopsies were obtained repeatedly from 11 patients with typical characteristics of the advanced gastric cancer under WLI, and pathological examination showed that all were low-grade intraepithelial neoplasia. Only 2 patients were treated and confirmed as EGC with advanced gastric cancer appearance. After cooperation with Department of Gastrointestinal Surgery, there are 10 patients with typical characteristics of the advanced gastric cancer under WLI, but pathological examination showed low-grade intraepithelial neoplasia. 6 patients were treated and confirmed as EGC with advanced gastric cancer appearance by consultation with Department of Gastrointestinal Surgery. The detection rate of EGC in the low-grade intraepithelial neoplasia was markedly increased from 0.7% to 1.6% before and after cooperation with Department of Gastrointestinal Surgery.

After high-risk patients of gastric cancer were screened by the gastroenterologists at outpatient service, endoscopists further made intensive gastroscopy for the high risk patients. The detection rate of EGC in high-risk patients by intensive gastroscopy was 3.3%, whereas the detection rate of EGC only by white light endoscopy was 0.5% (Fig. 4). Further results by univariate and multivariate logistic analyses showed that the cooperation with Department of Pathology (OR = 10.1, 95% CI 2.39–43.3, $P < 0.05$) and intensive gastroscopy for high-

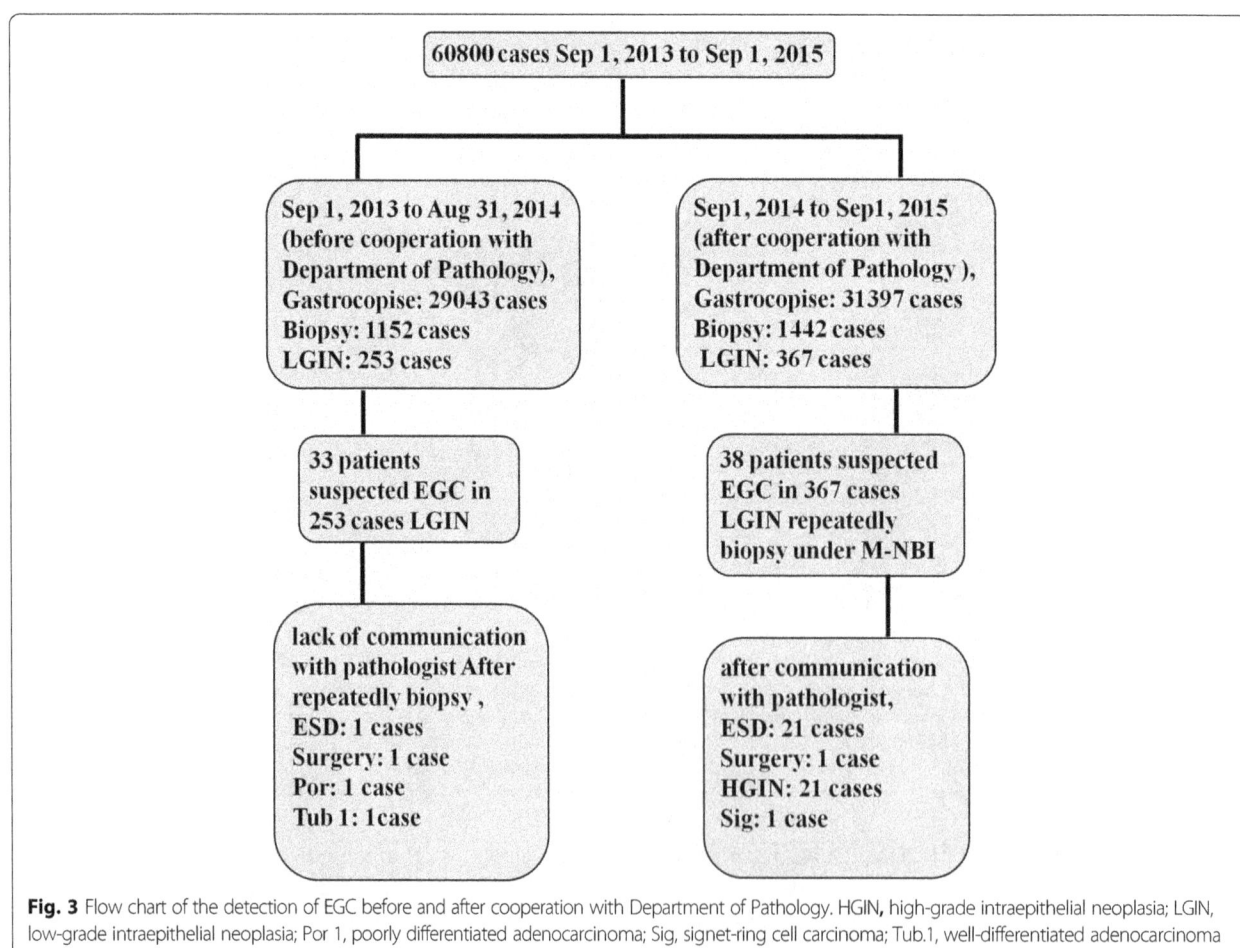

Fig. 3 Flow chart of the detection of EGC before and after cooperation with Department of Pathology. HGIN, high-grade intraepithelial neoplasia; LGIN, low-grade intraepithelial neoplasia; Por 1, poorly differentiated adenocarcinoma; Sig, signet-ring cell carcinoma; Tub.1, well-differentiated adenocarcinoma

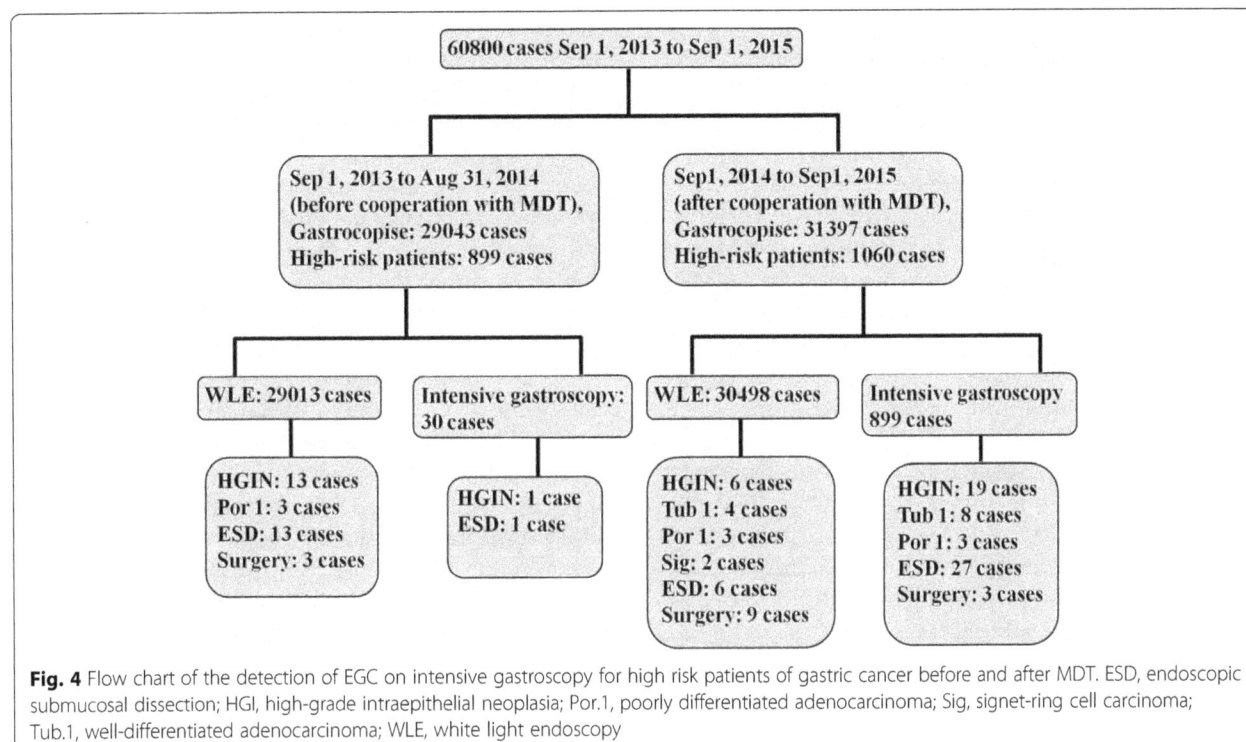

Fig. 4 Flow chart of the detection of EGC on intensive gastroscopy for high risk patients of gastric cancer before and after MDT. ESD, endoscopic submucosal dissection; HGI, high-grade intraepithelial neoplasia; Por.1, poorly differentiated adenocarcinoma; Sig, signet-ring cell carcinoma; Tub.1, well-differentiated adenocarcinoma; WLE, white light endoscopy

risk patients (OR = 28.3, 95% CI 19.6–40.7, $P < 0.001$) were independently associated with the detection of EGC. Intensive gastroscopy for high risk patients of gastric cancer enhanced the detection rate of EGC in cooperation with Department of Pathology. Moreover, 899 of 31,397 (2.8%) gastroscopies were performed under intensive gastroscopy during MDT, compared with 30 of 29,013 (0.1%) gastroscopies before MDT. There were no significant differences in gender and age of patients, tissue biopsy rate, the number of high-risk patients, and the number of painless gastroscopy before and during MDT (Table 3).

Discussion

The current study demonstrates that MDT for EGC diagnosis plays an important role in improving the detection rate of EGC. Enhancement of EGC detection rate needs not only the endoscopist's improvement of the ability to detect EGC, but also close cooperation and regular consultation with multidisplinary.

Table 3 Univariate and multivariate logistic analyses of related influencing factors on the detection of EGC

	Univariate Analysis			Multivariate analysis	
	Before MDT	During MDT	P value	OR	P value
Gender (male)	13,069/29043	14,599/31397	>0.05	—	—
Age, mean(SD)	43(8)	45(9)	>0.05	—	—
TBR	1152/29403	1442/31397	<0.001	—	—
High-risk patients	899/ 29,403	1060/31397	>0.05	—	—
CWDA	18,564/29403	19,665/31397	<0.05	—	—
CWDP	2/ 29,043	22/31397	<0.001	10.1 (2.39–43.3)	<0.05
CWDGS	2/29043	6/31397	>0.05	—	—
MDT	16/29043	45/31397	<0.001	2.60 (1.47–4.60)	<0.001
IG	30/29043	893/31397	<0.001	28.3 (19.6–40.7)	<0.001

Gender, number of male in total patients; TBR, number of patients with tissue biopsy in total patients; High-risk patients, number of high-risk patients in total patients; CWDA, cooperation with Department of Anesthsiology, number of painless gastroscopy in total gastroscopy; CWDP, cooperation with Department of Pathology, number of diagnosed patients with EGC in total patients; CWDGS, cooperation with Department of Gastroenterology surgery, number of diagnosed patients with EGC in total patients; MDT, number of diagnosed patients with EGC in total patients; IG, intensive gastroscopy for high-risk patients of gastric cancer, number of diagnosed patients with EGC in total patients

Gastroscopic diagnosis of EGC is difficult, because lesion of EGC is very complex or subtle so that it may be missed during gastroscopy. In addition, endoscopist's less attention and poor recognition ability for EGC, non-standardized biopsy, and lack of communication and cooperation between departments are also related to the missed diagnosis and misdiagnosis of EGC. Therefore, training for endoscopist, standardized endoscopic examination, and cooperation and communication of MDT should be done to enhance the detection rate of EGC.

Since MDT for EGC was established, we have been keeping on improving endoscopist's ability to detect EGC by regular consultation with multidisplinary, especially in cooperation with Department of Pathology. Endoscopist's awareness for EGC is strengthened and tissue biopsy rate and positive rate are increased. Meanwhile, pathologists also enhance their diagnostic level for EGC. During MTD (period 2), among 22 patients who were initially misdiagnosed as low-grade intraepithelial neoplasia, 21 were diagnosed as high-grade intraepithelial neoplasia and 1 was diagnosed as signet ring cell carcinoma after discussion with Department of Pathology. We think that the cause to result in initial pathological misdiagnosis may be related to the accuracy of pathological diagnosis, the judgment of tissue differentiation degree, pathologist's recognition ability for EGC, lack of standardized specimen processing and slice, and different diagnostic criteria. There are differences in pathological diagnosis between pathologists because of the lack of uniform diagnostic criteria, especially in the diagnosis for high-grade intraepithelial neoplasia and well-differentiated adenocarcinoma. Well-differentiated adenocarcinoma is misdiagnosed as high-grade intraepithelial neoplasia and severe dysplasia is misdiagnosed as moderate dysplasia. A study showed that 16% patients diagnosed as adenocarcinoma by Japanese pathologists were ascribed to dysplasia by the pathologists in western countries, whereas, in western countries, 90% patients diagnosed as dysplasia by pathologists were ascribed to gastric cancer by Japanese scholars [20]. For this situation, our center strengthens the cooperation with Department of Pathology and unifies diagnostic criteria for EGC. The detection rate of EGC is obviously improved.

High-risk patients of gastric cancer are recognized to have high risk suffering from gastric cancer. We made intensive gastroscopy on high-risk patients screened by gastroenterologists. The result showed that the detection rate of EGC in the high-risk patients by intensive gastroscopy was 3.3%, whereas the detection rate of EGC only by white light endoscopy was 0.5%, demonstrating that the intensive gastroscopy for the high risk patients could enhance the detection of EGC. The previous study also showed that targeted biopsy under M-NBI on doing intensive gastroscopy could improve the detection rate of EGC [21]. We think it is feasible and recommendable measure to make further intensive gastroscopy for high-risk patient of gastric cancer in China, because there are a large number of population and poor economic condition in China and it is impractical to make intensive gastroscopy for each patient.

Clinically, there are some patients with typical signs of advanced gastric cancer under WLE, but repeated biopsies show low-grade intraepithelial neoplasia. In this study, our result showed that the detection rate of EGC in the patients with endoscopic signs of gastric cancer, but pathological result of low-grade intraepithelial neoplasia, was enhanced from 0.7% to 1.6% after the cooperation with Department of Gastrointestinal Surgery. In addition, although univariate and multivariate analyses showed no statistical significance in the number of painless gastroscopy before and during MDT, we think that the painless and comfortable gastroscopy is important to detect EGC in cooperation with Department of Anesthesiology. The painless gastroscopy could make gastric peristalsis slow, without nausea and vomiting response, and eliminate the patient's fear, which is contributive to further intensive gastroscopy for suspicious lesions.

In general, our study showed that MDT could enhance the detection rate of EGC. Although it is a single-center study and a summary of the experience of a single endoscopy center, the study includes a large sample and it is applicable to other endoscopy centers, especially to those in which the detection rate of EGC by endoscopist is not satisfactory.

Conclusions
MDT for EGC can improve the detection rate of EGC by endoscopist. Intensive gastroscopy for high-risk patients of gastric cancer and cooperation with Department of Pathology contribute to the detection of EGC.

Abbreviations
CI: confidence interval; EGC: early gastric cancer; ESD: endoscopic submucosal dissection; MDT: multi-disciplinary team; M-NBI: magnifying endoscopy with narrow-band imaging; OR: odds ratio; WLE: white light endoscopy; WLI: white light imaging

Acknowledgements
Not applicable.

Funding
This study was supported by the grants from Engineering Center of Endoscopy Diagnosis and Treatment, Guizhou Province, China, and Clinical Medical Research Center for Digestive Diseases, Guizhou Province, China. The funding body had no role in the design of the study and collection, analysis, and interpretation of data and in writing this manuscript.

Authors' contributions

BT, study design, data analysis, and manuscript drafting and revision process; LD, data collection, data analysis, and manuscript drafting and revision process; HW, RZ, YL, XW, RX, HL, HW, HZ, HX, HC, HZ, KZ, XY, MX, data collection. All authors read and approved the final manuscript.

Competing interests

The authors declare that they have no financial competing interests.

Author details

[1]Department of Gastroenterology, Affiliated Hospital, Zunyi Medical College, Zunyi 563003, China. [2]Digestive Endoscopy Center, Affiliated Hospital, Zunyi Medical Colleage, Zunyi, China. [3]Department of Pathology, Affiliated Hospital, Zunyi Medical College, Zunyi, China. [4]Department of Anesthesiology, Affiliated Hospital, Zunyi Medical College, Zunyi, China. [5]Department of Gastrointestinal Surgery, Affiliated Hospital, Zunyi Medical College, Zunyi, China.

References

1. Ferlay J, Shin HR, Bray F, et al. Estimates of worldwide burden of cancer in 2008: GLOBOCAN 2008. Int J Cancer. 2010;127:2893–917.
2. Kamangar F, Dores GM, Anderson WF. Patterns of cancer Incidence,mortality,and prevalence across five continents: defining priorities to reduce cancer disparities in different geographic regions of the world. J Clin Oncol. 2006;24:2137–50.
3. Leung WK, MS W, Kakugawa Y, et al. Screening for gastric cancer in Asia: current evidence and practice. J. Lancet Oncol. 2008;9:279–87.
4. Bashash M, Hislop TG, Shah AM, et al. The prognostic effect of ethnicity for gastric and esophageal cancer: the population-based experience in British Columbia, Canada. BMC Cancer. 2011;11:164.
5. Rahman R, Asombang AW, Ibdah JA. Characteristics of gastric cancer in Asia. World J Gastroenterol. 2014;20:4483–90.
6. Yang L. Incidence and mortality of gastric cancer in China. World J Gastroenterol. 2006;12:17–20.
7. Matsuda A, Matsuda T, Shibata A, et al. Cancer incidence and incidence rates in Japan in 2007: a study of 21 population-based cancer registries for the monitoring of cancer incidence in Japan (MCIJ) project. J Clin Oncol. 2013;43:328–36.
8. Kim JY, Lee HS, Kim N, et al. Prevalence and clinicopathologic characteristics of gastric cardia cancer in South Korea. Helicobacter. 2012;17:358–68.
9. Fock KM, Ang TL. Epidemiology of helicobacter pylori infection and gastric cancer in Asia. J Gastroenterol Hepatol. 2010;25:479–86.
10. Khanderia E, Markar SR, Acharya A, et al. The influence of gastric cancer screening on the stage at diagnosis and survival: a meta-analysis of comparative studies in the Far East. J Clin Gastroenterol. 2016;50:190–7.
11. Japanese Gastric Cancer Association. Japanese classification of gastric carcinoma: 2nd English edition. Gastric Cancer. 1998;1:10–24.
12. Ajani JA, Bentrem DJ, Bosh S, et al. Gastric cancer ,version 2. 2013: featured updates to the NCCN guidelines. J Natl Compr Cancer Netw. 2013;11:531–46.
13. Isobe Y, Nashimoto A, Akazawa K. Et a1. Gastric cancer treatment in Japan: 2008 annual report of the JGCA nationwide registry. Gastric Cancer. 2011;14:301–16.
14. Shimizu S, Tada M, Kawai K. Early gastric cancer: its surveillance and natural course. Endoscopy. 1995;27:27–31.
15. Yamada M, Oda I, Taniguchi H, et al. Chronological trend in clinicopathological characteristics of gastric cancer. Nihon Rinsho. 2012;70:1681–5.
16. Zheng R, Zeng H, Zhang S, Chen W. Estimates of cancer incidence and mortality in China, 2013. Chin J Cancer. 2017;36:66.
17. Ajani JA, Bentrem DJ, Besh S, et al. National Comprehensive Cancer Network. Gastric cancer, version 2.2013: featured updates to the NCCN guidelines. J Natl Compr Cancer Netw. 2013;11:531–46.
18. Yao K, Anagnostopoulos GK, Ragunath K. Magnifying endoscopy for diagnosing and delineating early gastric cancer. Endoscopy. 2009;41:462–7.
19. Dixon MF. Gastrointestinal.Epithelial.Neoplasia: Vienna revisited. Gut. 2002;51:130–1.
20. Lansdown M, Quirke P, Dixon MF, et al. High grade dysplasia of the gastric mucosa: a marker for gastric carcinoma. Gut. 1990;31:977–83.
21. Yao K, Doyama H, Gotoda T, et al. Diagnostic performance and limitations of magnifying narrow-band imaging in screening endoscopy of early gastric cancer: a prospective multicenter feasibility study. Gastric Cancer. 2014;17:669–79.

5

Psychological wellbeing and physical activity in children and adolescents with inflammatory bowel disease compared to healthy controls

Laura Mählmann[1,4*] (iD), Markus Gerber[3], Raoul I. Furlano[2], Corinne Legeret[2], Nadeem Kalak[1], Edith Holsboer-Trachsler[1] and Serge Brand[1,3,5]

Abstract

Background: Children and adolescents with inflammatory bowel disease (IBD) report impairments in daily activities, social interactions and coping. Findings regarding psychological functioning are inconsistent, while limited information is available on objectively assessed physical activity (PA). The aims of the present study were therefore to compare anthropometric dimensions, blood values, psychological functioning and PA of children and adolescents with IBD with healthy controls.

Methods: Forty-seven children and adolescents took part in the study. Of these, 23 were diagnosed with IBD (mean age: 13.88 years, 44% females). The IBD group was divided into a medically well adjusted "remission-group" ($n = 14$; IBD-RE) and a group with an "active state" of disease ($n = 8$; IBD-AD). Healthy controls ($n = 24$; HC) were age- and gender-matched. Participants' anthropometric data, blood values and objective PA were assessed. Further, participants completed questionnaires covering socio-demographic data and psychological functioning.

Results: Participants with IBD-AD showed higher erythrocyte sedimentation rate (ESR), C-reactive protein (CRP) values, haemoglobin, and leukocyte values. IBD-AD had poorer psychological functioning and lower PA (average steps per day) compared to IBD-RE and HC. No mean differences were found between IBD-RE and HC.

Conclusions: The pattern of results suggests that effective medical treatment of IBD in children and adolescents is associated with favorable physiological parameters, psychological dimensions and PA. Psychological counselling of children and adolescents in an active state of IBD seem to be advised in addition to standard treatment schedules.

Keywords: Inflammatory bowel diseases, Pediatrics, Anthropometric dimensions, Psychological wellbeing, Physical activity, Blood values, Healthy controls

* Correspondence: laura.maehlmann@upkbs.ch
[1]Psychiatric Clinics of the University of Basel, Centre for Affective, Stress and Sleep Disorders, University of Basel, Wilhelm Klein-Strasse 27, Ch-4012 Basel, Switzerland
[4]United Nations University - Maastricht Economic and Social Research Institute on Innovation and Technology (UNU-MERIT), Maastricht University, Maastricht, The Netherlands
Full list of author information is available at the end of the article

Background

Inflammatory Bowel Disease (IBD) is a chronic, debilitating illness characterized by cycles of disease activity and quiescence. IBD is subdivided into Crohn's disease (CD), ulcerative colitis (UC) and atypical phenotypes as described by the Porto criteria (PIBD: Pediatric IBD) [1]. Although the ultimate aetiology of IBD remains unclear, three hypotheses are advanced: (1) A dysregulated inflammation emerges due to interactions between the gut luminal content (intestinal microflora) and the mucosa, especially in genetically predisposed hosts [2]. (2) Genetic factors seem to contribute slightly to the disease pathogenesis. (3) Microbial and environmental dimensions have been identified as possible contributing factors [3].

Worldwide it is estimated that 25% of all patients suffering from IBD are children and adolescents, with increasing incidence rates [4]. In children with IBD stunting of physical growth and delay in pubertal development are observed [5]. Furthermore, patients with active IBD are known to report increased erythrocyte-sedimentation rates (ESR) due to inflammation, decreased hemoglobin due to chronic blood loss in the gut, decreased albumin due to leaking gut at reduced intake and increased infection parameters such as leukocytes and C-reactive protein (CRP), when compared to healthy controls. Once the diagnosis is confirmed, the goals of medical therapy are to relieve symptoms, restore growth and bone health, normalize quality of life and psychosocial functioning, prevent complications and minimize the adverse effects of medications [6]. While the efficacy of anti-inflammatory pharmaceuticals are not 100% and the side effects might be severe, some young IBD patients might be in a symptom-free remission, while others are still in an active disease state. Accordingly, based on the regularly assessed PUCAI (Pediatric ulcerative colitis activity index) scores and pediatric Crohn's disease activity index (CDAI), participants in the present study were split into those with medically optimized treatment (IBD in remission, PUCAI <10; CDAI <150) the IBD – RE group, and those with not yet medically optimized treatment (active disease state), the IBD – AD group. As a result, our first hypothesis was that disease severity and the accompanying symptoms would be negatively associated with the physical development of children and adolescents with IBD. Specifically, we expected smaller and lighter body shapes and elevated inflammation markers in participants of the IBD-AD group, compared to IBD-RE and healthy controls.

In recent years, a plethora of studies have suggested that the prevalence of reduced health-related quality of life (HRQOL) and psychiatric disorders are significantly greater in young people with IBD than healthy controls [7–9]. More specifically, adolescents with IBD had higher levels of internalizing disorders such as anxiety and depression [7, 9], due to several factors such as unpredictable, unpleasant, and embarrassing symptoms, complex, demanding treatment regimens, treatment-related side effects, the ever-looming threat of exacerbations of the disease, and the need for surgical procedures in severe cases [10]. The rate of depression may be as high as 25%, and spreads among a broad variety of psychological and social difficulties. However, as reviewed by Ross et al. [8], the evidence these conclusions are based on, were inconsistent, included few paediatric samples, and used coarse-grained psychological instruments. As a result, recognition of the importance of mental wellbeing in young IBD patients is lacking in medical practice. If these psychological conditions are left untreated, mental disorders linked to more severe IBD symptoms might emerge, as well as more frequent IBD flares, higher hospitalization rates, increased health seeking behaviour and lower compliance with treatment [11, 12]. To counter this, in the present study, validated and reliable self-rating instruments were used to assess dimensions such as psychological wellbeing, social support and peer relationships. Consequently, the second aim of the present study was to expand upon existing research by assessing children's and adolescent's psychological functioning with self-rating questionnaires, investigating specific aspects of psychological functioning, along with a depression screener.

As regards physical activity and sports participation, research showed that children and adolescents with IBD participated less in sports activities and were less fit than their counterparts without IBD [13, 14]. In the specific case of paediatric IBD, reduced physical exertion during puberty might lead to impaired bone growth, strength and density, resulting in an increased risk for osteoporosis in the long term [10]. However, a large number of studies have proven the beneficial effect of PA for a diversity of health conditions: First, PA mitigates depressive symptoms while bolstering sleep [15] and cardiovascular fitness [16]. Second, sports participation (via clubs and sports associations) has the potential to increase and deepen children's and adolescents' social skills. So far, research on PA in children and adolescents with IBD has largely been based on rough estimates. Therefore, the third aim of the present study was to assess PA behavior in children and adolescents with IBD, both subjectively using an internationally established questionnaire, and objectively with three methods: First, to investigate participants' fitness, we used the Six-Minute-Walking-Test; second, for strength assessments, we applied a hydraulic grip strength test, and third, to generate long-term PA reports, a FitbitFlex® accelerometer was applied.

Taking into account the state-of-the-art regarding physical development, psychological functioning and physical activity among children and adolescents with IBD, the following three hypotheses were formulated: First, following others [5, 17], we expected impaired anthropometric development among children and adolescents suffering from IBD and increased inflammatory blood markers, and particularly among those in an active state of the disease. Second, on the basis of previous research [7–9], we expected poorer psychological functioning in children and adolescents with IBD, than in their healthy counterparts, and again, particularly among those in an active state of the disease. Third, previous findings [18] led us to expect lower levels of PA (both subjective and objective) in children and adolescents with IBD than in their healthy counterparts.

Methods
Procedure
All participants were invited to the hospital to measure height, weight, waist circumference (measured 4 cm above the navel using a standard anthropometry tape) compared to reference values established by Taylor et al. [19] and BMI (kg/m^2), which was compared to the WHO international growth references [20]. Following these anthropometric measurements, participants' blood values were collected and physical performance was examined; they also filled out a 30 min questionnaire with questions on psychological functioning and PA behaviour. All data were collected by two trained research assistants and supervised by a medical doctor.

The present study was approved by the local ethical committee (EKNZ: 2014:220), and was conducted in accordance to the ethical principles laid down in Declaration of Helsinki (Trial registration number: NCT02264275).

Sample
A total of 31 eligible children and adolescents with IBD were approached between April and November 2015 via the University Children's Hospital Basel (UKBB, Basel, Switzerland). Of these, 29 (93.5%) agreed to participate in the study, though five subsequently withdrew from the study because of time constraints, and three withdraw due to acute illness (flu). The final sample consisted of 23 children and adolescents with diagnosed IBD (mean age: 13.88 years, SD = 3.11, 10 females (43.5%), 7 UC, 12 CD and 3 UD). According to the regularly assessed PUCAI (Paediatric ulcerative colitis activity index) scores and Paediatric Crohn's disease activity index (clinical scores), eight participants were in an active disease state and 14 in remission at the time of the study [11]. Inclusion criteria were as follows: (1)

aged 6 to 20 years; (2) clinically and histologically confirmed diagnosis of IBD; (3) willing and able to take part in the study; (4) able to communicate and to complete questionnaires in German; (5) written informed consent from both the children/adolescents and their parents (or a legal caregiver). Exclusion criteria were: (1) severe physical diseases of the locomotor apparatus; (2) psychiatric disorders such as psychotic disorders, severe affective disorders, eating disorders, mental retardation, autism spectrum disorder; (3) unable to communicate and to complete questionnaires in German; (4) among female adolescents: pregnancy, breastfeeding, or intention to get pregnant during the study period; (5) refusal to give written informed consent. In parallel, 24 age- and gender-matched controls (mean age: 12.38 years, SD = 3.24, females $n = 15$ (62.5%)) were recruited by word of mouth recommendations. Inclusion criteria and exclusion criteria for healthy controls were the same as for patients with IBD except that they had to be physically healthy as reported from both participants and parents and as known from medical records. All participants were informed about the study aims and the voluntary and confidential basis of their participation. Written informed consent was signed both by participants and by their legal guardians.

Characteristics of the participants subdivided into three groups of IBD-AD, IBD-RE and healthy control are represented in Table 1.

Tools
Laboratory assessment
Using the finger prick technique, biochemical parameters were assessed involving inflammatory indices such as albumin [g/dl], CRP [g/dl], hemoglobin [g/dl], ESR [mm/h], hematocrit [%], thrombocyte [g/dl] and leucocyte [g/dl] count.

Assessing psychological functioning
To assess psychological functioning, participants completed the KIDSCREEN 27 [21]. The questionnaire

Table 1 Sample characteristics

	IBD-AD ($n = 8$)	IBD-RE ($n = 14$)	HC ($n = 24$)
Age in years	14.69 ± 3.25	13.23 ± 2.96	12.38 ± 3.24
Female	4 (50)	6 (42.9)	15 (62.5)
IBD			
Ulcerative colitis	3 (37.5)	4 (28.6)	
Crohn's disease	5 (62.5)	7 (50)	
Undefined colitis		3 (21.4)	
Time since diagnosis (in years)	3.67 ± 2.81	4.1 ± 2.9	

Notes: $N = 46$
IBD-AD IBD in an active state of the disease, *IBD-RE* IBD in remission, *HC* Healthy control

consists of 27 items covering five domains, physical wellbeing, psychological wellbeing, autonomy and relations with parents, social support and peers, and school environment. Answers were given on 5-point rating scales (1 = not at all, 5 = extremely/always). Higher mean scores reflect better functioning in a specific domain. Validity has been verified by Ravens-Sieberer et al. [21] (Cronbach's α = .91).

To assess symptoms of depression, the Child Depression Screener (ChilD-S) was completed [22]. The ChilD-S is a self-report screening instrument for pre-pubertal in- and out-patients in paediatric care. It consists of 8 items assessing how participants have felt for the last 2 weeks ("I am happy, I am doing fine, I feel exhausted, I worry a lot, I feel sad, I get upset quickly, I am not in the mood for anything, I often think I did something wrong"). Participants were asked to select from four alternative responses reflecting different levels of depressive symptomatology. The cut off value for clinically considerable depression is ≥11, with higher values indicating more marked depressive symptoms. Validity has been verified by Frühe et al. [22] (Cronbach's α = .78).

Assessing physical activity

Subjective assessment The short form of the IPAQ (IPAQ-S) questionnaire was applied as an internationally approved estimator of level of PA and sedentary behaviour [23]. It provides a comparison of vigorous- and moderate-intensity PA, walking, total PA and time spent sitting on weekdays over the past seven days. PA data are reported in hours and/or minutes per day and days per week. Where minutes of intense activity exceeded 180 per day, a cut-off of 180 min per day was applied as suggested by the guidelines of the IPAQ group. Data were transformed and summed using standardized IPAQ scoring protocols to indicate total metabolic equivalent minutes (MET-minutes) of PA per week. Total MET-minutes per week was calculated using the following formula [23]:

[Walking MET-minutes/week = 3.3 * walking minutes * walking days]

+[Moderate MET-minutes/week = 4.0

* moderate-intensity activity minutes * moderate days]

+[Vigorous MET-minutes/week = 8.0

* vigorous-intensity activity minutes * vigorous-intensity days]

= Total PA MET-minutes/week.

Furthermore, self-reported fitness was assessed on a 5-point Likert scale. Validity of the instrument has been established by Hagstömer et al. [24] Sitting time was reported as the amount of time in hours and/or minutes participants usually spent sitting on a weekday during the past 7 days.

Objective assessments *Grip force.* Maximum isometric grip force of the dominant hand was assessed using the hydraulic hand dynamometer. Participants made three attempts. Mean outcomes were compared to reference data [25].

Functional capacity. The 6-min walking test (6 MWT), a self-paced, submaximal exercise test, was employed [26]; the test is designed to assess functional exercise capacity in patients with chronic diseases. The 6 MWT is well-standardized and is increasingly being utilized in pediatric populations with chronic diseases [27]. Walking distance is accepted as the main outcome measure of the 6 MWT. Heart rate (HR) is continuously recorded during exercise using an elastic chest strap with heart rate sensor.

Daily PA. The Fitbit-Flex® (Fitbit Inc., San Francisco, CA, USA), a small and light wristband accelerometer which uses three-dimensional motion sensing technology to measure movement 24 h a day, was applied for a continuous assessment of 5 days (2 weekend days and 3 weekdays). It has a simple display of five LED lights which indicate the number of steps taken in a day. Fitbit data were recorded using the 1-min epoch setting and downloaded from the user website via the device's USB docking port in a raw data format. Validation studies have been conducted with children and adolescents [28].

Statistical analyses

Since normality was violated according to Shapiro-Wilk test, the groups IBD-AD, IBD-RE and HC were compared using the Kruskal-Wallis test with these diagnostic clusters as independent variable and anthropometric measures, psychological assessments and PA data as dependent variable. Due to heterogeneity of age distribution, Spearman's correlations were performed to determine whether significant correlations would be found beyond age and other dimensions. Accordingly, statistical calculations of anthropometric data, grip strength and 6 MWT were controlled for age. Post-hoc tests after Whitney-U for p-values were performed to examine differences between the three groups. The nominal level of statistical significance was set at alpha <.05. Further, effect sizes were reported as partial eta-squared [η_p^2]) and considered as follows: small (s) = $.01 \leq \eta_p^2 \leq .059$, medium (m) = $.06 \leq \eta_p^2 \leq .139$, or large (l) = $\eta_p^2 \geq .14$) [29]. All statistics were performed with SPSS® 24.0 (IBM Corporation, Armonk NY, USA) for Windows®.

Results

All descriptive and inferential statistical information is reported in the Tables and not repeated again in the written text. All Tables compare the three groups of IBD-AD, IBD-RE and HC.

Anthropometric and laboratory findings

As shown in Table 2, there was a statistically significant mean difference in thrombocytes ($p = .003$). According to Mann-Whitney-U Post-hoc test, differences between IBD-AD and HC were significant ($p = .003$). Further, there were no statistically significant mean differences between the three groups in the following dimensions: waist circumference, waist circumference difference from norm, height, weight to height percentage, weight, BMI, BMI z-score, percentile BMI vs age, z-score height vs age, percentile height vs age and the blood values albumin [g/l], CRP [mg/l], hemoglobin [g/l], ESR [mm/h, hematocrit [%] and leukocytes [×10^9/l]. Investigating effect sizes, the IBD-AD group scored moderately lower on BMI z-score, percentile BMI vs age, z-score height vs age and percentile height vs age.

Further, Table 2 shows higher C-reactive protein (CRP) values, hemoglobin values, and leukocyte values in the group of IBD-AD vs IBD-RE and HC. More specifically, six (75%) IBD-AD patients had low albumin levels, as did eight (61.54%) IBD-RE patients and 12 (50%) HC (reference 35 – 53 g/L). CRP was high in one (12.5%) IBD-AD and one (7.1%) IBD-RE patient (reference <10.0 mg/L). Two patients (25%) in the IBD-AD group, two IBD-RE (14.2%) and one control (4.2%) were anemic with mean hemoglobin scores of 101.5 g/L, 114 g/L and 100 g/L, respectively (reference 120 – 160 g/L).

Assessing the erythrocyte sedimentation rate (ERS) one IBD-AD (12.5%) was slightly above reference, as well as four (28.6%) IBD-RE and six (25%) HC (reference 4.1 – 5.1 × 10 ^12/L). One IBD-RE (7.1%) patient had results below reference.

Regarding hematocrit outcomes, two (25%) IBD-AD, four (28.6%) IBD-RE (mean 34.27%) and three (12.5%) HC had values below reference (36-46%). Thrombocytosis was present in two (25%) IBD-AD patients (reference 150 – 450 × 10^9/l). Leukocyte counts were high in two (25%) IBD-AD, three (21.4%) IBD-RE and one (4.2%) HC compared to reference (4.5 – 11 × 10^9/l).

Psychological functioning

As Table 3 shows, there were no statistically significant mean differences between the three groups (psychological wellbeing physical wellbeing, autonomy and parent relations,

Table 2 Anthropometrics and Blood values

	IBD-AD (N = 8) M ± SD	IBD-RE (N = 14) M ± SD	HC (N = 24) M ± SD	Statistical Analysis			
				H	p	np2	Interpretation of effect size
Waist circumference (cm)	67.63 ± 9.04	65.65 ± 7.17	64.48 ± 8.29	0.384	0.823	0.01	s
Difference from norm	−9.81 ± 6.15	−8.68 ± 4.95	−8.82 ± 6.0	0.521	0.783	0	s
Height (cm)	153.48 ± 17.53	152.69 ± 12.02	152.26 ± 18.0	0.212	0.903	0	s
Weight to height (%)	44.08 ± 3.07	42.94 ± 2.13	42.77 ± 3.49	1.108	0.585	0.02	s
Weight (kg)	45.28 ± 15.85	42.79 ± 12.83	44.37 ± 15.75	0.215	0.899	0	s
BMI	18.6 ± 3.37	17.91 ± 2.78	18.36 ± 3.16	0.074	0.965	0.12	m
BMI z-score	−0.588 ± 0.79	−0.34 ± 0.95	−0.19 ± 0.87	1.368	0.511	0.1	m
Percentile BMI vs Age	31.98 ± 24.31	39.82 ± 26.23	43.89 ± 26.43	1.386	0.516	0.1	m
z-score Height vs Age	−0.911 ± 1.73	0.02 ± 0.86	0.19 ± 1.01	2.234	0.334	0.1	m
Percentile Height vs Age	32.04 ± 32.99	52.91 ± 25.71	54.83 ± 31.53	2.236	0.333	0.07	m
Albumin [g/l]	23 ± 21.94	19.32 ± 19.20	20.79 ± 18.76	0.767	0.686	0	s
CRP [mg/l]	3.02 ± 4.56	3.28 ± 5.69	0.71 ± 0.85	4.159	0.125	0.13	m
Hemoglobin [g/l]	139.25 ± 8.62	134.92 ± 16.26	135.86 ± 12.33	1.423	0.493	0.01	s
ESR [mm/h]	4.83 ± 0.36	4.87 ± 0.54	4.88 ± 0.36	0.281	0.874	0	s
Hematocrit [%]	39.4 ± 2.11	38.09 ± 3.99	38.75 ± 3.17	0.359	0.837	0.02	s
Thrombocyts [×10^9/l]	323.25 ± 55.61	302.58 ± 56.15	271.55 ± 46.54	11.211	0.003	0.13	m
Leukocyten [×10^9/l]	10.16 ± 2.01	9.28 ± 2.83	8.25 ± 1.29	4.088	0.13	0.11	m

Notes: N = 46, degrees of freedom always = 2, 41, p < .05 statistically significant; effect sizes: small (s) = .01 > np2 < .059, medium (m) = .06 > np < .139, or large (l) = np ≥ .14

IBD-AD IBD in an active state of the disease, IBD-RE IBD in remission, HC Healthy Control, Waist circumference norm references is Taylor et al. [19], BMI Body Mass Index; CRP C-reactive protein, ESR Erythrocyte Sedimentation Rate

Table 3 Psychological functioning and depression

	IBD-AD (N = 8) M ± SD	IBD-RE (N = 14) M ± SD	HC (N = 24) M ± SD	Statistical Analysis			
				H	p	ηp2	Interpretation of effect sizes
Kidsscreen-27:							
Physical Wellbeing	17.71 ± 3.59	18.5 ± 3.61	19.38 ± 3.16	3.740	0.155	0.04	s
Psychological Wellbeing	28.14 ± 5.61	31.86 ± 2.28	31.46 ± 2.41	3.258	0.197	0.16	l
Parent & Autonomy	31.14 ± 3.53	31.57 ± 3.17	31.479 ± 2.95	0.238	0.89	0	s
Peers & Social Support	16.71 ± 2.43	17.43 ± 2.38	17.29 ± 2.24	0.705	0.719	0.01	s
School Environment	15.57 ± 3.41	17.07 ± 1.86	17.29 ± 2.35	1.033	0.599	0.06	m
ChilD-S	6.75 ± 5.78	4.07 ± 3.29	3.75 ± 2.75	1.895	0.395	0.09	m

Notes: $N = 46$; degrees of freedom always = 2.41; $p < .05$ statistically significant; effect sizes: small (s) = .01 > ηp2 < .059. medium (m) = .06 > ηp < .139. or large (l) = ηp ≥ .14

IBD-AD IBD in an active state of the disease, *IBD-RE* IBD in remission, *HC* Healthy Control, *ChilD-S* Child Depression Screener

social support and peers, school experience). Descriptively, IBD-AD had lower scores on the psychological wellbeing (PWB) dimension of the KIDSCREEN-27, while the other two groups did not differ from each other. The school dimension (SCH) showed a medium effect of .063, reflecting lower scores in the IBD-AD group.

Results of the depression scale indicated a medium effect size of .092, with the highest depression scores in the IBD-AD group and no differences between IBD-RE and HC.

Physical activity

Table 4 shows that results on a subjective scale assessing the last 7 days, the IPAQ questionnaire did not indicate any statistically significant mean differences in self-reported PA between the three groups IBD-AD, IBD-RE and HC. On a descriptive level, the IBD-AD group reported more vigorous physical activity (medium ES of .088) than the IBD-RE and HC groups. However, self-estimated fitness was lowest in the IBD-AD group (ES = .109).

Table 4 Subjective and objective physical activity

	IBD-AD (N = 8) M ± SD	IBD-RE (N = 14) M ± SD	HC (N = 24) M ± SD	Statistical Analysis			
				H	p	ηp2	Interpretation of effect sizes
MET min vigorous	2610 ± 2745.99	2202.86 ± 1832.39	1378.33 ± 1023.34	2.124	0.355	0.09	m
MET min moderate	710 ± 789.5	557.14 ± 406.85	1198.33 ± 2032.29	0.594	0.752	0.04	s
MET min walking	315.56 ± 136.19	321.16 ± 390.79	397.79 ± 330.5	1.878	0.409	0.02	s
Total MET	3635.56 ± 2819.76	3081.16 ± 1994.34	2974.45 ± 2354.31	0.546	0.768	0.01	s
Sitting Weekend	382.5 ± 198.84	407.14 ± 193.25	351.33 ± 163.72	0.504	0.779	0.02	s
Sitting Weekday	411.25 ± 132.23	408.21 ± 143.41	384.38 ± 107.55	1.022	0.608	0.01	s
Fitness	2.25 ± 1.17	2.93 ± 0.92	3.08 ± 0.78	3.501	0.177	0.11	m
Heart Rate pre 6 MWT	94.63 ± 15.91	101.69 ± 13.19	94.26 ± 11.25	3.357	0.189	0.11	m
Heart Rate post 6 MWT	142.88 ± 46.41	161.92 ± 28.19	163.13 ± 28.9	0.623	0.74	0.05	s
Heart Rate increase	48.25 ± 45.99	60.23 ± 26.47	68.87 ± 30.35	0.801	0.679	0.07	m
6 MWT Distance	655.38 ± 135.69	719.08 ± 84.91	687.78 ± 88.02	1.247	0.544	0.07	m
Borg 1-10	4 ± 1.31	4.31 ± 2.72	3.74 ± 2.4	0.689	0.715	0.02	s
Grip strength (kg)	28.72 ± 11.61	24.54 ± 8.66	24.12 ± 9.64	0.877	0.65	0.02	s
Difference from norm	1.42 ± 9.34	−3.2 ± 8.25	−2.08 ± 7.36	0.837	0.663	0.03	s
Average daily steps	8049 ± 3614	10.689 ± 3089	12.473 ± 4248	5.923	0.049	0.18	l

Notes: $N = 46$. degrees of freedom always = 2.41; $p < .05$ statistically significant; effect sizes: small (s) = .01 > ηp2 < .059. medium (m) = .06 > ηp < .139. or large (l) = ηp ≥ .14

IBD-AD IBD in an active state of the disease, *IBD-RE* IBD in remission, *HC* Healthy Control, *MET* Metabolic Equivalent, *6 MWT* 6-min walking test

Mean grip strength did not differ statistically significantly between the three groups IBD-AD, IBD-RE and HC.

Even though statistically non-significant, the mean 6MWT results indicated descriptive differences, with IBD-AD patients achieving the shortest distance compared to IBD-RE and HC (medium ES = .070). The IBD-AD also had less increase in heart rate (medium ES = .073), but still rated the intensity of the test as high as the other two groups (small ES = .018).

For the objective step counts as measured by the FitbitFlex®, a statistical significant mean difference ($p = .049$) and a large effect size of .183 were observed; the average count was 8049 steps per day in the IBD-AD group, 10,689 steps per day in IBD-RE and 12,473 steps per day in the HC group. According to Mann-Whitney-U post-hoc tests, comparisons between groups were not significant.

Discussion

The key findings of the present study were that children and adolescents with IBD-AD had poorer psychological functioning than children and adolescents with IBD-RE and HC. Furthermore, they had a lower functional capacity (6MWT) and engaged less in objectively assessed physical activity (average steps per day) compared to children and adolescents with IBD in remission or age- and gender-matched healthy controls. The present pattern of results adds to the current literature in an important way, showing that medically well-adjusted children and adolescents with IBD do not differ from healthy controls with regard to psychological functioning and objective and subjective PA.

Three hypotheses were tested and each of these is considered now in turn.

Our first hypothesis was that there would be anthropometric differences; specifically, we expected that participants with IBD were smaller, lighter and to have greater inflammation, especially among the more severe cases of IBD. Our data partly supported this hypothesis. The IBD-AD group had a moderately lower BMI z-score, BMI percentile, z-score height for age and percentile height for age when compared to both other groups. Therefore, the present data are in accordance with previous findings [14, 30]. In general, 10-40% of children with IBD are affected by growth failure [14, 30] and impaired nutritional status [31]. Underlying reasons are anorexia, malabsorption, intestinal inflammation and corticosteroid usage [32]. Given that the data available do not allow a deeper understanding of the pattern of results, we speculate that current treatment strategies lead to good disease control and less growth retardation [33].

With the first hypothesis, we also expected to detect indicators for inflammation and disease-related influences in the blood values of IBD patients. This hypothesis was partially supported; scores for the inflammatory markers ESR, CRP and leukocytes were higher among those with IBD-AD. Two patients with active IBD and two in remission were anemic, as well as one participant in the control group. In general, chronic anemia is prevalent and rapidly recurring in patients with IBD [34]. On the other hand, iron deficiency is a well-known phenomenon among many healthy female teenagers [35]. The small reported differences can be accounted to constant monitoring of blood values by the treating physician, who provides the patients with either oral or intravenous iron supplementation as soon as necessary. Looking at albumin values, it is not unusual to observe lower values in patients with IBD, as indicated by our findings. Patients with IBD might lose albumin due to increased gut permeability, even during symptom-free episodes [36]. However, we were unable to explain the low albumin values found in half of the healthy control participants. Common underlying reasons are undernourishment [37], decreased production due to liver disease [38] and increased excretion due to kidney problems [39], factors, which however could be ruled out by the supervising health professionals in the present study. Finally, the increased average hemoglobin among IBD-AD in comparison to HC was very surprising. The only possible explanation might be a blood clotting during blood sample taking since the hematocrit is elevated as well.

With the second hypothesis, we expected poorer psychological functioning in children and adolescents with IBD-AD compared to IBD-RE and healthy controls, and data did partially support this. Children and adolescents with increased disease activity had poorer psychological functioning in the area of psychological wellbeing. On the flipside, no other dimension of psychological functioning (physical functioning, autonomy and parent relations, social support and peers, and school experience) showed significant differences across the three groups, IBD-AD, IBD-RE and HC. Therefore, the present data do not match the study by Herzer et al. [40], showing a lower overall HRQOL among patients with IBD. Further, the present data do not accord with those studies reporting impaired physical functioning [41], impaired family functioning [40], limited participation in social activities [7], lower emotional functioning [42], and problematic school experience and performance.

Previous evidence can be explained by the association between increased disease activity and lower psychological functioning. One may claim that greater disease severity might be accompanied by an increasing presence of disruptive gastrointestinal symptoms and abdominal pain, which in turn need to be treated with more robust and invasive methods. Such increasing disease burden might result in psychological distress [43]. Two further hypotheses are the inflammation-depression hypothesis and the brain gut hypothesis. These two hypotheses claim that the increased production of pro-inflammatory cytokines (TNF alpha) is known to affect the brain both, directly and indirectly, thereby increasing symptoms of depression [44, 45]. Further, there is a bi-directional relationship, since psychological stress in turn increases the likelihood of inflammation, which again increases the occurrence of depressive symptoms [42]. The pro-inflammatory effect of experimental stress has been confirmed in human studies, and at the same time, inflammatory markers have been found to be raised in depressed patients [46]. To a wider extent, the inflammatory, unpredictable and disruptive nature of severe IBD, if not properly treated, could lead to an increase in internalizing symptoms (e.g., anxiety and depression). In particular, given that the long-term course of the disease is characterized by progressive deterioration [47], young patients might be at increased risk for psychological distress.

While comparing children and adolescents in remission with the healthy control group, we did not find differences on any of the HRQOL dimensions. This can be attributed to the fact that children in remission are by definition symptom-free [11]. A recent publication by the SWISS IBD Cohort even reported higher psychological functioning in IBD patients than in controls. The authors attributed this unexpected finding to the excellent social support in the young patients' environment [41]. Walter et al. [48], on the basis of a careful examination of the literature, noted that older studies (1989 – 2004) reported higher depression rates; subsequent advances in treatment may be responsible for the lower levels of psychological distress observed more recently. Therefore, we suggest that screening and treatment for mental wellbeing should be implemented especially for those with increased disease activity and potentially weaker social support.

Our third hypothesis, following others [18, 49], was that physical activity levels (subjective and objective) would be lower in children and adolescents with IBD than in their healthy counterparts. While the three groups did not differ regarding subjectively assessed PA in our study, lower objectively assessed PA was indicated by the number of steps per day, especially in the IBD-AD group. Thus, the present data are in account with previous results, however based on objective measurements. Werkstetter et al. [14] also reported reduced amounts of steps per day in children and adolescents with IBD, while studies of adult patients have found that suffering from IBD tended to lead to a sedentary lifestyle [50]. An explanation might be that patients with active IBD are restricted and discouraged by unpredictable symptoms, physical restriction, inconvenience and discomfort [49]. Furthermore, we found that children and adolescence with active IBD perceived physical strain to

be more vigorous as compared to IBD-RE and HC. This is reflected in their subjectively estimated greater intensity of the 6 MWT, while achieving less distance than the other groups and their extremely elevated self-reported vigorous PA levels over the last 7 days. This finding indicated a lower fitness in children and adolescents with active IBD, and was in line with findings of Ploeger et al. [13] Children with IBD exhibited impaired aerobic and anaerobic exercise capacity, compared to reference values.

However, a lower amount of PA might be an issue for the following reasons. Generally, regular low intensity exercise is beneficial in reducing distress and improving quality of life in young patients with IBD [51]. A UK survey revealed that PA made patients with IBD feel better and healthier, boosted energy, reduced IBD symptoms, provided an alternative focus and fostered feelings of normality [49]. On a physiological level, recent findings indicated that IBD patients could experience anti-inflammatory effects from the myokines released during skeletal muscle contraction while exercising, thereby inhibiting the release of protective heat shock proteins (Hsps), which help to regulate inflammation and immunity [52]. It was further asserted that PA is an anabolic stimulus, reducing inflammation and positively affecting growth factors, i.e., IGF-I [53]. Additionally, Robbins et al. [49] argued that regular PA should be undertaken in IBD to help maintain bone mineral density and prevent osteoporosis. We should note, however, that exaggerated amounts of (high-intensity) PA might lead to an increase in symptoms. Vigorous PA such as distance running and endurance exercise commonly might cause gastrointestinal discomfort including nausea, heartburn, and even gastrointestinal bleeding in patients with IBD [54]. By contrast, moderate PA seems to be useful in improving many aspects of the lives of patients with IBD. Nonetheless, a fear of symptoms exacerbation may be an indication that patients lack the impetus to start PA, and clinicians may be reluctant to prescribe PA, even though it might serve as a protective and preventive factor with respect to IBD. Collectively, we claim that regular moderate PA should receive greater attention in scientific intervention studies as adjuvant to prescribed pharmacotherapies.

Despite the novelty of the findings and the application of internationally validated and accepted questionnaires and objective measures, several limitations warrant against an overgeneralization of the present findings. First, the relatively small sample, especially the small number of children in an active disease state, created difficulties in detecting statistically significant effects. Though we also relied on effect sizes, which are not sensitive to sample size. Second, the recruitment of the sample was restricted to the German speaking part of

Switzerland. Of these patients, only participants willing and able to participate were assessed. Even though we tried to cover an extensive range of factors, it was not possible to control for all confounders, such as microbial or environmental conditions, which might have influenced two or more outcomes in the same or in opposite directions. In this context, one suggestion for future studies might be the assessment of objective disease severity, fecal calprotectin as another objective measure. Otherwise we would suggest extending the cross sectional design to include lifestyle intervention studies and their supportive effect in the disease coping process. Last, we did not distinguish between patients with CD and UC; whereas for diagnostic reasons such an approach would have been easy to follow and justify, we decided to split patients into IBD-AD and IBD-RE, as suggested by recent research such as Reigada et al. [42, 55].

Conclusion

The pattern of results suggests that effective medical treatment of IBD in children and adolescents is associated with favorable physiological parameters, psychological dimensions and PA. Psychological counselling of children and adolescents with severe IBD seem to be advised in addition to standard treatment schedules.

Abbreviations

6 MWT: Six minute walking test; CD: Crohn's disease; CDAI: Crohn's disease activity index; ChilD-S: Child Depression Screener; CRP: C-reactive protein; ERS: Erythrocyte sedimentation rate; ES: Effect size; HC: Healthy control; HR: Heart rate; HRQOL: Health related quality of life; Hsps: Heat shock proteins; IBD: Inflammatory bowel diseases; IBD-AD: IBD in an active state of the disease; IBD-RE: IBD in remission; MET: Metabolic equivalent; PA: Physical activity; PIBD: Pediatric IBD; PUCA: Pediatric ulcerative colitis activity index; UC: Undefined colitis

Acknowledgements
We thank the Kantonsspital Aarau for providing additional recruitment options. We are also grateful to Noe Stoll for support during data collection and data entry. Finally, we thank Nick Emler (Surrey, UK) for proofreading the manuscript and Harald Seelig for supporting the statistical analysis.

Funding
We thank the Freiwillige Akademische Gesellschaft Basel (FAG, Basel, Switzerland) for financially supporting the project.

Authors' contributions
Conception and Design, LM, MG, RIF, CL, NK, EHT, SB; Acquisition of data, LM, M.G, RIF, CL, NK; Analysis and interpretation of data: LM, MG, RF, CL, NK, EHT, SB; Drafting of manuscript: LM, MG, RIF, CL, NK, EHT, SB. All authors read and approved the final manuscript.

Competing interests
The authors declare that they have no competing interests.

Author details
[1]Psychiatric Clinics of the University of Basel, Centre for Affective, Stress and Sleep Disorders, University of Basel, Wilhelm Klein-Strasse 27, Ch-4012 Basel, Switzerland. [2]Pediatric Gastroenterology & Nutrition, University Children's Hospital Basel, Basel, Switzerland. [3]Department of Sport, Exercise and Health, Sport Science Section, University of Basel, Basel, Switzerland. [4]United Nations University - Maastricht Economic and Social Research Institute on Innovation and Technology (UNU-MERIT), Maastricht University, Maastricht, The Netherlands. [5]Substance Abuse Prevention Research Center; Sleep Disorders Research Center, Psychiatry Department, Kermanshah University of Medical Sciences, Kermanshah, Iran.

References
1. Levine A, de Bie CI, Turner D, et al. Atypical disease phenotypes in pediatric ulcerative colitis: 5-year analyses of the EUROKIDS registry. Inflamm Bowel Dis. 2013;19:370–7.
2. Lemberg DA, Day AS. Crohn disease and ulcerative colitis in children: an update for 2014. J Paediatr Child Health. 2015;51:266–70.
3. Loddo I, Romano C. Inflammatory bowel disease: genetics, epigenetics, and pathogenesis. Front Immunol. 2015;6 Available from: http://journal.frontiersin.org/Article/10.3389/fimmu.2015.00551/abstract. Cited 21 Mar 2016
4. Braegger CP, Ballabeni P, Rogler D, Vavricka SR, Friedt M, Pittet V, et al. Epidemiology of inflammatory bowel disease: is there a shift towards onset at a younger age? J Pediatr Gastroenterol Nutr. 2011;53:141–4.
5. Pappa H, Thayu M, Sylvester F, Leonard M, Zemel B, Gordon C. Skeletal health of children and adolescents with inflammatory bowel disease. J Pediatr Gastroenterol Nutr. 2011;53:11–25.
6. Rosen MJ, Dhawan A, Saeed SA. Inflammatory bowel disease in children and adolescents. JAMA Pediatr. 2015;169:1053.
7. Engstrom I. Mental-health and psychological functioning in children and adolescents with inflammatory bowel-disease: a comparison with children having other chronic illnesses and with healthy-children. J Child Psychol Psychiatry. 1992;3:563–82.
8. Ross SC, Strachan J, Russell RK, Wilson SL. Psychosocial functioning and health related quality of life in paediatric inflammatory bowel disease: a systematic review. J Pediatr Gastroenterol Nutr. 2011;53:480.
9. Vaisto T, Aronen ET, Simola P, Ashorn M, Kolho KL. Psychosocial symptoms and competence among adolescents with inflammatory bowel disease and their peers. Inflamm Bowel Dis. 2010;1:27–35.
10. Rabizadeh S, Dubinsky M. Update in pediatric inflammatory bowel disease. Rheum Dis Clin N Am. 2013;39:789–99.
11. Mikocka-Walus A, Knowles SR, Keefer L, Graff L. Controversies revisited: a systematic review of the comorbidity of depression and anxiety with inflammatory bowel diseases. Inflamm Bowel Dis. 2016;22:752–62.
12. Spekhorst LM, Hummel TZ, Benninga MA, van Rheenen PF, Kindermann A. Adherence to oral maintenance treatment in adolescents with inflammatory bowel disease. J Pediatr Gastroenterol Nutr. 2016;62:264–70.
13. Ploeger H, Obeid J, Nguyen T, Takken T, Issenman R, de Greef M, et al. Exercise and inflammation in pediatric Crohn's disease. Int J Sports Med. 2012;33:671–9.
14. Werkstetter KJ, Ullrich J, Schatz SB, Prell C, Koletzko B, Koletzko S. Lean body mass, physical activity and quality of life in paediatric patients

with inflammatory bowel disease and in healthy controls. J Crohns Colitis. 2012;6:665–73.

15. Loprinzi PD, Cardinal BJ. Association between objectively-measured physical activity and sleep, NHANES 2005–2006. Ment. Health and Phys Act. 2011;4:65–9.

16. Gerber M, Lindwall M, Lindegård A, Börjesson M, Jonsdottir IH. Cardiorespiratory fitness protects against stress-related symptoms of burnout and depression. Patient Educ Couns. 2013;93:146–52.

17. Hummel TZ, Tak E, Maurice-Stam H, Benninga MA, Kindermann A, Grootenhuis MA. Psychosocial developmental trajectory of adolescents with inflammatory bowel disease. J Pediatr Gastroenterol Nutr. 2013;57:219–24.

18. Chan D, Robbins H, Rogers S, Clark S, Poullis A. Inflammatory bowel disease and exercise: results of a Crohn's and Colitis UK survey. Frontline Gastroenterol. 2014;5:44–8.

19. Taylor RW, Jones IE, Williams SM, Goulding A. Evaluation of waist circumference, waist-to-hip ratio, and the conicity index as screening tools for high trunk fat mass, as measured by dual-energy X-ray absorptiometry, in children aged 3–19 y. Am J Clin Nutr. 2000;72:490–5.

20. WHO Multicentre Growth Reference Study Group. WHO Child growth standards: length/height-for-age, weight-for-age, weight-for-length, weight-for-height and body mass index-for-age: methods and development. Geneva: World Health Organization; 2006.

21. Ravens-Sieberer U, Herdman M, Devine J, Otto C, Bullinger M, Rose M, et al. The European KIDSCREEN approach to measure quality of life and well-being in children: development, current application, and future advances. Qual Life Res. 2014;23:791–803.

22. Frühe B, Allgaier A-K, Pietsch K, Baethmann M, Peters J, Kellnar S, et al. Children's Depression Screener (ChilD-S): development and validation of a depression screening instrument for children in pediatric care. Child Psychiatry Hum Dev. 2012;43:137–51.

23. IPAQ. Guidelines for data processing and analysis of the International Physical Activity Questionnaire (IPAQ) – short and long forms, revised on November 2005. 2005. Available from: http://www.ipaq.ki.se/scoring.pdf. Cited 15 Mar 2010.

24. Hagströmer M, Bergman P, De Bourdeaudhuij I, Ortega FB, Ruiz JR, Manios Y, et al. Concurrent validity of a modified version of the International Physical Activity Questionnaire (IPAQ-A) in European adolescents: the HELENA study. Int J Obes. 2008;32:S42–8.

25. Mathiowetz V, Wiemer DM, Federman SM. Grip and pinch strength: norms for 6-to 19-year-olds. Am J Occup Ther. 1986;40:705–11.

26. Solway S, Brooks D, Lacasse Y, Thomas S. A qualitative systematic overview of the measurement properties of functional walk tests used in the cardiorespiratory domain. Chest. 2001;119:256–70.

27. Hassan J, van der Net J, Helders PJM, Prakken BJ, Takken T. Six-minute walk test in children with chronic conditions. Br J Sports Med. 2010;44:270–4.

28. Meltzer LJ, Hiruma LS, Avis K, Montgomery-Downs H, Valentin J. Comparison of a commercial accelerometer with polysomnography and actigraphy in children and adolescents. Sleep. 2015;38:1323–30.

29. Cohen J. Statistical power analysis for the behavioral sciences. 2nd ed. Hillsdale: N.J: Routledge; 1988.

30. Dubinsky M. Special issues in pediatric inflammatory bowel disease. World J Gastroenterol. 2008;14:413.

31. Gasparetto M. Crohn's disease and growth deficiency in children and adolescents. World J Gastroenterol. 2014;20:13219.

32. Shamir R. Nutritional aspects in inflammatory bowel disease. J Pediatr Gastroenterol Nutr. 2009;48:S86–8.

33. De Greef E, Hoffman I, Smets F, Van Biervliet S, Bontems P, Hauser B, et al. Paediatric Crohn's disease: disease activity and growth in the BELCRO cohort after 3 years follow-up. J Pediatr Gastroenterol Nutr. 2016;63:253.

34. Kulnigg S, Teischinger L, Dejaco C, Waldhör T, Gasche C. Rapid recurrence of IBD-associated anemia and iron deficiency after intravenous iron sucrose and erythropoietin treatment. Am J Gastroenterol. 2009;12:1460–7.

35. Looker AC, Dallman PR, Carroll MD, Gunter EW, Johnson CL. Prevalence of iron deficiency in the United States. JAMA. 1997;12:973–6.

36. Michielan A, D'Incà R. Intestinal permeability in inflammatory bowel disease: pathogenesis, clinical evaluation, and therapy of leaky gut. Mediat Inflamm. 2015;2015:628157.

37. Vermeire S, Van Assche G, Rutgeerts P. Laboratory markers in IBD: useful, magic, or unnecessary toys? Gut. 2006;55:426–31.

38. Bernardi M, Maggioli C, Zaccherini G. Human albumin in the management of complications of liver cirrhosis. Crit Care. 2012;16:211.

39. Birn H, Christensen EI. Renal albumin absorption in physiology and pathology. Kidney Int. 2006;69:440–9.

40. Herzer M, Denson LA, Baldassano RN, Hommel KA. Patient and parent psychosocial factors associated with health-related quality of life in pediatric inflammatory bowel disease. J Pediatr Gastroenterol Nutr. 2011;52:295–9.

41. Rogler D, Fournier N, Pittet V, Bühr P, Heyland K, Friedt M, et al. Coping is excellent in Swiss children with inflammatory bowel disease: results from the Swiss IBD cohort study. J Crohns Colitis. 2014;8:409–20.

42. Goodhand JR, Wahed M, Mawdsley JE, Farmer AD, Aziz Q, Rampton DS. Mood disorders in inflammatory bowel disease: relation to diagnosis, disease activity, perceived stress, and other factors. Inflamm Bowel Dis. 2012;18:2301–9.

43. Gray WN, Denson LA, Baldassano RN, Hommel KA. Disease activity, behavioral dysfunction, and health-related quality of life in adolescents with inflammatory bowel disease. Inflamm Bowel Dis. 2011;17:1581–6.

44. Raison CL, Capuron L, Miller AH. Cytokines sing the blues: inflammation and the pathogenesis of depression. Trends Immunol. 2006;27:24–31.

45. van den Brink G, Stapersma L, El Marroun H, Henrichs J, Szigethy EM, Utens EM, et al. Effectiveness of disease-specific cognitive–behavioural therapy on depression, anxiety, quality of life and the clinical course of disease in adolescents with inflammatory bowel disease: study protocol of a multicentre randomised controlled trial (HAPPY-IBD). BMJ Open Gastroenterol. 2016;3:e000071.

46. Miller AH, Raison CL. The role of inflammation in depression: from evolutionary imperative to modern treatment target. Nat Rev Immunol. 2016;16:22–34.

47. Pittet V, Juillerat P, Mottet C, Felley C, Ballabeni P, Burnand B, et al. Cohort profile: the Swiss Inflammatory Bowel Disease Cohort Study (SIBDCS). Int J Epidemiol. 2009;38:922–31.

48. Walter JG, Kahn SA, Noe JD, Schurman JV, Miller SA, Greenley RN. Feeling fine: anxiety and depressive symptoms in youth with established IBD. Inflamm Bowel Dis. 2016;22:402–8.

49. Robbins H, Poullis A, Rogers S. Inflammatory bowel disease and exercise-preliminary results of a Crohn's and colitis UK survey. Gastroenterol Today. 2012;22:62–3.

50. Narula N, Fedorak RN. Exercise and inflammatory bowel disease. Can J Gastroenterol. 2008;22:497–504.

51. Ng V, Millard W, Lebrun C, Howard J. Low-intensity exercise improves quality of life in patients with Crohn's disease. Clin J Sport Med. 2007;17:384–8.

52. Chen Y, Noble EG. Is exercise beneficial to the inflammatory bowel diseases? An implication of heat shock proteins. Med Hypotheses. 2009;72:84–6.

53. Sanderson IR. Growth problems in children with IBD. Nat Rev Gastroenterol Hepatol. 2014;11:601.

54. Colditz GA, Cannuscio CC, Frazier AL. Physical activity and reduced risk of colon cancer: implications for prevention. Cancer Causes Control. 1997;8:649–67.

55. Reigada LC, Hoogendoorn CJ, Walsh LC, Lai J, Szigethy E, Cohen BH, et al. Anxiety symptoms and disease severity in children and adolescents with Crohn disease. J Pediatr Gastroenterol Nutr. 2015;60:30–5.

6

Design and validation of a German version of the GSRS-IBS - an analysis of its psychometric quality and factorial structure

Sarah K. Schäfer[1†], Kathrin Julia Weidner[2†], Jorge Hoppner[3], Nicolas Becker[1], Dana Friedrich[4], Caroline S. Stokes[4], Frank Lammert[4] and Volker Köllner[5,6*] (iD)

Abstract

Background: Currently, a suitable questionnaire in German language is not available to monitor the progression and evaluate the severity of irritable bowel syndrome (IBS). Therefore, this study aimed to translate the Gastrointestinal Symptom Rating Scale for Irritable Bowel Syndrome (GSRS-IBS) into German and to evaluate its psychometric qualities and factorial structure.

Methods: This study is based on a total sample of 372 participants [62.6% female, mean age = 41 years (SD = 17 years)]. 17.5% of the participants had a diagnosis of IBS, 19.9% were receiving treatment for chronic inflammatory bowel disease, 12.1% of the participants were recruited from a psychosomatic clinic, and 50.5% belonged to a control group. All participants completed the German version of GSRS-IBS (called Reizdarm-Fragebogen, RDF), as well as the Gießen Subjective Complaints List (GBB-24) and the Hospital Anxiety and Depression Scale - German version (HADS-D).

Results: The internal consistency of the RDF total scale was at least satisfactory in all subsamples (Cronbach's Alpha between .77 and .92), and for all subscales (Cronbach's Alpha between .79 and .91). The item difficulties (between .25 and .73) and the item-total correlations (between .48 and .83) were equally satisfactory. Principal axis analysis revealed a four-factorial structure of the RDF items, which mainly resembled the structure of the English original. Convergent validity was established based on substantial and significant correlations with the stomach-complaint scale of the GBB-24 ($r = .71$; $p < .01$) and the anxiety ($r = .42$; $p < .01$) and depression scales ($r = .43$; $p < .01$) of the HADS-D.

Conclusion: The German version of the GSRS-IBS RDF proves to be an effective, reliable, and valid questionnaire for the assessment of symptom severity in IBS, which can be used in clinical practice as well as in clinical studies.

Keywords: Irritable bowel syndrome, Questionnaire, Questionnaire design, Self-report, Colonic diseases

Background

Irritable bowel syndrome (IBS) is diagnosed on the basis of recurrent abdominal pain related to defecation or changes in stool frequency or form [1, 2]. The current prevalence of IBS ranges from 2.5 to 25%, depending on the diagnostic criteria used [3, 4]. For instance, the Manning criteria are associated with considerably higher prevalence rates when compared to the Rome I-III criteria. The prevalence of IBS is higher in women than in men. However, these gender differences decrease with increasing age [5, 6].

Patients with IBS experience a great degree of stress as a result of the condition. Several investigations with heterogeneous patient samples have illustrated that quality of life is perceived as being significantly impaired [7–10]. Further, adolescents suffering from IBS report a lower quality of life [11]. Moreover, IBS patients show considerably reduced health-related quality of life on all scales of the Short Form Health Survey (SF-36) [12] compared to other patient groups such as those with heart insufficiency [13]. A recent cross-sectional study from Norway

* Correspondence: volker.koellner@charite.de
†Equal contributors
[5]Department of Psychosomatic Medicine, Rehabilitation Clinic Seehof, Lichterfelder Allee 55, 14513 Teltow, Germany
[6]Psychosomatic Rehabilitation Research Group, Department of Psychosomatic Medicine, Center for Internal Medicine and Dermatology Charité – Universitätsmedizin Berlin, Berlin, Germany
Full list of author information is available at the end of the article

has shown that IBS is associated with poor outcomes, particularly in the presence of health complaints, organic diseases, and affective disorders [14].

Three validated scales are available to assess IBS severity, of which the IBS severity scoring system (IBS-SSS) is most frequently used [15]. However, the IBS-SSS is an external assessment tool which has to be administered by the treating physician.

Häuser [16] has produced a German translation of the Rome III criteria for IBS that allows for a categorical decision about the presence of IBS. However, none of these tools include a patient self-assessment which would provide valuable additional information to the external assessment, particularly with regard to the disruptions in quality of life frequently occuring [9, 17]. The validated Gastrointestinal Symptom Rating Scale for Irritable Bowel Syndrome (GSRS-IBS) by Wiklund et al. [18] firstly represents such a diagnostic tool, which is currently only available in the English language.

The instrument was first introduced in 2003 with the aim to establish a self-assessment tool specifically adapted to IBS patients [18]. The GSRS-IBS is based on the Gastrointestinal Symptom Rating Scale (GSRS-IBS, [19]) developed for IBS patients and the Health-Related Quality of Life Questionnaire (HRQL, [20]) which is disease independent.

Currently, there is no appropriate questionnaire available in the German language (spoken by approximately 100 million people) to assess self-perceived symptom severity in IBS. However, such an assessment tool would be useful in the context of clinical practice as it would aid formation of a diagnosis and the monitoring of the course of IBS and additionally, for clinical studies.

Objectives
Therefore, the aim of this study was to develop a German version of the GSRS-IBS (in the following called Reizdarm-Fragebogen, RDF) and to carry out a cross-cultural validation. For this purpose, the original questionnaire was translated into German and, in accordance with Wiklund et al. [18], was subsequently validated in a sample of IBS patients. Moreover, control groups were included to evaluate the specificity of the questionnaire.

Methods
The purpose of the following section is to provide a brief overview of the translation and design process of the German version of GSRS-IBS and to describe its validation in a sample of different subgroups.

Design of the German instrument
GSRS-IBS
The English version GSRS-IBS includes 13 items, which are rated on a seven-point scale ranging from "1 = no

discomfort at all" to "7 = very severe discomfort". All items exclusively capture IBS constructs. The questionnaire was neither designed to produce ceiling effects nor to assess redundant information. A factor-analytical examination of all items in a validation cohort provided the following five factors: pain, diarrhoea, satiety, constipation, and bloating. Based on these findings identically named subscales containing two to four items were defined and demonstrated satisfactory internal consistencies reflected in Cronbach's Alpha (α) ranging from .74 to .85.

Translation
In order to ensure a high quality translation process, a series of standards exists specifically for the cross-cultural translation of psychological and medical questionnaires [21]. The translation of the GSRS-IBS into German (RDF) was conducted in accordance with these recommended procedures. A preliminary version of the questionnaire was subsequently tested in a clinical sample. Contrary to the recommended standard specifications, no committee of experts was consulted concerning the quality of the questionnaire. Nonetheless, experienced gastroenterologists (including FL) confirmed its validity.

With regard to the specific process, two translators possessing the necessary knowledge of English and medical expertise independently translated the original questionnaire into their native German language. Both translations were then compared and the language was fine-tuned, which resulted in the translators agreeing on one version of the questionnaire. In order to assure the quality of the translation, the new version was retranslated back to English by two native English speakers who were not familiar with the original text. Except for some different choice of wording, the original English text did not differ from the retranslated version of the questionnaire, thus confirming the accuracy of the initial translation of the GSRS-IBS into German. Subsequently, the newly generated version of the questionnaire was given to a group of patients in a psychosomatic rehabilitation clinic in Blieskastel (MediClin Biestal-Kliniken), who were asked to check the comprehensibility of the items. None of these patients reported problems with comprehension. Therefore the German version was considered ready for implementation in the following validation study.

Study process
Sample recruitment
Validation cohorts Consecutive recruitment of the entire sample of 372 participants took place from April 2011 until June 2014. Out of these, 65 patients with a diagnosis of IBS were recruited from the department of Internal Medicine II at Saarland University Medical Centre in Homburg, Germany, and from an Internal Medicine private practice

in Neunkirchen, Germany. For quality control purposes, the Rome III-criteria was used to validate the IBS diagnosis in these patients, and only those with an appropriate diagnosis were included. A random selection of IBS patients was not possible due to difficulties in ensuring a sufficient sample size during recruitment. 45 patients with a psychosomatic disorder were recruited from the MediClin Bliestal clinic in Blieskastel, Germany. Further, 74 patients with chronic inflammatory bowel disease (IBD) who were treated at Saarland University Medical Centre, Homburg, Germany, took part. A control group of students and orthopaedic patients with no gastroenterological conditions was also included in the study. The students voluntarily completed the questionnaires during an introductory course of the elective course 'Medical case history' at Saarland University, and the orthopaedic patients were questioned in a radiology practice in Neustadt/Weinstraße, Germany, whilst awaiting an MRI scan. The mean age of the included subjects was $M = 41$ years ($SD = 17$ years) (for sample characteristics see Table 1). The mean age would be considerably higher, if the students were excluded from the sample.

Study procedure and instruments

Study procedure In addition to the RDF, a German version of the Hospital Anxiety and Depression Scale (HADS-D) [22] as well as a short version of the Gießen Subjective Complaints List (GBB-24) [23] were used to verify convergent validity.

GBB-24 The GBB-24 assesses the psychosomatic causes of physical complaints [23]. The 24-item short version was given to subjects instead of the longer 57-item long version [24]. GBB-24 assesses organ-specific, objective and subjective symptoms. The following physical complaints were documented: cardiac and gastric complaints, pain in the limbs, and fatigue. The total score represents the overall subjective complaints [25]. The split-half-reliabilities were situated in a satisfactory range between $r = .75$ (gastric discomfort) and $r = .94$ (general complaints, total score).

Table 1 Age and gender distribution of the entire sample

subsample	n	age (years)		women (percent)
		M	SD	
IBS patients	65	49	12	58.5
Chronic IBD patients	74	45	15	58.1
Psychosomatic patients	45	54	8	68.9
Orthopaedic patients and students	188	33	16	64.4
Total	372	41	17	62.6

IBD inflammatory bowel disease, *IBS* irritable bowel syndrome

HADS-D The HADS-D questionnaire contains 14 items and assesses symptoms of anxiety and depression (7 items per scale) based on somatic and physical complaints [22]. The HADS-D can therefore be applied as a screening tool as well as to assess the severity of anxiety and depressive symptoms. Both, the anxiety and the depression scale showed a good internal consistency of $\alpha = .80$.

Statistical analyses

Initially, according to Wiklund et al. [18] a total score of the RDF as well as the individual sub-scores for the five proposed subscales in the English version were calculated for each subject by summing the total of the 13 items. Moreover, sum scores were calculated for the identified subscales in the German version following the outcome of a subsequent factor analysis. Regarding both, the GBB-24 and the HADS-D, scoring was carried out according to the respective manual instructions. A total score as well as scores for the proposed subscales were calculated for the GBB-24. Additionally, a total score for anxiety and depression symptoms was calculated for the HADS-D. In case of missing data for a maximum of two of the 13 RDF items, the missing values were replaced by the subject's mean score. If three or more answers were missing, the subject was excluded from all analyses. The same principle was applied to the HADS-D and the GBB-24. However, in case of the latter a subject was excluded from analyses if five items or more were missing.

A new variable was created to compare presence versus absence of IBS. Thereafter, a binary logistic regression was calculated in order to verify if the IBS patients could be distinguished from the other groups based on their RDF results.

Internal consistencies (Cronbach's Alpha, α, [26]) were calculated for the entire questionnaire and for the subscales identified in the German version of the questionnaire, to determine the reliability of the RDF. Furthermore, the item difficulties and the item-total correlations were evaluated in order to assess item quality. To identify the factorial structure of the questionnaire, in comparison to the English validation, a slightly different procedure was employed: An exploratory principal axis analysis was performed with an oblique (Direct oblimin, Delta = 0) rotation. This analysis was chosen since exploratory factor analyses only consider item variance which is shared by at least two items. This was deemed to be more appropriate regarding measurement error [27]. Additionally, an oblique rotation appears to be more reasonable concerning the nature of IBS symptoms with respect to the chosen orthogonal rotation from Wiklund et al. [18]. To assume that those who suffer from severe constipation perceive the same amount of pain as those who do not suffer from constipation is implausible, which is why it seems appropriate to permit intercorrelations between factors.

The factor analyses were performed for the entire sample as well as separately for the subgroups (IBS, IBD, psychosomatic patients and control groups). Consequently, there is a factorial structure analysis for the entire sample (n = 372) from which 83% did not have a diagnosis of IBS. This can subsequently be compared to the factorial structure analysis in 65 patients with IBS. Moreover, this analysis in the IBS subsample can be compared with the IBS sample that was recruited for the validation of the original English version of the questionnaire. However, this comparison is limited due to the different types of factor analysis. Correlations with the GBB-24, its subscales and the HADS-scores were calculated to illustrate the questionnaire's convergent construct validity.

Results
Descriptive statistics
A comparison of the mean RDF scores between the different subgroups (see Table 2) revealed significant differences: The group of IBS patients had a significantly higher total score [$t(111)$ = –12.27, $p < .01$], corresponding to more severe symptoms related to IBS (see Fig. 1). Likewise, the student [$t(367)$ = 9.85, $p < .01$] and orthopaedic control groups [$t(367)$ = 2.65, $p = .004$] differed significantly from the mean scores of all clinical samples. These considerable differences could be demonstrated for all subscales of the questionnaire, irrespective of whether they were based on the German or English factor structure. Binary logistic regression analysis was used to differentiate IBS patients from the rest of the cohort (non-IBS patients) using the RDF items. Overall, 90.3% of IBS cases were correctly classified [$\chi^2(13)$ = 140.95, $p < .01$].

Assessment of item quality
Item quality
The item difficulties of the RDF ranged between $p = .25$ and $p = .73$ in the entire sample (see Table 3). As expected they were slightly lower ($p = .41$ to $p = .72$) in the IBS sample and had a lower range. The majority of the items were medium in difficulty with a few being very difficult or very easy. Such a distribution appears to be reasonable for differentiating IBS patients. The mean item-scale correlation

for the entire sample was $r = .65$. This corrected item-scale correlation is satisfactory. However, it was considerably lower for the IBS patients (mean $r = .40$). That is, however, to be evaluated in context to the later described diverging factorial structure.

Equally satisfactory are the results of the reliability analyses, with a Cronbach's Alpha in the entire sample of α = .92 for the RDF total scale (α = .77 in the IBS sample), and Cronbach's Alpha for the subscales of the German version within an acceptable range from α = .84 to α = .93 (α = .72 to α = .92 in the IBS sample) [28].

Factor analyses
The suitability of conducting a factorial analysis on the data derived from the entire sample was reflected in a KMO value (Kaiser-Meyer-Olkin measure of sample adequacy) of KMO = .88 and a significant Barlett test [$\chi^2(78)$ = 3457.68, $p < .01$]. The principal axis analysis with oblique rotation (Oblimin direct, Delta = 0) provided a two-factorial result for the overall sample according to Kaiser-Guttmann (Table 4). The first factor indicated an eigenvalue of 6.69 while the second factor lagged noticeably behind with an eigenvalue of 1.77. The KMO value of .68 for the IBS patients was not as strong, but nevertheless still appropriate for conducting a factor-analytical evaluation. The lower value might only reflect a significantly reduced sample size. The Barlett test of sphericity was also significant [$\chi^2(78)$ = 463.37, $p < .01$]. The principal axis analysis with an identical rotation provided a four-factorial structure for the IBS sample according to Kaiser-Guttman. The first factor is characterized principally by bloating-related sensations and the passing of gas, whereas the second factor mainly summarises symptoms of diarrhoea. The third factor is associated with constipation while the fourth factor is related to the urge to empty the bowel and the ensuing relief that the patients feel. In total, 64.5% of the item variance could be explained by these four extracted factors.

Intercorrelation of subscales
To determine the correlations between the various questionnaires, for RDF a total score with item 3 recoded was calculated. This process takes the negative sign of the factor scores into account. Subsequently, bivariate correlation analyses were conducted between the subscale scores and

Table 2 Mean values and standard deviations (in brackets) of the RDF scales for the various samples

Subgroups	Total (13 Items)	Pain (2)	Diarrhoea (4)	Constipation (2)	Satiety (2)	Bloating (3)
IBS	50.85 (12.86)	8.03 (2.92)	14.74 (5.93)	5.74 (3.83)	7.89 (3.80)	14.45 (4.60)
Chronic IBD	31.90 (13.57)	4.59 (2.85)	11.62 (6.01)	3.30 (2.20)	4.41 (2.76)	7.98 (4.55)
Psycho-somatic	29.85 (15.90)	3.86 (2.35)	8.54 (5.17)	4.36 (3.24)	4.38 (3.13)	8.72 (5.68)
Control group	21.84 (10.59)	3.61 (2.43)	6.10 (3.26)	2.85 (1.86)	3.44 (2.06)	5.84 (3.90)
Total	29.88 (16.18)	4.61 (3.05)	9.00 (5.75)	3.63 (2.77)	4.52 (3.14)	8.12 (5.37)

IBD inflammatory bowel disease, *IBS* irritable bowel syndrome

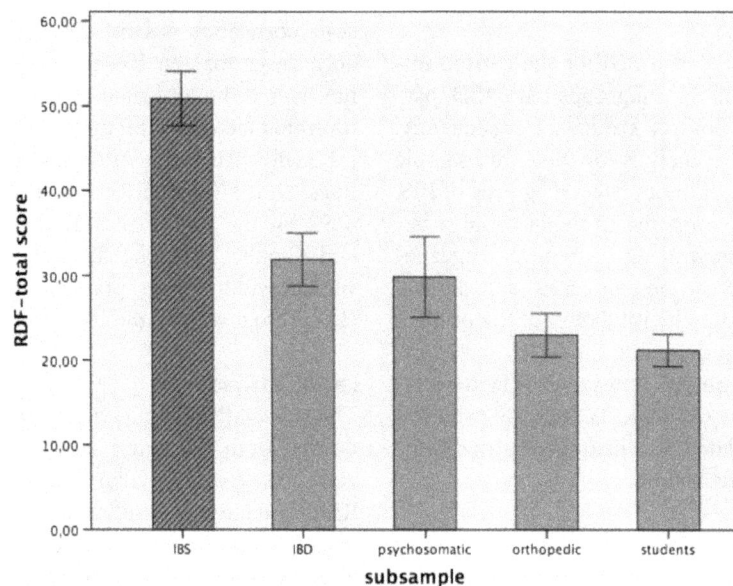

Fig. 1 Means of the GSRS-IBS/RDF total score for the different subgroups. Legend: The bars indicate the 95% confidence interval of the group mean. *GSRS-IBS* Gastrointestinal Symptom Rating Scale for Irritable Bowel Syndrome; *IBD* (chronic) inflammatory bowel disease; *IBS* irritable bowel syndrome; *RDF* Reizdarm-Fragebogen

the total score of the RDF, both for the entire sample and separately for patients with IBS (Table 5). This analysis revealed that the first subscale, 'bloating' (items 3 and 4), is the most independent. However, in IBS patients, a substantial association with constipation-related complaints was observed. Concerning the subscale 'diarrhoea' (items 6 and 7), significant correlations were shown for 'constipation' however not for IBS patients), 'pain and feelings of tension'. Significant correlations were identified between the subscale constipation (items 5, 8, 11, 12, and 13), and all other subscales. However, the correlations with 'diarrhoea' and 'pain and feelings of tension' are not significant for IBS patients. The subscales 'pain and feelings of tension' are considerably associated with the scales 'diarrhoea' and 'constipation' (but not for IBS patients). However, they were not correlated with 'bloating' in both, the IBS and the total sample. All subscales correlated significantly with the RDF total score (with the exception of the 'bloating' subscale in the entire sample).

Table 3 Item difficulties and item-total correlations for RDF in the entire sample and in the group of IBS patients

	IBS patients		Entire sample	
	Item difficulties	Item-total correlations	Item difficulties	Item-total correlations
1. Stomach pain	.62	.37	.36	.65
2. Relief through bowel movement	.52	.50	.30	.75
3. Passing gas	.71	.42	.41	.77
4. Stomach gas	.72	.68	.40	.83
5. Constipation	.41	.30	.25	.51
6. Diarrhoea or frequent bowel movement	.48	.18	.30	.57
7. Liquid stool	.41	.21	.73	.50
8. Hard stool	.41	.30	.26	.48
9. Urge to empty bowel	.59	.36	.37	.65
10. Feeling of complete emptying of the bowel	.62	.56	.34	.75
11. Feeling of fullness after meals	.55	.42	.31	.62
12. Prolonged feeling of fullness	.58	.39	.33	.65
13. Bloated stomach	.64	.51	.35	.77

IBS irritable bowel syndrome, *RDF* Reizdarm-Fragebogen

Table 4 Loading matrix (pattern matrix) of the oblique rotation (factor eigenvalue in brackets)

	Factor 1 Bloated stomach (2.48)	Factor 2 Diarrhoea (2.35)	Factor 3 Constipation (2.80)	Factor 4 Pain and feeling of tension (2.52)
1. Stomach pain	−.04	.06	.07	**.49**
2. Relief through bowel movement	.10	−.13	−.13	**.83**
3. Passing gas	**−.93**	.05	−.14	−.01
4. Stomach gas	**.87**	.08	.18	.05
5. Constipation	.06	−.39	**.44**	.12
6. Diarrhoea or frequent stool	.11	**.91**	.02	.09
7. Liquid stool	.05	**.83**	.10	.09
8. Hard stool	.03	−.40	**.45**	.13
9. Urge to empty bowel	−.05	.28	−.10	**.62**
10. Feeling of complete emptiness of the bowel	.13	−.09	.14	**.56**
11. Feeling of fullness after meals	−.12	.13	**.92**	−.01
12. Prolonged feeling of fullness	.03	−.03	**.85**	−.09
13. Bloated stomach	.23	.03	**.49**	.10

Note: Factor loadings > .40 in bold print

Convergent validity

The correlations between the HADS-D and GBB-24 total scores and RDF scores reflect the convergent validity for the latter (Table 6). All analysed samples showed significant and similar correlations between the responses on the RDF and those on the subscale for stomach pain in the GBB-24. As expected, the correlation was particulary strong in IBS patients ($r = .65$, $p < .01$). The same applies to the correlation of the GBB-total value that is associated with general abdominal pain and the total scores of the RDF. Correlations were significant for the entire sample ($r = .56$, $p < .01$) as well as for the group of IBS patients ($r = .44$, $p < .01$). Likewise, the correlations for the subscales of the HADS-D depression and anxiety were significant for the entire sample. It is, however, apparent that the correlations of RDF score and HADS scores are notably lower in the group of IBS patients than in the total sample.

Discussion

The results suggest that the RDF as the German version of the GSRS-IBS, can be used as a reliable and valid questionnaire to assess self-perceived severity and to monitor progress in IBS patients in German-speaking countries. The present analyses establish the RDF as a reliable and economical tool. This is evidenced by the sufficient psychometric quality of the tests, its plausible, factorial structure as well as its selective sensitivity for IBS symptoms. In line with this, significant differences in the total RDF score were reported for IBS patients in comparison to other clinical and non-clinical samples. Its suitability is further reflected by the convergent validity apparent in the correlations between the RDF and the GBB-24 and the HADS-D. The present study further demonstrates that the German version of the RDF is also suitable for subjective severity assessment of IBS and that the same IBS construct is consequently acquired in the English-speaking world as well as in Germany [29].

Table 5 Correlations and internal consistencies of the various dimensions in the entire sample (first correlation, $n = 372$) and the subsample of IBS patients (second correlation, $n = 65$)

	1	2	3	4	5
Bloating (1)	.93/.90	.01/.05	.13*/.32*	−.01/.07	.04/.25*
Diarrhoea (2)		.89/.92	.37**/−.11	.58**/.31*	.64**/.36**
Constipation (3)			.85/.82	.63**/.22	.82**/.64**
Pain and feeling of tension (4)				.84/.72	.91**/−.75**
RDF total (5)					.92/.77

The diagonal contains internal consistencies of each subscale, first for the entire sample and second for the IBS subsample
IBS irritable bowel syndrome, *RDF* Reizdarm-Fragebogen
*$p < .05$
**$p < .01$

56

Table 6 Correlations of RDF total scores and other instruments for the total sample (first correlation, n = 372) and the sample of IBS patients (second correlation, n = 65)

	1	2	3	4
RDF total (1)	–	.42**/.15	.26**/.12	.26**/.56**
HADS-D Anxiety (2)		–	.49**/.71**	.23**/.20
HADS-D Depression (3)			–	.55**/.12
GBB-24 stomach discomfort (4)				–

GBB-24 Gießen Subjective Complaints List 24, *HADS-D* Hospital Anxiety and Depression Scale - German Version, *IBS* irritable bowel syndrome, *RDF* Reizdarm-Fragebogen
*p < .05
**p < .01

However, it must be noted that the factorial structure of the German version does not perfectly match the original English version. The method of choice to prove the similarity of the factorial structure would certainly have to be a confirmatory factor analysis [30]. This method was deliberately not applied in the present study due to methodological reasons. A different exploratory approach was chosen that, on the one hand, seems to be more appropriate for the data - with respect to the inter-factor correlations and the considered variances - but, on the other hand, distinctly limits the comparison of the findings with the results from Wiklund et al. [18]. The employed factorial analysis resulted in four instead of five factors and raises concerns over whether the five-factorial structure found in the English original and the associated interpretation of the scales should be adjusted. It may be advisable to initially focus on the value of the entire RDF and to subsequently define the exact scale structure and compile indications of its interpretation, only after a further validation sample.

Despite the scale structure that still needs to be investigated, the RDF can certainly be recommended for its application in a screening procedure. However, in order to ensure a meaningful implementation in daily clinical practice or in general practitioner practices, it would be reasonable to define cut-off-values. This would require a larger sample of IBS patients, which would also be necessary to determine the extent to which the questionnaire is suitable to assess the subjective and additionally the objective degree of IBS. A comparison with the currently used severity scores in daily clinical practice would be particularly important. Such a comparison would also establish to what extent the RDF can be meaningfully implemented to document the (subjective) progression of IBS and if it should be included in the standard therapy plan.

Limitations
On a critical note, only 65 patients with IBS were recruited for this investigation, a small sample compared to the 234 IBS patients used in the validation of the original English version. This relatively small sample size is especially

associated with limitations in the interpretation of the factorial analytical results. Smaller samples (and thus samples with a greater range restriction) are more likely to be associated with a larger number of factors, which could present an alternative explanation for the diverse factorial structures in the total cohort and in the group of IBS patients. The fact that the IBS patients were less suitable for the factor analytic investigation is reflected in the significantly lower KMO coefficients, even when compared to the entire sample. Moreover, the control group comprising students is a further limitation, as characteristics such as age, years of education and socioeconomic status differed in the two groups, thus limiting their comparability. However, the inclusion of orthopaedic patients should have reduced such influences. Nevertheless, a replication and expansion of this study with a larger patient cohort and a matched control group would be desirable.

Additionally, not all aspects of the test quality could be taken in consideration. For instance, findings regarding stability of the results in terms of retest-reliability are lacking. The coherence of the HADS-D and the GBB-24 point towards a persuasive convergent construct validity, while a proof of a sufficient discriminant validity is indeed missing. Likewise, it seems reasonable to examine the extent to which the RDF scores correlate with other relevant variables within IBS.

Conclusion
The German version of the GSRS-IBS RDF proves to be an effective, reliable, and valid questionnaire for the assessment of self-perceived symptom severity in IBS, which can be used in clinical practice as well as in clinical studies.

Abbreviations
GBB-24: Gießen Subjective Complaints ListGießener Beschwerdebogen 24; GSRS-IBS: Gastrointestinal Symptom Rating Scale for Irritable Bowel Syndrome; HADS-D: Hospital Anxiety and Depression Scale - Deutsche Version (German Version) HRQLHealth-Related Quality of Life Questionnaire; IBD: (Chronic) inflammatory bowel disease; IBS: Irritable bowel syndrome; KMO: Kaiser-Meyer-Olkin measure of sample adequacy; RDF: Reizdarm-Fragebogen

Acknowledgements
We would like to sincerely thank Dr. Jutta Besch, who supported this project by helping us to recruit patients with IBS from her internal medicine practice in Neunkirchen. Further, we thank Marlene Staginnus for helping proof reading the manuscript.

Funding
There was no funding for this work.

Authors' contributions

CSS, DF, FL, JH, KJW and VK helped in study concept and design; DF, JH and KJW were responsible for acquisition of data; NB and SKS performed all statistical analyses and interpreted data; SKS drafted the manuscript. All authors contributed to the first version and the critical revision of the manuscript for important intellectual content. All authors read and approved the final version of the manuscript.

Competing interests

The authors declare that they have no competing interests.

Author details

[1]Department of Psychology, Saarland University, Saarbrücken, Germany. [2]University Mannheim, I. Medical Clinic-Cardiology, Pneumology and Angiology Mannheim, Mannheim, Germany. [3]University Heidelberg, Clinic for Diagnostic and Interventional Radiology Heidelberg, Heidelberg, Germany. [4]Saarland University, Department of Medicine II – Gastroenterology und Endocrinology, Homburg, Germany. [5]Department of Psychosomatic Medicine, Rehabilitation Clinic Seehof, Lichterfelder Allee 55, 14513 Teltow, Germany. [6]Psychosomatic Rehabilitation Research Group, Department of Psychosomatic Medicine, Center for Internal Medicine and Dermatology Charité – Universitätsmedizin Berlin, Berlin, Germany.

References

1. Ford AC, Lacy BE, Talley NJ. Irritable bowel syndrome. N Engl J Med. 2017; 376:2566–78.
2. Lacy BE, Mearin F, Chang L, Chey WD, Lembo AJ, Simren M, et al. Bowel disorders. Gastroenterology. 2016;150:1393–407.
3. Häuser W, Lempa M. Reizdarmsyndrom. Schmerz. 2004;18:130–5.
4. Spiller R, Aziz Q, Creed F, Emmanuel A, Houghton L, Hungin P, et al. Guidelines on the irritable bowel syndrome: mechanisms and practical management. Gut. 2007;56:1770.
5. Häuser W, Layer P, Henningsen P, Kruis W. Funktionelle Darmbeschwerden bei Erwachsenen. Dtsch Arztebl. 2012;109:83–93.
6. Layer P, Andresen V, Pehl C, Allescher H, Bischoff S, Classen M, et al. S3-Leitlinie Reizdarmsyndrom: Definition, Pathophysiologie, Diagnostik und Therapie. Gemeinsame Leitlinie der Deutschen Gesellschaft für Verdauungs-und Stoffwechselkrankheiten (DGVS) und der Deutschen Gesellschaft für Neurogastroenterologie und Motilität (DGNM). Z Für Gastroenterol. 2011;49:237–93.
7. Andrews E, Eaton S, Hollis K, Hopkins J, Ameen V, Hamm L, et al. Prevalence and demographics of irritable bowel syndrome: results from a large web-based survey. Aliment Pharmacol Ther. 2005;22:935–42.
8. Gulewitsch MD, Enck P, Hautzinger M, Schlarb AA. Irritable bowel syndrome symptoms among German students: prevalence, characteristics, and associations to somatic complaints, sleep, quality of life, and childhood abdominal pain. Eur J Gastroenterol Hepatol. 2011;23:311–6.
9. Hahn B, Kirchdoerfer L, Fullerton S, Mayer E. Patient-perceived severity of irritable bowel syndrome in relation to symptoms, health resource utilization and quality of life. Aliment Pharmacol Ther. 1997;11:553–9.
10. Jamali R, Jamali A, Poorrahnama M, Omidi A, Jamali B, Moslemi N, et al. Evaluation of health related quality of life in irritable bowel syndrome patients. Health Qual Life Outcomes. 2012;10:12.
11. Devanarayana NM, Rajindrajith S, Benninga MA. Quality of life and health care consultation in 13 to 18 year olds with abdominal pain predominant functional gastrointestinal diseases. BMC Gastroenterol. 2014;14:150.
12. Ware JE, Kosinski M, Dewey JE, Gandek B. SF-36 health survey: manual and interpretation guide: Quality Metric Inc.; 2000.
13. Whitehead WE, Burnett CK, Cook EW, Taub E. Impact of irritable bowel syndrome on quality of life. Dig Dis Sci. 1996;41:2248–53.
14. Michalsen VL, Vandvik PO, Farup PG. Predictors of health-related quality of life in patients with irritable bowel syndrome. A cross-sectional study in Norway. Health Qual Life Outcomes. 2015;13:113.
15. Francis CY, Morris J, Whorwell PJ. The irritable bowel severity scoring system: a simple method of monitoring irritable bowel syndrome and its progress. Aliment Pharmacol Ther. 1997;11:395–402.
16. Häuser W. Übersetzung der Rome III-RDS-Kriterien ins Deutsche. 2013.
17. Lembo A, Ameen VZ, Drossman DA. Irritable bowel syndrome: toward an understanding of severity. Clin Gastroenterol Hepatol. 2005;3:717–25.
18. Wiklund I, Fullerton S, Hawkey C, Jones R, Longstreth G, Mayer E, et al. An irritable bowel syndrome-specific symptom questionnaire: development and validation. Scand J Gastroenterol. 2003;
19. Svedlund J, Sjödin I, Dotevall G. GSRS—a clinical rating scale for gastrointestinal symptoms in patients with irritable bowel syndrome and peptic ulcer disease. Dig Dis Sci. 1988;33:129–34.
20. Guyatt GH. Measurement of health-related quality of life in heart failure. J Am Coll Cardiol. 1993;22:A185–91.
21. Beaton D, Bombardier C, Guillemin F, Ferraz MB. Recommendations for the cross-cultural adaptation of health status measures. N Y am Acad. Orthop Surg. 2002:1–9.
22. Herrmann-Lingen C, Buss U, Snaith RP. HADS-D: Hospital anxiety and depression scale: Deutsche Version. Huber; 2011.
23. Brähler E, Hinz A, Scheer JW. GBB-24. Der Giessener Beschwerdebogen. Manual, 3. überarbeitete und neu normierte Ausgabe. Bern: Hans Huber Verlag; 2008.
24. Brähler E, Hinz A, Scheer JW. GBB-24: der Giessener Beschwerdebogen: Manual. Bern: H. Huber; 2008.
25. Brähler E, Schumacher J, Brähler C. Erste gesamtdeutsche Normierung der Kurzform des Giessener Beschwerdebogens GBB-24. PPmP-Psychother Psychosom Med Psychol. 2000;50:14–21.
26. Cronbach LJ. Coefficient alpha and the internal structure of tests. Psychometrika. 1951;16:297–334.
27. Bryant FB, Yarnold PR. Principal-components analysis and exploratory and confirmatory factor analysis. In: Reading and understanding multivariate statistics. Washington, DC: American Psychological Association; 1995. p. 99–136.
28. Beaton DE, Bombardier C, Guillemin F, Ferraz MB. Guidelines for the process of cross-cultural adaptation of self-report measures. Spine. 2000;25:3186–91.
29. Stieglitz R-D. Diagnostik und Klassifikation psychischer Störungen: Konzeptuelle und methodische Beiträge zur Evaluierung psychiatrischer Diagnostikansätze. Verlag f. Psychologie: Hogrefe; 2000.
30. Thompson R. Exploring the link between maternal history of childhood victimization and child risk of maltreatment. J Trauma Pract. 2016;5:57–72.

7

Hepatic expression of Yin Yang 1 (YY1) is associated with the non-alcoholic fatty liver disease (NAFLD) progression in patients undergoing bariatric surgery

Xianwen Yuan[1,2†], Jun Chen[3†], Qi Cheng[1], Yinjuan Zhao[4], Pengzi Zhang[5], Xiaoyan Shao[1], Yan Bi[5], Xiaolei Shi[2], Yitao Ding[2*], Xitai Sun[2*] and Bin Xue[1,6,7*]

Abstract

Background: This study is to investigate the association between the hepatic expression of Yin Yang 1 (YY1) and the progression of non-alcoholic fatty liver disease (NAFLD) in patients undergoing bariatric surgery.

Methods: Obese patients undergoing bariatric surgery were included. Liver tissues were subjected to the quantitative real-time PCR, Western blot analysis, and immunohistochemical assay, to determine the expression levels of YY1.

Results: Totally 88 patients were included. According to the NAFLD activity score (NAS), these patients were divided into the control ($n = 12$), steatosis ($n = 20$), non-defining NASH ($n = 38$), and NASH ($n = 18$) groups. Significant differences in the serum glucose, insulin, ALT, AST, and HOMA-IR levels were observed among these different NAFLD groups. Hepatic YY1 expression had correlation with serum glucose, insulin, HOMA-IR, ALT, AST, triglycerides, HDL, and GGT. Immunohistochemical analysis showed that, compared with the control group, the expression levels of YY1 were significantly higher in the non-defining NASH and NASH groups. In addition, multivariate regression model showed that the serum ALT and YY1 levels were strongly associated with the NAFLD activity.

Conclusions: Several factors are associated with NAFLD progression, including the expression of YY1. Our findings contribute to understanding of the pathogenesis of NAFLD.

Keywords: Yin Yang 1(YY1), Non-alcoholic fatty liver disease (NAFLD), Bariatric surgery

Background

Non-alcoholic fatty liver disease (NAFLD) represents a liver disease spectrum characterized by excessive accumulation of fat in the liver, with no alcohol abuse [1, 2].

NAFLD could be classified into the non-alcoholic fatty liver (NAFL; which is simple steatosis) and the non-alcoholic steatohepatitis (NASH) [3]. Steatosis is a benign status with mild fat deposition, which could be reversed by the lifestyle modification (such as diet and exercise) [4]. On the other hand, for NASH, in addition to the fat deposition, there would be intralobular inflammation and hepatocyte ballooning. Moreover, NASH can progress into advanced liver fibrosis, cirrhosis, and ultimate hepatocellular carcinoma (HCC) [1, 5].

NAFLD is strongly associated with obesity, dyslipidemia, diabetes, and insulin resistance, which has been

---

* Correspondence: dytnanjing1983@126.com; sunxitai@sohu.com; xuebin@nju.edu.cn
†Yuan Xianwen and Chen Jun contributed equally to this work.
[2]Department of Hepatobiliary Surgery, the Affiliated Drum Tower Hospital of Nanjing University Medical School, Nanjing 210008, Jiangsu Province, China
[1]State Key Laboratory of Pharmaceutical Biotechnology, Jiangsu Key Laboratory of Molecular Medicine and School of Medicine, Nanjing University, Nanjing, Jiangsu Province, China
Full list of author information is available at the end of the article

therefore regarded as the hepatic manifestation of metabolic syndromes [6]. Despite massive advances in elucidating the genetic mechanism in NAFLD development, understanding of the disease pathogenesis remains incomplete [1]. Recently, the *two-hit* theory has been widely accepted to elucidate the pathogenesis of NAFL and NASH. The first *hit* refers to the accumulation of triglyceride (TG) in hepatocytes, i.e., the simple steatosis. This process is closely associated with abnormal lipid metabolism involved in central obesity and insulin resistance. The second *hit* includes mechanisms contributing to the development of inflammation and fibrosis, such as oxidative stress and mitochondrial dysfunction [7, 8].

Patients with NAFLD are always asymptomatic in clinic. The disease is often diagnosed when there is evidence for liver steatosis on imaging modality, which is associated with the metabolic syndromes, including obesity (high body mass index, BMI, and waist circumference) and diabetes (high blood glucose with hypertriglyceridemia) [5, 6]. Ultrasonography is a non-invasive method frequently used in the assessment of hepatic lipid accumulation [9, 10], so as other imaging techniques like computed tomography (CT) and nuclear magnetic resonance (NMR) [10, 11]. In addition, the blood biochemistry results could also give a hint on the diagnosis of NAFLD, such as the elevated transaminase level [12].

Recently, there are advances in the non-invasive techniques intending to assess the NASH/fibrosis level, including the NAFLD fibrosis score (NFS) [5], Fibro Meter [13, 14], and Fibro Scan [15], with, however, relatively low accuracy. Up to now, the liver biopsy is still considered to be the gold standard for the diagnosis of stages of NASH, as well as distinguishing NAFL, NASH, and liver fibrosis [16]. However, no factors against NAFLD have been elucidated to date.

Yin Yang 1 (YY1), a ubiquitous, is a multifunctional zinc-finger transcription factor from the protein family, which can work as transcriptional repressor, activator, or initiator element binding protein [17]. A myriad of potential YY1 target genes have already been identified, important for cell proliferation and differentiation process. YY1 has been shown to play an important role in regulating proliferation and apoptosis of tumor cells [18]. Moreover, YY1 promotes the triglyceride accumulation in the adipocytes via repressing Chop10 transcription, implying its potential role in the development of obesity [19]. Furthermore, YY1 has also been found to be able to repress the genes associated with the insulin/insulin-like growth factor (IGF) signaling pathway, such as IGF1–2, IRS1–2, and Akt1–3 in skeletal muscles [20]. A recent study has also found that YY1 might be related to the body weight, glucose level, and cholesterol or free fatty acid level [21]. In addition, compared with control subjects, the YY1 levels are significantly down-regulated in the liver tissues in NAFLD

patients [22]. However, the association between the YY1 expression and the NAFLD progression has not completely elucidated.

In this study, the obese patients undergoing bariatric surgery were divided into four groups according to the liver pathogenesis. The mRNA and protein expression levels of YY1 were determined, and the association between the YY1 expression and the NAFLD progression was investigated.

Methods
Study subjects
This study was approved by the Ethics Committee of the Affiliated Drum Tower Hospital of the Medical School of Nanjing University (Permit Number: 2017–030-02). This study was registered in International Clinical Trial Registry Platform (ICTRP), with the clinical trial number NCT03296605. Patients were selected from a cohort undergoing laparoscopic Roux-en-Y gastric bypass surgery at the Department of Hepatobiliary Surgery of the Affiliated Drum Tower Hospital of the Medical School of Nanjing University. Exclusion criteria were included the patients with evidence for viral hepatitis, hemochromatosis, or alcohol consumption (> 20 g/d for females and > 30 g/d for males) [23]. The participants were recruited from April 2017 to February 2018. Written informed consent was obtained from all subjects.

Data collection
Liver tissue samples were obtained during surgery. One half was put into lipid nitrogen and stored at − 80 °C; and the other half was fixed by 10% formaldehyde, embedded in paraffin, and subjected to the hematoxylin-eosin (H&E) staining. Specimen was stored in the Nanjing Multicenter Biobank, the Biobank of Nanjing Drum Tower Hospital, and the Affiliated Hospital of Nanjing University Medical School. We conducted this study from February 2018. We had access to information that could identify individual participants during or after data collection. Histological characteristics were determined according to the Kleiner scoring system [24]. Steatosis was assessed and scored in a scale of 0–3, inflammation grades of 0–3, and hepatocellular ballooning of 0–2. These histopathological features were used to estimate the NAFLD activity score (NAS). These subjects were classified into the control (without steatosis), hepatic steatosis (NAS of 1–2), non-defining NASH (NAS of 3–4), and NASH (NAS of ≥5) groups [25]. Fibrosis was staged in based on the grades of 0–4. For biochemical measurement, blood samples were taken after an overnight (10-h) fast. Samples were analyzed and tested for the liver function, insulin level, C-reactive protein level, glucose level, and lipid panels (including total cholesterol, LDL, HDL, and triglycerides). Insulin activity

was determined by the homeostatic model assessment for insulin resistance (HOMA-IR) index [26, 27].

Quantitative real-time PCR

Total RNA was extracted from the liver tissue using Trizol (Invitrogen, Carlsbad, CA, USA). RNA (500 ng) was used for cDNA synthesis using random primers and Primescriptreverse transcriptase (Takara, Dalian, Liaoning, China). Quantitative real-time PCR was carried out using the SYBR Green qPCR kit (Takara), on a fluorescent temperature cycler. Primer sequences were as follows: YY1, forward 5′-ACGG CTTCGAGGATCAGATTC-3′ and reverse 5′-TGAC CAGCGTTTGTTCAATGT-3′; and GAPDH, forward 5′-TGACTTCAACAGCGACACCCA-3′ and reverse5′-- CACCCTGTTGCTGTAGCCAAA-3′. Reaction conditions were set as: 95 °C for 30 s, followed by 40 cycles of 95 °C for 5 s and 60 °C for 34 s. Target gene expression was calculated with semi-quantitative method. GAPDH was used as internal reference.

Western blot analysis

Tissues were lysed with the RIPA buffer containing phosphatase inhibitors. The protein concentration was determined using the BCA method (Pierce, Rockford, IL, USA). Totally 24 mg protein was separated on 10% SDS-PAGE, and then electronically transferred onto a PVDF membrane. After blocking with 3% BSA in 10 mM Tris-HCl (pH 7.4) containing 0.05% Tween-20, the membrane was incubated with the mouse anti-YY1 (Abcam, Cambridge, MA, USA) and anti-β-actin primary antibody (1:1000 dilution; Key GEN Bio TECH, Nanjing, Jiangsu, China) at 4 °C overnight.

After washing, the membrane was incubated with the peroxidase-conjugated secondary antibody (Santa Cruz, Santa Cruz, CA, USA), and developed in the Super Signal West Pico Chemiluminescent Substrate (Pierce). The protein was visualized and quantified with the Imagine J software.

Immunohistochemistry analysis

Formalin-fixed liver tissue samples were subjected to the immunohistochemistry analysis. Briefly, liver sections were deparaffinized and treated by citrate, and then blocked with Immuno Detector Peroxidase Blocker (Bios SB, Santa Barbara, CA, USA). Sections were incubated with the rabbit anti-YY1 primary antibody (1:250dilution; Abcam, Cambridge, MA, USA) at 4 °C overnight. Liver sections were then treated with peroxidase-conjugated secondary antibody (Santa Cruz) and DAB chromogen. Then the samples were counterstained with hematoxylin, and observed under light microscope.

Statistical analysis

Data were expressed as mean ± SD. Statistical analysis was performed using the SPSS 19.0 software (SPSS Inc., Chicago, IL, USA). Group comparison of numeric variables was performed using the ANOVA or Kruskal-Wallis test, depending on the variables' distribution. The χ^2test was used for comparison of nominal categorical variables. Correlation analysis was conducted with the Spearman's test. Multivariate logistic regression model was used to identify the significant clinical and metabolic factors that predicted the NAFLD absence, after adjusting for other factors such as BMI.

Table 1 Anthropometric and biochemical parameters of the study subjects

	Control (n = 12)	Steatosis (n = 20)	Non-defining NASH (n = 38)	NASH (n = 18)	P
Age (years)	33.4 ± 12.9	39.1 ± 12.1	34.2 ± 10.4	34.2 ± 13.1	NS
BMI (kg/m²)	38.1 ± 8.5	37.7 ± 5.02	40.4 ± 7.3	39.4 ± 5.9	NS
Glucose (mmol/L)	4.9 (4.6–5.3)	5.5 (4.8–7.3)	5.5 (5.2–6.5)	6.6 (5.7–8.8)	< 0.05#, Δ, &, +
Insulin (μIU/mL)	15.3 (12.9–23.1)	19.6 (12.9–31.4)	26.5 (19.6–41.5)	33.4 (20.0–50.8)	< 0.05#, Δ, §, &
HOMA-IR	3.6 (3.1–4.4)	4.9 (3.9–8.2)	7.3 (5.2–10.6)	11.5 (5.8–16.9)	< 0.05*, #, Δ, §, &
C reactive protein (mg/L)	4.95 (2.75–6.85)	5.9 (4.1–7.4)	6.7 (5.5–11.3)	6.8 (5.1–10.3)	NS
Triglycerides (mmol/L)	1.59 (0.96–2.45)	1.43 (1.18–2.04)	1.90 (1.23–2.34)	1.95 (1.52–6.29)	NS
Total Cholesterol (mmol/L)	4.7 ± 0.9	4.8 ± 0.9	4.8 ± 0.6	5.4 ± 1.0	NS
HDL-C (mmol/L)	1.05 (0.96–1.50)	1.12 (0.99–1.27)	1.01 (0.83–1.10)	0.92 (0.75–1.02)	NS
LDL-C (mmol/L)	3.09 (1.83–3.36)	2.94 (2.15–3.12)	2.71 (2.16–3.35)	2.53 (2.29–3.51)	NS
ALT (IU/mL)	19.4 (14.0–28.6)	25.2 (21.0–37.5)	35.8 (27.3–60.2)	76.5 (50.3–128.8)	< 0.05#, Δ, &, +
AST (IU/mL)	19.5 (15.0–25.4)	20.2 (14.7–25.9)	24.1 (18.5–35.2)	50.5 (29.2–90.7)	< 0.05Δ, §, &, +
GGT (IU/mL)	35.4 (21.6–53.3)	39.5 (20.2–66.5)	43.5 (26.5–64.0)	55.8 (37.5–90.5)	NS

Note: BMI body mass index, HOMA-IR homeostasis model assessment for insulin resistance, HDL-C high-density lipoprotein cholesterol, LDL-C low-density lipoprotein cholesterol, ALT alanine transaminase, AST aspartate transaminase, and GGT gamma glutamyltranspeptidase. *, P < 0.05 between the control and steatosis groups; #, P < 0.05 between the control and non-defining NASH groups; Δ, P < 0.05 between the control and NASH groups; §, P < 0.05 between the steatosis and non-defining NASH groups; &, P < 0.05 between the steatosis and NASH groups; +, P < 0.05 between the non-defining NASH and NASH groups; and NS, none significance

Results

Clinical characteristics of study population

Totally 88 patients were included in this study. Clinical and biochemical characteristics of these patients were shown in Table 1. In these subjects, there were 12 cases without steatosis (13.6%), 20 cases of steatosis (22.7%), 38 cases of non-defining NASH (43.2%), and 18 cases of NASH (20.5%). Our results showed that the glucose levels were significantly changed along with the NAFLD progression. Significant differences were observed between the control and non-defining NASH groups, the control and NASH groups, and the non-defining NASH and NASH groups (all $P < 0.05$). Moreover, the insulin level was significantly changed along with the NAFLD progression. Significant differences were observed between the control and non-defining NASH groups, the control and NASH groups, the steatosis and non-defining NASH groups, and then steatosis and NASH groups (all $P < 0.05$). Furthermore, the HOMA-IR was significantly changed along with the NAFLD progression. Significant differences were observed between all these groups ($P < 0.05$), except for the non-defining NASH and NASH groups. In addition, the ALT levels were significantly changed along with the NAFLD progression. Significant differences were observed between all the groups ($P < 0.05$), except for the control and steatosis groups, and the steatosis and non-defining NASH groups. Besides, the AST levels were significantly changed along with the NAFLD progression. Significant differences were observed between all the groups (all $P < 0.05$), except for the control and steatosis groups, and the control and non-defining NASH groups. However, no significant differences were observed in other biochemical parameters between these groups. Taken together, these results suggest significantly different serum ALT, AST, glucose, insulin, and HOMA-IR levels at different NAFLD stages.

Pathological characteristics of study population

Before surgery, the included patients subjected to the liver spy, and the pathological sections were evaluated and analyzed by pathologists. As shown in Table 2, the results of liver histology showed that, there were 20 case of grade 0 steatosis, 32 cases of grade 1 steatosis, 17 cases of grade 2 steatosis, and 19 cases of grade 3 steatosis. For the fibrosis score, there were 25, 46, 14, 2, and 1 cases of scores 0–4, respectively. Moreover, there were 33 cases with lobular inflammation score 0, 47 cases with score 1, and only 8 cases with score 2. Furthermore, there were 22 cases with hepatocyte ballooning score 0, 45 cases with score 1, and 21 cases with score 2. The NAS activity was based on the above scores, and these patients could be divided into four groups accordingly. A representative slice was shown in Fig. 1. Taken together, these results suggest that, NAFLD is very common in obese population.

Table 2 Histological characteristics of liver in the study subjects

	Patients ($n = 88$) n (%)
Steatosis grade	
0	20 (22.7)
1	32 (36.4)
2	17 (19.3)
3	19 (21.6)
Fibrosis stage	
0	25 (28.4)
1	46 (52.3)
2	14 (15.9)
3	2 (2.3)
4	1 (1.1)
Lobular inflammation	
0	33 (37.5)
1	47 (53.4)
2	8 (9.1)
3	0 (0)
Hepatocyte ballooning	
0	22 (25.0)
1	45 (51.1)
2	21 (23.9)
NASH activity score (NAS)	
0	12 (13.6)
1–2	20 (22.7)
3–4	38 (43.2)
5–8	18 (20.5)

YY1 expression and association with exact NAFLD progression

Although YY1 expression is high in the NAFLD patients, the association between YY1 and the exact NAFLD progression has not yet been explored. To investigate the expression of YY1 at different NAFLD stages, the quantitative real-time PCR and Western blot analysis were performed. Our results showed that, compared with the control group, the mRNA and protein level of YY1 in the NASH groups was significantly elevated (Fig. 2). As shown in the Table 3, the YY1 mRNA level was significantly correlated with the serum ALT ($r = 0.339$, $P = 0.001$), AST ($r = 0.216$, $P = 0.043$), glucose ($r = 0.274$, $P = 0.01$), insulin ($r = 0.313$, $P = 0.003$), and HOMA-IR ($r = 0.355$, $P = 0.001$) levels. As shown in Table 4, statistical analysis indicated that the YY1 protein expression level was significantly correlated with the serum ALT ($r = 0.459$, $P = 0.001$), glucose ($r = 0.438$, $P = 0.001$), insulin ($r = 0.369$, $P = 0.001$), and HOMA-IR ($r = 0.463$, $P = 0.001$) levels. On the other hand, for the hepatic sections, our

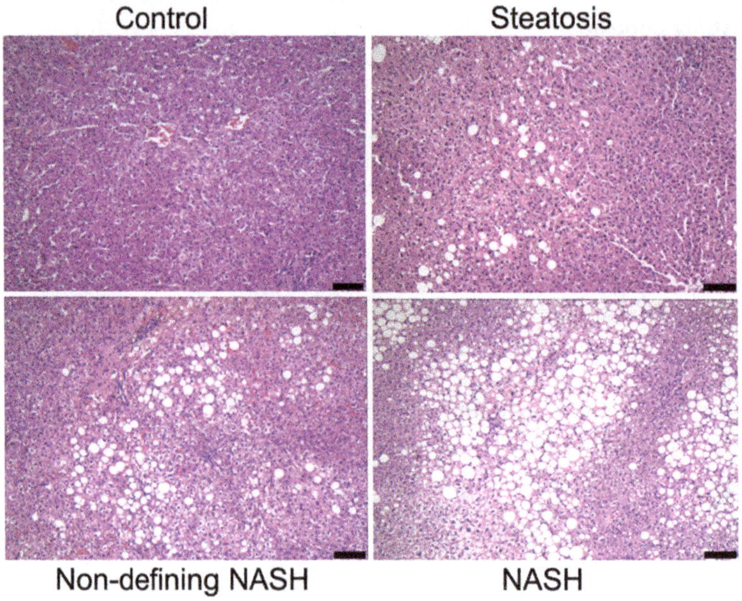

Fig. 1 H&E staining for NAFLD at different stages. Representative pictures from the H&E staining of the control, steatosis, non-defining NASH, and NASH groups, respectively. Scale bar, 100 μm

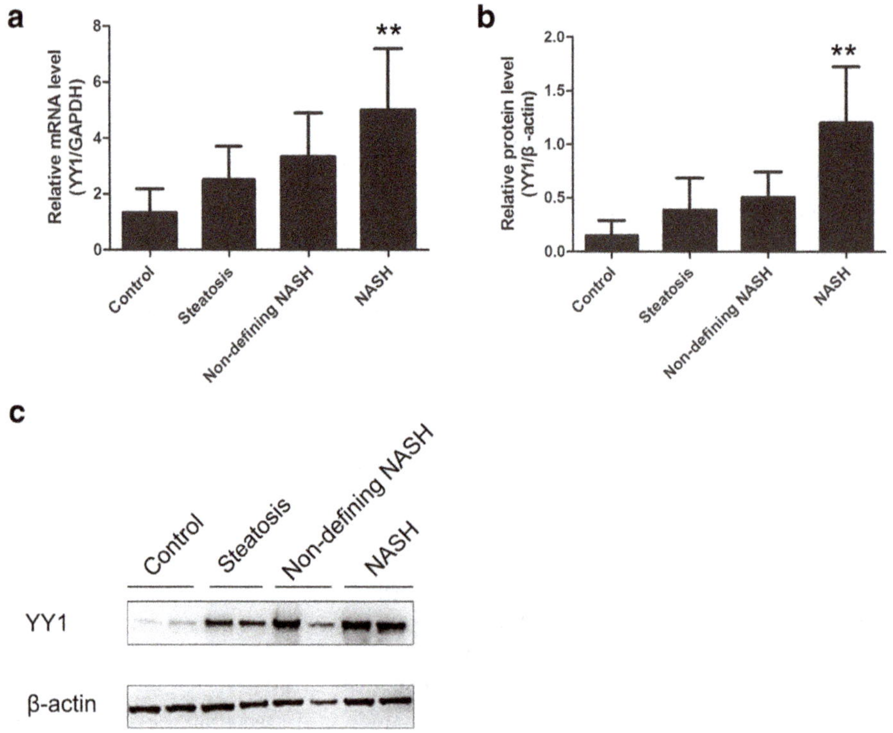

Fig. 2 YY1 expression for NAFLD at different stages. **a** The YY1 mRNA levels in the control, steatosis, non-defining NASH, and NASH groups were detected with the quantitative real-time PCR. **p < 0.01 compared with control group. **b** The YY1 protein levels in the control, steatosis, non-defining NASH, and NASH groups were detected with western blot analysis, respectively. **p < 0.01 compared with control group. **c** Representative image of western blot in different groups

Table 3 Correlation between hepatic YY1 mRNA levels and biochemical parameters

| | Association with YY1 mRNA levels | |
	Correlation coefficient	P
Age (years)	0.2	0.578
BMI (kg/m^2)	0.1	0.515
Glucose (mmol/L)	0.3	0.010
Insulin (μIU/mL)	0.2	0.003
HOMA-IR	0.4	0.001
C reactive protein (mg/L)	0.3	0.165
Triglycerides (mmol/L)	0.1	0.977
Total cholesterol (mmol/L)	0.3	0.768
HDL (mmol/L)	0.1	0.965
LDL (mmol/L)	0.1	0.841
ALT (IU/mL)	0.1	0.001
AST (IU/mL)	0.1	0.043
GGT (IU/mL)	0.3	0.808

results showed that the YY1 expression was associated with the NAFLD progression. In the control group, there were 8 patients negative for YY1 and 4 patients positive for YY1. In the steatosis group, there were 5 patients negative for YY1 and 15 patients positive for YY1. In non-defining NASH group, there were patients negative for YY1 and 28 patients positive for YY1. In the NASH group, all the 18 patients were positive for YY1. Compared with the control group, the expression of YY1 was significantly higher in the NASH and non-defining NASH groups (Fig. 3). Taken together, these results suggest that, YY1 expression levels are not the same at different NAFLD stages.

Table 4 Correlation between hepatic YY1 protein levels and biochemical parameters

| | Association with YY1 protein levels | |
	Correlation coefficient	P
Age (years)	0.2	0.519
BMI (kg/m^2)	0.4	0.080
Glucose (mmol/L)	0.3	0.001
Insulin (μIU/mL)	0.5	0.001
HOMA-IR	0.3	0.001
C reactive protein (mg/L)	0.2	0.106
Triglycerides (mmol/L)	0.1	0.043
Total cholesterol (mmol/L)	0.1	0.273
HDL (mmol/L)	0.2	0.009
LDL (mmol/L)	0.2	0.423
ALT (IU/mL)	0.3	0.001
AST (IU/mL)	0.3	0.001
GGT (IU/mL)	0.2	0.049

NAFLD activity predicting factors

To investigate the relationship between NAFLD and YY1, multivariable linear regression model was used. Our results showed that glucose, insulin, HOMA-IR, ALT, and AST were associated with the NAFLD progression. Therefore, a multivariate linear regression model was constructed to predict NAFLD activity score (NAS). According to this model, the ALT and hepatic YY1 protein content were independent predictive factors associated with NAS Table 5. The following equation was obtained based on these results, i.e., NAS activity = 0.181 (Glucose) + 0.023 (Insulin) - 0.024 (HOMA-IR) + 0.018 (ALT) - 0.013 (AST) + 2.259 (YY1) - 0.242. Taken together, these results suggest that, the NAS activity is significantly associated with the serum ALT level and hepatic YY1 protein level.

Discussion

In the present study, the factors associated with normal liver histology in patients with obesity were identified and investigated. Our findings identifying the protective factors could help guide the NAFLD screening among the patients with high risk, as well as further understand the disease pathogenesis. Patients undergoing weight-loss surgery offered insights into the unique patient subset. This cohort allowed for the identification of the protective factors against the development of NAFLD confirmed by histology in the high risk group. Our results showed that YY1 was associated with the NAFLD progression. Furthermore, YY1 had strong association with glucose, insulin, HOMA-IR, ALT, and AST. These findings suggest that besides NAFLD, YY1 is also associated with the hepatic metabolism.

Recently, it has been shown that the hepatic YY1 expression level is increased in the diabetic rats [28]. Moreover, YY1 promotes the hepatosteatosis and insulin resistance, mainly via FXR, in the animal model [22]. FXR is a metabolic nuclear receptor, abundantly expressed in the liver, intestine, and kidney, which has been first identified as a key regulator in the cholesterol and bile acid homeostasis [29]. Moreover, FXR is also a major transcriptional factor participating in the regulation of the glucose and lipid metabolism in liver. In line with this, our results showed that YY1 might influence the liver metabolism. Moreover, YY1 and ALT were most important factors to predict the NAFLD activity, further supporting the important interaction between the YY1 and NAFLD progression. The more severe NAFLD was, the higher the YY1 expression level would be. Taken together, these results suggest that the hepatic YY1 expression is an important factor involved in the progression of NAFLD. This study has important clinical significance for diagnose and treatment of NAFLD. And combination of YY1 and NAS scores can serve as a more accurate diagnostic indicator for NAFLD.

There are also limitations about this study. The data was derived from the cohort of patient undergoing bariatric

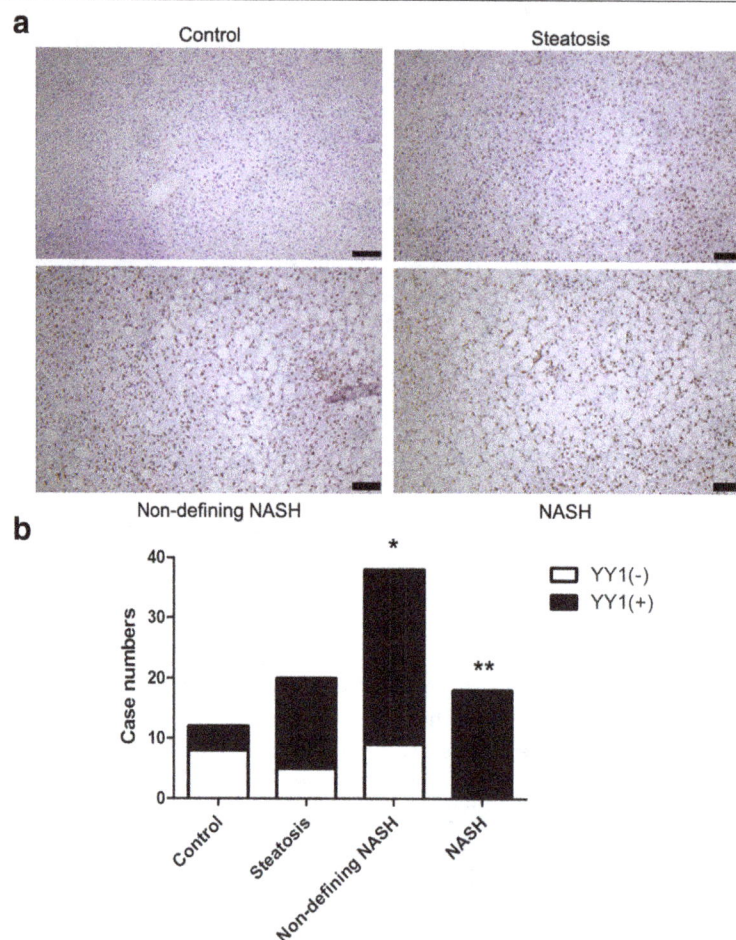

Fig. 3 Immunohistochemistry detection of YY1 for NAFLD at different stages (**a**) Immunohistochemistry analysis was performed to detect the expression of YY1 in the control, steatosis, non-defining NASH, and NASH groups.Scale bar, 100 μm. **b** The cases positive or negative for YY1 expression were analyzed. *$p < 0.05$ compared with control group, **$p < 0.01$ compared with control group

surgery. However, there is need for confirmation in an additional cohort which including patients selected at daily routine in a hepatological setting for NASH, outside the setting for bariatric surgery, and it should be evaluated more broadly in healthy people. Actually, the data is difficult to collect because healthy people and patients without NASH usually reject invasive testing especially in China, so it's not feasible to confirm our conclusion in another cohort in this study. Of course, further in-depth studies are still needed to investigate the correlation between YY1 and NAFLD progression in broader populations in the future.

Conclusion

In conclusion, this study identified factors associated with the development of NAFLD in obese patients undergoing bariatric surgery. Our results showed that YY1 had strong association with the NAFLD progression, which contributed to understanding the underlying mechanisms of NAFLD. This is the first study reporting the association between the hepatic YY1 expression and NAFLD at different stages. Our findings suggest that YY1 may be a promising therapeutic target for fatty liver diseases and related metabolic disorders in clinic.

Table 5 Multivariate regression model predicting NAS

	B	SE	P
Constant	−0.242	0.809	0.765
Glucose	0.181	0.119	0.131
Insulin	0.023	0.030	0.446
HOMA-IR	−0.024	0.093	0.800
ALT	0.018	0.006	0.007
AST	−0.013	0.012	0.270
Hepatic YY1 protein	2.259	0.317	0.000

Abbreviations
ALT: Alanine transaminase; AST: Aspartate transaminase; CT: Computed tomography; H&E: Hematoxylin-eosin; HCC: Hepatocellular carcinoma; HOMA-IR: Homeostatic model assessment for insulin resistance; ICTRP: International Clinical Trial Registry Platform; IGF: Insulin/insulin-like

growth factor; NAFL: Non-alcoholic fatty liver; NAFLD: Non-alcoholic fatty liver disease; NAS: NAFLD activity score; NASH: Non-alcoholic steatohepatitis; NFS: NAFLD fibrosis score; NMR: Nuclear magnetic resonance; TG: Triglyceride; YY1: Yin Yang 1

Acknowledgements
We thank Dr. Biyun Xu for the kind assistant in statistical analysis.

Funding
This study was supported by the National Natural Science Foundation of China (No. 31300103, 31371373, 31771572), the Nature Science Foundation of Jiangsu Province (BK20151395), the Open Fund of State Key Laboratory of Natural Medicines (No. SKLNMKF201606), the Fundamental Research Funds for the Central Universities (021414380330), Research of Institute of hospital management Nanjing University (NDYG2017016), the Innovation Capability Development Project of Jiangsu Province (No. BM2015004), the Nanjing Healthy and Family Planning Commission Medical Science Technology Innovation Platform Project (ZDX16006), and the National Human Genetic Resources Sharing Service Platform (2005DKA21300).

Authors' contributions
XB, SXT and DY conceived and designed this study. YX, CJ, ZY, CQ, ZP, SXY, BY and SXL performed the experiments. YX and CJ analyzed the data. YX and XB drafted the manuscript. All authors read and approved the final manuscript.

Competing interests
The authors declare that they have no competing interests.

Author details
[1]State Key Laboratory of Pharmaceutical Biotechnology, Jiangsu Key Laboratory of Molecular Medicine and School of Medicine, Nanjing University, Nanjing, Jiangsu Province, China. [2]Department of Hepatobiliary Surgery, the Affiliated Drum Tower Hospital of Nanjing University Medical School, Nanjing 210008, Jiangsu Province, China. [3]Department of Pathology, the Affiliated Drum Tower Hospital of Nanjing University Medical School, Nanjing, Jiangsu Province, China. [4]Collaborative Innovation Center of Sustainable Forestry in Southern China, College of Forestry, Nanjing Forestry University, Nanjing, China. [5]Department of Endocrinology, the Affiliated Drum Tower Hospital of Nanjing University Medical School, Nanjing, Jiangsu Province, China. [6]State Key Laboratory of Natural Medicines, Nanjing Pharmaceutical University, Nanjing, Jiangsu Province, China. [7]Liver Disease Collaborative Research Platform of Medical School of Nanjing University, 22 Hankou Road, Gulou District, Nanjing 210093, Jiangsu Province, China.

References
1. Cohen JC, Horton JD, Hobbs HH. Human fatty liver disease: old questions and new insights. Science. 2011;332:1519–23.
2. Angulo P. Nonalcoholic fatty liver disease. N Engl J Med. 2002;346:1221–31.
3. Lau JK, Zhang X, Yu J. Animal models of non-alcoholic fatty liver disease: current perspectives and recent advances. J Pathol. 2017;241:36–44.
4. Schwenger KJ, Allard JP. Clinical approaches to non-alcoholic fatty liver disease. World J Gastroenterol. 2014;20:1712–23.
5. Issa D, Alkhouri N. Nonalcoholic fatty liver disease and hepatocellular carcinoma: new insights on presentation and natural history. Hepatobiliary Surg Nutr. 2017;6:401–3.
6. Marchesini G, Bugianesi E, Forlani G, Cerrelli F, Lenzi M, Manini R, Natale S, Vanni E, Villanova N, et al. Nonalcoholic fatty liver, steatohepatitis, and the metabolic syndrome. Hepatology. 2003;37:917–23.
7. Day CP, James OF. Steatohepatitis: a tale of two "hits"? Gastroenterology. 1998;114:842–5.
8. Day CP. Pathogenesis of steatohepatitis. Best Pract Res Clin Gastroenterol. 2002;16:663–78.
9. Dowman JK, Tomlinson JW, Newsome PN. Systematic review: the diagnosis and staging of non-alcoholic fatty liver disease and non-alcoholic steatohepatitis. Aliment Pharmacol Ther. 2011;33:525–40.
10. Festi D, Schiumerini R, Marzi L, Di Biase AR, Mandolesi D, Montrone L, Scaioli E, Bonato G, Marchesini-Reggiani G, et al. Review article: the diagnosis of non-alcoholic fatty liver disease - availability and accuracy of non-invasive methods. Aliment Pharmacol Ther. 2013;37:392–400.
11. Federico A, Trappoliere M, Loguercio C. Treatment of patients with non-alcoholic fatty liver disease: current views and perspectives. Dig Liver Dis. 2006;38:789–801.
12. Yan E, Durazo F, Tong M, Hong K. Nonalcoholic fatty liver disease: pathogenesis, identification, progression, and management. Nutr Rev. 2007;65:376–84.
13. Wong VW, Vergniol J, Wong GL, Foucher J, Chan HL, Le Bail B, Choi PC, Kowo M, Chan AW, et al. Diagnosis of fibrosis and cirrhosis using liver stiffness measurement in nonalcoholic fatty liver disease. Hepatology. 2010;51:454–62.
14. Cales P, Laine F, Boursier J, Deugnier Y, Moal V, Oberti F, Hunault G, Rousselet MC, Hubert I, et al. Comparison of blood tests for liver fibrosis specific or not to NAFLD. J Hepatol. 2009;50:165–73.
15. Yoneda M, Yoneda M, Mawatari H, Fujita K, Endo H, Iida H, Nozaki Y, Yonemitsu K, Higurashi T, et al. Noninvasive assessment of liver fibrosis by measurement of stiffness in patients with nonalcoholic fatty liver disease (NAFLD). Dig Liver Dis. 2008;40:371–8.
16. Adams LA, Feldstein AE. Non-invasive diagnosis of nonalcoholic fatty liver and nonalcoholic steatohepatitis. J Dig Dis. 2011;12:10–6.
17. Liu L, Wang JF, Fan J, Rao YS, Liu F, Yan YE, Wang H. Nicotine suppressed fetal adrenal StAR expression via YY1 mediated-histone deacetylation modification mechanism. Int J Mol Sci. 2016;17:E1477.
18. López-Perrote A, Alatwi HE, Torreira E, Ismail A, Ayora S, Downs JA, Llorca O. Structure of yin Yang 1 oligomers that cooperate with RuvBL1-RuvBL2 ATPases. J Biol Chem. 2014;289:22614–29.
19. Huang HY, Li X, Liu M, Song TJ, He Q, Ma CG, Tang QQ, et al. Transcription factor YY1 promotes adipogenesis via inhibiting CHOP-10 expression. Biochem Biophys Res Commun. 2008;375:496–500.
20. Blattler SM, Cunningham JT, Verdeguer F, Chim H, Haas W, Liu H, Romanino K, Rüegg MA, Gygi SP, et al. Yin Yang 1 deficiency in skeletal muscle protects against rapamycin-induced diabetic-like symptoms through activation of insulin/IGF signaling. Cell Metab. 2012;15:505–17.
21. Logsdon BA, Hoffman GE, Mezey JG. Mouse obesity network reconstruction with a variational Bayes algorithm to employ aggressive false positive control. BMC Bioinformatics. 2012;13:53.
22. Lu Y, Ma Z, Zhang Z, Xiong X, Wang X, Zhang H, Shi G, Xia X, Ning G, et al. Yin Yang 1 promotes hepatic steatosis through repression of farnesoid X receptor in obese mice. Gut. 2014;63:170–8.
23. Ahrens M, Ammerpohl O, von Schonfels W, Kolarova J, Bens S, Itzel T, Teufel A, Herrmann A, Brosch M, et al. DNA methylation analysis in nonalcoholic fatty liver disease suggests distinct disease-specific and remodeling signatures after bariatric surgery. Cell Metab. 2013;18:296–302.
24. Kleiner DE, Brunt EM, Van Natta M, Behling C, Contos MJ, Cummings OW, Ferrell LD, Liu YC, Torbenson MS, et al. Design and validation of a histological scoring system for nonalcoholic fatty liver disease. Hepatology. 2005;41:1313–21.
25. Gutiérrez-Vidal R, Vega-Badillo J, Reyes-Fermín LM, Hernández-Pérez HA, Sánchez-Muñoz F, López-Álvarez GS, Larrieta-Carrasco E, Fernández-Silva I, Méndez-Sánchez N, et al. SFRP5 hepatic expression is associated with non-alcoholic liver disease in morbidly obese women. Ann Hepatol. 2015;14:666–74.
26. Matthews DR, Hosker JP, Rudenski AS, Naylor BA, Treacher DF, Turner RC. Homeostasis model assessment: insulin resistance and beta-cell function from fasting plasma glucose and insulin concentrations in man. Diabetologia. 1985;28:412–9.

27. Weng J, Li Y, Xu W, Shi L, Zhang Q, Zhu D, Hu Y, Zhou Z, Yan X, et al. Effect of intensive insulin therapy on beta-cell function and glycaemic control in patients with newly diagnosed type 2 diabetes: a multicentre randomised parallel-group trial. Lancet. 2008;371:1753–60.

28. Kloting N, Follak N, Kloting I. Diabetes per se and metabolic state influence gene expression in tissue-dependent manner of BB/OK rats. Diabetes Metab Res Rev. 2005;21:281–7.

29. Makishima M, Okamoto AY, Repa JJ, Tu H, Learned RM, Luk A, Hull MV, Lustig KD, Mangelsdorf DJ, et al. Identification of a nuclear receptor for bile acids. Science. 1999;284:1362–5.

8

Self-reported dietary adherence, disease-specific symptoms, and quality of life are associated with healthcare provider follow-up in celiac disease

Jacob J. Hughey[1]*(iD), Bonnie K. Ray[2], Anne R. Lee[3], Kristin N. Voorhees[4], Ciaran P. Kelly[5] and Detlef Schuppan[5,6]

Abstract

Background: The only treatment for celiac disease (CeD) is a lifelong gluten-free diet (GFD). The restrictive nature of the GFD makes adherence a challenge. As an integral part of CeD management, multiple professional organizations recommend regular follow-up with a healthcare provider (HCP). Many CeD patients also participate in patient advocacy groups (PAGs) for education and support. Previous work found that follow-up of CeD patients is highly variable. Here we investigated the self-reported factors associated with HCP follow-up among individuals diagnosed with CeD who participate in a PAG.

Methods: We conducted a survey of members of Beyond Celiac (a PAG), collecting responses from 1832 U.S. adults ages 19–65 who reported having CeD. The survey queried HCP follow-up related to CeD and included validated instruments for dietary adherence (CDAT), disease-specific symptoms (CSI), and quality of life (CD-QOL).

Results: Overall, 27% of respondents diagnosed with CeD at least five years ago reported that they had not visited an HCP about CeD in the last five years. The most frequent reason for not visiting an HCP was "doing fine on my own" (47.6%). Using multiple logistic regression, we identified significant associations between whether a respondent reported visiting an HCP about CeD in the last five years and the scores for all three validated instruments. In particular, as disease-specific symptoms and quality of life worsened, the probability of having visited an HCP increased. Conversely, as dietary adherence worsened, the probability decreased.

Conclusions: Our results suggest that many individuals with CeD manage their disease without ongoing support from an HCP. Our results thus emphasize the need for greater access to high quality CeD care, and highlight an opportunity for PAGs to bring together patients and HCPs to improve management of CeD.

Keywords: Celiac disease, Diagnosis, Disease management, Genetic testing, Gluten-free diet, Healthcare provider, Patient-reported factors, Quality of life, Symptoms, Well-being

Background

Celiac disease (CeD) is a chronic condition with auto-immune features driven by dietary consumption of gluten (a group of proteins present in wheat, barley, and rye) in genetically susceptible individuals [1]. The prevalence of CeD is estimated to be approximately 1% in most Western countries, although many individuals with CeD remain undiagnosed [2, 3]. Currently, the only treatment for CeD is a strict, lifelong gluten-free diet (GFD). Although the prognosis for most CeD patients on the GFD is good, the ubiquity of gluten in the Western diet and the need to avoid even minor contamination of otherwise gluten-free foods make adherence to the GFD a severe challenge [4–6]. Adherence to the GFD is highly variable and many CeD patients report a treatment burden that is comparable to patients with end-stage renal disease on dialysis [7, 8].

* Correspondence: jakejhughey@gmail.com
[1]Department of Biomedical Informatics, Vanderbilt University School of Medicine, Nashville, TN, USA
Full list of author information is available at the end of the article

As an integral part of CeD management, guidelines from the American Gastroenterological Association (AGA) and the American College of Gastroenterology (ACG) and a consensus statement from the U.S. National Institutes of Health recommend regular follow-up with a healthcare provider (HCP) [9–11]. Such follow-up with a doctor and/or dietitian is essential for providing accurate information about the GFD, improving adherence to the GFD, verifying normalization of serology and other abnormalities found during diagnosis, monitoring symptoms, and checking for complications. The NIH consensus statement also recommends participation in a patient advocacy group (PAG) as a means to improve dietary adherence and to obtain emotional and social support. Unfortunately, a previous study found that HCP follow-up for many CeD patients is inadequate by multiple measures [12]. Overall, only 35% of patients followed for more than four years after diagnosis received care consistent with AGA recommendations.

Although improved HCP follow-up could enable improved CeD management, the factors that influence variation in HCP follow-up in CeD remain unknown. Importantly, several improved questionnaires have now been developed and validated to assess various aspects of life with CeD [13–15]. To our knowledge, however, these questionnaires have not yet been applied to understand how HCP follow-up is related to factors such as an individual's CeD-related symptoms and quality of life. The aim of this study was to identify the patient-specific factors associated with HCP follow-up among adults diagnosed with CeD who participate in the online network of a national PAG.

Methods

Survey design and distribution

The survey was designed by a committee of CeD physicians and researchers, as well as patient representatives from Beyond Celiac. The committee identified validated instruments to include and developed new questions to capture information regarding patients' healthcare utilization as well as personal and family medical history. The survey was reviewed by individuals with CeD for readability, clarity, and comprehensiveness before being sent to participants.

The survey was divided into five categories: Demographics, Emotional Well-Being, Celiac Disease-Specific Health, Gluten-Free Diet, Natural Course of Celiac Disease and Celiac Disease Diagnosis and Management. The survey comprised a total of 51 questions, with 15 including multiple sub-questions. The total number of questions a participant was asked to answer was dependent on the participant's age (12 years old and under, 13–18 years old, and 19 years old and above).

The study population consisted of individuals active in the online community of Beyond Celiac, a national PAG in the United States. Beyond Celiac disseminated announcements about the survey to over 49,000 people using email and shared the survey among a network of more than 114,000 Facebook followers from March 19 to March 31, 2015. The announcements included a description of the survey and a link to complete the survey.

For this paper, we analyzed data from respondents who were 19–65 years old, living in the United States, and personally diagnosed with CeD. Analysis of the survey data was approved as non-human subjects research by the Vanderbilt University IRB (#161349).

Validated instruments

The survey included validated instruments for dietary adherence (CDAT), CeD-specific symptoms (CSI), and quality of life (CD-QOL) [13–15]. Higher CDAT and CSI scores correspond to worse dietary adherence and CeD-specific symptoms, respectively, whereas a higher CD-QOL score corresponds to better quality of life. Two questions are common to both the CDAT and CSI ("Have you been bothered by headaches during the past 4 weeks?" and "Have you been bothered by low energy levels during the past 4 weeks?"). These two questions were each asked only once in the survey and unless noted otherwise, were used to calculate the score for both instruments. One question in the CSI ("How much physical pain have you had during the past 4 weeks?") and one element in the CD-QOL ("I have trouble socializing because of my disease.") were inadvertently omitted from the survey.

All elements of the CD-QOL have negative valence, with one exception ("I feel the diet is sufficient treatment for my disease"). For consistency with previous work, we calculated the CD-QOL score as the sum of scores from the individual elements after first reversing the scores of elements with negative valence. For example, since the score for each element could go from 1 to 5, a score of 4 ("quite a bit") for the element "I feel frightened by having this disease" was converted to a 2.

Analysis and visualization

Analysis was performed in R 3.4.0 [16]. Venn diagrams were generated using the VennDiagram package [17]. For multiple logistic regression, we first divided the score of each instrument by the number of elements in the instrument, resulting in a scaled score that could range between 1 and 5. This has no effect on statistical significance and makes the coefficients easier to compare to each other. In addition, age group was converted to an integer value. Coefficients for the multiple logistic regression based on all three instruments (Fig. 1) were

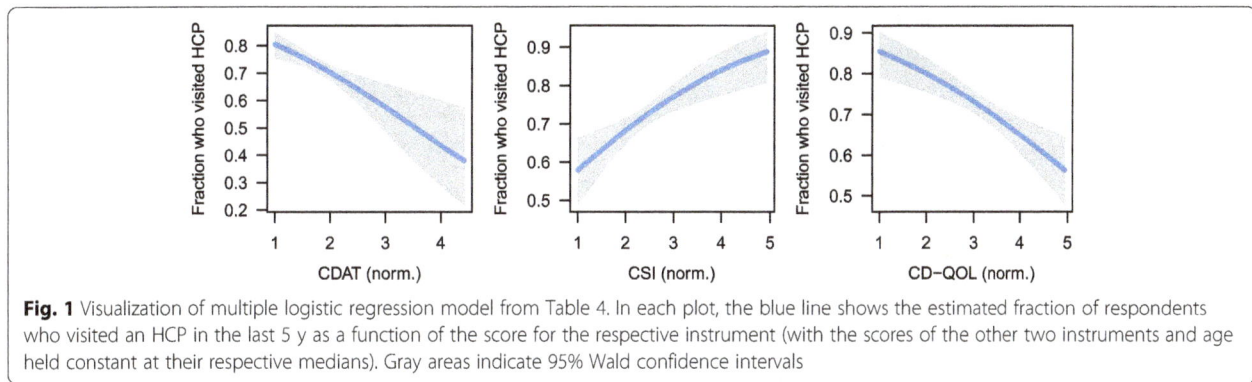

Fig. 1 Visualization of multiple logistic regression model from Table 4. In each plot, the blue line shows the estimated fraction of respondents who visited an HCP in the last 5 y as a function of the score for the respective instrument (with the scores of the other two instruments and age held constant at their respective medians). Gray areas indicate 95% Wald confidence intervals

visualized using the visreg package [18]. For multiple logistic regression based on individual elements in each instrument, *p*-values were converted to *q*-values (controlling the false discovery rate) using the method of Benjamini and Hochberg [19].

Results

The survey was made available to members of Beyond Celiac and responses were collected from 1832 U.S. adults ages 19–65 who reported having CeD. The survey was designed to query multiple aspects of life with CeD. We first examined the respondents' demographics (Table 1). Overall, 89% of respondents were female, which is somewhat higher than previous studies [12–15].

The vast majority of respondents (95%) reported their race as "White or Caucasian," which is similar to a previous study based on individuals from an academic medical center and celiac support groups [15] and which could be a result of the higher frequency of CeD in non-Hispanic whites than in Hispanics or non-Hispanic blacks [20]. Respondents came from every age group and region of the U.S.

We next examined how and by whom the respondents reported being diagnosed with CeD (Table 2). Overall, 83% of respondents were diagnosed by a pediatrician, primary care provider, or gastroenterologist (80% of respondents also considered one of these their main provider for CeD; Additional file 1: Figure S1). In addition, similar to previous work [15], 95% were diagnosed based on a blood test (83%), small intestinal biopsy (79%), or both (67%; Additional file 1: Figure S2). Although these distributions were similar in each age group, we did observe higher frequencies of blood test and gluten challenge in younger age groups and a lower frequency of small intestinal biopsy in the youngest age group (19–25 y.o.; Additional file 1: Figure S3). Respondents reported an

Table 1 Demographics of survey respondents (*n* = 1832)

Gender	
Female	89.0%
Male	11.0%
Age (y)	
19–25	7.9%
26–35	18.8%
36–45	23.7%
46–55	26.0%
56–65	23.6%
Race/ethnicity	
White or Caucasian	95.2%
Hispanic or Latino	2.2%
Black or African American	0.7%
Asian or Pacific Islander	0.2%
Other[a]	1.6%
Region of the U.S.	
Midwest	23.6%
Northeast	30.0%
South	28.9%
West	17.6%

[a]Includes Native American or American Indian, Indian, and prefer not to say

Table 2 Self-reported information on how and by whom respondents were diagnosed with CeD

Person who made diagnosis	
Gastroenterologist	57.0%
Primary care provider	24.1%
Pediatrician	2.0%
Dietitian or nutritionist	0.8%
Self-diagnosed	2.1%
Other	13.9%
Methods of diagnosis[a]	
Blood test	83.0%
Small intestinal biopsy	78.8%
Gluten challenge	14.8%
Genetic test (e.g., HLA)	14.1%
Not sure	1.9%

[a]Not mutually exclusive

array of other autoimmune or CeD-related conditions (Additional file 1: Figure S4), although the prevalence of type 1 diabetes was less than expected [21]. Taken together, these results suggest that the respondents are reasonably representative of U.S. adults diagnosed with CeD.

We then analyzed the respondents' reported HCP follow-up. Of 1493 respondents diagnosed at least five years ago, 27% reported that they had not visited an HCP about CeD in the last five years (Table 3). Although we do not have additional data (e.g., medical records) to evaluate the follow-up care received by those individuals who did report visiting an HCP, these results suggest that many U.S. adults diagnosed with CeD are managing their disease without ongoing support from an HCP. We next quantified the reasons that respondents gave for not visiting an HCP. The most frequent reason was "doing fine on my own" (47.6%), followed by "haven't needed to," "provider was not knowledgeable," and "previous visits were not helpful" (Table 3, Additional file 1: Figure S5). Financial reasons ("co-pay is too high" and "uninsured") and general distrust of HCPs were less common.

To better understand the factors related to HCP follow-up, we used the survey responses from the validated instruments for dietary adherence (CDAT), disease-specific symptoms (CSI), and quality of life (CD-QOL) (Additional file 1: Figure S6) [13–15]. Scores from all three instruments were significantly better in respondents diagnosed at least five years ago than in respondents diagnosed more recently (Additional file 1: Figure S7). For those respondents diagnosed at least five years ago, we then used their age group and CDAT, CSI, and CD-QOL scores in multiple logistic regression to predict whether an individual reported visiting an HCP about CeD in the last five years (Table 4). Scores from all three

Table 3 Self-reported information on HCP follow-up among respondents diagnosed at least 5 y ago

Visited HCP in last 5 y	n = 1493
Yes	65.6%
No	27.1%
Not sure	7.4%
Reasons for not visiting HCP[a]	n = 479
Doing fine on my own	47.6%
Haven't needed to	28.0%
Provider not knowledgeable	27.6%
Previous visits not helpful	23.6%
Co-pay is too high	7.9%
Don't trust healthcare providers	5.0%
Uninsured	3.5%

[a]Not mutually exclusive

Table 4 Multiple logistic regression to predict whether respondent has visited an HCP about CeD in last 5 years (assuming he or she was diagnosed at least 5 years ago)

	Coefficient	Std. error	P-value
Age group	0.081	0.049	0.098
CDAT score	−0.56	0.16	$3.6*10^{-4}$
CSI score	0.45	0.13	$4.2*10^{-4}$
CD-QOL score	−0.38	0.096	$5.8*10^{-5}$

Positive coefficient means that as age or score increases, probability of visiting an HCP increases. Coefficients and standard errors for CDAT, CSI, and CD-QOL are normalized by the number of questions in the instrument. A higher CD-QOL corresponds to better quality of life, whereas higher CDAT and CSI scores correspond to worse dietary adherence and disease-specific symptoms, respectively

instruments, but not age group, were significantly associated with having visited an HCP. In particular, as celiac-specific symptoms and quality of life worsened (indicated by higher CSI and lower CD-QOL scores, respectively), the probability of having visited an HCP increased (Fig. 1). Conversely, as dietary adherence worsened (indicated by a higher CDAT score), the probability decreased. These results suggest that although scores from the three instruments are moderately correlated with each other (Additional file 1: Table S1), each instrument captures a unique aspect of life with CeD.

Finally, we determined which individual questions or statements in each instrument were the most strongly associated with having visited an HCP. For each instrument, we performed multiple logistic regression using age group, scores from the other two instruments, and the response to one question of the selected instrument (Fig. 2). The three instruments varied in the fraction of questions or statements that were significantly associated with visiting an HCP. In each instrument, we observed the strongest associations with questions or statements that referred to more general aspects of life with CeD. In the CDAT, the strongest association was with the statement "Before I do something I carefully consider the consequences" (stronger agreement indicated higher probability of having visited an HCP). In the CSI, the strongest association was with the question "Related to celiac disease, how is your health?" (worse health indicated higher probability of having visited an HCP). In the CD-QOL, the strongest association was with the statement "I feel frightened by having this disease" (stronger agreement indicated higher probability of having visited an HCP).

Discussion

Celiac disease is a complex condition with autoimmune characteristics for which the only current treatment is a strict, lifelong, gluten-free diet. Although recommendations for managing CeD include regular follow-up with an HCP, follow-up is often inadequate [12]. Here we studied the factors associated with patient-reported

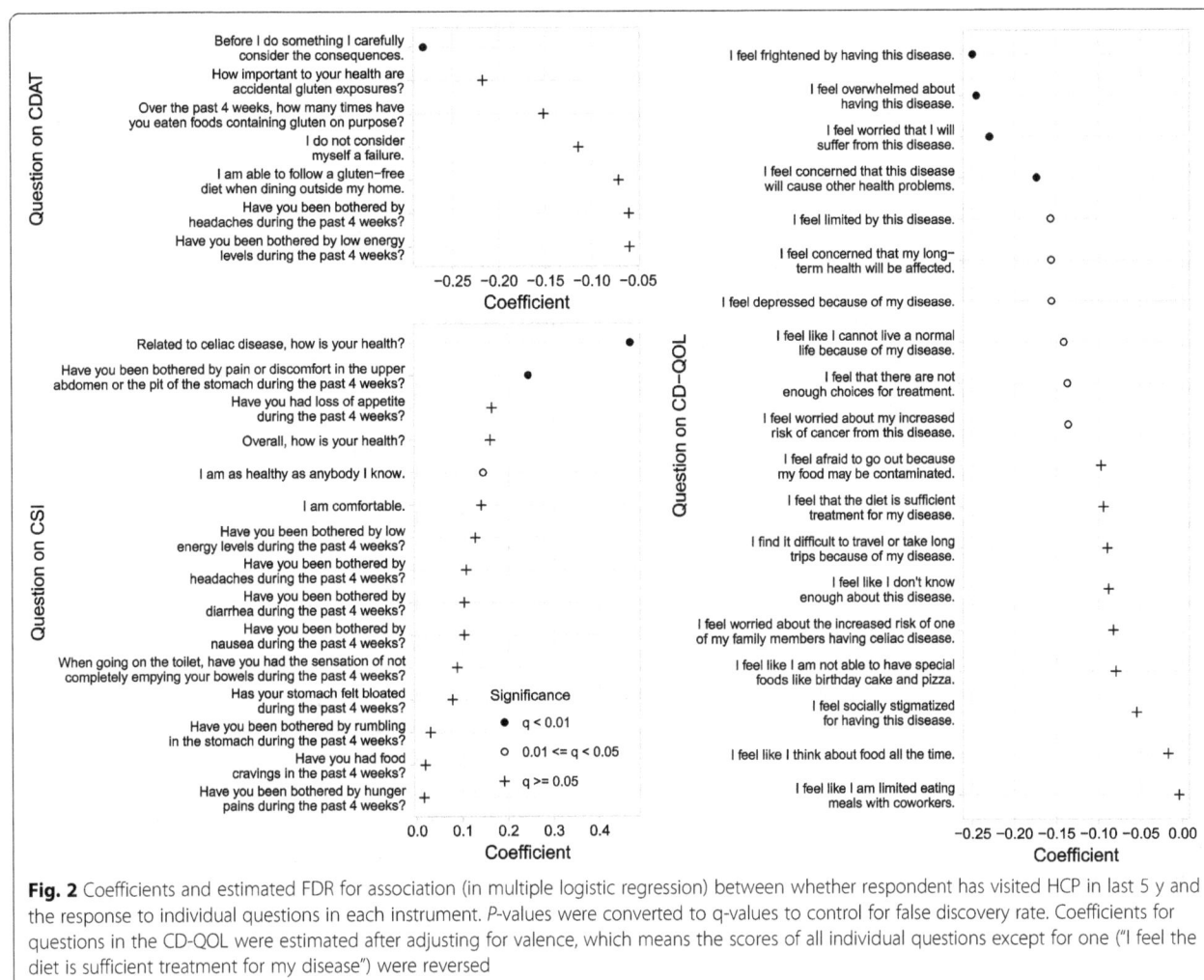

Fig. 2 Coefficients and estimated FDR for association (in multiple logistic regression) between whether respondent has visited HCP in last 5 y and the response to individual questions in each instrument. P-values were converted to q-values to control for false discovery rate. Coefficients for questions in the CD-QOL were estimated after adjusting for valence, which means the scores of all individual questions except for one ("I feel the diet is sufficient treatment for my disease") were reversed

follow-up related to CeD in a large group of U.S. adults. Over a quarter of our survey respondents who were diagnosed at least five years ago reported not having visited an HCP about CeD in the last 5 years. In addition, individuals who have visited an HCP about CeD generally have better dietary adherence, worse symptoms, and worse quality of life than those who have not.

The survey question about HCP follow-up was designed to be broad and straightforward to answer. The limitation is that our metric for HCP follow-up is necessarily coarse and does not account for all the variation in the quantity, and more importantly the quality, of care. Thus, even for the 66% of respondents who reported having visited in HCP about CeD in the last five years, it is likely that the level of follow-up often does not meet AGA recommendations [12].

Individuals with CeD face high rates of underdiagnosis and misdiagnosis and often endure 5–10 years of symptoms before being correctly diagnosed [22–24]. Such a long and frustrating "diagnostic odyssey" could negatively influence patients' opinions of the healthcare system and reduce the likelihood that they continue to interact with it after diagnosis. Notably, 37.8% of respondents to our survey reported not visiting an HCP in the last five years because their provider was not knowledgeable and/or previous visits were not helpful. If this is the case, then increasing the speed of an accurate diagnosis could contribute to improved CeD management after diagnosis.

To our knowledge, this is the first study to collect responses from the same individuals for three validated, CeD-related, instruments. Although the inadvertent omission of one element each from two of the instruments prevents strict comparison with previous studies, we reproduced the correlation between dietary adherence and symptoms [14] and between dietary adherence and quality of life [25]. Furthermore, our analysis allowed us to disentangle the effects of the three instruments on CeD-related follow-up. For example, even though better dietary adherence is positively correlated with better symptoms, a higher probability of visiting an HCP is associated with better adherence and worse symptoms. In addition, by analyzing the responses to individual elements of each instrument, we discovered that the correlates of having visited an HCP follow a hierarchy, at the top of which are more general concerns related to CeD, such as one's overall perception of health related to CeD and feeling frightened by CeD.

We observed multiple trends in the frequency of diagnosis methods between age groups. Individuals aged 19–25 reported the lowest frequency of small intestinal biopsy, which may reflect the growing willingness of HCPs to diagnose CeD without a biopsy [26, 27]. For example, the most recent European Society for Pediatric Gastroenterology, Hepatology, and Nutrition (ESPGHAN) guidelines omit the need for a small intestinal biopsy, as long as IgA anti-transglutaminase (TG2) antibody titers are >10× the upper limit of normal and other clinical criteria are met [28]. We also found that younger age groups reported higher frequencies of gluten challenge. For example, 25% of respondents aged 19–25 reported that a gluten challenge was part of their diagnostic workup. Although our survey was not designed to address this issue, we speculate that this result may be related to the increasing prevalence of the GFD among people not diagnosed with CeD, especially among younger people [29]. Because the blood tests and small intestinal biopsy currently used for diagnosis are markers of active disease, a person who has been following a GFD will typically have to resume gluten consumption for 2–6 weeks (the gluten challenge) in order to be definitively diagnosed [11]. The gluten challenge is often accompanied by the return of symptoms, making this method of diagnosis burdensome and making patients reluctant to obtain a definitive diagnosis [30]. Notably, the need for a gluten challenge is obviated by a negative genetic test for HLA-DQ2 or -DQ8 [11], which excludes CeD, and we speculate that for most survey participants who underwent both genetic testing and a gluten challenge, the former was used to rule in (but not necessarily confirm) CeD. Our findings thus highlight the need for diagnostic tools that do not depend on ongoing gluten consumption.

Our study has several limitations. First, although our sample size is large, it is non-random and could suffer from self-selection bias based on who received notification of the survey (those who had previously interacted with the online community of Beyond Celiac) and who chose to respond. For example, involvement in support groups has been associated with less severe CeD-related symptoms [14] and involvement in face-to-face social support networks has been associated with higher CeD-related quality of life [31]. However, we observed considerable variation in the

scores for all three instruments, which indicates that our respondents cover a wide range of lifestyles with respect to managing CeD. Second, our study is based only on self-reported data, and we do not have the respondents' medical records to confirm their diagnosis or their follow-up with an HCP. However, the frequency of various diagnostic methods in our data is consistent with previous studies, which suggests that the self-reported data from our respondents is accurate. Moreover, the high level of self-management required of CeD patients (often before and after diagnosis) means that they are typically well informed about their disease and diagnostic workup.

A third limitation is that our study is cross-sectional and observational, so it is not possible to determine causality in the associations we observe. That said, we find it unlikely that visiting an HCP about CeD causes worse symptoms and quality of life. We believe the more likely scenario is that symptoms and quality of life influence how a person manages CeD, in particular, whether a person seeks support from an HCP. Individuals who are satisfied with or who can tolerate their symptoms and quality of life may be less likely to visit an HCP, possibly because they feel that the lack of non-dietary treatment options means that HCPs have little to offer. The association between dietary adherence and having visited an HCP also has multiple interpretations. One is that visiting an HCP causes improved adherence, perhaps because HCPs provide patients with a better understanding of how to implement the diet or a better appreciation of the diet's importance. Another interpretation is that both dietary adherence and visits to an HCP are indirect measures for how conscientiously a patient manages his or her disease. These interpretations are not mutually exclusive, and it is likely that both are valid to varying extents among CeD patients.

Conclusions

Our results suggest that many adults with CeD manage their disease without ongoing follow-up care from an HCP. This study also demonstrates the ability of PAGs to rapidly engage CeD patients for research, which is encouraging for future efforts using patient input to drive clinical research directed at a better understanding of cofactors that trigger CeD, improved disease management, and non-dietary therapies [32]. Finally, our results emphasize the need for greater access to high quality CeD care, and highlight an opportunity for HCPs and PAGs to work collaboratively to achieve improved disease management by raising levels of awareness and education.

Abbreviations
ACG: American College of Gastroenterology; AGA: American Gastroenterological Association; CDAT: celiac dietary adherence test; CD-QOL: celiac disease-related quality of life; CeD: celiac disease; CSI: celiac symptom index; FDR: false discovery rate; GFD: gluten-free diet; HCP: healthcare provider; PAG: patient advocacy group

Acknowledgments
The authors thank the celiac disease patient community for sharing their experiences in pursuit of advancing research.

Funding
The study was funded by Beyond Celiac.

Authors' contributions
Conceived and designed the study: JJH, BKR, KNV, DS. Performed analysis: JJH. Interpreted results: JJH, BKR, ARL, KNV, CPK, DS. Wrote the paper: JJH. Reviewed drafts of the paper: JJH, BKR, ARL, KNV, CPK, DS. All authors read and approved the final manuscript.

Competing interests
At the time of the study, KNV was an employee of Beyond Celiac and contributed to the study as described in the Authors' Contributions section. All the other authors declare that they have no competing interests.

Author details
[1]Department of Biomedical Informatics, Vanderbilt University School of Medicine, Nashville, TN, USA. [2]Talkspace, New York, NY, USA. [3]Celiac Disease Center, Columbia University Medical Center, New York, NY, USA. [4]Beyond Celiac, Ambler, PA, USA. [5]Division of Gastroenterology, Beth Israel Deaconess Medical Center, Boston, MA, USA. [6]Institute of Translational Immunology, University Medical Center, Mainz, Germany.

References
1. Di Sabatino A, Corazza GR. Coeliac disease. Lancet. 2009;373:1480–93.
2. Choung RS, Larson SA, Khaleghi S, Rubio-Tapia A, Ovsyannikova IG, King KS, et al. Prevalence and Morbidity of Undiagnosed Celiac Disease From a Community-Based Study. Gastroenterology. 2017;152:830–9.e5.
3. Choung RS, Unalp-Arida A, Ruhl CE, Brantner TL, Everhart JE, Murray JA. Less Hidden Celiac Disease But Increased Gluten Avoidance Without a Diagnosis in the United States. Mayo Clin. Proc. Elsevier. 2017;92:30–8.
4. Ciacci C, Cirillo M, Cavallaro R, Mazzacca G. Long-term follow-up of celiac adults on gluten-free diet: prevalence and correlates of intestinal damage. Digestion. 2002;66:178–85.
5. Pietzak MM. Follow-up of patients with celiac disease: achieving compliance with treatment. Gastroenterology. 2005;128:S135–41.
6. Hollon JR, Cureton PA, Martin ML, Puppa ELL, Fasano A. Trace gluten contamination may play a role in mucosal and clinical recovery in a subgroup of diet-adherent non-responsive celiac disease patients. BMC Gastroenterol. 2013;13:40.
7. Hall NJ, Rubin G, Charnock A. Systematic review: adherence to a gluten-free diet in adult patients with coeliac disease. Aliment. Pharmacol. Ther. 2009;30:315 30.
8. Shah S, Akbari M, Vanga R, Kelly CP, Hansen J, Theethira T, et al. Patient perception of treatment burden is high in celiac disease compared with other common conditions. Am. J. Gastroenterol. 2014;109:1304–11.
9. National Institutes of Health Consensus Development Conference Statement on Celiac Disease. June 28-30, 2004. Gastroenterology. 2005;128:S1–9.
10. Rostom A, Murray JA, Kagnoff MF. American Gastroenterological Association (AGA) Institute technical review on the diagnosis and management of celiac disease. Gastroenterology. 2006;131:1981–2002.
11. Rubio-Tapia A, Hill ID, Kelly CP, Calderwood AH, Murray JA. American College of Gastroenterology. ACG clinical guidelines: diagnosis and management of celiac disease. Am. J. Gastroenterol. 2013;108:656–76. quiz 677
12. Herman ML, Rubio-Tapia A, Lahr BD, Larson JJ, Van Dyke CT, Murray JA. Patients with celiac disease are not followed up adequately. Clin. Gastroenterol. Hepatol. 2012;10:893–9.e1.
13. Leffler DA, Dennis M, Edwards George JB, Jamma S, Magge S, Cook EF, et al. A simple validated gluten-free diet adherence survey for adults with celiac disease. Clin. Gastroenterol. Hepatol. 2009;7:530–6–536.e1–2.
14. Leffler DA, Dennis M, Edwards George J, Jamma S, Cook EF, Schuppan D, et al. A validated disease-specific symptom index for adults with celiac disease. Clin. Gastroenterol. Hepatol. 2009;7:1328–34–1334.e1–3.
15. Dorn SD, Hernandez L, Minaya MT, Morris CB, Hu Y, Leserman J, et al. The development and validation of a new coeliac disease quality of life survey (CD-QOL). Aliment. Pharmacol. Ther. 2010;31:666–75.
16. R Core Team. R: A Language and Environment for Statistical Computing [Internet]. Vienna, Austria: R Foundation for Statistical Computing; 2017. Available from: https://www.R-project.org
17. Chen H, Boutros PC. VennDiagram: a package for the generation of highly-customizable Venn and Euler diagrams in R. BMC Bioinformatics. 2011;12:35.
18. Breheny P, Burchett W. Visualization of Regression Models Using visreg [Internet]. 2016 [cited 2017 Apr 17]. Available from: http://myweb.uiowa.edu/pbreheny/publications/visreg.pdf
19. Benjamini Y, Hochberg Y. Controlling the False Discovery Rate: A Practical and Powerful Approach to Multiple Testing. J. R. Stat. Soc. Series B Stat. Methodol. [Royal Statistical Society, Wiley]; 1995;57:289–300.
20. Mardini HE, Westgate P, Grigorian AY. Racial Differences in the Prevalence of Celiac Disease in the US Population: National Health and Nutrition Examination Survey (NHANES) 2009-2012. Dig. Dis. Sci. 2015;60:1738–42.
21. Holmes GKT. Screening for coeliac disease in type 1 diabetes. Arch. Dis. Child. 2002;87:495–8.
22. Green PHR, Stavropoulos SN, Panagi SG, Goldstein SL, Mcmahon DJ, Absan H, et al. Characteristics of adult celiac disease in the USA: results of a national survey. Am. J. Gastroenterol. 2001;96:126–31.
23. Cranney A, Zarkadas M, Graham ID, Butzner JD, Rashid M, Warren R, et al. The Canadian Celiac Health Survey. Dig. Dis. Sci. 2007;52:1087–95.
24. Gray AM, Papanicolas IN. Impact of symptoms on quality of life before and after diagnosis of coeliac disease: results from a UK population survey. BMC Health Serv. Res. 2010;10:105.
25. Nachman F, del Campo MP, González A, Corzo L, Vázquez H, Sfoggia C, et al. Long-term deterioration of quality of life in adult patients with celiac disease is associated with treatment noncompliance. Dig. Liver Dis. 2010;42:685–91.
26. Barker CC, Mitton C, Jevon G, Mock T. Can tissue transglutaminase antibody titers replace small-bowel biopsy to diagnose celiac disease in select pediatric populations? Pediatrics. 2005;115:1341–6.
27. Hill PG, Holmes GKT. Coeliac disease: a biopsy is not always necessary for diagnosis. Aliment. Pharmacol. Ther. 2008;27:572–7.
28. Husby S, Koletzko S, Korponay-Szabó IR, Mearin ML, Phillips A, Shamir R, et al. European Society for Pediatric Gastroenterology, Hepatology, and Nutrition guidelines for the diagnosis of coeliac disease. J. Pediatr. Gastroenterol. Nutr. 2012;54:136 60.
29. Kim H-S, Patel KG, Orosz E, Kothari N, Demyen MF, Pyrsopoulos N, et al. Time Trends in the Prevalence of Celiac Disease and Gluten-Free Diet in the US Population: Results From the National Health and Nutrition Examination Surveys 2009-2014. JAMA Intern. Med. 2016;176:1716–7.
30. Leffler D, Schuppan D, Pallav K, Najarian R, Goldsmith JD, Hansen J, et al. Kinetics of the histological, serological and symptomatic responses to gluten challenge in adults with coeliac disease. Gut. 2013;62:996–1004.

9

Quantifying the effects of aging and urbanization on major gastrointestinal diseases to guide preventative strategies

Liu Hui

Abstract

Background: This study aimed to quantify the effects of aging and urbanization on major gastrointestinal disease (liver cirrhosis, hepatitis B, diarrhea, liver cancer, stomach cancer, pancreas cancer, hepatitis C, esophagus cancer, colon/rectum cancer, gastrointestinal ulcers, diabetes, and appendicitis).

Methods: We accessed 2004 and 2011 mortality statistics from the most developed cities and least developed rural areas in China using a retrospective design. The relative risk of death associated with urbanization and age was quantified using Generalized linear model (the exp.(B) from model is interpreted as the risk ratio; the greater the B, the greater the impact of urbanized factors or aging factor or effect of aging factor with urbanization). The interaction between region (cities and rural areas) and age was considered as indicator to assess role of age in mortality with urbanization.

Results: Greater risk of disease with urbanization were, in ascending order, for diabetes, colon/rectum cancer, hepatitis C and pancreas cancer. Stronger the effect of aging with urbanization were, in ascending order, for stomach cancer, ulcer, liver cancer, colon/rectum cancer, pancreas cancer, diabetes, hepatitis C, appendicitis and diarrhea. When the effects of aging and urbanization on diseases were taken together as the dividing value, we were able to further divide the 12 gastrointestinal diseases into three groups to guide the development of medical strategies.

Conclusions: It was suggested that mortality rate for most gastrointestinal diseases was sensitive to urbanization and control of external risk factors could lead to the conversion of most gastrointestinal disease.

Keywords: Gastrointestinal disease, Cancer, Aging, Urbanization, Categorization, Epidemiology

Background

Gastrointestinal disease refers to disease involving the gastrointestinal tract, including disease of the esophagus, stomach, small intestine, large intestine and rectum, and the accessory organs of digestion, liver, gallbladder and pancreas. Gastrointestinal disease may have many pathomechanisms can be infectious or chronic, and involve acute or chronic inflammation, or cancer.

Global urbanization, which has continued to increase since the arrival of the industrial revolution, results in alteration to and loss of natural habitats. A sedentary lifestyle, higher-kilojoule food intake, a decrease in exposure

to sunlight, and increasingly stressful conditions have all been associated with increasing urbanization, which, in turn, may be impacting on prevalence of gastrointestinal disease. Urbanization leads to many challenges, not only for global health, but also specifically to the field of gastrointestinal disease [1–3]. To identify and implement medical strategies, it is necessary to explore how rapid urbanization may be affecting the burden of gastrointestinal disease in growing economies. To date, there have been no comprehensive studies into the quantitative effects of urbanization on gastrointestinal disease.

China has a relatively simple ethnic composition and a large land area, and is presently undergoing rapid urbanization [4–6]. Economic growth has had a profound impact on the health of its citizens and levels of

Correspondence: liuhui60@sina.com; liuhui60@dmu.edu.cn
Department of Clinical Immunology, Dalian Medical University, Dalian
116044, People's Republic of China

medical care; however, because of an unbalanced economy, there is considerable disparity between regions. China, therefore, is an ideal model for assessing patterns of disease occurrence, development and changes with this modernization process [7–9].

Life expectancy will increase with urbanization [10–12]. Greater human longevity and an increasingly elderly population might also be important reasons for changes in the spectrum of gastrointestinal disease. Therefore, this study focused on the impact of urbanization and the aging process on gastrointestinal disease. We found that these two properties varied significantly in different gastrointestinal diseases (diarrhea, viral hepatitis B, viral hepatitis C, esophagus cancer, stomach cancer, colon/rectum cancer, liver cancer, pancreas cancer, diabetes, gastrointestinal ulcers, liver cirrhosis and appendicitis). To inform medical strategies, we also categorized the 12 major gastrointestinal diseases listed above, based on the quantitative effects of age and urbanization.

Methods

Original data

We obtained raw data from the 2004 and 2011 data sets of the National Disease Mortality Surveillance System [13, 14]. These data were obtained from people living in the most undeveloped rural areas (rural) in 2004 and the most developed cities (urban) in 2011 for keeping considerable disparity between regions. The definition of urbanization and rural areas was according to administrative regions of China; name with city or district in city (a large majority of the population is not engaged in agriculture and/or fishing) was defined as urban and others were rural areas (Table 1) [13, 14]. The causes of death must be recorded in patient's place of household registration. The mortality due to nutritional deficiencies was 1.32/0.1 million individuals (standard rate) in the rural population and 0.80/0.1 million individuals (standard rate) in the urban population and; the life expectancy at birth was 73.90 years in the rural areas and 79.53 years in the urban areas, respectively [13, 14]. The underlying causes of death (the disease which initiated the train of morbid events leading directly to death) were classified according to International Classification of Diseases (ICD)-10 codes [15] to determine the mortality statistics. Rate of objective diagnosis (as evidenced by laboratory, pathologic, imaging and/or surgical intervention findings) was 90.76% in rural areas and that was 92.00% in urban areas [13, 14]. The raw data are presented in Table 2 and Table 3.

Assessment of the role of urbanization and age in death caused by gastrointestinal disease

From the 2004 and 2011 data, we collected the age-stratified number of deaths from different gastrointestinal diseases (death group) and the age-stratified number of survivors (survival group) in the monitored urban and rural populations (Table 2 & Table 3). A generalized linear model (Poisson loglinear method) was used to assess the mortality risk from aging and urbanization with covariates of categorical age (age < 60 and age ≥ 60 for death group and survival group) and region (urban and rural); the cut-off of age was 65 years for appendicitis, because of the zeros for people aged under 60 in urbanised areas. The B coefficients for both age and region and interaction between region and age were obtained from the model: here the exp.(B) is interpreted as the risk ratio (RR). B = 0 indicated that given cause had no effect on the death; the greater (positive) the B, the greater the impact of urbanized factors or aging factor or effect of aging factor with urbanization on the gastrointestinal diseases.

Data were considered statistically significant when the probability of a type I error was 0.05 or less. Calculations were performed using the Windows version of SPSS 17.0 (SPSS Inc., Chicago, IL, US).

Characteristics of the effects of aging and urbanized factors on gastrointestinal disease

The B value of interaction between region (cities and rural areas) and age was considered as indicator to assess role of age in mortality from gastrointestinal disease with urbanization, where a larger B value of interaction between region and age indicated a stronger effect of aging or a weaker effect of other risk factors in death with urbanization.

The quantitative values (B) of the impact of age on disease with urbanization were plotted against those for urbanized factors to form a scatter diagram. We used the locations of the various gastrointestinal diseases in this coordinate system to sort them according to the effects of aging and urbanization.

The group in the upper right quadrant represents old disease associated with the old population and developed urbanized disease; the group in the upper left quadrant shows disease associated with the other factor and developed urbanized disease; the group in the lower left quadrant, was termed other factor and undeveloped rural disease; the group in the lower right quadrant represents disease associated with the old population and undeveloped rural disease.

Results

Generalized linear model was used to assess mortality risk from major gastrointestinal diseases with urbanization and aging as shown in Table 4. The contribution of urbanization to different gastrointestinal diseases varied; the B for the 12 gastrointestinal diseases ranged from – 5.760 to 1.216. A higher B indicated greater risk of disease with urbanization (negative value implied a protective

Table 1 The name of urban and rural area/regions where data collected in China

Cities	Cities	Rural areas	Rural areas
Dongcheng in Beijing	Tongxiang	Balimyouqi	Xiangyunxian
Tongzou in Beijing	Wucheng Jinhua	Kailuxian	Lanpingxian
Hongqiao in Tianjin	Meijie in Sanming	Suniteyouqi	Milinxian
Kaiping in Tangshan	Jianou	Binyangxiang	Naidongxian
Haigang in Qinhuangdao	Jiaocheng in Ningde	Hepuxian	Jiangzixian
Wuan	Shibei in Qingdao	Lingyunxian	Meixian
Qiaodong in Zhangjiakou	Xuecheng in Zaozhang	Luochengxian	Luochuanxia
Xinceng in Shenyang	Zifu in Yantai	Dazuxian	Hanyinxiangn
Shahekou in Dalian	Penglai	Zizhongxian	Jingtaixian
Qianshan in Anshan	Gaomi	Xichongxian	Lintanxian
Fengcheng	Laicheng in Laiwu	Shuangyuanxian	Pinganxian
Luwan in Shanghai	Lichang inQingdao	Kangdingxian	Menyuanxian
Songjiang in Shanghai	Xiuyue in Guangzhou	Yuexixian	Xinhexian
Pukou in Nanjing	Nanxiong	Meitanxian	Shachexian
Yunlong in Xuzou	Sihui	Yupingxian	Hetianxian
Wuzhong in Suzhou	Shanwei	Dushanxian	Xinyuanxian
Zhangjiagang	Yunfu	Tonghaixian	–
Xiacheng in Hangzou	Meilian in haikou	Guangnanxian	–
Fenghua	–	Menglaxian	–

Table 2 Age-stratified number of deaths from major gastrointestinal diseases in 2004 in underdeveloped rural areas of China [13]

Age	Gastrointestinal diseases												All cause	Survival
	A	B	C	D	E	F	G	H	I	J	K	L		
0-	180	0	0	0	0	0	1	0	0	0	2	0	3038	173,744
1-	88	6	0	0	0	0	2	0	2	0	1	1	1186	792,643
5-	11	4	0	0	0	1	3	0	2	0	3	1	597	1,145,068
10-	3	5	0	0	0	1	6	0	2	1	2	0	557	1,437,804
15-	6	2	0	0	1	4	8	1	1	1	3	2	948	1,247,497
20-	3	5	0	4	5	8	15	0	1	5	8	3	1213	1,161,369
25-	2	13	0	2	17	17	46	2	8	15	19	3	1438	1,355,108
30-	10	35	1	8	34	18	111	3	14	15	38	4	2038	1,339,658
35-	6	39	0	19	66	22	180	9	26	20	81	5	2590	1,153,155
40-	3	51	0	41	94	19	239	4	15	28	84	3	2580	846,773
45-	4	75	0	78	170	49	314	11	39	35	98	2	3352	855,146
50-	3	85	0	147	265	65	383	17	66	45	136	1	4671	688,043
55-	7	73	1	199	394	75	399	17	65	55	154	1	5681	563,297
60-	16	91	0	285	459	102	411	16	116	88	175	7	7464	484,754
65-	21	95	2	259	470	100	410	23	111	119	156	7	9432	382,483
70-	32	79	0	280	512	92	338	17	121	141	144	15	11,439	281,429
75-	39	39	0	180	352	82	213	17	110	128	101	6	10,555	179,351
80-	39	29	0	109	222	57	137	5	79	103	63	4	8864	109,024
>85	33	15	0	65	127	54	70	0	62	57	33	7	7700	66,137

Diseases classified by ICD-10 code: A: diarrhea (A00, A01, A03, A04, A06-A09); B: viral hepatitis B (B16–B19 excluding B17.1, B18.2); C: viral hepatitis C (B17.1, B18.2); D: esophageal cancer (C15); E: stomach cancer (C16); F: colon/rectum cancer (C18–C21); G: liver cancer (C22); H: pancreatic cancer (C25); I: diabetes (E10–E14); J: ulcer (K25–K27); K: liver cirrhosis (K70, K74); L: appendicitis (K35–K37)

Table 3 Age-stratified number of deaths from major gastrointestinal diseases in 2011 in developed cities in China [14]

Age	Gastrointestinal diseases												All cause	Survival
	A	B	C	D	E	F	G	H	I	J	K	L		
0-	0	0	0	0	0	0	1	0	0	1	0	0	453	104,883
1-	1	0	0	0	0	0	0	0	0	0	0	0	123	404,828
5-	0	0	0	0	0	0	0	0	0	0	0	0	88	493,202
10-	0	0	0	0	0	0	0	0	1	0	0	0	85	516,918
15-	0	0	0	0	0	1	0	0	0	0	1	0	184	925,854
20-	0	0	0	0	4	0	2	1	2	1	1	0	363	1,024,382
25-	0	2	0	0	4	4	7	1	3	0	2	0	358	1,245,437
30-	0	3	0	0	12	9	26	3	13	0	5	0	463	1,049,958
35-	0	5	0	2	15	8	58	7	15	2	15	0	793	1,298,489
40-	0	14	0	10	44	31	119	12	15	3	35	0	1374	1,350,515
45-	0	20	1	46	107	63	212	35	43	5	72	0	2500	1,357,587
50-	0	31	1	67	154	92	288	54	65	7	81	0	3251	1,422,892
55-	0	32	2	125	242	157	359	97	101	14	82	0	4656	1,235,044
60-	1	27	2	114	252	170	353	92	147	12	64	1	4811	747,831
65-	0	12	2	138	270	145	270	107	167	11	57	0	5309	424,295
70-	1	21	5	137	339	239	285	133	284	25	50	1	8120	378,526
75-	1	31	3	162	469	335	354	151	433	24	63	2	11,978	279,355
80-	0	11	1	115	314	263	273	102	353	40	50	3	12,527	151,104
>85	3	13	0	91	198	191	167	76	283	43	32	2	14,624	50,773

Diseases classified by ICD-10 code: A: diarrhea (A00, A01, A03, A04, A06-A09); B: viral hepatitis B (B16-B19 excluding B17.1, B18.2); C: viral hepatitis C (B17.1, B18.2); D: esophageal cancer (C15); E: stomach cancer (C16); F: colon/rectum cancer (C18–C21); G: liver cancer (C22); H: pancreatic cancer (C25); I: diabetes (E10-E14); J: ulcer (K25–K27); K: liver cirrhosis (K70, K74); L: appendicitis (K35–K37)

effect). The Bs were, in ascending order, for gastrointestinal diseases of the diarrhea, appendicitis, ulcer, hepatitis B, liver cirrhosis, esophagus cancer, stomach cancer, liver cancer, diabetes, colon/rectum cancer, hepatitis C and pancreas cancer.

The quantitative values of the impact of age with urbanization on diseases also varied. The value of B (interaction between region and age) for the 12 gastrointestinal diseases ranged from −0.314 to 2.065 as shown in Table 4. The larger the B value, the stronger

Table 4 Mortality risk from major gastrointestinal diseases with urbanization and aging

Diseases	Effect of region			Effect of age			Age*Region		
	B	Confidence interval(95%)	p	B	Confidence interval(95%)	p	B	Confidence interval(95%)	p
Diarrhea	−5.760	−7.723~ − 3.797	< 0.001	1.511	1.329~ 1.693	< 0.001	2.065	− 0.059~ 4.190	0.057
Hepatitis B	−1.274	−1.487~ − 1.060	< 0.001	1.983	1.839~ 2.129	< 0.001	− 0.127	− 0.427~ 0.174	0.409
Hepatitis C	0.720	−0.977~ 2.418	0.405	2.105	0.145~ 4.065	0.035	0.858	−1.399~ 3.116	0.456
Esophagus Ca.	−0.662	− 0.841~ − 0.510	< 0.001	2.966	2.861~ 3.071	< 0.001	− 0.073	− 0.251~ 0.104	0.417
Stomach Ca.	−0.559	−0.660~ − 0.458	< 0.001	2.822	2.748~ 2.895	< 0.001	0.115	−0.004~ 0.234	0.058
Colon/rectum Ca.	0.296	0.140~ 0.452	< 0.001	2.662	2.515~ 2.809	< 0.001	0.425	0.238~ 0.613	< 0.001
Liver Ca.	−0.438	− 0.514~ − 0.362	< 0.001	2.027	1.958~ 2.095	< 0.001	0.220	0.117~ 0.323	< 0.001
Pancreas Ca.	1.216	0.936~ 1.495	< 0.001	2.303	1.972~ 2.633	< 0.001	0.629	0.263~ 0.994	0.001
Diabetes	0.095	−0.080~ 0.271	0.287	3.015	2.866~ 3.165	< 0.001	0.635	0.436~ 0.834	< 0.001
Ulcer	−1.870	−2.236~ − 1.504	< 0.001	3.166	3.013~ 3.320	< 0.001	0.165	−0.241~ 0.571	0.425
Liver cirrhosis	−0.733	−0.872~ − 0.595	< 0.001	2.171	2.062~ 2.280	< 0.001	− 0.314	−0.507~ − 0.122	0.001
Appendicitis	−3.490	−5.480~ − 1.501	0.001	2.689	2.226~ 3.153	< 0.001	1.680	−0.450~ 3.810	0.122

Age*Region represents interaction between age and region; Ca. represents cancer

the effect of aging with urbanization (negative value implied a protective effect from aging). The B values were, in ascending order, for liver cirrhosis, hepatitis B, esophagus cancer, stomach cancer, ulcer, liver cancer, colon/rectum cancer, pancreas cancer, diabetes, hepatitis C, appendicitis and diarrhea.

The effects of age and urbanization on gastrointestinal disease are summarized and quantified in Fig. 1. According to their location on the scatter diagram, the 12 gastrointestinal diseases could be divided into three groups. In the upper right quadrant is what we termed old and developed urbanized disease, which had 4 diseases. The second group, closer to the lower left quadrant, was termed other factor and undeveloped rural disease, and had 3 diseases. The third group close to the lower right quadrant, was termed old and undeveloped rural disease and had 5 diseases.

Discussion

In our study, the life expectancy at birth was 79.43 years in urban areas and 73.90 years in rural areas, implying that data from urban areas and rural areas can be used for determining sensitivity to urbanization. Urbanization is associated with elongated life expectancy and thus higher rate of diseases that occur in elderly group; that aging and urbanization were included in one model as covariates could be eliminated the influence of elongated life expectancy for analyzing effects of urbanization on diseases.

Nutritional deficiencies could be referred to as an undeveloped rural disease. In present study, the mortality due to nutritional deficiencies was higher in rural areas than that in urban areas, implying that data sets were reliable. Although the diagnostic technique could be improved with urbanization, the rates of objective diagnosis (as evidenced by laboratory, pathologic, imaging and/or surgical intervention findings) were almost same in two regions, suggesting that bias from the improved diagnostic technique could be limited.

The B value was used to quantify the contribution of changes in urbanization to mortality from gastrointestinal disease revealed that these contributions varied. A higher B indicated greater risk of disease with urbanization (negative value implied a protective effect). We defined gastrointestinal diseases with a value of B (region) greater than zero as the "developed urbanized disease", and from our analysis, four gastrointestinal diseases (diabetes, colon/rectum cancer, hepatitis C and pancreas cancer) were developed urbanized disease. Urbanization may be a protective factor for other gastrointestinal diseases.

It is well known that the incidence of diabetes mellitus increases greatly with the development of a society [16–18]. Therefore, diabetes mellitus could be referred to as a developed urbanized disease. In the present study, diabetes mellitus was included in a group of developed urbanized disease, implying that statistical method was appropriate in our study.

As aging is a key observed variable for noncommunicable diseases [19] and an uncontrollable factor in mortality, it is important to evaluate the effects of aging on gastrointestinal disease with urbanization. The

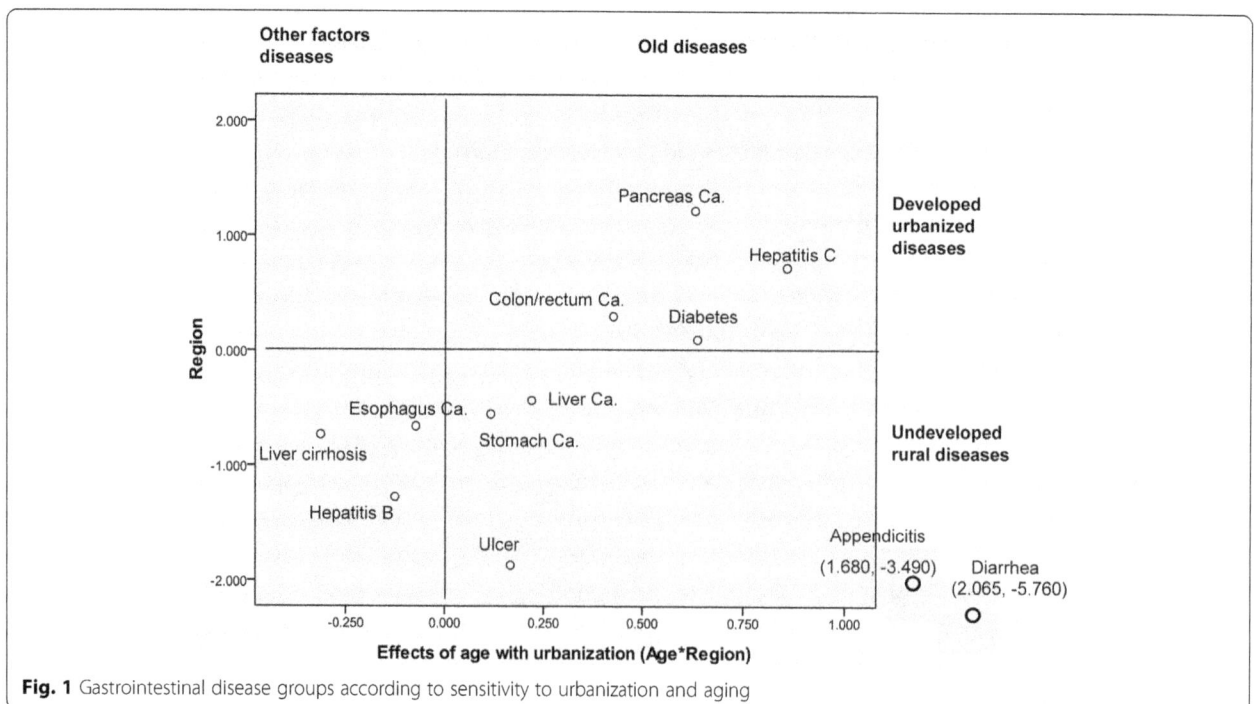

Fig. 1 Gastrointestinal disease groups according to sensitivity to urbanization and aging

B value of interaction between age and region (cities and rural areas) could be considered as indicator to assess role of age in mortality from gastrointestinal disease with urbanization, where a larger B value implied a stronger effect of aging with urbanization; the negative B value implied a stronger effect of other urbanized factors except aging in death with urbanization. We found that the value of B (interaction between region and age) for the 12 gastrointestinal diseases also varied.

We defined gastrointestinal diseases with a value of B (interaction between region and age) greater than zero as the "old diseases", and from our analysis, nine gastrointestinal diseases (stomach cancer, ulcer, liver cancer, colon/rectum cancer, pancreas cancer, diabetes, hepatitis C, appendicitis and diarrhea) were old diseases; for these diseases, aging could become a major cause of death with urbanization. This indicates that common protective interventions for health or aging process have an important role.

The scatter diagram represented the effects of aging and urbanization on gastrointestinal disease together as the dividing value. We divided the 12 gastrointestinal diseases into three groups according to their location on the diagram; each group represented gastrointestinal diseases with different attributes.

The group in the lower left quadrant, was termed other factor and undeveloped rural disease and includes esophageal cancer, liver cirrhosis and hepatitis B. Urbanization may be a protective factor for this group of diseases. We also clearly saw a tendency toward other factor (non-aging factors) with the development of society and the increase in the life expectancy, suggesting a independent of aging and a characteristic of programmed onset (occurrence of disease in a certain life stage) [20]. Accordingly, an emphasis on increasing basal health status may contribute to disease preventative strategies in this group.

The group in the lower right quadrant represents disease associated with the old population and undeveloped rural areas and includes stomach cancer, liver cancer, gastrointestinal ulcers, diarrhea and appendicitis. Urbanization may also be a protective factor for this group of diseases. Undeveloped rural risk factors for this disease group appear to be eliminated with urbanization. Therefore, aging will be a major causes of death with urbanization for this group of diseases. Accordingly, an emphasis on public health may contribute to disease preventative strategies in this group.

The group in the upper right quadrant shows disease associated with the relative-old onset and developed urbanized disease and included pancreas cancer, colon/rectum cancer, hepatitis C, and diabetes. That disease occurs relative-old implies the increase of age at disease onset is so many as the increase of life expectancy. The

aging and increase of life expectancy may be major causes for mortality, suggesting this group of diseases should be prevented by delaying aging, although it may be difficult.

The group in the upper left quadrant shows disease associated with the other factor and developed urbanized disease; unexpectedly, there is not major gastrointestinal diseases in this group. This group disease implies the increase of age at death is not so many as the increase of life expectancy. The other risk factors (non-aging factors) from urbanization, such as sedentary lifestyle and higher-kilojoule food intake [21–23], may be major causes for mortality, suggesting this group of diseases could be prevented by avoiding these urbanization associated risk factors. Further study is needed to explore whether these risk factors from urbanization have important role in occurrence of some gastrointestinal diseases or not.

Conclusion

Most gastrointestinal diseases were sensitive or protective to change of socioenvironmental factors; death from gastrointestinal disease would increase with the urbanization for some of the types and would decrease with the urbanization for the other types. Since the aging factors leading to disease are relatively uncontrollable, the study and control of external risk factors could lead to the conversion of most gastrointestinal disease. Common protective interventions for public health and quality of life, which include quality of social life and nutritional status, have the potential to eliminate the undeveloped rural diseases. Understanding the categorization of gastrointestinal disease according to urbanization and age will aid in its primary prevention.

Acknowledgments
I thank professor Liu Qigui, a statistician at my university, for providing support on generalized linear model analysis.

Authors' contributions
LH conceived the analysis and wrote the final version of the manuscript. The author read and approved the final manuscript.

Competing interests
The author declares that he/she has no competing interests.

References

1. Zeng Z, Zhu Z, Yang Y, Ruan W, Peng X, Su Y, Peng L, Chen J, Yin Q, Zhao C, Zhou H, Yuan S, Hao Y, Qian J, Ng SC, Chen M, Hu P. Incidence and clinical characteristics of inflammatory bowel disease in a developed region of Guangdong Province, China: a prospective population-based study. J Gastroenterol Hepatol. 2013;28(7):1148–53.
2. Amorim CA, Moreira JP, Rial L, Carneiro AJ, HS FÃ§a, Elia C, Luiz RR, de Souza HS. Ecological study of gastric cancer in Brazil: geographic and time trend analysis. World J Gastroenterol. 2014;20(17):5036–44.
3. Wong SH, Ng SC. What can we learn from inflammatory bowel disease in developing countries? Curr Gastroenterol Rep. 2013;15(3):313.
4. Liang Y, Li S. Landless female peasants living in resettlement residential areas in China have poorer quality of life than males: results from a household study in the Yangtze River Delta region. Health Qual Life Outcomes. 2014;12:71.
5. Chen J. Chronic conditions and receipt of treatment among urbanized rural residents in China. Biomed Res Int. 2013;2013:568959.
6. Wu N, Tang X, Wu Y, Qin X, He L, Wang J, Li N, Li J, Zhang Z, Dou H, Liu J, Yu L, Xu H, Zhang J, Hu Y, Iso H. Cohort profile: the Fangshan cohort study of cardiovascular epidemiology in Beijing, China. J Epidemiol. 2014;24(1):84–93.
7. Ma L, Mai J, Jing J, Liu Z, Zhu Y, Jin Y, Chen Y. Empirical change in the prevalence of overweight and obesity in adolescents from 2007 to 2011 in Guangzhou, China. Eur J Pediatr. 2014;173(6):787–91.
8. Zhang Y, Mo J, Weschler CJ. Reducing health risks from indoor exposures in rapidly developing urban China. Environ Health Perspect. 2013;121(7):751–5.
9. Chan F, Adamo S, Coxson P, Goldman L, Gu D, Zhao D, Chen CS, He J, Mara V, Moran A. Projected impact of urbanization on cardiovascular disease in China. Int J Public Health. 2012;57(5):849–54.
10. Hui L. Chronic diseases and societal development, based on the death-risk index. Epidemiology. 2015;26(1):e9–e10.
11. Gong P, Liang S, Carlton EJ, Jiang Q, Wu J, Wang L, Remais JV. Urbanisation and health in China. Lancet. 2012;379(9818):843–52.
12. Idrovo AJ. Physical environment and life expectancy at birth in Mexico: an eco-epidemiological study. Cad Saude Publica. 2011;27(6):1175–84.
13. Chinese Center for Disease Control and Prevention. National Disease Mortality Surveillance System, 2004. Military Medical Science Press, 2009:102–107.
14. Chinese Center for Disease Control and Prevention. National Disease Mortality Surveillance System, 2011. People's Medical Publishing House, 2013:171–405.
15. World Health Organization. International statistical classification of diseases and related health problems, tenth revision. Geneva: World Health Organization; 1992.
16. Xin G, Yang G, Hui L. Study to assess whether waist circumference and changes in serum glucose and lipid profile are independent variables for the CETP gene. Diabetes Res Clin Pract. 2014;106(1):95–100.
17. Sherwin R, Jastreboff AM. Year in diabetes 2012: the diabetes tsunami. J Clin Endocrinol Metab. 2012;97(12):4293–301.
18. Xin G, Shong L, Hui L. Effect of genetic and non-genetic factors, including aging, on waist circumference and BMI, and inter-indicator differences in risk assessment. Exp Gerontol. 2014;60:83–6.
19. Hui L. Assessment of the role of ageing and non-ageing factors in death from non-communicable diseases based on a cumulative frequency model. Sci Rep. 2017;7(1):8159.
20. Hui L. Aging and chronic disease as independent causative factors for death and a programmed onset for chronic disease. Arch Gerontol Geriatr. 2015; 60:178–82.
21. Doherty ML, Owusu-Dabo E, Kantanka OS, Brawer RO, Plumb JD. Type 2 diabetes in a rapidly urbanizing region of Ghana, West Africa: a qualitative study of dietary preferences, knowledge and practices. BMC Public Health. 2014;14:1069.
22. Ng SW, Howard AG, Wang HJ, Su C, Zhang B. The physical activity transition among adults in China: 1991-2011. Obes Rev. 2014;15(Suppl 1):27–36.
23. Du SF, Wang HJ, Zhang B, Zhai FY, Popkin BM. China in the period of transition from scarcity and extensive undernutrition to emerging nutrition-related non-communicable diseases, 1949-1992. Obes Rev. 2014;15(Suppl 1):8–15.

10

Clinicopathologic and endoscopic features of early-stage colorectal serrated adenocarcinoma

Daiki Hirano[1], Shiro Oka[1*], Shinji Tanaka[2], Kyoku Sumimoto[1], Yuki Ninomiya[1], Yuzuru Tamaru[1], Kenjiro Shigita[1], Nana Hayashi[2], Yuji Urabe[1], Yasuhiko Kitadai[4], Fumio Shimamoto[5], Koji Arihiro[3] and Kazuaki Chayama[1]

Abstract

Background: Serrated adenocarcinoma (SAC) is a distinct colorectal carcinoma variant that accounts for approximately 7.5% of all advanced colorectal carcinomas. While its prognosis is worse than conventional carcinoma, its early-stage clinicopathologic features are unclear. We therefore aimed to clarify the clinicopathologic and endoscopic characteristics of early-stage SACs.

Methods: Forty consecutive early-stage SAC patients at Hiroshima University Hospital were enrolled; SACs were classified into epithelial serration (Group A, $n = 17$) and non-epithelial serration (Group B, $n = 23$) groups. Additionally, we classified serrated adenoma into 4 types: sessile serrated adenoma (SSA), traditional serrated adenoma (TSA), unclassified, and non-serrated adenoma type.

Results: There were significant differences between Groups A and B in terms of tumor size (27.6 vs. 43.1 mm), incidences of T1 carcinoma (71% vs. 13%), and having the same color as normal mucosa (47% vs. 17%), respectively ($p < 0.01$). In SACs >20 mm, the incidence of T1 carcinoma in Group A (70%) was significantly greater than that in Group B (13%) ($p < 0.05$). There were significant differences in 'Japan NBI Expert Team' type 3 and type V pit pattern classifications between the 2 groups. The average TSA-type tumor size (42.6 mm) was significantly larger than that of the SSA (17.2 mm) and non-serrated component types (18.3 mm). The incidences of submucosal invasion in SSA- (80%), unclassified- (100%), and non-serrated-type (100%) tumors were significantly higher than that in the TSA type (11%).

Conclusions: Epithelial serration in the cancerous area and a non-TSA background indicated aggressive behavior in early-stage SACs.

Keywords: Serrated adenocarcinoma, Colorectal cancer, Narrow band imaging, Pit pattern

Background

Colorectal carcinoma is one of the most common malignancies in the world. The classical genetic model for colorectal tumorigenesis described by Fearon and Vogelstein is the adenoma-adenocarcinoma sequence, which is driven by the progressive accumulation of critical mutations [1]. In this model, the adenomatous polyp is the principal precursor of colorectal carcinomas [1, 2]. More than 90% of colorectal carcinomas are medullary, micropapillary, mucinous, serrated, or signet ring cell [3]. Serrated adenocarcinomas (SACs) were first described by Jass and Smith [4] and represent the malignant progression of dysplastic serrated lesions, most commonly serrated adenomas. SAC is considered to be one of several end-points of a progression pattern known as the serrated neoplasia pathway [5, 6], which is a major contributor to colorectal carcinoma; approximately 25% of cases arise through this pathway [7, 8]. Such carcinomas originate in serrated polyps such as sessile serrated adenomas (SSAs) and traditional serrated adenomas (TSAs) [9]. SACs arising from SSAs have molecular profiles that are CpG island methylator phenotype-high and *BRAF* mutation-positive, with high microsatellite instability (MSI). SACs arising from TSAs are CpG island methylator phenotype-low, KRAS mutation-positive, and

* Correspondence: oka4683@hiroshima-u.ac.jp
[1]Department of Gastroenterology and Metabolism, Hiroshima University Hospital, 1-2-3 Kasumi, Minami-ku, Hiroshima 734-8551, Japan
Full list of author information is available at the end of the article

exhibit microsatellite stability or low microsatellite instability [10–12]. Recently, SACs have been described as having less favorable 5-year survival outcomes than conventional colorectal carcinomas [5]. However, there are no reports on the clinicopathologic and endoscopic features in early-stage SACs. Therefore, the aim of this study was to investigate and clarify these features in early-stage SACs.

Methods

Forty consecutive early-stage colorectal SACs were extracted from 1142 colorectal carcinoma patients (895 with Tis carcinoma and 247 with T1 carcinoma) who were treated at Hiroshima University Hospital between January 2009 and January 2016. Patients with familiar adenomatous polyposis, inflammatory bowel disease, or serrated polyposis syndrome were excluded. The lesions were resected using polypectomy, endoscopic mucosal resection, endoscopic submucosal dissection, or surgical resection.

Endoscopic examination

Upon detection of a lesion by standard colonoscopy, the surface mucus was washed away with lukewarm water and indigo carmine dye was spread over the lesion. When it was not possible to adequately stain the surface with indigo carmine for diagnosis, crystal violet dye was used instead, and magnifying observation was performed. All images were obtained with magnifying colonoscopies (CF-Q240ZI, CF-H260AZI, and CF-H290ZI; Olympus, Tokyo, Japan) with up to 80-fold magnification in combination with a standard video processor system (EVIS LUCERA system, EVIS EXERA system; Olympus Inc., Tokyo, Japan). Pit pattern diagnosis was

based on the dominant pit pattern according to the Kudo and Tsuruta classification [13, 14] as well as the dominant narrow-band imaging (NBI) findings as proposed by the Japan NBI Expert Team (JNET) classification [15, 16]. The JNET classification divides vessel and surface patterns into 4 categories: types 1, 2A, 2B, and 3, which are consistent with the histopathological findings of hyperplastic polyp/sessile serrated polyp, low-grade intramucosal neoplasia, high-grade intramucosal neoplasia/shallow submucosal invasive cancer, and deep submucosal invasive cancer, respectively.

Pathological examination

Resected specimens were fixed in a 10% buffered formalin solution. Paraffin-embedded samples were then sliced into 2–3-mm sections and stained with hematoxylin and eosin.

The subjects were diagnosed by 2 pathologists (K.A. and F.S.) who were blinded to the endoscopic features of the lesion. Histologic type, depth of tumor, venous invasion, and lymphatic invasion were also categorized according to the Japanese Classification of Colorectal Carcinoma [17]. For submucosal (SM) invasive cancer, we measured the SM depth and budding grade. According to the JSCCR guidelines [18], the method used for measuring the SM depth was as follows: When it was possible to identify or estimate the location of the muscularis mucosae, the depth of SM invasion was measured from the lower border of the muscularis mucosae of the lesion, irrespective of macroscopic type. When it was not possible to identify or estimate the location of the muscularis mucosae, the depth of SM invasion was measured from the surface of the lesion.

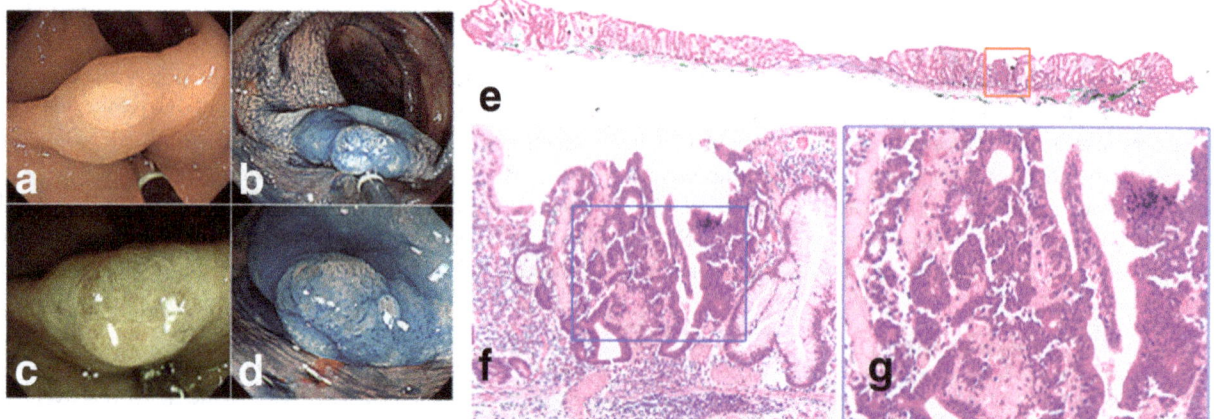

Fig. 1 A case of Tis serrated adenocarcinoma with a serrated adenoma. **a** Colonoscopic view of a serrated adenocarcinoma lesion in the ascending colon. **b** Endoscopic findings after indigo carmine spraying; the small elevated nodule in the tumor can be observed. **c** Magnifying narrow-band imaging (NBI) observation. In the tumor lesion, mucosa with a Japan NBI Expert Team classification type B can be observed. **d** Magnifying endoscopic finding after indigo carmine dye spraying. Type II-open-containing normal type II pits are observed in the tumor. **e** Hematoxylin and eosin (HE) staining of the whole specimen. **f, g** High-power view of the HE-stain specimen; a section of adenocarcinoma is shown

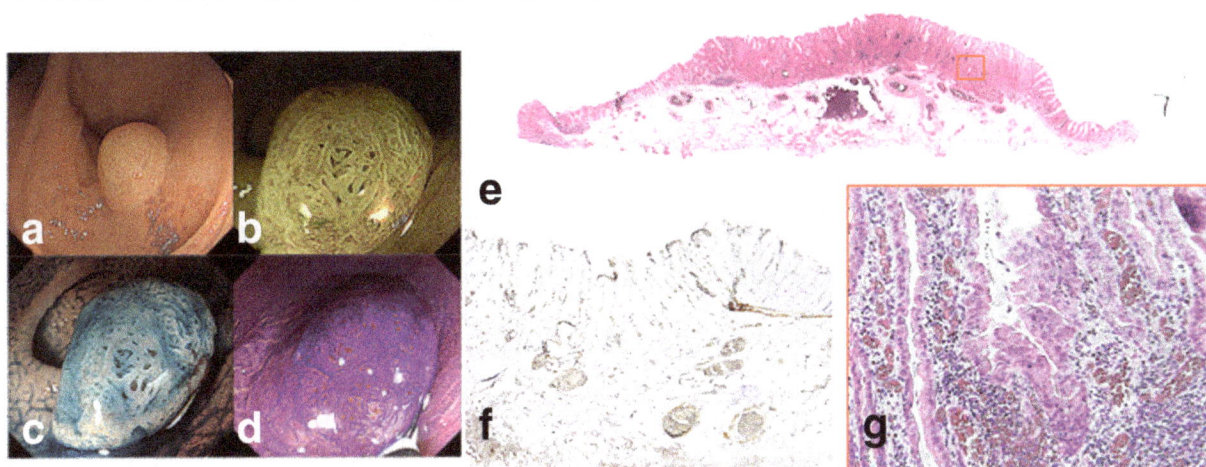

Fig. 2 A case of T1 serrated adenocarcinoma without a serrated adenoma. **a** Colonoscopic view of serrated adenocarcinoma in the cecum. **b** Endoscopic view after indigo carmine dye spraying. A 0-Is lesion is clearly delineated. **c** Magnifying narrow-band imaging (NBI) observation; a Japan NBI Expert Team classification type 2B lesion can be observed. **d** Magnifying view of a crystal violet-stained section. **e** Hematoxylin and eosin (HE) staining of the whole specimen. **f** Immunostaining of the specimen with anti-desmin antibody; the muscle fibers are no longer visible. **g** High-power view of HE-stained specimen; epithelial serration is visible, and adenocarcinoma can be observed invading the submucosa

Budding is defined as a single cancer cell or a cluster of 5 cells along the invasion margin, and was graded per microscopic field at 200× magnification (i.e., grade 1, 0–4 buds; grade 2, 5–9 buds; and grade 3, ≥10 buds) [19].

Tumors that contained more than one histologic type of carcinoma were classified based on the predominant histologic type. Well-differentiated tubular adenocarcinoma (tub1) was characterized by distinct and large gland formation; moderately differentiated tubular adenocarcinoma (tub2) was composed of medium-to-small glands with a cribriform structure, and poorly differentiated adenocarcinoma (Por) had little tendency to form glands or tubules; however, intracellular mucus production was observed [17].

The current diagnostic criteria for SAC are based on the recognition of a serrated polyp (hyperplastic polyp, SSA, or TSA) next to the carcinoma or of a characteristic carcinoma histology.

The morphological characteristics of SAC were defined using Mäkinen's criteria, and include epithelial serrations, clear or eosinophilic cytoplasm, abundant cytoplasm, vesicular nuclei, distinct nucleoli, scarceness (<10%) of necrosis, mucin production, and cell balls or papillary rods in the mucin. However, the pathological general definition of SAC is tubular adenocarcinoma with serration. A diagnosis of SAC was considered when the carcinoma met at least 6 of the first 7 features listed above [5] or when the carcinoma was adjacent to a serrated adenoma [20–22]. SACs were diagnosed by 2 pathologists (K.A. and F.S.) and 1 gastroenterologist (D.H.).

Evaluation

We classified SACs into the 2 groups: those with epithelial serration (Group A, $n = 17$) and those with non-epithelial serration (Group B, $n = 23$); examples are shown in Figs. 1 and 2, respectively. SACs were categorized as having epithelial serration if more than 5% of the cancerous area exhibited such morphology.

We compared the following clinicopathologic characteristics between the 2 groups: sex, age, location, tumor size, and invasion depth (Tis/T1). Lesion location was divided into proximal colon (i.e., proximal to the splenic flexure), distal colon (i.e., distal to the splenic flexure) and rectum. We also compared the following endoscopic findings between the 2 groups: tumor surface color (same as normal mucosa vs. discolored vs. reddish), macroscopic type (protruded vs. superficial), pineconelike status, varicose microvascular vessels (VMVs) vs. pit pattern, and JNET classification [15, 16]. We also classified the serrated adenoma close to the carcinoma into 4

Table 1 Characteristics of serrated adenocarcinoma

Variables	Epithelial serration		p-value
	Present ($n = 17$)	Absent ($n = 23$)	
Sex (male/female)	9/8	14/9	N.S.
Average age (years)	70.5	68.5	N.S.
Location (proximal colon/distal colon/rectum)	8/1/8	8/1/14	N.S.
Average size (mm)	27.6	43.1	<0.05
Invasion depth (Tis/T1)	5/12	20/3	<0.05

N.S. not significant

Table 2 Endoscopic features of serrated adenocarcinoma

Variables	Epithelial serration		p-value
	Present ($n = 17$)	Absent ($n = 23$)	
Color			
Same as normal mucosa	8 (47)	4 (17)	<0.05
Discolored	1 (6)	4 (17)	N.S.
Reddish	8 (47)	15 (66)	N.S.
Macroscopic type			
Protruded	14 (82)	20 (87)	N.S.
Superficial	3 (18)	3 (13)	N.S.
Pinecone like findings (+)	2 (12)	6 (26)	N.S.
Varicose microvesicular (+)	3 (18)	1 (4)	N.S.

Values in parentheses are percentages (%)
N.S. not significant

types: SSA, TSA, unclassified, and non-serrated adenoma type, and compared clinicopathologic and endoscopic features between these 4 types. This study was conducted in accordance with the Declaration of Helsinki and was approved by the Institutional Review Board of our hospital. Written informed consent was obtained from all patients who participated in this study.

Statistical analysis

Each continuous variable was presented as the mean ± standard deviation. Comparisons of continuous variables were performed using Student's t-test, and comparisons of dichotomous variables were based on the chi-square and Fisher's exact tests. JMP version 8 (SAS Institute, Cary, NC) was used to analyze the data. The significance level was set at 5% for each analysis; $p < 0.05$ was considered statistically significant.

This study was conducted in accordance with the Declaration of Helsinki and was approved by the Institutional Review Board of our hospital. Written informed consent was obtained from all patients who participated in this study.

Results

With respect to clinicopathologic characteristics, there were significant differences in average tumor size, incidence of

Table 3 Narrow band imaging magnification findings in the carcinoma area of serrated adenocarcinoma

Epithelial serration	JNET classification			
	1	2A	2B	3
Present ($n = 17$)	1 (6)	6 (35)	7 (41)	3 (18)[a]
Absent ($n = 23$)	1 (4)	13 (57)	9 (39)	0 (0)[b]
Total ($n = 40$)	2 (5)	19 (48)	16 (40)	3 (7)

a vs. b: $p < 0.01$. Values in parentheses are percentages (%). JNET: Japan NBI [narrow-band imaging] Expert Team

Table 4 Pit pattern classification in the carcinoma area of serrated adenocarcinoma

Epithelial serration	Pit pattern				
	II	Open-II	III$_L$	IV	V
Present ($n = 17$)	0 (0)	1 (6)	2 (12)	2 (12)[a]	12 (70)[c]
Absent ($n = 23$)	1 (4)	0 (0)	3 (13)	10 (44)[b]	9 (39)[d]
Total ($n = 40$)	1 (3)	1 (3)	5 (13)	12 (30)	21 (53)

a vs. b, c vs. d: $p < 0.01$. Values in parentheses are percentages (%)

T1 carcinoma, and incidence of tumor color being the same as normal mucosa between Groups A and B ($p < 0.01$); however, there were no significant differences in sex, age, and tumor location. Furthermore, there were no significant differences in macroscopic type, pinecone-like findings, and VMVs regardless of epithelial serration (Tables 1, 2).

Endoscopic findings revealed that there were significant differences in the incidence of JNET Type 3 and type V pit pattern between Groups A and B, respectively (Tables 3, 4).

In SACs smaller than 10 mm, there were no cases with submucosal invasion; however, in SACs larger than 20 mm, the incidence of T1 carcinoma in Group A (71%) was significantly higher than that in Group B (13%) ($p < 0.05$) (Table 5). Serrated adenocarcinoma characteristics listed according to their serrated adenoma are shown in Table 6.

TSA-type tumors were significantly larger than SSA and non-serrated adenoma type lesions. The TSA type SACs were mainly located in the rectum. The SSA type SACs were located in the proximal colon in all cases. The incidences of submucosal invasion in SSA type (80%), unclassified type (100%) and non-serrated adenoma type (100%) lesions were significantly greater than those of the TSA type (11%) (Table 6). T1 SACs were observed in 15 patients (12 in Group A and 3 in Group B). For T1 SACs, vessel invasion was observed in 4 Group A patients. Among surgical patients, lymph node metastasis was observed in 2 patients in Group A; none of the patients in group B had vessel invasion or lymph node metastasis (Table 7).

Table 5 Incidence of submucosal invasion in serrated adenocarcinoma according to size and epithelial serration

Size (mm)	Epithelial serration		p-value
	Present ($n = 17$)	Absent ($n = 23$)	
<10	0% (0/0)	0% (0/1)	N.S.
11–20	67% (4/6)	17% (1/6)	N.S.
>20	73% (8/11)	13% (2/16)	<0.05
Total	70% (12/17)	13% (3/23)	<0.05

N.S. not significant

Table 6 Characteristics of serrated adenocarcinomas according to the serrated adenoma type

Variables	TSA (n = 27)	SSA/P (n = 5)	Unclassified (n = 5)	Non-serrated adenoma (n = 3)
Sex (male/female)	16/11	3/2	3/2	1/2
Average age (years)	69.1	69.0	68.6	73.3
Location (proximal colon/distal colon/rectum)	7/1/19	5/0/0	2/1/2	2/0/1
Average size (mm)	42.6[a]	17.2[b]	34.0	18.3[c]
Invasion depth (Tis/T1)	24/3[d]	1/4[e]	0/5[f]	0/3[g]
Epithelial serration (+/−)	6/21	3/2	5/0	3/0

TSA traditional serrated adenoma, *SSA/P* serrated adenoma/polyp
a vs. b and c, d vs. e, f, and g: $p < 0.01$

Discussion

To our knowledge, this is the first study of the clinico-pathologic and endoscopic features of early-stage SAC. The discovery of SAC was anticipated by the recognition of high-grade dysplasia or Tis carcinoma in TSA in several studies [23–28]. The ages and sexes of our SAC patients were consistent with those reported previously [29, 30]. SACs were observed predominantly in the proximal colon and the rectum. Those in the proximal colon appear to be more related to SSAs; however, most distal SACs likely originate from TSAs since SSAs were located predominantly in the right colon whereas TSAs were located in the left colon [24, 29, 30]. The diagnosis of SACs with poorly differentiated carcinoma or without an adjacent serrated adenoma is difficult in advanced

stages. In SACs with mucinous components, the serrated growth pattern is well presented; however, displacement may compress the epithelium so that the serrated projections are not apparent, or an abundance of mucus in combination with poor differentiation may render the serrated pattern unrecognizable. We were able to detect minute changes in serrated morphology and in the serrated components close to the carcinoma.

Our study also showed that group A tumors exhibited more aggressive behavior and malignant potential, even though the average size of SACs with epithelial serration was smaller than that of SACs with non-epithelial serration. Of the T1 carcinomas in Group A, 67% were 11–20 mm in size. Molecularly distinct subtypes of colorectal carcinomas, including those that develop from serrated precursor lesions, are considered to have poor prognoses [31]. Carcinomas of the serrated pathway without MSI are aggressive; SACs with epithelial serration tend to exhibit submucosal invasion, even during early stages. The incidences of vessel invasion in SACs with epithelial serration were significantly higher than those in SACs with non-epithelial serration. Therefore, epithelial serration appears to be a predictor of aggressive carcinoma.

Endoscopic findings revealed that the incidence of type V pit pattern in SACs with epithelial serration was significantly higher than that in SACs with non-epithelial serration. Recently, the JNET established a universal NBI magnifying endoscopic classification system for colorectal tumors [15, 16], according to which submucosal deep invasive colorectal carcinomas were classified as type 3. The incidences of JNET type 3 lesions in SACs with

Table 7 Fifteen cases of T1 serrated adenocarcinoma

Case No.	Sex	Age (decade years)	Location	Size (mm)	Epithelial serration	Serrated adenoma	SM invasion depth (μm)	Budding grade	Vessel invasion	Lymph node metastasis
1.	Female	50s	C/C	30	+	+	200	1	ly0, v0	−
2.	Female	70s	Rb	40	+	+	1000	2	ly0, v0	−
3.	Male	70s	Rb	40	+	+	1100	3	ly0, v0	−
4.	Male	70s	D/C	30	+	+	1400	2	ly0, v0	−
5.	Male	60s	C/C	10	+	+	1500	1	ly0, v0	−
6.	Male	60s	A/C	30	+	+	1500	1	ly3, v1	+
7.	Female	80s	C/C	20	+	+	1500	1	ly0, v0	−
8.	Male	70s	A/C	15	+	−	1900	3	ly1, v1	−
9.	Female	80s	C/C	10	+	−	2000	3	ly0, v0	−
10.	Female	60s	Ra	30	+	−	2500	3	ly3, v0	+
11.	Female	80s	Rb	50	+	+	2600	1	ly1, v0	−
12.	Male	60s	T/C	30	+	+	3000	1	ly0, v0	−
13.	Male	60s	A/C	20	−	+	170	1	ly0, v0	−
14.	Male	50s	Rb	90	−	+	3000	3	ly0, v0	−
15.	Male	50s	Ra	40	−	+	5200	2	ly0, v0	−

C/C Cecum, *A/C* Ascending colon, *T/C* Transverse colon, *D/C* Descending colon, *Ra* Rectum above the peritoneal reflection, *Rb* Rectum below the peritoneal reflection, *SM* submucosal

epithelial serration were significantly higher than those in SACs with non-epithelial serration. NBI magnification is also useful to predict the depths for SACs. The latest WHO classification categorizes SACs into 3 groups: HP, SSA/polyps (SSA/P), and TSA; the endoscopic features of conventional SSA/P have a pale color similar to HPs. When observed with crystal violet staining under magnification, the orifices are observed to be widely open, and are referred to as type II-open pit [32]. SSAs are also classified as type 1 according to the JNET classification when observed with NBI magnification [15, 16]. VMVs are defined as vessels thicker than meshed capillary ducts that have meander-like flow resembling varicose veins; this is distinct from the capillary pattern of the mucosal vascular network [33]. The endoscopic features of protruded-type TSAs include enhanced-reddish villous lesions [34]. As for macroscopic features, Sano et al. documented the pinecone-like appearance as characteristic of TSA [35]; when observed with crystal violet staining under magnification, the type IV pit pattern is often present, and is associated with the type II pit pattern at the base [36]. When observed with magnifying NBI, TSAs were consequently classified as type 2A according to the JNET guidelines [15, 16]; therefore, it is possible to distinguish between TSA and SSA endoscopically using magnification. There were no significant differences in pinecone-like findings and VMVs between Group A and Group B, even though Group A tended to exhibit more of the latter while Group B had more of the former. Moreover, distinct areas or transition points in which the pit pattern changes from type II to type III or IV suggest the development of a dysplasic area [37]. Therefore, determining the origins of SACs remains challenging.

There were some limitations in this study, including its retrospective, single-center nature and the relatively small number of SACs owing to the rarity of such lesions. A large, multicenter prospective trial is required for further validation of our findings.

Conclusions

We found that epithelial serration in the cancerous area of early-stage SACs and a non-TSA serrated adenoma background are independent predictors of aggressive behavior. Our results may be helpful for determining indications of endoscopic resection in patients with serrated lesions. Further research ought to elucidate the molecular or genetic mechanisms behind the aggressive behavior of early-stage SACs.

Abbreviations
HP: Hyperplastic polyp; JNET: Japan NBI Expert Team; MSI: Microsatellite instability; NBI: Narrow-band imaging; SAC: Serrated adenocarcinoma; SSA: Sessile serrated adenoma; SSA/P: SSA/polyps; TSA: Traditional serrated adenoma; VMV: Varicose microvascular vessels; WHO: World Health Organization

Acknowledgements
Not applicable.

Funding
This study was not funded by any external sources.

Authors' contributions
DH designed the study and wrote the initial draft of the manuscript. SO contributed to the analysis and interpretation of the data, and assisted in the preparation of the manuscript. ST, K Sumimoto, YN, YT, K Shigita, NH, YU, YK, FS, KA, and KC contributed to data collection and interpretation, and critically reviewed the manuscript. The final version of the manuscript was read and approved by all authors.

Competing interests
The authors declare that they have no competing interest.

Author details
[1]Department of Gastroenterology and Metabolism, Hiroshima University Hospital, 1-2-3 Kasumi, Minami-ku, Hiroshima 734-8551, Japan. [2]Department of Endoscopy, Hiroshima University Hospital, Hiroshima, Japan. [3]Department of Anatomical Pathology, Hiroshima University Hospital, Hiroshima, Japan. [4]Department of the Faculty of Human Culture and Science, Prefectural University of Hiroshima, Hiroshima, Japan. [5]The Faculty of Humanities and Human Sciences, Hiroshima Shudo University Hiroshima, Hiroshima, Japan.

References
1. Ferlay J, Shin HR, Bray F, Forman D, Mathers C, Parkin DM. Estimates of worldwide burden of cancer in 2008: GLOBOCAN 2008. Int J Cancer. 2010; 127:2893–917.
2. Pino MS, Chung DC. The chromosomal instability pathway in colon cancer. Gastroenterology. 2010;138:2059–72.
3. Bosman FT, Hruban RH, Theise ND. WHO classification of tumors of the digestive system. Lyon, France: International Agency for Research on Cancer; 2010.
4. Jass JR, Smith M. Sialic acid and epithelial differentiation in colorectal polyps and cancer—a morphological, mucin and lectin histochemical study. Pathology. 1992;24:233–42.
5. García-Solano J, Pérez-Guillermo M, Conesa-Zamora P, Acosta-Ortega J, Trujillo-Santos J, Cerezuela-Fuentes P, et al. Clinicopathologic study of 85 colorectal serrated adenocarcinomas: further insights into the full recognition of a new subset of colorectal carcinoma. Hum Pathol. 2010;41: 1359–68.
6. Yao T, Nishiyama K, Oya M, Kouzuki T, Kajiwara M, Tsuneyoshi M. Multiple 'serrated adenocarcinomas' of the colon with a cell lineage common to metaplastic polyp and serrated adenoma: case report of a new subtype of colonic adenocarcinoma with gastric differentiation. J Pathol. 2000;190:444–9.
7. Leggett B, Whitehall V. Role of the serrated pathway in colorectal cancer pathogenesis. Gastroenterology. 2010;138:2088–100.
8. Snover DC. Update on the serrated pathway to colorectal carcinoma. Hum Pathol. 2011;42:110.

9. Bettington M, Walker N, Clouston A, Brown I, Leggett B, Whitehall V. The serrated pathway to colorectal carcinoma: current concepts and challenges. Histopathology. 2013;62:367–86.

10. Sheridan TB, Fenton H, Lewin MR, Burkart AL, Iacobuzio-Donahue CA, Frankel WL, et al. Sessile serrated adenomas with low-and high-grade dysplasia and early carcinomas: an immunohistochemical study of serrated lesions "caught in the act". Am J Clin Pathol. 2006;126:564–71.

11. East JE, Saunders BP, Jass JR. Sporadic and syndromic hyperplastic polyps and serrated adenomas of the colon: classification, molecular genetics, natural history, and clinical management. Gastroenterol Clin N Am. 2008;37:25–46.

12. Hinoue T, Weisenberger DJ, Lange CP, Shen H, Byun HM, Van Den Berg D, et al. Genome- scale analysis of aberrant DNA methylation in colorectal cancer. Genome Res. 2012;22:271–82.

13. Kudo S, Hirota S, Nakajima T, Hosobe S, Kusaka H, Kobayashi T, et al. Colorectal tumours and pit pattern. J Clin Pathol. 1994;47:880–5.

14. Tanaka S, Kaltenbach T, Chayama K, Soetikno R. High- magnification colonoscopy. Gastrointest Endosc. 2006;64:604–13.

15. Sano Y, Tanaka S, Kudo SE, Saito S, Matsuda T, Wada Y, et al. Narrow-band imaging (NBI) magnifying endoscopic classification of colorectal tumors proposed by the Japan NBI expert team. Dig Endosc. 2016;28:526–33.

16. Sumimoto K, Tanaka S, Shigita K, Hirano D, Tamaru Y, Ninomiya Y, et al. Clinical impact and characteristics of the narrow-band imaging magnifying endoscopic classification of colorectal tumors proposed by the Japan NBI expert team. Gastrointest Endosc. 2016; https://doi.org/10.1016/j.gie.2016.07.035.

17. Sugihara K, Kusunoki M, Watanabe T, Sakai Y, Sekimoto M, Ajioka Y. Guidelines for classification; in Japanese Society for Cancer of the colon and Rectum (ed): Japanese classification of colorectal carcinoma. Kanehara: Tokyo; 2009. p. 1–34.

18. Watanabe T, Itabashi M, Shimada Y, Tanaka S, Ito Y, Ajioka Y, et al. Japanese Society for Cancer of the colon and Rectum (JSCCR) guidelines 2014 for treatment of colorectal cancer. Int J Clin Oncol. 2015;20:207–39.

19. Ueno H, Mochizuki H, Hashiguchi Y, Shimazaki H, Aida S, Hase K, et al. Risk factors for an adverse outcome in early invasive colorectal carcinoma. Gastroenterology. 2004;127:385–94.

20. Snover D, Ahnen D, Burt R, Odze R. Serrated polyps of the colon and rectum and serrated ("hyperplastic") polyposis. In: Bozman FT, Carneiro F, Hruban RH, editors. WHO classification of Tumours pathology and genetics Tumours of the digestive system. 4th ed. Berlin: Germany, Springer-Verlag; 2010.

21. Mäkinen MJ, George SM, Jernvall P, Mäkelä J, Vihko P, Karttunen TJ. Colorectal carcinoma associated with serrated adenoma—prevalence, histological features, and prognosis. J Pathol. 2001;193:286–94.

22. Tuppurainen K, Mäkinen JM, Junttila O, Liakka A, Kyllönen AP, Tuominen H, et al. Morphology and microsatellite instability in sporadic serrated and non-serrated colorectal cancer. J Pathol. 2005;207:285–94.

23. Longacre TA, Fenoglio-Preiser CM. Mixed hyperplastic adenomatous polyps/ serrated adenomas. A distinct form of colorectal neoplasia. Am J Surg Pathol. 1990;14:524–37.

24. Goldstein NS. Small colonic microsatellite unstable adenocarcinomas and high-grade epithelial dysplasias in sessile serrated adenoma polypectomy specimens: a study of eight cases. Am J Clin Pathol. 2006;125:132–45.

25. Oka S, Tanaka S, Hiyama T, Ito M, Kitadai Y, Yoshihara M, et al. Clinicopathologic and endoscopic features of colorectal serrated adenoma: differences between polypoid and superficial types. Gastrointest Endosc. 2004;59:213–9.

26. Tanaka M, Kusumi T, Sasaki Y, Yamagata K, Ichinohe H, Nishida J, et al. Colonic intra-epithelial carcinoma occurring in a hyperplastic polyp via a serrated adenoma. Pathol Int. 2001;51:215–20.

27. Ajioka Y, Watanabe H, Jass JR, Yokota Y, Kobayashi M, Nishikura K. Infrequent K-Ras codon 12 mutation in serrated adenomas of human colorectum. Gut. 1998;42:680–4.

28. Hiyama T, Yokozaki H, Shimamoto F, Haruma K, Yasui W, Kajiyama G, et al. Frequent p53 gene mutations in serrated adenomas of the colorectum. J Pathol. 1998;186:131–9.

29. Torlakovic E, Skovlund E, Snover DC, Torlakovic G, Nesland JM. Morphologic reappraisal of serrated colorectal polyps. Am J Surg Pathol. 2003;27:65–81.

30. Hasegawa S, Mitsuyama K, Kawano H, Arita K, Maeyama Y, Akagi Y, et al. Endoscopic discrimination of sessile serrated adenomas from other serrated lesions. Oncol Lett. 2011;2:785–9.

31. De Sousa E, Melo F, Wang X, Jansen M, Fessler E, Trinh A, de Rooij LP, et al. Poor-prognosis colon cancer is defined by a molecularly distinct subtype and develops from serrated precursor lesions. Nat Med. 2013;19:614–8.

32. Ishigooka S, Nomoto M, Obinata N, Oishi Y, Sato Y, Nakatsu S, et al. Evaluation of magnifying colonoscopy in the diagnosis of serrated polyps. World J Gastroenterol. 2012;18:4308–16.

33. Uraoka T, Higashi R, Horii J, Harada K, Hori K, Okada H, et al. Prospective evaluation of endoscopic criteria characteristic of sessile serrated adenomas/polyps. J Gastroenterol. 2015;50:555–63.

34. Saito S, Ikegami M, Ono M, Sato Y, Ichinose M, Sasaki T, et al. Clinicopathological study of serrated adenoma and mixed hyperplastic adenomatous polyp (MHAP). Gastroenterol Endosc. 1998;40:12–21.

35. Sano Y, Saito Y, KI F, Matsuda T, Uraoka T, Kobayashi N, et al. Efficacy of magnifying chromoendoscopy for the differential diagnosis of colorectal lesions. Dig Endosc. 2005;17:105–16.

36. Saito S, Tajiri H, Ikegami M. Serrated polyps of the colon and rectum: endoscopic features including image enhanced endoscopy. World J Gastrointest Endosc. 2015;7:860–71.

37. Burgess NG, Pellise M, Nanda KS, Hourigan LF, Zanati SA, Brown GJ, et al. Clinical and endoscopic predictors of cytological dysplasia or cancer in a prospective multicentre study of large sessile serrated adenomas/polyps. Gut. 2016;65:437–46.

11

Faecal bacterial microbiota in patients with cirrhosis and the effect of lactulose administration

Aditya Narayan Sarangi[1,2†], Amit Goel[1†], Ankur Singh[1], Avani Sasi[1] and Rakesh Aggarwal[1,2*] (iD)

Abstract

Background: Gut microbiota may be altered in patients with cirrhosis, and may further change after administration of lactulose. We studied the composition of gut microbiota in patients with cirrhosis and assessed the effect on it of lactulose administration.

Methods: Stool specimens were collected from 35 patients with cirrhosis (male 26; median [range] age: 42 [29–65] years) and 18 healthy controls (male 14; 44.5 [24–67] years); 21 patients provided another specimen after lactulose administration for 55 [42–77] days. For each, a DNA library of V3 region of bacterial 16S ribosomal RNA was subjected to paired-end Illumina sequencing. Inter-specimen relationship was studied using principal co-ordinate analysis. Abundances of various bacterial taxa, and indices of alpha and beta diversity were compared, between patients and controls, and between specimens collected before and after lactulose.

Results: Gut microbiota from cirrhosis patients and controls showed differential clustering, and microbiota from patients with cirrhosis had less marked alpha diversity. Abundances of dominant phyla (Bacteroidetes, Firmicutes and Proteobacteria) were similar. However, patients with cirrhosis had lower abundances of five phyla, namely Tenericutes, Cyanobacteria, Spirochaetes, Elusimicrobia and Lentisphaerae, and differences in abundances of several families and genera than in controls. Lactulose administration did not lead to any change in alpha and beta diversities, species richness and abundances of various bacterial taxa in gut microbiota.

Conclusions: Gut microbiota in cirrhosis differ from healthy persons and do not change following lactulose administration. The latter suggests that the effect of lactulose on hepatic encephalopathy may not be related to alteration in gut microbiota.

Keywords: Cirrhosis, Dysbiosis, Gut microbiota, Hepatic encephalopathy, Lactulose

Background

Cirrhosis is characterized by fibrosis leading to altered liver architecture, resulting in marked reduction in its function and in portal hypertension. Patients with cirrhosis are prone to serious complications, such as variceal gastrointestinal bleeding, hepatic encephalopathy (HE), ascites, spontaneous bacterial peritonitis, hepatorenal syndrome, hepatocellular carcinoma, and an increased mortality.

Normal human gut is inhabited by several microorganisms, in particular bacteria. The number of bacterial cells in the intestinal lumen of an individual is of the order of that of human cells in the body. These bacteria perform several important physiologic functions, such as digestion of complex carbohydrates leading to energy salvage, synthesis of essential substances such as vitamin K, and modulation of mucosal and systemic immune responses [1]. With its strategic placement between the bowel and the systemic circulation, liver acts as a filter and removes any bacteria and their harmful products that may enter the blood from the gut [2]; the loss of this function in patients with cirrhosis may play a role in

* Correspondence: aggarwal.ra@gmail.com
†Equal contributors
[1]Department of Gastroenterology, Sanjay Gandhi Postgraduate Institute of Medical Sciences, Lucknow 226014, India
[2]Biomedical Informatics Center, Sanjay Gandhi Postgraduate Institute of Medical Sciences, Lucknow, India

the occurrence of complications such as spontaneous bacterial peritonitis, sepsis and hepatorenal syndrome [3].

Modulation of gut microbiota using antimicrobial agents [4] and probiotic preparations [5] has been shown to improve HE; this suggests that intestinal bacteria play a role in the causation of HE. Lactulose, a non-absorbable disaccharide, is another drug used for the prevention and treatment of HE. It cannot be digested by human intestinal enzymes, and reaches the colon unchanged where it is degraded by bacteria. It is believed that the resultant acidic environment changes the composition of the gut microbiota [6, 7], with a reduction in the bacteria that produce ammonia and an increase in those that trap and use ammonia for their metabolism [7], ameliorating HE. In fact, in studies using stool culture, lactulose administration has been shown to alter the abundance of certain gut bacteria [8, 9]. However, culture-based techniques have several limitations. In particular, a majority of bacterial species inhabiting the gut can either not be cultured or not be reliably distinguished from other related bacteria. Further, these techniques are only qualitative or, at best, semi-quantitative. Thus, there is a need to study the effect of lactulose on the composition of gut microbiota using better techniques.

In recent years, high-throughput sequencing of gene for bacterial 16S ribosomal RNA has emerged as a useful method for studying the composition of complex bacterial mixtures [10]. These techniques exploit the differences in this gene between various bacteria, such that their sequences accurately identify various bacterial groups, often up to the species level. Further, these techniques can sequence several DNA molecules in parallel, providing data on relative abundance of different bacteria in a mixture. In the current study, we applied high-throughput sequencing to determine whether gut microbiota in patients with cirrhosis differed from those of healthy controls, and whether lactulose treatment leads to a change in the composition of gut microbiota in patients with cirrhosis.

Methods
Subjects
Patients with cirrhosis, irrespective of the cause or severity of liver dysfunction, measured using Child-Turcotte-Pugh (CTP) class, and with no co-existing disease, were enrolled from the outpatient clinic of our institution between October 2013 and April 2014. Diagnosis of cirrhosis was based on a combination of typical clinical, biochemical, endoscopic and radiological findings. Patients who had taken drugs that can influence the gut microbiota, such as gastric acid suppressants, antimicrobial agents, probiotics, non-absorbable disaccharides (such as lactulose) or those that alter gastrointestinal motility, or complementary or alternative medicines, in

the previous 6 weeks, were excluded. Since we also aimed to study the effect of lactulose on gut microbiota, we particularly included those patients who were likely to be prescribed lactulose, as a prophylaxis against HE in view of CTP class B or C disease.

For each patient, one stool specimen was collected at enrollment. For patients who received lactulose, a second specimen was collected after 6 weeks of lactulose administration (in a dose of 30–60 ml/day, adjusted to obtain 2–3 semisolid stools daily); any patient who had worsening of clinical condition, or received another medication or required hospitalization was excluded.

In addition, a group of healthy adult volunteers, with similar age and gender distribution, were recruited as controls from among family members of other patients presenting with minor illnesses (so that they were similar to the patients in terms of socioeconomic status, diet, lifestyle, habits, etc). The prospective control subjects underwent recording of clinical history and a physical examination by a physician, and those with any current symptom/illness or any significant previous illness, and those receiving any drug likely to affect gut microbiota were excluded. Each control subject provided one stool specimen.

The subjects, both patients and controls, collected a stool specimen in a wide-mouthed container at site (in the hospital) and placed it immediately in a box containing cool-packs which had been frozen at –80 °C. The study was approved by the Ethics Committee of Sanjay Gandhi Postgraduate Institute of Medical Sciences, Lucknow and each participant provided informed consent.

Sequencing of gut microbiota
DNA was extracted from approximately 0.5 g of stool using standard phenol-chloroform method, and V3 hypervariable region of 16S rRNA gene was amplified [11]. These primers, in addition to the V3-specific priming sequences, contained sequences complementary to Illumina forward, reverse and multiplex sequencing primers. Different reverse primers, each with a unique six-nucleotide index, were used for different stool specimens to enable multiplexing (Table 1).

Illumina sequencing libraries were prepared using a one-step polymerase chain reaction in a 50-µl reaction mixture that contained 200 ng of input DNA, 6.25 pmol each of forward and reverse primers and KAPA Hi-Fi PCR master mix (Kapa Biosystems, Boston, MA, USA). The PCR conditions were: an initial denaturation at 95 ° C for 5 min, followed by 20 cycles of 95 °C, 65 °C, and 72 °C for 1 min each, and a final extension at 72 °C for 5 min. The amplification products were purified using 2% agarose (in tris-borate-ethylenediaminetetraacetic acid) gel electrophoresis, followed by recovery of amplicons of desired length (GenElute Gel extraction kit;

Table 1 Custom primers used for generation of Illumina DNA libraries

Primer name	Primer nucleotide sequence
V3F	5'-aatgatacggcgaccaccgagatct<u>acactctttccctacacgacgctcttccgatct</u>**NNNN**CCTACGGGAGGCAGCAG-3'
V3R	5'-caagcagaagacggcatacgagat**XXXXX**<u>gtgactggagttcagacgtgtgctcttccgatct</u>ATTACCGCGGCTGCTGG-3'

Lower case letters represent adapter sequences necessary for binding to Illumina flow cell, underlined lowercase letters represent binding site for Illumina sequencing primers, and upper case letters represent V3 region primers (341F on the forward and 518R on the reverse primer). NNNN represents degenerate bases for adding sequence diversity necessary for proper cluster identification by the sequencer, and XXXXXX represents the 6-nucleotide index region for multiplexing

Sigma-Aldrich). Purified libraries were checked for size distribution, quantitated (Agilent Bioanalyser DNA1000) and normalized to 10 nM. The normalized libraries were pooled in sets of 8–12 specimens each and sequenced in one lane of an Illumina HiScan SQ sequencing flow cell using standard 2 X 101-cycle paired-end multiplex sequencing format. Library pool was spiked with 30% Illumina PhiX control library to enhance sequence diversity for efficient base calling. Data were then demultiplexed using Illumina CASAVA software.

Processing of sequence data

The raw reads in opposite directions were merged using PANDAseq software [12], and primer sequences were trimmed out. Sequences shorter than 100 nucleotides, with any ambiguous nucleotide, or with an overlap of fewer than 20 nucleotides in paired reads were purged. The merged reads were subjected to quality control using NGSQC Toolkit [13], to exclude those with average Phred quality score below 30. The selected high-quality reads were processed using Quantitative Insights into Microbial Ecology (QIIME V1.8) software package [14]. Any chimeric sequences, identified using Usearch61, were purged. The remaining reads were assigned to operational taxonomic units (OTUs) using UCLUST-based sub-sampled open-reference OTU picking protocol [15]. A representative sequence for each OTU was aligned with the Greengenes core set alignment using the PyNAST tool [16]; any sequences that failed to align were purged. Based on alignment of the representative OTU sequences, a phylogenetic tree was constructed using the FastTree tool [17]. Taxonomy was assigned to each OTU using the QIIME's UCLUST Consensus Taxonomy Assigner against the Greengenes v13.8 reference OTUs, using the software's default parameters. Thereafter, to reduce noise, OTUs that were observed in fewer than 10% of stool specimens ($n = 5$) or accounted for fewer than 0.002% of reads in all the specimens taken together were purged out. Sample-wise observation count of each OTU was tabulated as an OTU table in 'biom' format. The filtered OTU table was then used for determination of bacterial composition of each sample.

Alpha diversity analysis

OTU table was rarefied, using PhyloSeq [18], to equalize the sampling depth of all the specimens to the one with the fewest reads. For each specimen, alpha diversity was estimated using Chao1 and Abundance-based Coverage Estimator indices, which measure the species richness, and using Shannon and Simpson indices, which measure the richness and distribution of taxa [19]. These indices were compared between groups using the compare_alpha_diversity.py script of QIIME 1.8, with Bonferroni correction.

Beta diversity analysis

The filtered data were assembled into a table where each row represented an OTU and each column represented a faecal specimen. The cells contained observation counts for a particular OTU in a particular specimen, normalized using a log-frequency transformation, as follows:

$$\text{Normalized value} = \text{Log}_{10}\left(\frac{OC}{n} \times \frac{\sum X}{N} + 1\right)$$

Where 'OC' represents the actual observed count of a particular OTU in a specimen, 'n' is the sum of observed counts for all OTUs in the particular specimen, Σx is the sum of 'n' across all specimens in the table and N is the total number of specimens in the table.

Beta diversity was assessed using principal co-ordinate analysis (PCoA) on weighted UniFrac distance matrices generated from the normalized OTU tables.

Comparison of gut microbiota composition between groups

Abundances of various bacterial taxa at different taxonomic levels in patients and controls were compared using Mann-Whitney U test, and those before and after lactulose were compared using paired t test. In either case, Benjamini-Hochberg false discovery rate correction was used to account for multiple comparisons, using $p < 0.05$ as the cut-off.

Cirrhosis-dysbiosis ratio

This ratio, a previously-described quantitative index of microbiota alterations accompanying cirrhosis progression, was computed as the natural log (ln) of the ratio of aggregated abundance of autochthonous (Lachnospiraceae, Ruminococcaceae and Veillonellaceae) and non-autochthonous (Enterobacteriaceae and Bacteroidaceae) taxa [20]. Data from patients and controls were compared using Mann-Whitney U test, and those before and after lactulose using Wilcoxon's signed-rank test.

PICRUSt analysis

Putative metabolic functions of the microbial communities in each specimen were predicted using PICRUSt (Phylogenetic Investigation of Communities by Reconstruction of Unobserved States) [21]. This tool compares the identified 16S rRNA gene sequences with the annotated genome sequences of known species, thereby estimating the possible gene content of a particular microbial community. In brief, OTUs were picked using the closed-reference OTU picking approach at ≥97% identity against the Greengenes database (version 13.5) using QIIME 1.8. The OTU table was then normalized for 16S rRNA gene copy numbers and the corresponding metagenomes were predicted. In addition, the proportions of bacteria that would be expected to contain the glutamine gene, and alpha, beta and gamma subunits of the urease gene were also estimated. Putative metabolic functions of the microbial communities in each specimen were compared between patients and controls using Mann-Whitney U test, and those before and after lactulose were compared using Wilcoxon's signed-rank test.

Statistical analysis

Clinical and laboratory variables were compared between groups using chi-squared test for categorical data, and unpaired t-test or Mann-Whitney U test for numerical data. P values <0.05 were considered significant.

Results

Baseline stool specimens were collected from 35 patients with cirrhosis (median [range] age: 42 [29–65] years; 26 male; body mass index: 22.8 [17.3–32.3] Kg/m^2) and 18 controls (44.5 [24–67] y; male 14; 23.3 [20.0–25.0] Kg/m^2); the clinical and laboratory findings for patients are summarized in Table 2. Thirty of them received regular lactulose administration as a part of standard of care, and 21 of these 30 patients provided repeat stool specimens after lactulose administration for a median of 55 (42–77) days. The baseline characteristics of these 21 patients were similar to those of 14 patients for whom repeat specimens were not available, because they did not receive lactulose, were lost to follow-up, received a proton-pump inhibitor or an antibiotic during the intervening period, or had a clinical worsening or required hospitalization (Additional file 1: Table S1).

The 74 stool specimens studied (18 controls; 35 pre-lactulose and 21 post-lactulose) yielded a total of 40,023,099 high-quality reads (median [range] = 474,267 [131,802–1,267,206]), their rarefaction curves are shown in Additional file 2: Fig. S1.

Table 2 Laboratory parameters and disease severity indices in patients with cirrhosis (n = 35)

Parameter	Value	
Hemoglobin (g/dL) (reference: >13.0)	11.0	(6.6–14.7)
Leucocyte count (×1000/μL) (reference: 4.0–7.0)	4.5	(1.9–9.2)
Platelet count (×1000/μL) (reference: 150–400)	75.0	(22–184)
Serum bilirubin (mg/dL) (reference: <1.2)	2.0	(0.5–8.0)
Serum aspartate transaminase (IU/L) (reference: <40)	68.0	(26–273)
Serum alanine transaminase (IU/L) (reference: <40)	40.0	(17–162)
Serum alkaline phosphatase (IU/L) (reference: <150)	141.0	(36–455)
Serum albumin (g/dL) (reference: 3.5–5.0)	3.4	(2.1–4.5)
Serum creatinine (mg/dL) (reference: <1.2)	0.9	(0.6–1.8)
Prothrombin time (International normalized ratio)	1.3	(0.9–2.8)
Child-Turcotte-Pugh score	7.0	(5–11)
Model for end-stage liver disease (MELD) score	13.0	(6–25)
Cause of liver disease		
Hepatitis C	9	
Hepatitis B	7	
Alcohol	7	
Autoimmune	1	
Cryptogenic	11	
Child-Pugh class		
A	10	(29%)
B	21	(60%)
C	4	(11%)
Clinical history		
Ascites	19	(54%)
Spontaneous bacterial peritonitis	6	(32%)
Hepatic encephalopathy	4	(11%)
Variceal bleed	8	(23%)

Data are shown as median (range) or as number (%)

Gut microbiota in healthy controls versus patients with cirrhosis

The patients and controls were comparable in age, gender distribution, and BMI. All the participants consumed predominantly vegetarian diet.

In PCoA, faecal specimens from patients showed a wider spread than those from control subjects, indicating a more marked intra-group diversity of microbiota among patients. Further, the specimens from controls showed differential clustering than those from patients with cirrhosis (Fig. 1a). The patient specimens also showed lower alpha diversity and species richness than those from controls (Fig. 1b, Additional file 3: Table S2).

Median [range] number of high-quality reads for 18 controls and 35 baseline cirrhosis specimens were 407,482 (316,749–1,139,360; total reads 9,388,696) and 504,182 (131,802–1,267,206; total 19,466,867), respectively. These reads belonged to 16,357 non-singleton OTUs. Of these, 855 OTUs belonging to 11 phyla were identified in at least five specimens each and formed >0.002% of the total reads, and were analyzed further. Abundances of the dominant phyla, namely Bacteroidetes (71.91% [0.11–90.01] vs 66.82% [30.35–88.99]), Firmicutes (21.95% [6.95–74.56] vs. 18.65% [3.95–43.47]) and Proteobacteria (4.37% [0.61–50.64] vs. 8.20% [1.34–48.35]) were comparable in patients and controls. However, five phyla, namely Tenericutes [0% vs 0.07%], Cyanobacteria [0% vs 0.53%], Spirochaetes [0.00065% vs 0.0014%], Elusimicrobia [0% vs 0.0013%] and Lentisphaerae [0% vs 0.007%] were less abundant in patients than in controls (Benjamini-Hochberg corrected p-values <0.05 for each) (Fig. 2a, Additional File 4: Table S3). Similarly, some specific classes, orders, families and genera had significantly different abundances in patients and controls (Fig. 2b; Additional file 5: Figure S2a, S2b and S2c; Additional file 4: Table S3).

Cirrhosis-dysbiosis ratio was significantly lower in patients with cirrhosis than in controls (1.55 ± 1.86 versus 2.71 ± 1.48; p = 0.019, Mann-Whitney U test). The abundances of bacteria that are predicted to contain the glutaminase gene or genes for alpha, beta or gamma subunits of urease were more widely distributed and

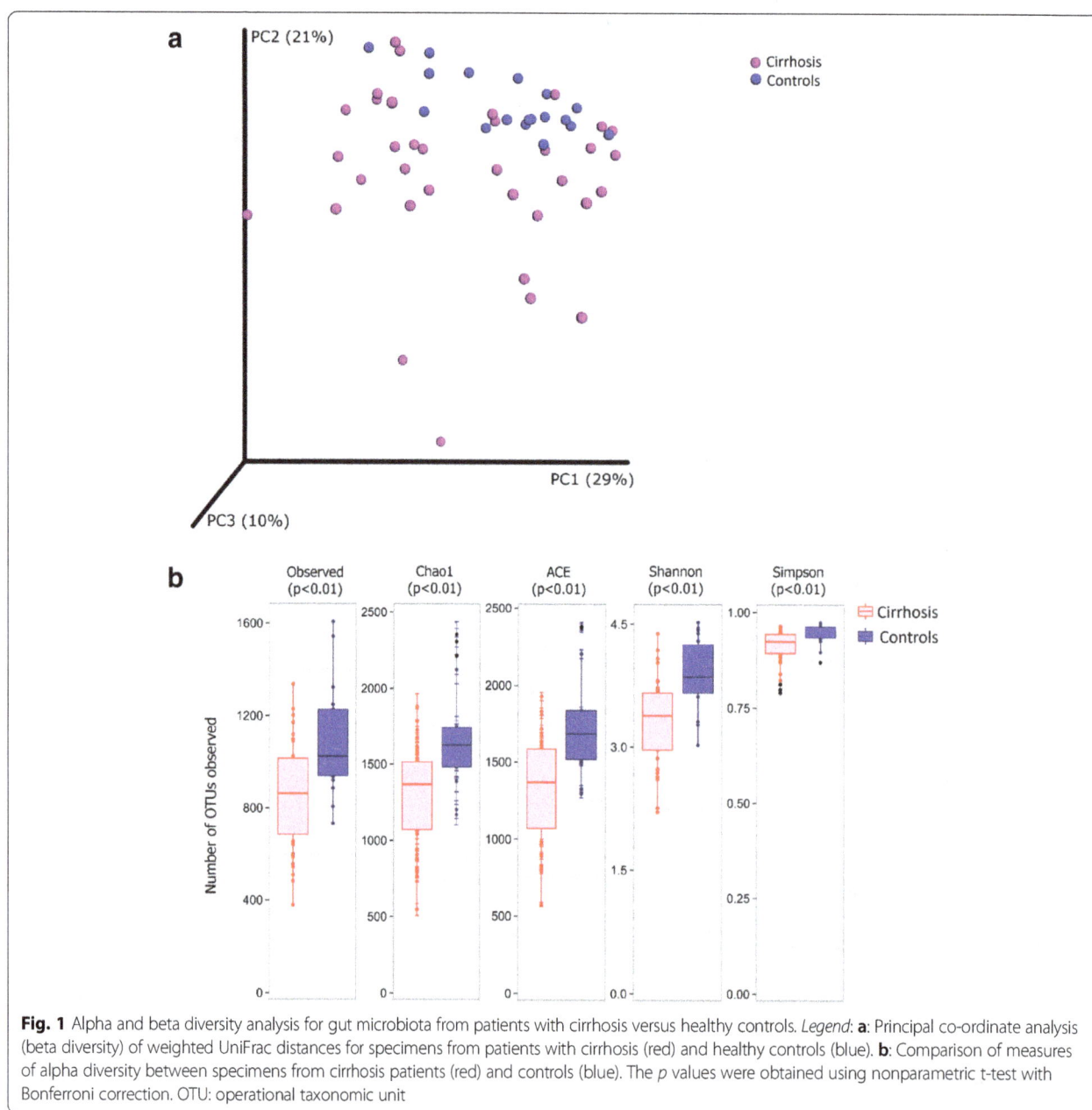

Fig. 1 Alpha and beta diversity analysis for gut microbiota from patients with cirrhosis versus healthy controls. *Legend*: **a**: Principal co-ordinate analysis (beta diversity) of weighted UniFrac distances for specimens from patients with cirrhosis (red) and healthy controls (blue). **b**: Comparison of measures of alpha diversity between specimens from cirrhosis patients (red) and controls (blue). The p values were obtained using nonparametric t-test with Bonferroni correction. OTU: operational taxonomic unit

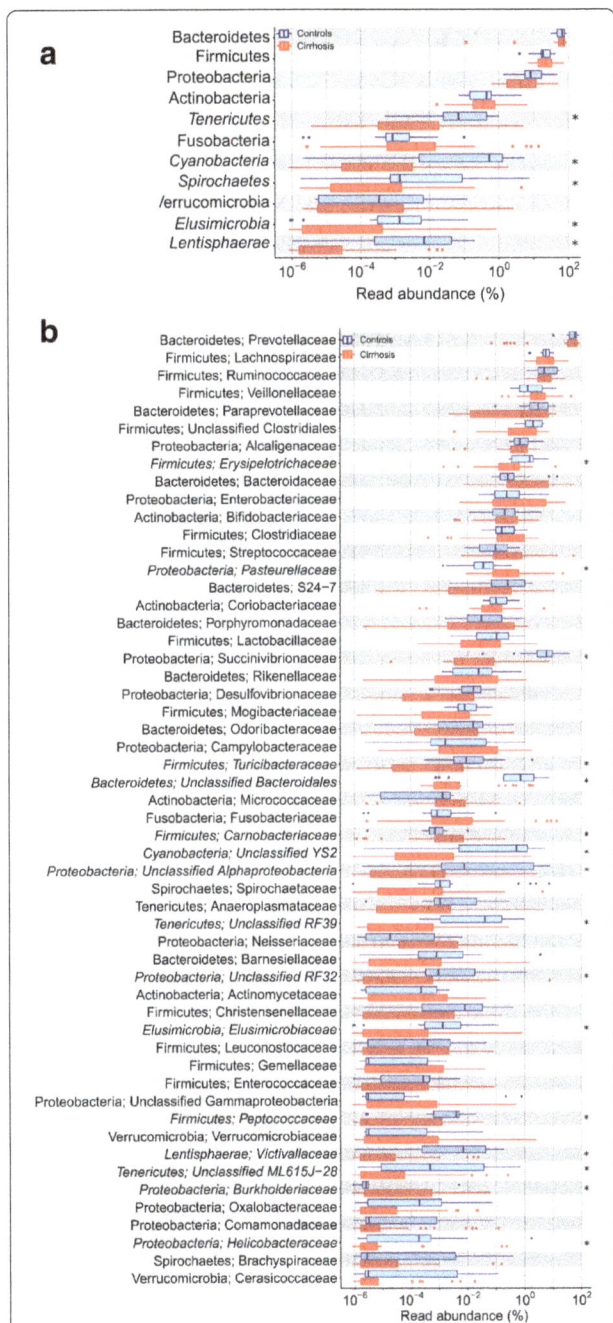

Fig. 2 Abundances of various bacterial phyla and families among gut microbiota in cirrhosis and controls. *Legend:* **a**: Abundances of various phyla in patients with cirrhosis (red) and healthy controls (blue). **b**: Abundances of selected families in patients with cirrhosis (red) and healthy controls (blue). All data are shown using box-plots (25th to 75th percentiles) and percent values on a $\log_{10}$ scale. Any dots to the left or right of the boxes indicate outliers. Asterix marks indicate values with significant difference between patients and controls ($p < 0.05$; Mann-Whitney U test with Benjamini-Hochberg correction

somewhat higher in patients than in controls (Fig. 3), but the inter-group comparisons did not show a significant difference (Fig. 3).

Gut microbiota in patients with liver cirrhosis before and after lactulose use

Paired stool specimens, before and after lactulose, were available for 21 patients (median age: 45 [29–64] years; male 13; Child-Pugh class A: 7, B: 13, C: 1). Median [range] number of high-quality reads in their specimens before and after lactulose were similar (465,630 [131,802–1,231,311] versus 446,762 [159,321–1,022,517]). On PCoA, the distributions of data points for specimens collected before or after lactulose overlapped. Data points for specimens collected before and after lactulose for individual subjects were located close to each other (Fig. 4a); the weighted UniFrac distances between paired specimens were smaller than those between individual pre-lactulose specimens (Fig. 4b). None of the indices of alpha diversity showed a significant change following lactulose (Fig. 4c).

High-quality reads from the 42 paired specimens belonged to 15,209 non-singleton OTUs; of these, 741 OTUs which were identified in at least 10% specimens (four specimens) each and formed >0.002% of the total

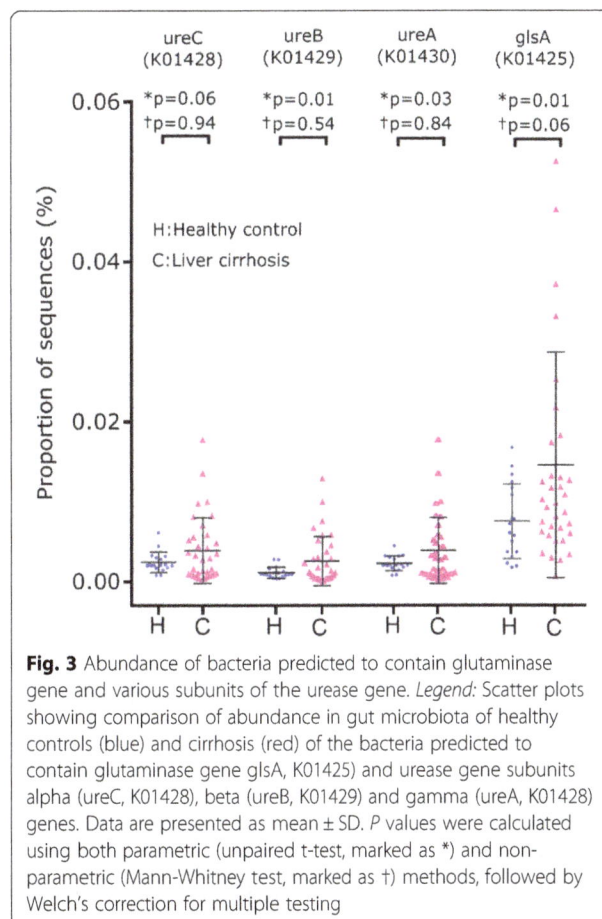

Fig. 3 Abundance of bacteria predicted to contain glutaminase gene and various subunits of the urease gene. *Legend:* Scatter plots showing comparison of abundance in gut microbiota of healthy controls (blue) and cirrhosis (red) of the bacteria predicted to contain glutaminase gene glsA, K01425) and urease gene subunits alpha (ureC, K01428), beta (ureB, K01429) and gamma (ureA, K01428) genes. Data are presented as mean ± SD. *P* values were calculated using both parametric (unpaired t-test, marked as *) and non-parametric (Mann-Whitney test, marked as †) methods, followed by Welch's correction for multiple testing

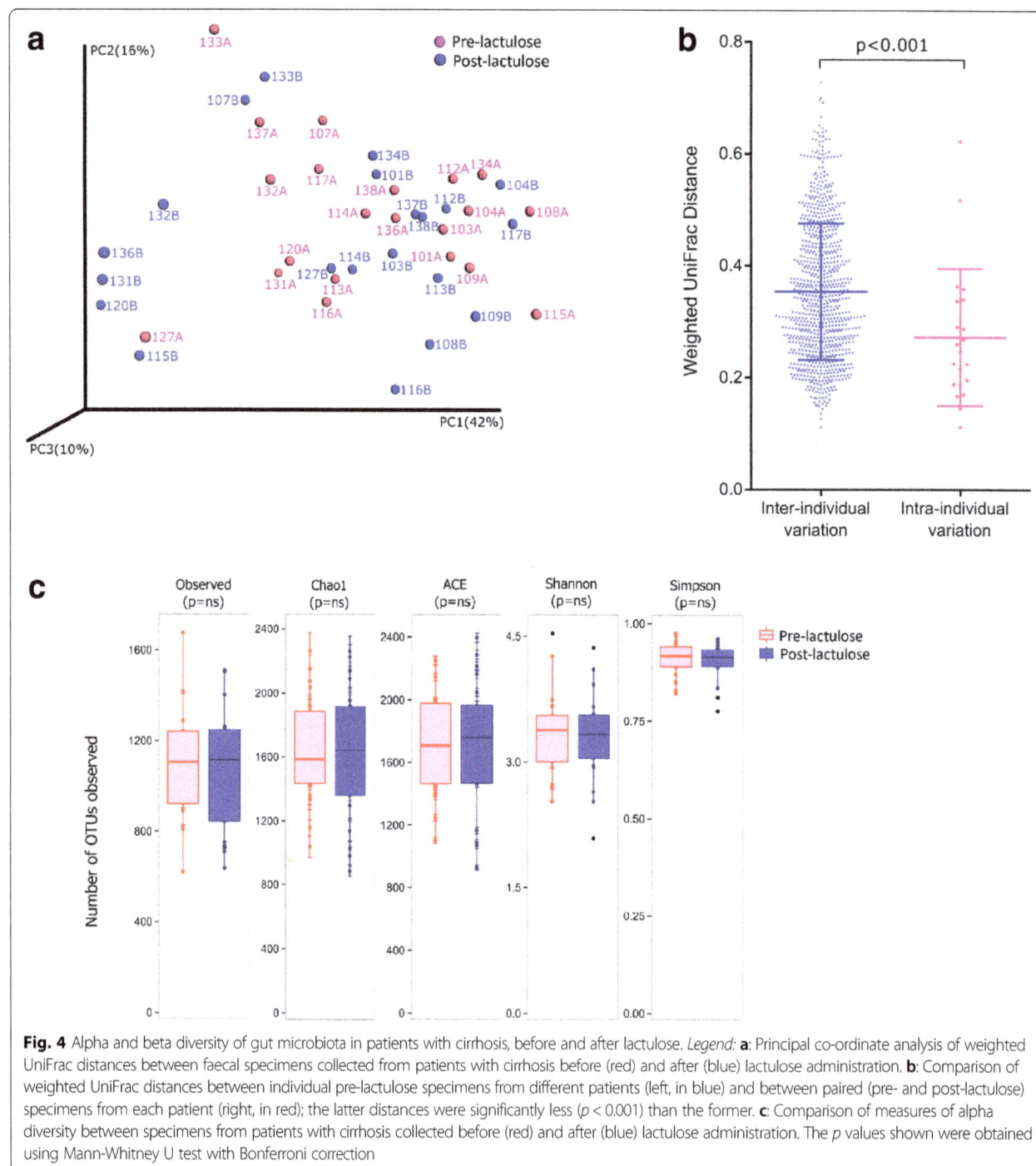

Fig. 4 Alpha and beta diversity of gut microbiota in patients with cirrhosis, before and after lactulose. *Legend:* **a**: Principal co-ordinate analysis of weighted UniFrac distances between faecal specimens collected from patients with cirrhosis before (red) and after (blue) lactulose administration. **b**: Comparison of weighted UniFrac distances between individual pre-lactulose specimens from different patients (left, in blue) and between paired (pre- and post-lactulose) specimens from each patient (right, in red); the latter distances were significantly less ($p < 0.001$) than the former. **c**: Comparison of measures of alpha diversity between specimens from patients with cirrhosis collected before (red) and after (blue) lactulose administration. The p values shown were obtained using Mann-Whitney U test with Bonferroni correction

reads were analysed further. The abundances of four major phyla were similar in the specimens collected before and after lactulose, namely Bacteroidetes (75.55% [2.86–84.49] versus 61.79% [3.16–90.99]), Firmicutes (20.27% [6.93–74.93] versus 21.72% [4.62–86.93]), Proteobacteria (4.37% [1.08–20.37] versus 6.82% [1.27–25.45]) and Actinobacteria (0.33% [0.02–6.74] versus 0.87% [0.03–11.92]). Further, no difference was found in abundances of various phyla, classes, orders, families or

genera between the specimens collected before and after lactulose (Fig. 5a and b; Additional file 6: Figure S3a, S3b and S3c).

Cirrhosis-dysbiosis ratios of faecal specimens before and after lactulose were similar (1.75 ± 1.98 and 2.01 ± 1.70, respectively; $p = 0.337$). The abundances of bacteria predicted to contain genes for glutaminase, or genes for alpha, beta or gamma subunits of urease gene also did not change after lactulose (Fig. 6).

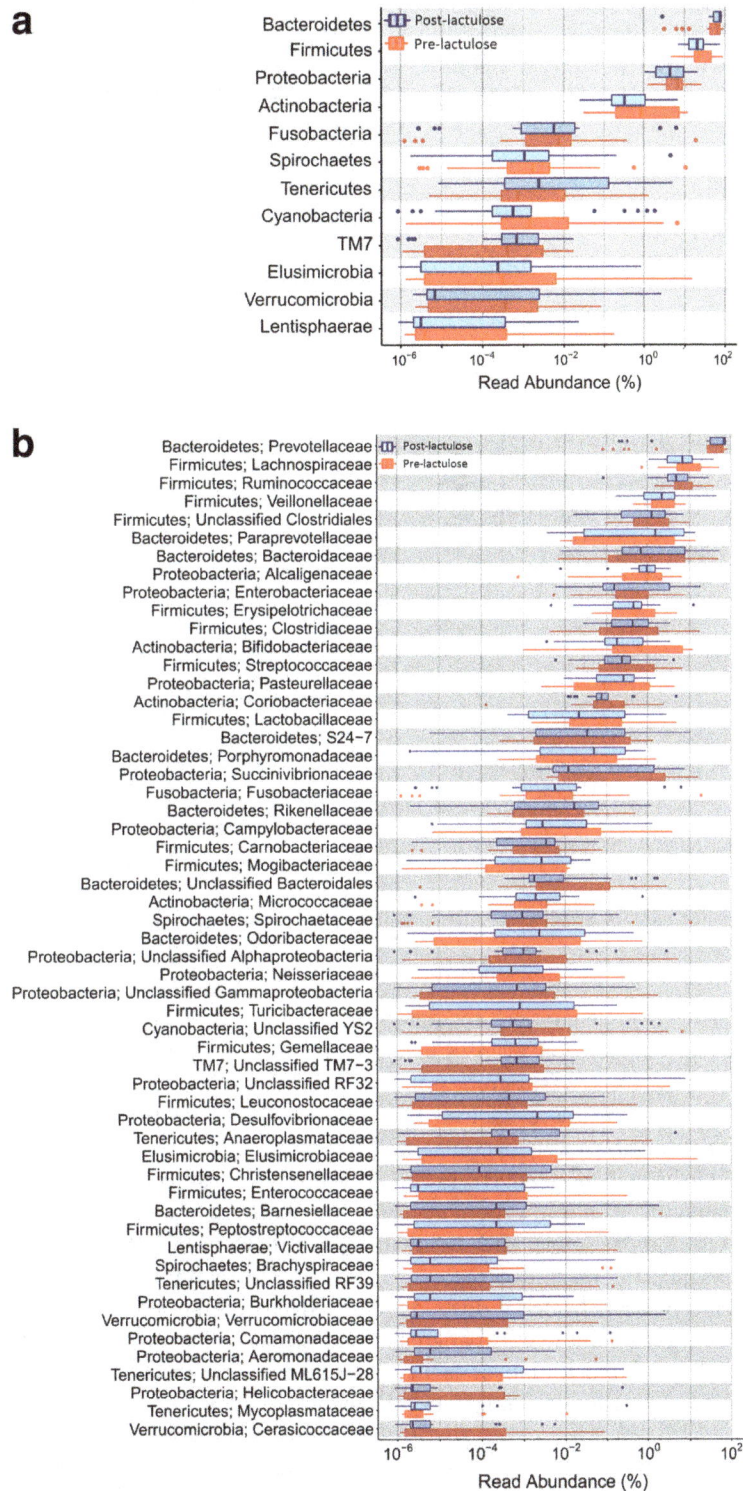

Fig. 5 Abundances of various bacterial groups in gut microbiota before and after lactulose administration. *Legend:* Abundances of various bacterial groups among gut microbiota from in patients with liver cirrhosis before (red) and after lactulose (blue) at phylum (**a**) and family (**b**) levels. Data are shown using box-plots (25th to 75th percentiles) and percent values on a log$_{10}$ scale. Any dots to the left or right of the boxes indicate outliers. No bacterial groups showed a significant difference (p value cut-off = 0.05; paired t test with Benjamini-Hochberg correction)

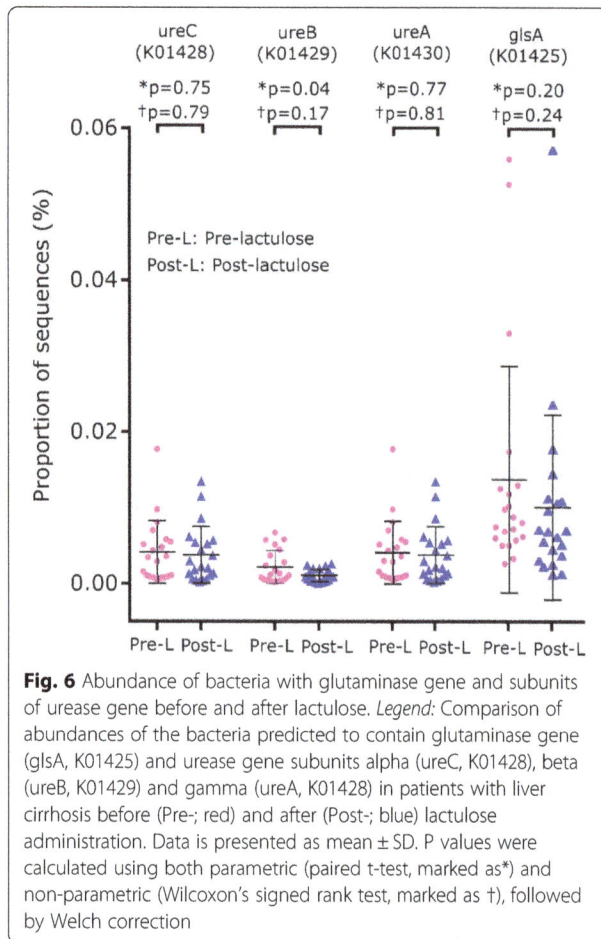

Fig. 6 Abundance of bacteria with glutaminase gene and subunits of urease gene before and after lactulose. *Legend:* Comparison of abundances of the bacteria predicted to contain glutaminase gene (glsA, K01425) and urease gene subunits alpha (ureC, K01428), beta (ureB, K01429) and gamma (ureA, K01428) in patients with liver cirrhosis before (Pre-; red) and after (Post-; blue) lactulose administration. Data is presented as mean ± SD. P values were calculated using both parametric (paired t-test, marked as*) and non-parametric (Wilcoxon's signed rank test, marked as †), followed by Welch correction

Discussion

Using a culture-independent, next-generation sequencing technique, we found that composition of intestinal microbiota in patients with cirrhosis was significantly different from that in healthy persons, as evidenced by differential clustering of patients and healthy persons on PCoA. The patients with cirrhosis had relatively lower abundances of bacteria belonging to phyla Tenericutes, Cyanobacteria, Spirochaetes, Elusimicrobia and Lentisphaerae, and to some specific families and genera. In addition, their gut microbiota had less bacterial diversity and species richness. Further, gut microbiota in patients with cirrhosis before and after administration of lactulose for 6 weeks, showed no difference in composition or diversity.

Healthy human intestine, contains several bacterial species, with a fair degree of inter-individual diversity [21]. For instance, in a study of 124 European individuals, though their faecal specimens taken together harboured between 1000 and 1150 bacterial species, each individual specimen was found to contain only about 160 bacterial species. Several species were shared across individuals, with nearly 75 being common to more than

half the subjects; however, the other species were highly variable between individuals. In most people, nearly 90% of the gut bacteria belong to two phyla – Bacteroidetes and Firmicutes, whereas the remaining belong mostly to phyla Proteobacteria, Actinobacteria, Verrucomicrobia and Fusobacteria [22]. The mixture of bacteria and other organisms (such as archaea and fungi) present in an individual's gut – collectively referred to as the 'gut microbiota' – behaves as a metabolic organ and plays an intimate role in regulation and maintenance of normal physiology, metabolism and immune functions. In recent years, changes in gut microbiota – the so-called gut 'dysbiosis' – has been implicated in the pathogenesis of several diseases, such as hepatic and gastrointestinal diseases [3], obesity [23], diabetes mellitus [24] and hypertension [25].

We found a difference in the profile of gut microbiota in patients with cirrhosis and healthy persons, as shown by differential clustering on PCoA. Further, the patients with cirrhosis had less diverse gut microbiota than healthy persons. Previous studies, based on sequencing of V2 region of 16S rRNA gene [26] and quantitative metagenomics [27] have also shown a trend towards reduction of bacterial diversity and of bacterial gene richness, respectively, in patients with cirrhosis from other geographic regions. Reduced microbial diversity has also been reported in patients with many diseases, including Crohn's disease [28], obesity, insulin resistance and dyslipidemia [29]. The mechanism underlying this reduced diversity of gut bacteria in human disease remains unknown. It is possible that this reduced bacterial diversity is associated with the absence of some specific bacteria, producing a metabolic imbalance due to the unopposed action of the other bacteria.

Despite a difference in the overall composition of gut microbiota in patients with cirrhosis compared to healthy persons, the most abundant phyla in the two group were similar, i.e. Bacteroidetes, Firmicutes and Proteobacteria. Results of the previous studies on this subject have been conflicting. In two of the three previous studies from China, with 98 and 36 patients, respectively, the abundance of Bacteroidetes was reduced, and those of Proteobacteria and Fusobacteria were increased in cirrhosis [27, 30], whereas the third study with 26 patients showed no difference in phylum-level abundances [26]. At lower taxonomic levels, we found that abundances of several bacterial families and genera differed in cirrhosis patients from those in healthy persons, as has been reported previously [31]. However, the bacterial taxa showing such difference in our study were different from those reported in the previous Chinese studies. These differences between studies could be related to differences in several factors, e.g. (i) prevalent microbiota in healthy Chinese and Indian population;

(ii) cause of liver disease, with hepatitis B being commoner in China; (iii) dietary habits in the two countries; (iv) severity of liver disease; and, (v) techniques for specimen processing and data analysis between studies.

In particular, we found that abundances of the bacterial groups which are involved in nitrogen metabolism and possess the capability to produce ammonia did not show any difference between the patients and controls. Such a comparison has not been reported previously. This finding suggests that even though the gut microbiota in patients with cirrhosis differs from that in healthy persons, this alteration may not impact the production of nitrogenous substances, which may play a role in causation of HE.

Lactulose is extensively used for the treatment of HE in several parts of the world. On reaching the colon, lactulose is broken down by colonic bacteria (primarily bifidobacteria, lactobacilli and streptococci) into lactic acid, acetic acid and other short-chain fatty acids. Several mechanisms have been proposed for the beneficial effects of lactulose in HE, including (i) its laxative action which reduces the contact time between luminal contents and the intestinal mucosa, reducing the absorption of ammonia; (ii) creation of an acidic environment in the colonic lumen, which traps ammonia by enhancing its conversion into polar and less-absorbable ammonium ions; and, (iii) change in the composition of colonic microbiota, with reduced density of bacteria that produce ammonia and an increased density of those that utilize ammonia for their metabolism [32, 33].

Data on the effect of lactulose on gut microbiota are quite scanty and conflicting [8, 34, 35]. In previous studies, lactulose was shown to facilitate the growth of acidophilic, urease-deficient bacteria, such as lactobacilli and bifidobacteria, in the colon [8, 36]. Another study reported an increase in the number of anaerobic lactobacilli and a decrease in that of Bacteroides spp. after lactulose [37]. However, in yet another study, no association was found between clinical improvement following lactulose and reduction in the number of ammonia-producing bacteria [9]. However, all these studies were based on stool culture, a technique with several inherent limitations, such as the failure of a large majority of colonic bacteria to grow in vitro, and an inability to reliably distinguish between various bacterial groups or to provide a quantitative measure of the relative abundance of various species in a bacterial mixture.

High-throughput 16S rRNA sequencing has a major advantage in that it not only permits accurate species-level identification of various bacterial species present in a complex mixture, but also estimates their relative abundances. This technique has not previously been used to assess the effect of lactulose on intestinal microbiota. Our study, using this technique, failed to show any change in gut microbiota after lactulose

administration. This lack of effect was found on analysis at different levels of phylogenetic organization, i.e. from phylum to species level. Further, we also did not find any change in the alpha diversity of the gut microbiota, or of the abundance of bacteria that can produce ammonia. This indicates that the beneficial effect of lactulose on HE may not be related to a change in the composition of gut microbiota, and may instead be mediated by another mechanism. Our findings support a recent report in which Bajaj et al. [38] found no major change, except for a reduction in the abundance in Faecalibacterium spp. (from 6% to 1%), in gut microbiota 14 days after lactulose withdrawal in seven patients with cirrhosis. In our study, bacteria belonging to this genus had an abundance of ~0.1% in both pre- and post-lactulose specimens, with no change after lactulose. Furthermore, we observed a closer similarity of paired (before and after lactulose) specimens from each individual with each other than with specimens from other patients collected at a similar time point; this too supports the conclusion that lactulose did not have a major effect on gut microbiota.

In a recent randomized controlled study, Rahimi et al. compared the effect of lactulose on HE with that of polyethylene glycol, which has a laxative effect but is not expected to alter the gut microbiota. They found the two treatments to be equally effective. This is in consonance with our finding that the effect of lactulose is not mediated by a modulation of gut microbiota and may be related simply to its laxative action [39].

Our data have some limitations. First, we used faecal specimens to study the gut microbiota. Bacterial composition of faeces may differ somewhat from luminal contents of the colon, particularly in the proximal colon, where most of the ammonia or other toxic substances may be produced [40]. However, sampling the colonic luminal contents, e.g., using an endoscope, requires prior cleansing of the gut, which would disrupt the luminal microbiota per se. Second, the diet of patients with cirrhosis may differ from that in healthy persons; this may by itself influence the gut microbiota [41]. Also, alcohol consumption is known to alter gut microbiota [42]. To obviate this, we excluded persons with recent alcohol intake from our study. Third, our study included patients with liver disease of varied causes and severity; this variability may have limited its ability to detect differences between patients with liver cirrhosis and controls. To obviate this problem, it may be useful in the future studies to include a more homogeneous patient group. And, finally, it may be argued that the number of patients in whom we studied the effect of lactulose on gut microbiota was small. However, this component of our study had a paired design, in which each patient serves as his own control, with a higher sensitivity for detecting even minor changes. Also, on a positive note, we ensured that the dose and duration of lactulose administration were adequate.

It would have been interesting to compare the gut flora in patients developing HE despite lactulose treatment versus those who did not develop this complication. However, this was not possible since we did not encounter HE in any of our patients receiving lactulose.

Finally, our data do not rule out the possibility that lactulose may affect the balance of production and utilization of ammonia without changing the species composition of gut microbiota. For instance, lactulose or one of its breakdown products could alter the expression or activity of enzymes in one or more bacterial species without affecting their density or number. The 16S rRNA gene sequencing technique which we used is not able to pick up such changes. This aspect may be studied further in future studies using either shot-gun sequencing of gut bacterial transcriptome or using a metabolomic analysis of fecal water or urine.

Conclusion

In conclusion, our data indicate that intestinal bacterial microbiota in patients with cirrhosis is different from that in healthy persons; however, whether these changes are primary or are a consequence of liver disease remains unclear. Lactulose administration does not lead to any change in the nature and relative abundance of various bacteria resident in human colon. This suggests that the effect of this drug on HE is possibly mediated by mechanisms other than a change in the composition of gut microbiota.

Additional files

Additional file 1: Table S1. Comparison of cirrhosis patients who provided paired stool specimens and those who did not provide a post-lactulose specimen. Numerical data are expressed as median (range) and have been compared using Mann-Whitney U test; categorical data are expressed as numbers or proportions and have been compared using Fisher's exact test. (DOC 36 kb)

Additional file 2: Fig. S1. Results of rarefaction analysis of 16S rRNA sequence reads from 74 stool specimens included in the study. OTUs, operational taxonomic units; the color of each line represents the source of the corresponding specimen. (TIFF 803 kb)

Additional file 3: Table S2. Measures of alpha diversity for gut flora in stool specimens from patients with liver cirrhosis and healthy controls. (DOC 118 kb)

Additional file 4: Table S3. Comparison of abundances of various bacterial groups at different levels of taxonomy (phyla, classes, orders, genera and species). The rows for groups showing significant differences (after Benjamini-Hochberg correction) are shaded pink. (DOC 289 kb)

Additional file 5: Figure S2. Comparison of abundances of different bacteria in gut microbiota, between healthy controls and liver cirrhosis, at the level of class (a), order (b) and genus (c). Data are shown using boxplots and percent values on a log10 scale. Asterix marks and italic font point to the groups where the values for patients and controls showed significant differences. (TIFF 4056 kb)

Additional file 6: Figure S3. Comparison of abundances of gut microbiome bacteria, in patients with liver cirrhosis before and after 6 weeks of lactulose use, at the level of (a) class (b) order and (c) genus on a log10 scale. None of the bacterial groups showed any significant difference. (TIFF 6332 kb)

Abbreviations
CPT: Child-Turcotte-Pugh; HE: Hepatic encephalopathy; PCoA: Principal co-ordinate analysis

Acknowledgements
The Biomedical Informatics Center at the authors' institution is supported by the Indian Council of Medical Research (ICMR), New Delhi.

Funding
This work was supported by a grant from the Department of Biotechnology, Government of India. Award number: BT/PR4642/Med/29/630/20127.

Authors' contributions
Study concept and design RA, AG: Acquisition of data: RA, AG, AS2, AS3 Analysis and interpretation of data: RA, AS1, AG,AS2,AS3 Drafting of the manuscript RA, AG, AS1 Critical revision of the manuscript for important intellectual content: RA, AG,AS2,AS3 Statistical analysis: RA, AS1, AG Study supervision: RA, AG Approval of the final manuscript: RA,AG,AS1,AS2,AS3.

Competing interest
The authors declare that they have no competing interests.

References
1. Sekirov I, Russell SL, Antunes LC, Finlay BB. Gut microbiota in health and disease. Physiol Rev. 2010;90:859–904.
2. Gao B, JeongWI TZ. Liver: an organ with predominant innate immunity. Hepatology. 2008;47:729–36.
3. Goel A, Gupta M, Aggarwal R. Gut microbiota and liver disease. J Gastroenterol Hepatol. 2014;29:1139–48.
4. Bass NM, Mullen KD, Sanyal A, Poordad F, Neff G, Leevy CB, et al. Rifaximin treatment in hepatic encephalopathy. N Engl J Med. 2010;362:1071–81.
5. Saab S, Suraweera D, Au J, Saab E, Alper T, Tong MJ. Probiotics are helpful in hepatic encephalopathy: a meta-analysis of randomized trials. Liver Int. 2016;36:986–93.
6. Chen C, Li L, Wu Z, Chen H, Fu S. Effects of lactitol on intestinal microflora and plasma endotoxin in patients with chronic viral hepatitis. J Inf Secur. 2007;54:98–102.
7. Mortensen PB. The effect of oral-administered lactulose on colonic nitrogen metabolism and excretion. Hepatology. 1992;16:1350–6.
8. Riggio O, Varriale M, Testore GP, Di Rosa R, Di Rosa E, Merli M, et al. Effect of lactitol and lactulose administration on the fecal flora in cirrhotic patients. J Clin Gastroenterol. 1990;12:433–6.

9. Vince A, Zeegen R, Drinkwater JE, O'Grady F, Dawson AM. The effect of lactulose on the faecal flora of patients with hepatic encephalopathy. J Med Microbiol. 1974;7:163–8.

10. Fraher MH, O'Toole PW, Quigley EM. Techniques used to characterize the gut microbiota: a guide for the clinician. Nat Rev Gastroenterol Hepatol. 2012;9:312–22.

11. Bartram AK, Lynch MD, Stearns JC, Moreno-Hagelsieb G, Neufeld JD. Generation of multimillion-sequence 16S rRNA gene libraries from complex microbial communities by assembling paired-end illumina reads. Appl Environ Microbiol. 2011;77:3846–52.

12. Masella AP, BartramAK TJM, Brown DG. Neufeld JD PANDAseq: paired-end assembler for illumina sequences. BMC Bioinformatics. 2012;13:31.

13. Dai M, Thompson RC, Maher C, Contreras-Galindo R, Kaplan MH, Markovitz DM, et al. NGSQC: cross-platform quality analysis pipeline for deep sequencing data. BMC Genomics. 2010;11(Suppl 4):S7.

14. Navas-Molina JA, Peralta-Sanchez JM, Gonzalez A, McMurdie PJ, Vazquez-Baeza Y, Xu Z, et al. Advancing our understanding of the human microbiome using QIIME. Methods Enzymol. 2013;531:371–444.

15. Rideout JR, He Y, Navas-Molina JA, Walters WA, Ursell LK, Gibbons SM, et al. Subsampled open-reference clustering creates consistent, comprehensive OTU definitions and scales to billions of sequences. PeerJ. 2014;2:e545.

16. Caporaso JG, Bittinger K, Bushman FD, DeSantis TZ, Andersen GL, Knight R. PyNAST: a flexible tool for aligning sequences to a template alignment. Bioinformatics. 2010;26:266–7.

17. Price MN, Dehal PS, Arkin AP. FastTree 2–approximately maximum-likelihood trees for large alignments. PLoS One. 2010;5:e9490.

18. McMurdie PJ, Holmes S. Phyloseq: an R package for reproducible interactive analysis and graphics of microbiome census data. PLoS One. 2013;8:e61217.

19. Gotelli NJ, Anne C. Measuring and estimating species richness, species diversity, and biotic similarity from sampling data. In: Levin SA, editor. Encyclopedia of biodiversity. 2nd ed. Waltham, MA: Academic Press; 2013. p. 195–211.

20. Bajaj JS, Heuman DM, Hylemon PB, Sanyal AJ, White MB, Monteith P, et al. Altered profile of human gut microbiome is associated with cirrhosis and its complications. J Hepatol. 2014;60:940–7.

21. Ley RE, Peterson DA, Gordon JI. Ecological and evolutionary forces shaping microbial diversity in the human intestine. Cell. 2006;124:837–48.

22. Qin J, Li R, Raes J, Arumugam M, Burgdorf KS, Manichanh C, et al. A human gut microbial gene catalogue established by metagenomic sequencing. Nature. 2010;464:59–65.

23. Turnbaugh PJ, Hamady M, Yatsunenko T, Cantarel BL, Duncan A, Ley RE, et al. A core gut microbiome in obese and lean twins. Nature. 2009;457:480–4.

24. Qin J, Li Y, Cai Z, Li S, Zhu J, Zhang F, et al. A metagenome-wide association study of gut microbiota in type 2 diabetes. Nature. 2012;490:55–60.

25. Yang T, Santisteban MM, Rodriguez V, Li E, Ahmari N, Carvajal JM, et al. Gut dysbiosis is linked to hypertension. Hypertension. 2015;65:1331–40.

26. Zhang Z, Zhai H, Geng J, Yu R, Ren H, Fan H, et al. Large-scale survey of gut microbiota associated with MHE via 16S rRNA-based pyrosequencing. Am J Gastroenterol. 2013;108:1601–11.

27. Qin N, Yang F, Li A, Prifti E, Chen Y, Shao L, et al. Alterations of the human gut microbiome in liver cirrhosis. Nature. 2014;513:59–64.

28. Manichanh C, Rigottier-Gois L, Bonnaud E, Gloux K, Pelletier E, Frangeul L, et al. Reduced diversity of faecal microbiota in Crohn's disease revealed by a metagenomic approach. Gut. 2006;55:205–11.

29. Le Chatelier E, Nielsen T, Qin J, Prifti E, Hildebrand F, Falony G, et al. Richness of human gut microbiome correlates with metabolic markers. Nature. 2013;500:541–6.

30. Chen Y, Yang F, Lu H, Wang B, Chen Y, Lei D, et al. Characterization of fecal microbial communities in patients with liver cirrhosis. Hepatology. 2011;54:562–72.

31. Bajaj JS. The role of microbiota in hepatic encephalopathy. Gut Microbes. 2014;5:397–403.

32. Elkington SG. Lactulose. Gut. 1970;11:1043–8.

33. Avery GS, Davies EF, Brogden RN. Lactulose: a review of its therapeutic and pharmacological properties with particular reference to ammonia metabolism and its mode of action of portal systemic encephalopathy. Drugs. 1972;4:7–48.

34. Macgillivray PC, Finlay HV, Binns TB. Use of lactulose to create a preponderance of lactobacilli in the intestine of bottle-fed infants. Scott Med J. 1959;4:182–9.

35. Elkington SG, Floch MH, Conn HO. Lactulose in the treatment of chronic portal-systemic encephalopathy. A double-blind clinical trial. N Engl J Med. 1969;281:408–12.

36. Conn HO, Floch MH. Effects of lactulose and lactobacillus acidophilus on the fecal flora. Am J Clin Nutr. 1970;23:1588–94.

37. Bircher J, Scollo-Lavizzari G, Hoffmann K, Haemmerli UP. Treatment of chronic porto-systemic encephalopathy with lactulose. Schweiz Med Wochenschr. 1969;99:584.

38. Bajaj JS, Ridlon JM, Hylemon PB, Thacker LR, Heuman DM, Smith S, et al. Linkage of gut microbiome with cognition in hepatic encephalopathy. Am J Physiol Gastrointest Liver Physiol. 2012;302:G168–75.

39. Rahimi RS, Singal AG, Cuthbert JA, Rockey DC. Lactulose vs polyethylene glycol 3350–electrolyte solution for treatment of overt hepatic encephalopathy: the HELP randomized clinical trial. JAMA Intern Med. 2014;174:1727–33.

40. Bajaj JS, Hylemon PB, Ridlon JM, Heuman DM, Daita K, White MB, et al. Colonic mucosal microbiome differs from stool microbiome in cirrhosis and hepatic encephalopathy and is linked to cognition and inflammation. Am J Physiol Gastrointest Liver Physiol. 2012;303:G675–85.

41. Xu Z, Knight R. Dietary effects on human gut microbiome diversity. Br J Nutr. 2015;113(Suppl):S1–5.

42. Mutlu EA, Gillevet PM, Rangwala H, Sikaroodi M, Naqvi A, Engen PA, et al. Colonic microbiome is altered in alcoholism. Am J Physiol Gastrointest Liver Physiol. 2012;302:G966–78.

12

Epidemiology of Paediatric constipation in Indonesia and its association with exposure to stressful life events

Hanifah Oswari[1]*[iD], Fatima Safira Alatas[1], Badriul Hegar[1], William Cheng[1], Arnesya Pramadyani[1], Marc Alexander Benninga[2] and Shaman Rajindrajith[3]

Abstract

Background: We aimed to study the epidemiology and risk factors, including exposure to emotional stress, for constipation in Indonesian children and adolescents of 10–17 year age group.

Methods: A cross-sectional survey using a validated, self-administered questionnaire was conducted in randomly selected children and adolescents in nine state junior high schools from five districts of Jakarta. All of them were from urban areas. Constipation was defined as a diagnosis by using the Rome III criteria.

Results: Of 1796 children included in the analysis, 328 (18.3%; 95% CI 016–0.2) had constipation. Females and those residing in North Jakarta showed risks associated with constipation in school-age children and adolescents. Symptoms independently associated with constipation were abdominal pain (64% vs 43.3% of control) and straining (22.9% vs 6.3%). The prevalence of constipation was significantly higher in those with stressful life events such as father's alcoholism (adjusted OR 1.91, 95% CI 1.27–2.89, $P = 0.002$), severe illness of a close family member (adjusted OR 1.77, 95% CI 1.12–2.80, $P = 0.014$), hospitalization of the child for another illness (adjusted OR 1.68, 95% CI 1.22–2.31, $P < 0.001$), being bullied at school (adjusted OR 1.67, 95% CI 1.01–2.76, $P = 0.047$) and loss of a parent's job (adjusted OR 1.39, 95% CI 1.03–1.88, $P = 0.034$).

Conclusions: Constipation in children and adolescent is a significant health problem, affecting almost 20% of Indonesian school-age children and adolescents. Common school and home related stressful life events appear to have predisposed these children to develop constipation.

Keywords: Functional constipation, Prevalence, Risk factor, Symptom, Children, Adolescent

Background

Childhood constipation is considered to be an emerging global public health problem [1]. The prevalence varies among countries from 0.7 to 29.6% [2, 3]. It is estimated that approximately one third of children with constipation suffer from psychological maladjustment [4]. In addition, childhood constipation leads to significant healthcare costs and poor health-related quality of life [5–8]. The aetiology of constipation in children and young adults is not clear. Studies suggest that psychological stress, childhood maltreatment and abnormal childhood personality traits such as hostility, aggression, and negative self-esteem, are associated with functional constipation in children [4, 9, 10]. Some studies have evaluated potential socio-demographic factors, including social class and living area (urban/rural), that may play a role in the development of constipation in children [10–12].

A few studies in Asia have shown that the prevalence of childhood constipation vary between 0.3% in Japan to 32.2% in Taiwan [11–13]. However, there is still a dearth of studies and information to fully understand the clinical epidemiology of this important health problem in Asia [11]. Indonesia has a multi-cultural, multi-lingual and multi-ethnic society. Population of Indonesia is estimated to be over 261 million people. It is the world's 4th most populous country and the most populous country in the Austronesian region. About 53% of the population

* Correspondence: hoswari@gmail.com
[1]Department of Child Health, Gastrohepatology Division, Cipto Mangunkusumo Hospital, Faculty of Medicine, Universitas Indonesia, Jakarta, Indonesia
Full list of author information is available at the end of the article

live in urban areas. Indonesia has 17,504 islands with over 300 different native languages [14].

We hypothesized that studying the socio-demographic factors, stressful events and bowel habits of the Indonesian children and adolescents would contribute towards the provision of a novel insight into the epidemiology and precipitating factors of constipation in children and adolescents. Therefore, we aimed to study epidemiology, and risk factors, including exposure to emotional stress, for constipation in Indonesian children and adolescents of the 10–17 year age group.

Methods
Study design and setting
A cross-sectional study was conducted in all five administrative cities (Municipalities) of Jakarta, Indonesia. Jakarta is the capital of the country and all the selected cities are therefore classified as urban. The inhabitants of these areas are predominantly regular employees (67.2%) and self-employed workers (19.8%) [15].

This study was conducted in 9 state junior high schools in these five administrative cities districts. Data were collected from July 2016 to December 2016 after obtaining consent from School Principals of each school. Informed written consent was obtained from the parents and assent was obtained from children and adolescents before commencement of the study.

This data was secured through 2 collection methods: take-home test (July to August 2016) and examination setting (November–December 2016). In the first method, participants filled the questionnaires at home while in the second, children were asked to fill the questionnaires at school in the presence of a research assistant and in a virtual examination setting. Sensitivity analysis was carried out to identify differences, if any, regarding the collection methods.

Participants
Nine schools from five districts of Jakarta were selected for this study with convenient sampling and requiring each district to have at least one school. Study participants were gathered consecutively in each school with inclusion criteria: age 10 to 16 years of age and generally in a good health condition. Data included into this study was obtained using the self-administered Questionnaire on Paediatric Gastrointestinal Symptoms which was modified from that used in previous studies [11].

To be eligible to be in the study, participants data regarding subjects' bowel habits and defecation behaviour, demographic data, family characteristics and other symptoms should have been completed. This study was approved by the Medical Ethics Committee of the Universitas Indonesia.

Study size
A previous study about constipation in adolescent population conducted in Sri Lanka had reported a prevalence of 15.3% [11]. Since Indonesia and Sri Lanka have some similarities in diet and socio-demographic factors, an anticipated prevalence rate of 15% with 80% of power, 5% significance and 20% of attrition were used for the sample size collection. Based on the above, the minimum sample size for each study site was calculated to be 245.

Variables
The Rome III criteria were used to define constipation [16]. They include,

1. Defecation frequency of less than three stools/week
2. At least one episode of faecal incontinence
3. A history of retentive posturing or excessive stool retention
4. A history of painful or hard bowel movements
5. A history of a large diameter stool that may obstruct the toilet

Children were considered to have constipation, if they fulfilled at least 2 of the above 5 criteria for at least 2 months. Although the Rome criteria state the presence of palpable faecal mass in the abdomen or rectum as a criterion, we could not practically use this in our epidemiological survey as it was not possible to conduct a physical examination in the setup that was used. Rectal examination was not approved because of limited examination facilities and for ethical reasons.

Stress events included in this study, with reference to the previous study from Sri Lanka were: change in school, suspension from school, frequent punishment in school, separation from the best friend, sitting for a national school examination, failure in school examinations, being bullied at school, severe illness in a close family member, death of a close family member, loss of a parent's job, divorce or separation of parents, remarriage of divorced parents, birth of a sibling, frequent domestic fights, frequent punishment by the parents, father's alcoholism, hospitalization of the child for another illness, and exposure to at least 1 stressful event. Each stress event was asked for in the questionnaires given and then separately analysed for association with constipation.

Data analysis
Data were analysed using SPSS version 23 (IBM Corp. Armonk, NY, USA). $P < 0.05$ was considered statistically significant and 95% confidence interval (CI) was calculated to describe the odd ratio for each variable. Multiple logistic regression analysis was performed on socio-demographic factors and stressful life events that were found to have significant association with

constipation during univariate analysis (Chi-squared test or Fisher's exact test). The 95% CI was measured and attuned to obtain the adjusted odd ratio.

Results

Three thousand five hundred and seventy-two (3572) questionnaires were distributed in total through the first and second methods listed in the Methods. In the first round (July to August 2016), 2718 questionnaires were distributed and only 1196 (44%), were returned. Then out of that, 1007 (37.1%) questionnaires had all the necessary data to be included into the analysis. In the second round (November–December 2016), 854 questionnaires were distributed, and children were asked to fill the questionnaires at school in the presence of a research assistant. From that, 811 (95%) questionnaires were collected, and 789(92.4%) questionnaires had complete data to be included into the analysis. Therefore, 2007 questionnaires were collected, of which 1796 (89.5%) were included in the analysis; males 732 (40.8%), mean age 13.58 years, SD 0.992 years. Two hundred and eleven (211) questionnaires were excluded due to incomplete socio-demographic details and bowel habit descriptions that would affect the result. In the context that participants recruited by the second method had higher proportion of the return rate compared to the first method, it is possible that this might have resulted in some bias. Therefore, sensitivity analysis was carried out and that showed that there was no difference in the results for the two methods.

Epidemiology and risk factors

Three hundred and twenty-eight children and adolescents (18.3%; 95% CI 0.16–0.2) met the Rome III criteria for constipation. Table 1 shows the distribution of subjects according to socio-demographic characteristics and prevalence of constipation in each category. Following multivariate analysis, only female gender (adjusted odd ratio 1.319, 95%CI 1.018–1.709, $p = 0.036$) and those residing in North Jakarta (adjusted odd ratio 1.832, 95%CI 1.199–2.799, $p = 0.005$) showed a higher risk of developing constipation .

Bowel habits of children with constipation

Bowel habits of children with constipation are depicted in Table 2. Withholding behaviour was present in 68.3% of subjects with constipation. Defecation less than 3 times per week was found in 64.6% of subjects. Presence of hard stools was seen in 63.4%.

Concerning the most common other bowel related symptoms associated with constipation, Table 3 shows that abdominal pain (OR 2.33, 95% CI 1.82–2.98; $P < 0.001$), loss of appetite (OR 1.51 95% CI 1.16–1.97; $P = 0.002$) and straining during defecation (OR 3.87, 95% CI

3.14–6.11; $P < 0.001$) were associated with constipation. However, following multiple logistic regression analysis, only abdominal pain (adjusted OR 2.14, CI 1.66 to 2.77 $P < 0.001$) and straining (adjusted OR 3.87, CI 2.744 to 5.446; $P < 0.001$) were found to be independently associated with constipation.

Association between constipation and stressful life events

Table 4 depicts the association between constipation and exposure to stressful life events. Although several stressful events were significantly associated with constipation during the univariate analysis, following multivariate analysis, father's alcoholism showed the strongest risk associated with constipation in school aged children (adjusted OR 1.91, 95% CI 1.27–2.89, $P = 0.002$), severe illness of a close family member (adjusted OR 1.77, 95% CI 1.12–2.80, $P = 0.014$), hospitalization of the child for another illness (adjusted OR 1.68, 95% CI 1.22–2.31, $P < 0.001$), being bullied at school (adjusted OR 1.67, 95% CI 1.01–2.76, $P = 0.047$) and loss of parent's job (adjusted OR 1.39, 95% CI 1.03–1.88, $P = 0.034$) also showed a significant association with constipation.

Discussion

This large epidemiological survey describes the prevalence and risk factors for constipation of children and adolescents in Jakarta, Indonesia [17]. Nearly one fifth (18.3%) of Indonesian school children and adolescents aged 10–17 years fulfil the Rome III criteria for constipation. Constipation was more common in girls and adolescents who were exposed to both home and school related stressful life events had higher odds of developing constipation.

The prevalence rate of constipation in Indonesia (18.3%) is slightly higher than most of the studies from the Western world, [US (12.9%) [18], Greece (13.9%) [19]], South-East Asia, [Sri Lanka (15.3%) [11]] and South America, [Mexico (12.6%) [20], and Panama (15.9%) [21]]. In contrast, the prevalence rate of constipation in Taiwan (32.2%) [12] was nearly twice as high as in the current study. However, the prevalence of constipation in Indonesia was markedly higher than China where the prevalence rates range from 3.1 to 12.2% [22–25]. The reason for these differences are not entirely clear. It may have been due to many reasons such as differences in sample selection (community samples vs. school samples), differences in methods of data collection (parental vs. child questionnaires), differences in data collection instruments including subtle alterations in translations, differences in cultural and regional interpretation of bowel habits and other GI symptoms together with differences in diet and behavioural patterns. In addition, there could be a true difference in genetic potential in developing constipation in these populations.

Table 1 Distribution of subjects according to sociodemographic characteristics and prevalence of constipation in each category

Variable		Distribution of subjects		Prevalence of constipation in each category (%)	Crude OR (CI 95%)	p value	Adjusted OR (95%CI)	Adjusted p value
		Controls N = 1468, n(%)	Children with constipation N = 328, n(%)					
Age	10–12 y.o	186 (12.7)	31 (9.5)	14.3	1.00 (ref)	–	1.00 (ref.)	–
	13–15 y.o	1268 (86.4)	292 (89.0)	18.7	1.382 (0.925–2.063)	0.114	1.466 (0.944–2.276)	0.089
	16–17 y.o	14 (1)	5 (1.5)	26.3	2.143 (0.721–6.371)	0.17	2.229 (0.727–6.834)	0.161
					p = 0.188			
Sex	Male	617 (42)	115 (35.1)	15.7	1.00 (ref)	–	1.00 (ref.)	–
	Female	851 (58)	213 (64.9)	20	1.343 (1.047–1.723)	0.02	1.319 (1.018–1.709)	0.036
					p = 0.02			
Family size	Only child	116 (7.9)	18 (5.5)	13.4	1.00 (ref)	–	1.00 (ref.)	–
	2–3 children	1083 (73.8)	235 (71.6)	17.8	1.398 (0.835–2.343)	0.203	4.736×10^8 (0)	1
	≥4 children	269 (18.3)	75 (22.9)	21.8	1.797 (1.028–3.141)	0.04	6.282×10^8 (0)	1
					p = 0.076			
Birth order[a]	Eldest	509 (37.6)	122 (39.4)	19.3	1.00 (ref)	–	1.00 (ref.)	–
	Youngest	490 (36.2)	104 (33.5)	17.5	0.886 (0.663–1.183)	0.41	0.854 (0.634–1.151)	0.3
	Other	354 (26.2)	84 (27.1)	19.2	0.990 (0.727–1.349)	0.949	0.867 (0.613–1.226)	0.419
					p = 0.675			
Mother[b]	Housewife	1058 (72.3)	246 (75.0)	18.9	1.00 (ref)	–	1.00 (ref.)	–
	Employed	405 (27.7)	82 (25.0)	16.8	0.871 (0.661–1.146)	0.324	1.880 (0.853–4.145)	0.117
					p = 0.324			
Father's employment	Leading profession (eg. Doctor, engineer)	16 (1.1)	4 (1.2)	20	1.00 (ref)	–	1.00 (ref.)	–
	Lesser profession (eg. Nurse, teacher)	451 (30.7)	100 (30.5)	18.1	0.887 (0.290–2.710)	0.833	0.790 (0.252–2.477)	0.686
	Skilled non-manual (eg. Clerk)	653 (44.5)	132 (40.2)	16.8	0.809 (0.266–2.457)	0.708	0.767 (0.247–2.382)	0.646
	Skilled manual	207 (14.1)	56 (17.1)	21.3	1.082 (0.348–3.366)	0.892	0.901 (0.282–2.880)	0.861
	Unskilled/unemployed	141 (9.6)	36 (11)	20.3	1.021 (0.322–3.242)	0.972	0.886 (0.267–2.939)	0.843
					p = 0.513			
Maternal employment	Leading profession (eg. Doctor, engineer)	12 (0.8)	3 (0.9)	20	1.00 (ref)	–	1.00 (ref.)	–
	Lesser profession (eg. Nurse, teacher)	168 (11.4)	36 (11)	17.6	0.857 (0.230–3.194)	0.818	0.682 (0.176–2.635)	0.578
	Skilled non-manual	179 (12.2)	28 (8.5)	13.5	0.626 (0.166–2.357)	0.488	0.539 (0.137–2.125)	0.377

Table 1 Distribution of subjects according to sociodemographic characteristics and prevalence of constipation in each category *(Continued)*

Variable		Distribution of subjects		Prevalence of constipation in each category (%)	Crude OR (CI 95%)	p value	Adjusted OR (95%CI)	Adjusted p value
		Controls N = 1468, n(%)	Children with constipation N = 328, n(%)					
	(eg. Clerk)							
	Skilled manual	16 (1.1)	2 (0.6)	11.1	0.500 (0.072–3.477)	0.484	0.32 (0.044–2.354)	0.263
	Unskilled/unemployed	1093 (74.5)	259 (79.0)	19.2	0.948 (0.266–3.383)	0.934	1.332 (0.293–6.059)	0.711
					p = 0.339			
Location of school	South Jakarta	370 (25.2)	67 (20.4)	15.3	1.00 (ref)	–	1.00 (ref.)	–
	North Jakarta	162 (11)	58 (17.7)	26.4	1.977 (1.329–2.941)	0.001	1.832 (1.199–2.799)	0.005
	Central Jakarta	264 (18.0)	73 (22.3)	21.7	1.527 (1.058–2.205)	0.024	1.469 (0.989–2.181)	0.057
	East Jakarta	349 (23.8)	70 (21.3)	16.7	1.108 (0.769–1.596)	0.584	0.959 (0.650–1.413)	0.831
	West Jakarta	323 (22)	60 (18.3)	15.7	1.026 (0.702–1.499)	0.895	0.984 (0.662–1.465)	0.938
					p = 0.002			

[a]Family with more than one child
[b]Living mother

Table 2 Bowel habits of children with constipation

Bowel habits	Category	n (Percentage)
Defecation frequency	< 3 per week	212 (64.6)
	3–6 per week	24 (7.3)
	Once daily	56 (17.1)
	> One per day	36 (11.0)
Stool Consistency	Hard	206 (63.4)
	Normal	107 (32.9)
	Soft	15 (4.5)
Large diameter stools	Yes	88 (26.8)
	No	240 (73.2)
Withholding posture	Yes	224 (68.3)
	No	104 (31.7)
Painful bowel motions	Yes	180 (54.9)
	No	148 (45.1)
Fecal incontinence	Yes	100 (30.6)
	No	228 (69.4)

Predominance of a gender in constipation is still far from conclusive. Studies from Panama and Sri Lanka reported no difference between males and females [11, 21]. Whereas Lewis et al. found constipation more prevalent in males than females in the US [18]. In contrast to the latter study we found a higher prevalence in females. Similar to our findings, Wu et al noted a significantly higher prevalence of constipation in females in Taiwan [12]. Adult studies have also shown that constipation was more common in females than males [26]. When we looked further into our data, the predominance of constipation in females might be related to more stressful events in females than males in our study (data not shown). Socio-demographic factors did not show any significant difference between children with constipation and controls in our study.

Only a few studies describe bowel habits of children with constipation. Compared to children with constipation in Sri Lanka and Iran, children and adolescents included in this study had higher occurrence of infrequent stools (< 3/ per week), and hard stools [11, 27]. They were also noted to have higher frequency of posturing and having more faecal incontinence. The frequency of

faecal incontinence was higher than that of Brazilian children with constipation [28]. However, pain while passing stools and large diameter stools were less frequent in Indonesian children with constipation compared to Sri Lankan and Iranian children [11, 27]. Of the other symptoms studied, abdominal pain was the only symptom that was independently associated with constipation. A similar observation was noted in the study conducted among Sri Lankan adolescents [11].

Many factors could contribute to the development of constipation in children, such as abnormal personality traits [4], stressful life events [9], child maltreatment [10], dietary habits [29] and obesity [30]. Pressure at home and school could transform into stressful events that lead to constipation. In our study, father's alcoholism, severe illness in a close family member, hospitalization of the child for another illness, being bullied at school and loss of a parent's job were clearly associated with constipation. Similarly, another study reported the association between stress and constipation [9]. In that study, separation from the best friend, failure in exam, severe illness among family members, and frequent punishments by parents were associated with constipation. Although there are subtle variations in the findings of that study and the current study, it is evident that home and school related stressful events predispose children to develop constipation. In contrast, a study from Nigeria, using the same list of stressful events, did not find a significant association between constipation and stressful life events. A smaller sample size could have contributed to this lack of difference in the Nigerian study. It had been shown that poor quality of interactions due to marital disharmony, verbal/emotional abuse of children etc., between the child and the caregiver before the age of 18 years could lead to the development of functional gastrointestinal disorders [31].

There are several strengths of this study. We included a large number of children in the study which conferred adequate power to our findings. We also used standard Rome III criteria for the diagnosis of constipation and therefore were able to compare our findings with other studies to draw meaningful conclusions. However, as many of the other epidemiological surveys across the world on this topic, we did not conduct a physical

Table 3 Symptoms associated to constipation

Symptoms	Groups		Constipation versus controls	
	Constipation, n(%)	Controls, n(%)	OR (95% CI)	p value[*]
Abdominal pain	210 (64)	636 (43.3)	2.33 (1.82–2.98)	< 0.0001
Nausea	1 (0.3)	9 (0.6)	0.49 (0.06–3.93)	0.7[**]
Vomiting	14 (4.3)	36 (2.5)	1.77 (0.95–3.33)	0.07
Loss of appetite	97 (29.7)	320 (21.8)	1.51 (1.16–1.97)	0.002
Straining	75 (22.9)	93 (6.3)	4.38 (3.14–6.11)	< 0.0001

[*]Chi-squared test and [**]Fisher's Exact test

Table 4 Distribution of respondent according to exposure to stressful life events

Stressful event	Constipation n(%)	Controls n(%)	OR (95% CI)	P Value[*]
Change in school	38 (11.6)	107 (7.3)	1.67 (1.13–2.47)	0.01
Suspension from school	42 (12.8)	145 (9.9)	1.34 (0.93–1.94)	0.114
Frequent punishment in school	22 (15.4)	63 (4.3)	1.62 (0.98–2.67)	0.058
Separation from best friend	21 (6.5)	66 (4.5)	1.46 (0.88–2.43)	0.138
Sitting for a national school examination	12 (3.7)	42 (2.9)	1.3 (0.68–2.49)	0.43
Failure in school examination	15 (4.6)	44 (3)	1.56 (0.86–2.85)	0.14
Being bullied at school	39 (12)	78 (5.3)	2.43 (1.62–3.64)	< 0.0001
Severe illness in a close family member	46 (14.2)	91 (6.2)	2.49 (1.71–3.63)	< 0.0001
Death of a close family member	29 (11.9)	89 (9.1)	1.36 (0.87–2.11)	0.179
Loss of a parent's job	180 (55)	606 (41.3)	1.74 (1.36–2.21)	< 0.0001
Divorce or separation of parents	106 (32.4)	264 (20.6)	2.18 (1.67–2.85)	< 0.0001
Remarriage of divorced parents	38 (11.6)	142 (9.7)	1.23 (0.84–1.79)	0.293
Birth of a sibling	3 (0.9)	9 (0.6)	1.51 (0.41–5.59)	0.465[**]
Frequent domestic fights	185 (56.6)	622 (42.4)	1.77 (1.39–2.25)	< 0.0001
Frequent punishment by the parents	130 (39.8)	457 (31.2)	1.46 (1.14–1.87)	0.003
Father's alcoholism	52 (15.9)	108 (7.4)	2.38 (1.66–3.39)	< 0.0001
Hospitalization of the child for another illness	124 (37.9)	332 (22.6)	2.09 (1.62–2.69)	< 0.0001
Exposure to at least 1 stressful event	82 (25.1)	285 (19.4)	1.39 (1.05–1.84)	0.022

[*]Chi-squared test and [**]Fisher exact test

examination on these children nor did we investigate them to rule out the possibility of organic disorders. However, most of the studies have failed to find significant organic disorders in children who have fulfilled Rome criteria for functional gastrointestinal disorders [32, 33] and current guidelines also do not recommend investigating children who fulfil standard criteria for constipation [34].

As an observational study, data were obtained using questionnaires which may be subject to information bias, including recall bias. As this study was conducted using two different methods for data collection (questionnaires filled at home and questionnaires filled in the school), sensitivity analysis was performed between the two methods. In sociodemographic factor, gender was found to be not significant in the second method ($p = 0.378$) while the first method showed the same result with the total participants ($p = 0.027$). This could have occurred because of differences in gender proportion (60.7% subjects are girls). We did not find any other significant differences in the sensitivity analysis.

Our findings have noteworthy implications both at national and global levels for clinical and research practices. According to Unicef estimates, Indonesia has around 85 million children, which represents one-third of the national population [17]. Therefore, allocation of healthcare resources for this growing problem of constipation would be an uphill task for policymakers. Our data also provide

the understanding of epidemiological distribution of constipation in children at the global level and provide an insight towards predisposing factors. We believe that these findings could contribute to the development of preventive strategies for constipation in children.

Conclusions

The present study shows that almost 20% of children and adolescents in Indonesia suffer from constipation. This functional gastrointestinal disorder is more common in girls. Some common school and home related stressful live events predispose children to develop constipation and therefore, national, regional and global policymakers need to pay attention to the growing problem of constipation in Indonesian children.

Acknowledgements
We are grateful to Dr. B.J.C.Perera for editing the manuscript.

Authors' contributions
HO: Planning the research project, analysis, writing, edited the manuscript FSA: Data collection, analysis, and writing the manuscript. BH: Planning the research project, edited the manuscript WC: Data collection and analysis, AP: Data collection and analysis, MAB: Conceptualised the study, critically analysed the manuscript with significant intellectual contribution, and approved the final script, SR: Helped to develop the study protocol, edited the manuscript with a significant intellectual contribution and approved the final manuscript. All the authors have read and approved the manuscript.

Competing interests

The authors declare that they have no competing interests.

Author details

[1]Department of Child Health, Gastrohepatology Division, Cipto Mangunkusumo Hospital, Faculty of Medicine, Universitas Indonesia, Jakarta, Indonesia. [2]Department of Pediatric Gastroenterology and Nutrition, Emma Children's, Hospital, Academic Medical Centre, Amsterdam, The Netherlands. [3]Department of Paediatrics, University of Kelaniya, Ragama 11010, Sri Lanka.

References

1. Rajindrajith S, Devanarayana NM, Crispus Perera BJ, Benninga MA. Childhood constipation as an emerging public health problem. World J Gastroenterol. 2016;22:6864–75.
2. van den Berg MM, Benninga MA, Di Lorenzo C. Epidemiology of childhood constipation: a systematic review. Am J Gastroenterol. 2006;101:2401–9.
3. Mugie SM, Benninga MA, Di Lorenzo C. Epidemiology of constipation in children and adults: a systematic review. Best Pract Res Clin Gastroenterol. 2011;25:3–18.
4. Ranasinghe N, Devanarayana NM, Benninga MA, van Dijk M, Rajindrajith S. Psychological maladjustment and quality of life in adolescents with constipation. Arch Dis Child. 2017;102:268–73.
5. Clarke MC, Chow CS, Chase JW, Gibb S, Hutson JM, Southwell BR. Quality of life in children with slow transit constipation. J Pediatr Surg. 2008;43:320–4.
6. Rajindrajith S, Devanarayana NM, Weerasooriya L, Hathagoda W, Benninga MA. Quality of life and somatic symptoms in children with constipation: a school-based study. J Pediatr. 2013;163:1069–72 e1.
7. Youssef NN, Langseder AL, Verga BJ, Mones RL, Rosh JR. Chronic childhood constipation is associated with impaired quality of life: a case-controlled study. J Pediatr Gastroenterol Nutr. 2005;41:56–60.
8. Choung RS, Shah ND, Chitkara D, Branda ME, Van Tilburg MA, Whitehead WE, et al. Direct medical costs of constipation from childhood to early adulthood: a population-based birth cohort study. J Pediatr Gastroenterol Nutr. 2011;52:47–54.
9. Devanarayana NM, Rajindrajith S. Association between constipation and stressful life events in a cohort of Sri Lankan children and adolescents. J Trop Pediatr. 2010;56:144–8.
10. Rajindrajith S, Devanarayana NM, Lakmini C, Subasinghe V, de Silva DG, Benninga MA. Association between child maltreatment and constipation: a school-based survey using Rome III criteria. J Pediatr Gastroenterol Nutr. 2014;58:486–90.
11. Rajindrajith S, Devanarayana NM, Adhikari C, Pannala W, Benninga MA. Constipation in children: an epidemiological study in Sri Lanka using Rome III criteria. Arch Dis Child. 2012;97:43–5.
12. Wu TC, Chen LK, Pan WH, Tang RB, Hwang SJ, Wu L, et al. Constipation in Taiwan elementary school students: a nationwide survey. J Chin Med Assoc. 2011;74:57–61.
13. Sagawa T, Okamura S, Kakizaki S, Zhang Y, Morita K, Mori M. Functional gastrointestinal disorders in adolescents and quality of school life. J Gastroenterol Hepatol. 2013;28:285–90.
14. Wikipedia. Indonesia. https://en.wikipedia.org/wiki/Indonesia#cite_note-IslandPop-14. Accessed 15 Aug 2018.
15. Statistik BP. Population of 15 years of age and over who are working by region nad employment status of main job-DKI Jakarta Provice. http://

sp2010.bps.go.id/index.php/site/tabel?wid=3100000000&tid=270&fi1=58&fi2=3. Accessed 15 Aug 2018.
16. Waker LS, Caplan A, Rasquin A. Manual for the questionnaire on paediatric gastrointestinal symptoms. Nashville: Department of Pediatrics, Vanderbilt University Medical Centre; 2000.
17. Unicef-Indonesia. The big picture. https://www.unicef.org/indonesia/children.html. Accessed 9 Jan 2017.
18. Lewis ML, Palsson OS, Whitehead WE, van Tilburg MAL. Prevalence of functional gastrointestinal disorders in children and adolescents. J Pediatr. 2016;177:39–43.e3.
19. Bouzios I, Chouliaras G, Chrousos GP, Roma E, Gemou-Engesaeth V. Functional gastrointestinal disorders in Greek children based on ROME III criteria: identifying the child at risk. Neurogastroenterol Motil. 2017;29:e12951-n/a.
20. Dhroove G, Saps M, Garcia-Bueno C, Leyva Jimenez A, Rodriguez-Reynosa LL, Velasco-Benitez CA. Prevalence of functional gastrointestinal disorders in Mexican schoolchildren. Rev Gastroenterol Mex. 2017;82:13–8.
21. Lu PL, Saps M, Chanis RA, Velasco-Benítez CA. The prevalence of functional gastrointestinal disorders in children in Panama: a school-based study. Acta Paediatr. 2016;105:e232–e6.
22. Tam YH, Li AM, So HK, Shit KY, Pang KK, Wong YS, et al. Socioenvironmental factors associated with constipation in Hong Kong children and Rome III criteria. J Pediatr Gastroenterol Nutr. 2012;55:56–61.
23. Xu HL, Lin SH, Lin LR, Ni MY, Ji XF, XI W. Epidemiologic survey of children with functional constipation in Jieyang City. Hainan Med J. 2008;19:103–4.
24. Zhang SC, Wang WL, Qu RB, Su PJ, Zhang SW, Zhang HR. et al. [Epidemiologic survey on the prevalence and distribution of childhood functional constipation in the northern areas of China: a population-based study. Zhonghua Liu Xing Bing Xue Za Zhi. 2010;31:751–4.
25. Zhou HQ, Li DG, Song YY, Zhong CH, Hu Y, Xu XX, et al. An epidemiologic study of functional bowel disorders in adolescents in China. Zhonghua Yi Xue Za Zhi. 2007;87:657–60.
26. Chang L. Review article: epidemiology and quality of life in functional gastrointestinal disorders. Aliment Pharmacol Ther. 2004;20(Suppl 7):31–9.
27. Dehghani SM, Kulouee N, Honar N, Imanieh MH, Haghighat M, Javaherizadeh H. Clinical manifestations among children with chronic functional constipation. Middle East J Dig Dis. 2015;7:31–5.
28. De Araujo Sant'Anna AM, Calcado AC. Constipation in school-aged children at public schools in Rio de Janeiro, Brazil. J Pediatr Gastroenterol Nutr. 1999;29:190–3.
29. Kranz S, Brauchla M, Slavin JL, Miller KB. What do we know about dietary fiber intake in children and health? The effects of fiber intake on constipation, obesity, and diabetes in children. Adv Nutr. 2012;3:47–53.
30. Pashankar DS, Loening-Baucke V. Increased prevalence of obesity in children with functional constipation evaluated in an academic medical center. Pediatrics. 2005;116:e377–80.
31. Felitti VJ, Anda RF, Nordenberg D, Williamson DF, Spitz AM, Edwards V, et al. Relationship of childhood abuse and household dysfunction to many of the leading causes of death in adults. The Adverse Childhood Experiences (ACE) Study. Am J Prev Med. 1998;14:245–58.
32. Devanarayana NM, de Silva DG, de Silva HJ. Aetiology of recurrent abdominal pain in a cohort of Sri Lankan children. J Paediatr Child Health. 2008;44:195–200.
33. Dhroove G, Chogle A, Saps M. A million-dollar work-up for abdominal pain: is it worth it? J Pediatr Gastroenterol Nutr. 2010;51:579–83.
34. Tabbers MM, DiLorenzo C, Berger MY, Faure C, Langendam MW, Nurko S, et al. Evaluation and treatment of functional constipation in infants and children: evidence-based recommendations from ESPGHAN and NASPGHAN. J Pediatr Gastroenterol Nutr. 2014;58:258–74.

13

Distinct patterns of serum hepatitis B core-related antigen during the natural history of chronic hepatitis B

Zhan-Qing Zhang[1*†], Xiao-Nan Zhang[2*†] (ID), Wei Lu[1], Yan-Bing Wang[1], Qi-Cheng Weng[3] and Yan-Ling Feng[4]

Abstract

Background: The current clinical practice on chronic hepatitis B (CHB) requires better on-treatment monitoring of viral persistence. Quantified assays for hepatitis B surface antigen (HBsAg) and core-related antigen (HBcrAg) hold promise for further optimization of therapy. Here, we aimed to characterize HBcrAg during the natural course of CHB.

Methods: Four-hundred and forty four treatment naïve CHB patients, who all underwent liver histology examination, were enrolled in this cross-sectional study. Their HBV DNA, HBsAg, HBeAg and HBcrAg titres were quantified and analyzed in the context of four distinct clinical phases. Correlation of HBcrAg and HBsAg with other markers were performed. The relationship between liver and serum antigen levels were also assessed.

Results: HBcrAg, like HBsAg, exhibited high degree of correlation with HBV DNA. However, a more significant linear relationship was found between HBcrAg and HBeAg titre in immune tolerant (IT) and immune clearance (IC) phases, while in HBeAg negative hepatitis (ENH) group, HBV DNA is a major determinant of HBcrAg. Significant difference was observed in liver HBcAg score and HBcrAg level in both IT and IC phases whereas barely significant positive correlations between liver HBsAg score and HBsAg titre was documented.

Conclusion: HBcrAg titre exhibited distinct correlative profile in a phase-specific manner. In addition, its level is well-related to the intrahepatic expression of core antigen. It has a considerable utility in monitoring and refining antiviral therapy.

Keywords: HBcrAg, HBV, HBsAg

Background

The hepatitis B virus continues to be a global public health issue with over 240 million chronically infected individuals worldwide. Chronic hepatitis B virus (CHB) infection is connected with a high risk of developing liver fibrosis, cirrhosis and hepatocellular carcinoma, which results in over 780,000 deaths annually [1]. The natural history of CHB is commonly regarded as consisting of four phases [2]; immune-tolerant (IT), immune-clearance (IC), non/low-replicative (LR), and hepatitis B

e antigen negative hepatitis (ENH). These phases have been classified by specific biochemical, serological and virological characteristics, including serum ALT levels, hepatitis B e antigen (HBeAg) serostatus, and hepatitis B virus DNA (HBVDNA) titre.

A deeper understanding of the pathogenesis and natural history of CHB has been facilitated by the improved sensitivity of HBV DNA viral load assays, reliable assays for serum hepatitis B surface antigen (HBsAg) and HBeAg [2, 3] and the development of assays for the detection and measurement of HBV intrahepatic reservoir, covalently closed circular DNA (cccDNA) [4]. As a relatively new serum immunoassay, quantification of hepatitis B core-related antigen (HBcrAg) provided additional virological information regarding the status of chronic HBV infection [5]. The HBcrAg assay detects the sum of hepatitis B core

* Correspondence: doctorzzqsphc@163.com; zhangxiaonan@shaphc.org
†Equal contributors
[1]Department of Hepatology, Shanghai Public Health Clinical Center, Fudan University, Caolang Road 2901, Shanghai 201508, China
[2]Research Unit, Shanghai Public Health Clinical Center, Fudan University, Caolang Road 2901, Shanghai 201508, China
Full list of author information is available at the end of the article

antigen (HBcAg), e antigen (HBeAg) and its related byproduct, 22-kDa precore protein (p22cr) [6]. It has been shown to have close correlation with HBV DNA but exhibit less decline after antiviral therapy [7]. Thus it was proposed as a surrogate marker for HBV persistence [8].

In this study, we aimed to further evaluate the HBcrAg assay in 444 treatment naïve CHB patients spanning all four phases of its natural history, all of whom underwent liver histological examinations. The relationships between HBcrAg and serum, liver markers were analyzed in a phase-specific manner.

Methods

Patients

This study included 444 Chinese patients with CHB who were hospitalized at the Shanghai Public Health Clinical Center of Fudan University between January 2012 and September 2015. The diagnosis of all the patients were made according to with the "Guideline on the prevention and treatment for chronic hepatitis B" (2010 version) jointly released by the Chinese Society of Hepatology and the Chinese Society of Infectious Diseases, Chinese Medical Association. The detailed inclusion and exclusion criteria were previously described [9].

Patients were classified into one of four phases of CHB based on HBeAg serostatus, HBV DNA and serum ALT levels. The Immune tolerant (IT) phase was defined as: HBeAg positive, HBV DNA > 20,000 IU/mL, serum ALT ≤ 2 × upper limit of normal (ULN). The Immune clearance (IC) phase was defined as: HBeAg positive, HBV DNA > 20,000 IU/mL, serum ALT > 2 × ULN. The low replicative (LR) group was defined as: HBeAg negative, HBV DNA < 2000 IU/mL and normal serum ALT. The E negative hepatitis (ENH) phase was defined as: HBeAg negative, HBV DNA > 2000 IU/mL, serum ALT >2 × ULN.

Liver biopsy and pathological diagnosis

The detailed procedures for ultrasound-assisted liver biopsy and pathological evaluations of necro-inflammatory activity and fibrosis were previously described [9]. The pathological diagnosis referred to the Scheuer standard, in which grade is used to describe the intensity of necro-inflammatory activity, and stage is a measure of fibrosis and architectural alteration. The grades include five levels, G0–G4, and the stages include five levels, S0–S4 [10].

For immunohistochemistry (IHC), formalin-fixed paraffin embedded sections were routinely dewaxed and rehydrated. After heat induced antigen retrieval in sodium citrate (pH 6.0) buffer, sections were incubated with the primary monoclonal antibody against HBsAg (clone

1044/341, Novocastra) and rabbit polyclonal anti-HBcAg antibodies (Dako). After washing, the polymer detection system (Polink-1 HRP, GBI Labs) was incubated for 30 min at room temperature and developed with 3, 3'-diaminobezdine (DAB). The expression of liver HBsAg and HBcAg was evaluated by semiquantitative scoring method. The scores include four levels: 0 (no positive cells), 1 (positive cells <25%), 2 (positive cells 25% -49%), 3 (positive cells ≥ 50%).

Laboratory assays

Measurement of serum HBcrAg was performed using a CLEIA Lumipulse G1200 automated analyzer (Fujirebio Inc., Tokyo, Japan) and the reagents were provided by Fujirebio Inc., lot number: SAX5031 (Japan) [5]. Serum HBsAg and HBeAg were measured using a chemiluminescence microparticle immunoassay Abbott Architect I2000 automated analyzer (Abbott Laboratories, Chicago, IL, USA) [11, 12]. The detailed measurement procedures were previously described [9]. Serum HBV DNA levels were measured using a Bio-Rad Icycler PCR System (Bio-Rad Laboratories, Inc., California, USA), and the PCR kits were obtained from Qiagen Shenzhen Co. Ltd. (China). The linear detection range was 5×10^2 IU/mL to 5×10^7 IU/mL.

Statistical analyses

Statistical analyses were performed using PASW version 18.0 (SPSS Inc., Chicago, Illinois, USA). The Mann-Whitney U test and Kruskall-Wallis ANOVA test were used for non-parametric continuous data. Prearson's correlation coefficient was used for analyzing the correlation among logarithmized serum HBcrAg, HBsAg, HBeAg and HBV DNA values. Multiple linear regression analysis was employed to evaluate the contribution of HBeAg and HBV DNA to the overall readout of HBcrAg.

Results

Basic characteristics of enrolled patients

The basic characteristics of enrolled patients are presented in Table 1. Based on the criteria described above, they were classified into four distinct groups: i.e., IT ($n = 158$), IC ($n = 133$), LR, ($n = 99$) and ENH ($n = 54$). The male-to-female ratios in these four groups were generally comparable ($p = 0.053$). As expected, HBeAg negative patients (LR and ENH group) were older than HBeAg positive patients (IT and IC group, $p < 0.001$). In terms of liver histology, significant lower scores of necro-inflammation and fibrosis were documented in IT and LR groups compared with IC and ENH groups ($p < 0.001$), which agreed well with their phase classification.

Table 1 Baseline characteristics of enrolled patients

	Immune Tolerant (n = 158)	Immune clearance (n = 133)	Low Replicative (n = 99)	HBeAg negativ hepatitis (n = 54)	p value
Age	34 (28–42)	31 (26–39)	42 (32/49)	43 (37–52)	<0.001[a]
Gender M/F	92/66	94/39	58/41	39/15	0.053[b]
ALT IU/L	40.5 (24–58.5)	175 (103–356)	22 (14–30)	160 (112–391)	<0.001[a]
HBV DNA log IU/ml	7.65(6.45–7.70)	7.50 (6.65–7.69)	<2.70 (<2.70–2.73)	5.81 (5.10–6.74)	<0.001[a]
HBsAg log IU/ml	4.43 (3.54–4.76)	3.96 (3.55–4.52)	3.96 (3.56–4.51)	3.28 (2.78–3.69)	<0.001[a]
HBeAg log COI	2.97 (1.93–3.13)	2.80 (2.12–3.08)	Negative	negative	–
Necro-inflammation (G1:G2:G3)	109:23:26	36:50:47	82:10:7	18:17:19	<0.001[a]
Fibrosis: (S1, S2, S3, S4)	84:38:16:20	33:48:20:32	65:13:10:11	13:15:12:14	<0.001[a]
Liver HBsAg (0:1:2:3)	1:29:71:57	3:30:44:56	20:38:25:16	2:13:22:17	<0.001[a]
Liver HBcAg (0:1:2)	78:50:30	85:38:10	96:2:1	49:5:0	<0.001[a]

Data expressed as the median (interquartile range)
[a]Kruskall–Wallis analysis
[b]chi square test

The level of HBcrAg and its relationship with other markers

The levels of HBcrAg across four phases of diseases were evaluated (Fig. 1a). Highest level of HBcrAg was observed in IT (median 5.00 log kU/ml) and IC (4.94 log kU/ml) whereas lowest level was found in LR group, in which 61 of 99 patients tested negative for HBcrAg. The median level of HBcrAg in ENH group is 2.58 log kU/ml with three tested negative. The general feature of HBcrAg distribution is similar to that of HBV DNA (Fig. 1b) and

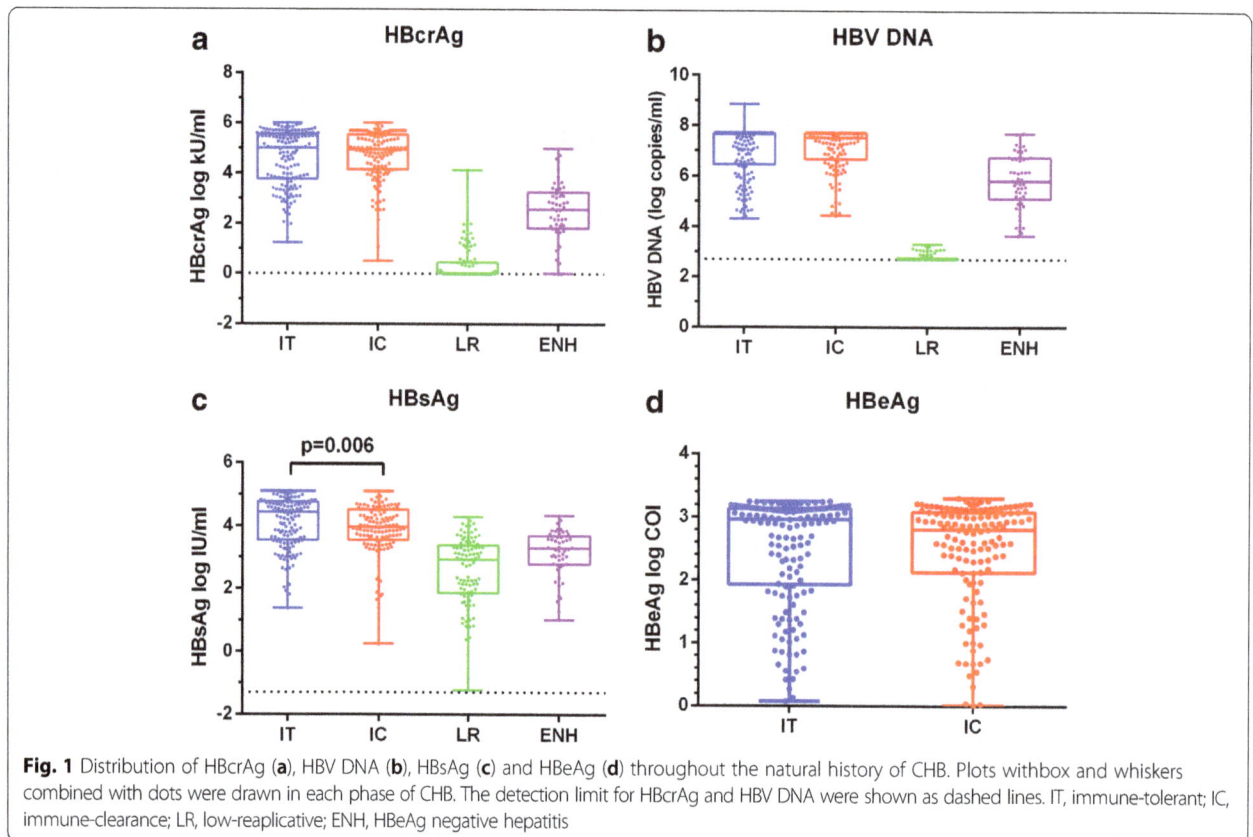

Fig. 1 Distribution of HBcrAg (**a**), HBV DNA (**b**), HBsAg (**c**) and HBeAg (**d**) throughout the natural history of CHB. Plots withbox and whiskers combined with dots were drawn in each phase of CHB. The detection limit for HBcrAg and HBV DNA were shown as dashed lines. IT, immune-tolerant; IC, immune-clearance; LR, low-reaplicative; ENH, HBeAg negative hepatitis

HBsAg (Fig. 1c). However, the HBsAg titre exhibited less dramatic changes across four phases, and the HBcrAg titre did not show significant difference between IT and IC group as opposed to HBsAg ($p = 0.006$, Mann-Whitney U test). The HBeAg titre between IT and IC group were generally comparable (Fig. 1d).

We next evaluated the correlation patterns among levels of major viral antigens and nucleic acid in a phase-specific manner. In agreement with a large body of literature, HBV viral antigen and DNA levels exhibited high degree of correlation in IT and IC phases (Fig. 2a-h). However, we noticed that HBcrAg and HBeAg showed highest correlation coefficient in IT ($r = 0.761$) and IC group ($r = 0.652$) (Fig. 2d, h and Table 2). In ENH group, HBcrAg and HBV DNA showed higher level of correlation ($r = 0.583$, Fig. 2j) compared with HBsAg and HBcrAg ($r = 0.296$, $p = 0.03$, Fig. 2i, Table 2). In LR group, a lack of correlation was found between HBV DNA and HBsAg/HBcrAg (data now shown) mainly because a relatively less sensitive qPCR assay was used (detection limit 500 copies/ml). However, statistically significant correlation was found between HBsAg and HBcrAg titre ($p < 0.001$, $r = 0.368$, Table 2).

Multiple linear regression analysis of HBcrAg

As the HBcrAg titre is actually the sum of HBcAg, HBeAg and its related byproduct, and the amount of HBcAg can be approximated with HBV viral load, we reasoned that HBcrAg readout can be decomposed into two major elements, i.e., HBV DNA and HBeAg titre. Thus, we performed multiple linear regression of HBcrAg titre using HBV viral load and HBeAg titre as variables (Table 3). Interestingly, we found that in HBeAg positive patients (IT and IC group), HBeAg titre is the major factor for HBcrAg ($r = 0.751$, $p = 1.99E-11$ in IT group, $r = 0.697$, $p = 3.35E-13$ in IC group) whereas HBV DNA level had a minor effect ($r = 0.262$, $p = 0.004$ in IT group, $r = 0.164$, $p = 0.057$ in IC group). In ENH group however, with HBeAg absent, HBV DNA exhibit significant linear relationship with HBcrAg ($p = 0.635$, $p = 3.68E-6$).

The relationship between circulating antigens and their intrahepatic status

We then tried to evaluate whether the levels of circulating HBsAg, HBcrAg corresponded to the intrahepatic abundance of their counterparts, i.e., HBsAg and HBcAg. We grouped the IT and IC patients according to their HBsAg or HBcAg immunohistochemistry scores and analyzed their corresponding serum antigens. It was found that there was a barely significant difference in HBsAg titre when grouped with liver HBsAg score in IT ($p = 0.10$, Fig. 3a) and IC group ($p = 0.04$, Fig. 3b). However, a gradual increase in HBsAg titre was found in

accordance with higher HBsAg score in liver biopsy of LR group ($p < 0.0001$, Fig. 3c) whereas no difference was found in ENH group ($p = 0.196$, Fig. 3d). In terms of HBcrAg, significant differences were observed in HBcrAg level when grouped with liver HBcAg score in both IT ($p < 0.0001$, Fig. 3e) and IC group ($p = 0.002$, Fig. 3f). In LR and ENH group, due to the very limited cases positive for intrahepatic HBcAg (3 in LR and 5 in ENH group, Table 1), no meaningful statistical analysis was possible.

Discussion

The hepatitis B virus exploits its limited genome for transcription of various messenger RNAs and pregnomic RNA. In addition, it utilizes alternative translation initiation to express various polypeptide products from a single messenger. HBV encodes two core-related open reading frames (ORFs), i.e., precore and core ORF. The precore ORF express a 25-kDa polypeptide containing an N terminal 19-aa signal peptide, which is cleaved during translocation into the ER lumen [11]. After its subsequent cleavage of its carboxy terminus by furin endopeptidase [12], a 17-kDa mature HBeAg is secreted. In addition, a 22-kDa precore protein (p22cr) was reported, whose N-terminal signal peptide was not cleaved and lacked arginine-rich C terminal domain critical for nucleic acid binding. It was found to be assembled into Dane-like particles but devoid of HBV genome [6]. The core ORF expresses the 21.5-kDa HBcAg which assembles into dimers and form the capsid. In serum of HBV patients, HBV capsids were believed to be encapsidated by HBV surfaces antigens to form Dane particles although naked capsids were reported in hepatoma cell lines [13].

Since HBcAg is encapsidated by viral envelope and high activity of HBcAg neutralizing antibody in the serum, its level cannot be easily quantified. Kimura et al. reported a sensitive enzyme immunoassay for quantifying HBV core-related antigens using monoclonal antibodies reactive to denatured HBcAg and HBeAg. This assay exhibited a detection limit of 4 pg/ml and was insensitive to interfering anti-HBc and anti-HBe antibodies in specimens. Clinical evaluation of the HBcrAg assay found that, although it was highly correlated with HBV viral load, its decline after antiviral therapy was less pronounced compared with HBV DNA [7]. Hence, HBcrAg was proposed to be a marker for viral persistence. Indeed, van Campenhout et al. reported that HBcrAg levels were associated with response to entecavir and Peginterferon add-on therapy in HBeAg positive patients [14]. Furthermore, Honda et al. reported that HBcrAg is related to intra-hepatic HBV replication and development of hepatocellular carcinoma [15].

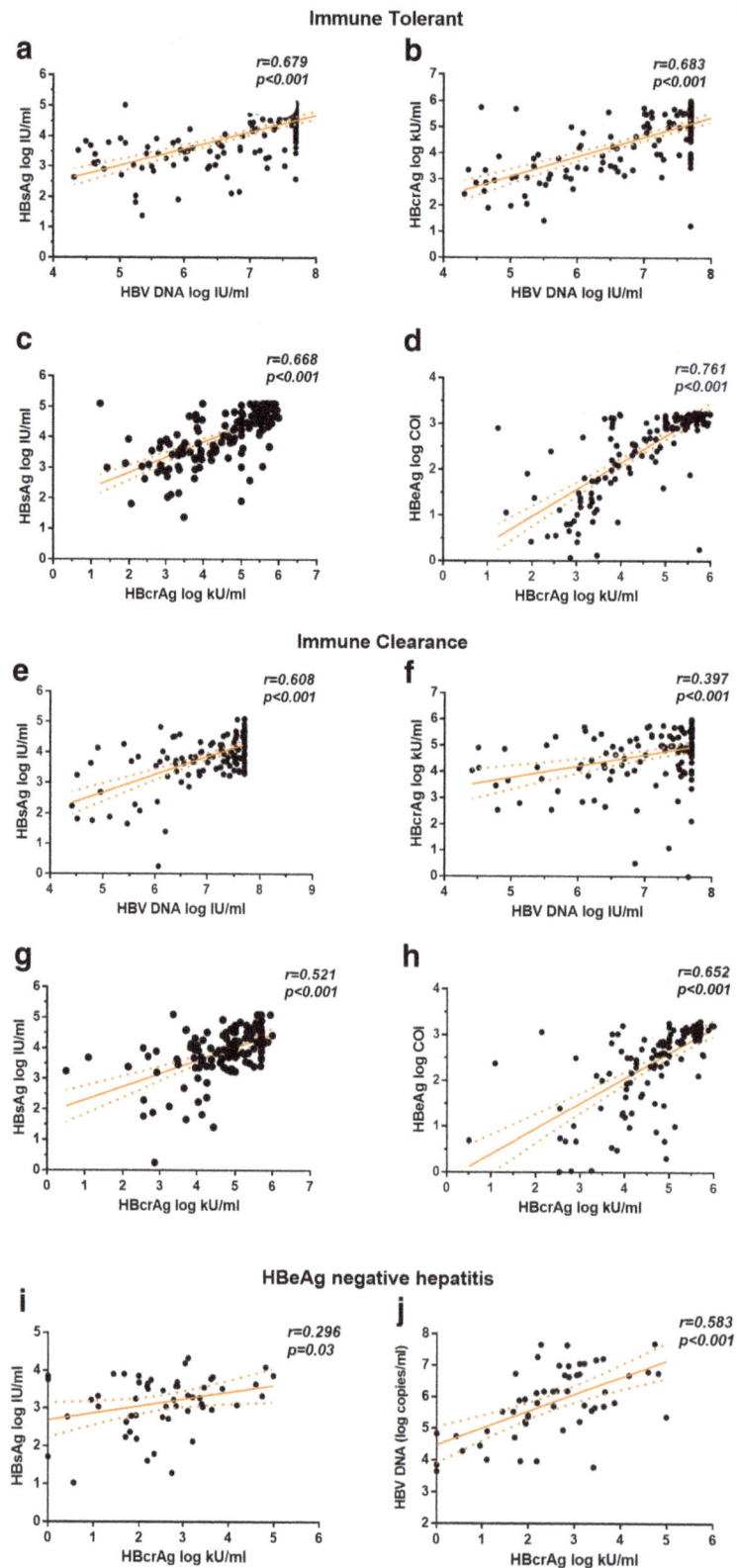

Fig. 2 Correlation of major viral markers in immune-tolerant (**a-d**), Immune-clearance (**e-h**) and HBeAg negative hepatitis (**i, j**) groups.Pearson's correlation coefficient, *p* value and estimate of linear regression curve were shown in each plot

Table 2 Phase-specific correlation of HBcrAg and HBsAg with various biomarkers

	Immune Tolerant (n = 159)		Immune clearance (n = 134)		Low Replicative (n = 99)		HBeAg negativ hepatitis (n = 54)	
	r	P	r	P	r	P	r	P
HBcrAg								
HBV DNA (log IU/ml)	**0.683**	**<0.001**	**0.397**	**<0.001**	0.023	0.822	**0.583**	**<0.001**
HBeAg (log COI)	**0.761**	**<0.001**	**0.652**	**<0.001**	NA	NA	NA	NA
HBsAg (log IU/ml)	**0.668**	**<0.001**	**0.521**	**<0.001**	**0.368**	**<0.001**	0.296	0.03
ALT IU/L	−0.78	0.330	0.082	0.133	0.06	0.555	0.126	0.365
HBsAg								
HBV DNA (log IU/ml)	**0.679**	**<0.001**	**0.608**	**<0.001**	0.224	0.026	0.380	0.005
HBeAg (log COI)	**0.624**	**<0.001**	**0.456**	**<0.001**	NA	NA	NA	NA
HBcrAg (log IU/ml)	**0.668**	**<0.001**	**0.521**	**<0.001**	**0.368**	**<0.001**	0.296	0.030
ALT IU/L	−0.08	0.271	0.104	0.231	0.015	0.879	−0.092	0.509

The r and P values of the correlation analyses were in bold if statistical significance is prominent (p<0.001)

Previously, in a total of 205 Chinese CHB patients, all of whom underwent liver histology examination, we found that HBcrAg is useful in predicting the necro-inflammation and advanced fibrosis [9]. In this study, we analyzed the relationship between HBcrAg and other viral markers in more detail, based on basic molecular biology of HBV precore and core proteins, in 444 CHB patients spanning all four phases of CHB natural history. It should be noted, that European Association for the Study of Liver recently issued a updated guideline for management of hepatitis B virus [16], in which a new nomenclature is used to describe these four phases, i.e., HBeAg-positive chronic infection, HBeAg-positive chronic hepatitis, HBeAg-negative chronic infection and HBeAg-negative chronic hepatitis. Nevertheless, the criteria for patient classification is essentially unchanged and will not affect the statistical analysis in this study.

We found, by multiple linear regression, that the major variance of HBcrAg can be attributed to HBeAg in IT and IC groups, while in ENH group, HBV DNA is a major determinant of HBcrAg. It should be noted that these linear regression analyses were by no means intended to formulate an accurate quantitative relationship between HBcrAg and HBVDNA/HBeAg. They were utilized to better elucidate the major contributors of HBcrAg in different stages of diseases. Indeed, these results could well explain the less pronounced decline of HBcrAg level during antiviral therapy compared with HBV DNA [7]. However, it should be acknowledged that this analysis still did not fully reflect the real picture since genome-free HBV virions containing HBcAg were reported to exist in high molar ratio to Dane particles [13] and p22cr, which can assemble into Dane-like particles devoid of HBV DNA, also exists [6]. Nevertheless, our analysis revealed that HBcrAg titre exhibited a phase-specific relationship with serum viral biomarkers such as HBeAg, HBsAg and HBV DNA.

Apart from circulating biomarkers, our analysis also looked into the abundance of viral antigens (HBsAg, HBcAg) in different compartments (serum and liver). A significant positive relationship was observed in liver HBcAg-IHC scores and HBcrAg level. Since most of the

Table 3 Multiple linear regression analysis of HBcrAg

Clinical Variables	Regression Coefficient	SE of Regression Coefficient	95% CI		P value	Multiple Regression Coefficient (R)
			Lower	Upper		
Immune tolerant						**0.776**
logHBV DNA	**0.262**	**0.089**	**0.087**	**0.437**	**0.004**	
logHBeAg	**0.751**	**0.104**	**0.546**	**0.956**	**1.99E-11**	
Immune clearance						**0.664**
logHBV DNA	0.164	0.085	−0.005	0.333	0.057	
LogHBeAg	**0.697**	**0.086**	**0.527**	**0.867**	**3.35E-13**	
E negative hepatitis						**0.583**
LogHBV DNA	**0.635**	**0.123**	**0.389**	**0.881**	**3.68E-6**	

The r and P values of the correlation analyses were in bold if statistical significance is prominent (p<0.001)

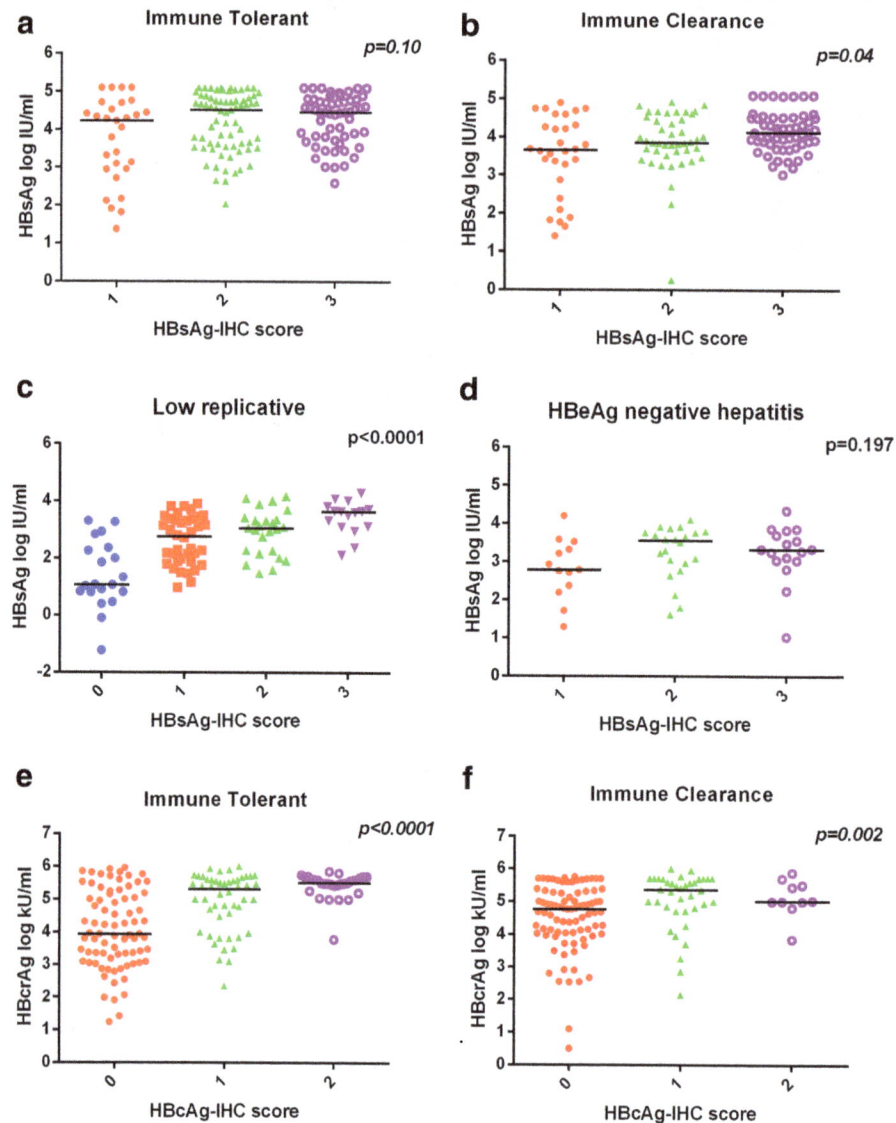

Fig. 3 Relationship between circulating antigens and their intrahepatic status. The HBsAg (**a-d**) and HBcrAg (**e**, **f**) titres in each phases were grouped according to immunohistochemistry scores of HBsAg and HBcAg respectively and plotted

core antigen staining was found within hepatocyte nuclei [4], it is conceivable that over-production of precore and core antigens would lead to core antigen nuclear transport and accumulation. As to the surface antigen, it was reported that the major intrahepatic S protein is large surface antigen, while circulating S protein was dominated by small surface antigen [17]. These large S protein can even accumulate in high levels which induces ground-glass morphology [18]. It is possible that these differences lead to the lack of correlation between liver and serum surface antigens in IT, IC and ENH groups. Nevertheless, the existence of around 20% HBsAg-IHC negative cases in LR group may be responsible for the statistical significance in this particular phase.

Conclusions

In conclusion, although several articles have already been published on the features of HBcrAg during the natural course of CHB [19, 20], our analyses provided additional information. First, HBcrAg titre were statistically related to HBeAg and HBV DNA which exhibited a phase-specific dominance pattern. This pattern can be well explained by the basic virology of hepatitis B virus. Second, the histological examinations on all enrolled 444 patients revealed a clear correlation between HBcrAg and intrahepatic HBcAg. Indeed, quantitative assays for core-related antigen has shown its utility in monitoring and refining antiviral therapy. It would be most desirable that novel precision assays could be developed to quantify all major products of precore and core ORF (HBcAg, p22cr, HBeAg etc) which would allow detailed analyses on their dynamics in the natural course of disease and their immune-modulatory roles leading to life-time persistent infection.

Abbreviations

CHB: Chronic hepatitis B; ENH: HBeAg negative hepatitis; HBcAg: Hepatitis B core antigen; HBcrAg: Hepatitis B core-related antigen; HBeAg: Hepatitis B e antigen; HBsAg: Hepatitis B surface antigen; HBV: Hepatitis B virus; IC: Immune clearance; IT: Immune tolerance; LR: Low replicative; ULN: Upper limit of normal

Acknowledgements

Not applicable.

Funding

This work was supported by the "12th Five-year" National Science and Technology Major Project of China (2013ZX10002005), National Natural Science Foundation (81671998), Shanghai Science and Technology Commission (16411960100) and key scientific research project of Shanghai municipal health and Family Planning Commission (20134032). The funders had no role in study design, data collection and analysis, decision to publish, or preparation of the manuscript.

Authors' contributions

ZZ conceived and designed the study; QW and YF conducted experiments; ZZ and XZ analyzed the data, WL, YW and ZZ coordinated and provided the collection of human materials, ZZ wrote the manuscript, ZZ and XZ performed critical revision of the manuscript. All authors have read and approved the manuscript.

Competing interests

The authors declare that they have no competing interests.

Author details

[1]Department of Hepatology, Shanghai Public Health Clinical Center, Fudan University, Caolang Road 2901, Shanghai 201508, China. [2]Research Unit, Shanghai Public Health Clinical Center, Fudan University, Caolang Road 2901, Shanghai 201508, China. [3]Shanghai Representative Office, Fujirebio Inc., Shanghai, China. [4]Department of Clinical Pathology, Shanghai Public Health Clinical Center, Fudan University, Shanghai, China.

References

1. WHO: Guidelines for the prevention, care and treatment of persons with chronic hepatitis B infection.; 2015.
2. Nguyen T, Thompson AJ, Bowden S, Croagh C, Bell S, Desmond PV, Levy M, Locarnini SA, Hepatitis B. Surface antigen levels during the natural history of chronic hepatitis B: a perspective on Asia. J Hepatol. 2010;52(4):508–13.
3. Thompson AJ, Nguyen T, Iser D, Ayres A, Jackson K, Littlejohn M, Slavin J, Bowden S, Gane EJ, Abbott W, et al. Serum hepatitis B surface antigen and hepatitis B e antigen titers: disease phase influences correlation with viral load and intrahepatic hepatitis B virus markers. Hepatology. 2010;51(6):1933–44.
4. Zhang X, Lu W, Zheng Y, Wang W, Bai L, Chen L, Feng Y, Zhang Z, Yuan Z. In Situ analysis of intrahepatic virological events in chronic hepatitis B virus infection. J Clin Invest. 2016;126(3):1079–92.
5. Kimura T, Rokuhara A, Sakamoto Y, Yagi S, Tanaka E, Kiyosawa K, Maki N. Sensitive enzyme immunoassay for hepatitis B virus core-related antigens and their correlation to virus load. J Clin Microbiol. 2002;40(2):439–45.
6. Kimura T, Ohno N, Terada N, Rokuhara A, Matsumoto A, Yagi S, Tanaka E, Kiyosawa K, Ohno S, Maki N, Hepatitis B. Virus DNA-negative dane particles lack core protein but contain a 22-kDa precore protein without C-terminal arginine-rich domain. J Biol Chem. 2005;280(23):21713–9.
7. Rokuhara A, Tanaka E, Matsumoto A, Kimura T, Yamaura T, Orii K, Sun X, Yagi S, Maki N, Kiyosawa K. Clinical evaluation of a new enzyme immunoassay for hepatitis B virus core-related antigen; a marker distinct from viral DNA for monitoring lamivudine treatment. J Viral Hepat. 2003; 10(4):324–30.
8. Suzuki F, Miyakoshi H, Kobayashi M, Kumada H. Correlation between serum hepatitis B virus core-related antigen and intrahepatic covalently closed circular DNA in chronic hepatitis B patients. J Med Virol. 2009;81(1):27–33.
9. Zhang ZQ, Lu W, Wang YB, Weng QC, Zhang ZY, Yang ZQ, Feng YL. Measurement of the hepatitis B core-related antigen is valuable for predicting the pathological status of liver tissues in chronic hepatitis B patients. J Virol Methods. 2016;235:92–8.
10. Goodman ZD. Grading and staging systems for inflammation and fibrosis in chronic liver diseases. J Hepatol. 2007;47(4):598–607.
11. Garcia PD, JH O, Rutter WJ, Walter P. Targeting of the hepatitis B virus precore protein to the endoplasmic reticulum membrane: after signal peptide cleavage translocation can be aborted and the product released into the cytoplasm. J Cell Biol. 1988;106(4):1093–104.
12. Ito K, Kim KH, Lok AS, Tong S. Characterization of genotype-specific carboxyl-terminal cleavage sites of hepatitis B virus e antigen precursor and identification of furin as the candidate enzyme. J Virol. 2009;83(8):3507–17.
13. Ning X, Nguyen D, Mentzer L, Adams C, Lee H, Ashley R, Hafenstein S, Hu J. Secretion of genome-free hepatitis B virus–single strand blocking model for virion morphogenesis of para-retrovirus. PLoS Pathog. 2011;7(9):e1002255.
14. van Campenhout MJ, Brouwer WP, van Oord GW, Xie Q, Zhang Q, Zhang N, Guo S, Tabak F, Streinu-Cercel A, Wang J, et al. Hepatitis B core-related antigen levels are associated with response to entecavir and Peginterferon add-on therapy in Hbeag-positive chronic hepatitis B patients. Clin Microbiol Infect. 2016;22(6):571.e5–9.
15. Honda M, Shirasaki T, Terashima T, Kawaguchi K, Nakamura M, Oishi N, Wang X, Shimakami T, Okada H, Arai K, et al. Hepatitis B virus (HBV) Core-related antigen during Nucleos(t)ide analog therapy is related to intra-hepatic HBV replication and development of hepatocellular carcinoma. J Infect Dis. 2016;213(7):1096–106.
16. European Association for the Study of the Liver. Electronic address eee, European Association for the Study of the L: EASL 2017 clinical practice guidelines on the management of hepatitis B virus infection. J Hepatol. 2017;67(2):370–98.
17. Gerken G, Manns M, Gerlich WH, Hess G, Meyer zum Buschenfelde KH. Immune blot analysis of viral surface proteins in serum and liver of patients with chronic hepatitis B virus infection. J Med Virol. 1989;29(4):261–5.
18. Hadziyannis S, Gerber MA, Vissoulis C, Popper H, Cytoplasmic h B. Antigen in "ground-glass" hepatocytes of carriers. Arch Pathol. 1973;96(5):327–30.
19. Maasoumy B, Wiegand SB, Jaroszewicz J, Bremer B, Lehmann P, Deterding K, Taranta A, Manns MP, Wedemeyer H, Glebe D, et al. Hepatitis B core-related antigen (HBcrAg) levels in the natural history of hepatitis B virus infection in a large European cohort predominantly infected with genotypes A and D. Clin Microbiol Infect. 2015;21(6) 606 e601–610
20. Seto WK, Wong DK, Fung J, Huang FY, Liu KS, Lai CL, Yuen MF, Linearized h B. Surface antigen and hepatitis B core-related antigen in the natural history of chronic hepatitis B. Clin Microbiol Infect. 2014;20(11):1173–80.

14

Attenuating the rate of total body fat accumulation and alleviating liver damage by oral administration of vitamin D-enriched edible mushrooms in a diet-induced obesity murine model is mediated by an anti-inflammatory paradigm shift

A. Drori[1], D. Rotnemer-Golinkin[1], S. Avni[2], A. Drori[3], O. Danay[2], D. Levanon[2], J. Tam[3], L. Zolotarev[1] and Y. Ilan[1]*

Abstract

Background: Hypovitaminosis D is associated with many features of the metabolic syndrome, including non-alcoholic fatty liver disease. Vitamin D-enriched mushrooms extracts exert a synergistic anti-inflammatory effect. The aim of the present study is to determine the immunomodulatory effect of oral administration of vitamin D-enriched mushrooms extracts on high-fat diet (HFD) animal model of non-alcoholic steatohepatitis (NASH).

Methods: C57BL/6 mice on HFD were orally administered with vitamin D supplement, *Lentinula edodes* (LE) mushrooms extract, or vitamin D-enriched mushrooms extract for 25 weeks. Mice were studied for the effect of the treatment on the immune system, liver functions and histology, insulin resistance and lipid profile.

Results: Treatment with vitamin D-enriched LE extracts was associated with significant attenuation of the rate of total body fat accumulation, along with a decrease in hepatic fat content as measured by an EchoMRI. Significant alleviation of liver damage manifested by a marked decrease in ALT, and AST serum levels (from 900 and 1021 U/L in the control group to 313 and 340; 294 and 292; and 366 and 321 U/L for ALT and AST, in Vit D, LE and LE + Vit D treated groups, respectively). A corresponding effect on hepatocyte ballooning were also noted. A significant decrease in serum triglycerides (from 103 to 75, 69 and 72 mg/dL), total cholesterol (from 267 to 160, 157 and 184 mg/dL), and LDL cholesterol (from 193 mg/dL to 133, 115 and 124 mg/dL) along with an increase in the HDL/LDL ratio, and improved glucose levels were documented. These beneficial effects were associated with a systemic immunomodulatory effect associated with an increased CD4/CD8 lymphocyte ratio (from 1.38 in the control group to 1.69, 1.71 and 1.63), and a pro- to an anti-inflammatory cytokine shift.

Conclusions: Oral administration of vitamin-D enriched mushrooms extracts exerts an immune modulatory hepato-protective effect in NASH model.

Keywords: Vitamin D, *Lentinula edodes*, Shiitake, NASH

* Correspondence: ilan@hadassah.org.il
[1]Gastroenterology and Liver Units, Department of Medicine,
Hadassah-Hebrew University Medical Center, P.O.B 12000, -91120 Jerusalem,
IL, Israel
Full list of author information is available at the end of the article

Background

Non-alcoholic fatty liver disease (NAFLD) is the most common form of chronic liver disease in western countries [1]. The immune system plays an important role in the pathogenesis of the liver damage as well as in the development of liver fibrosis [2–5]. Epidemiologic data show that NAFLD and vitamin D deficiency often coexist [6], and both conditions are considered as cardio-metabolic risk factors [7]. Several studies have linked vitamin D, NAFLD, and diabetes [8]. The hypovitaminosis D is associated with central obesity, impaired glucose homeostasis, insulin resistance, hypertension, and dyslipidemia [8]. High serum levels of 25(OH)D3 were shown to protect against the development of NAFLD, and a negative correlation was shown between vitamin D levels and visceral fat area [9]. Vitamin D was found earlier to possess an anti-fibrotic property in the onset of fibrosis in specific genotypes for vitamin D receptor (VDR) [10].

Vitamin D through its active form 1α-25-dihydroxy vitamin D [1,25(OH)2D] is a secosteroid hormone that plays a key role in mineral metabolism [6]. Recent data suggest its role in immune regulation [11, 12]. Biologically active vitamin D, 1,25-dihydroxylvitamin D3, is synthesized by the classic two-step hydroxylation in the liver and kidneys. The 1,25-dihydroxylvitamin D3 can also be produced locally by immune cells in response to infection [13]. Several immune regulatory function of vitamin D were shown to include the induction of antimicrobial peptides, suppression of innate immune response, induction of Th2 cytokines, and promotion of T-regulatory T cells (Tregs) [13].

Hypovitaminosis D is common worldwide with a prevalence of 30% to 50%. This is mainly attributed to inadequate exposure to ultraviolet radiation and insufficient consumption of the vitamin [8]. An association between hypovitaminosis D and the metabolic syndrome has been described earlier. Patients with a serum 25-hydroxy vitamin D concentration < 10 ng/mL had an increased risk of abdominal obesity and a higher prevalence of the metabolic syndrome. In an intervention program, weight loss was strongly related to increased serum vitamin D concentration [14].

Extracts derived from *Lentinula edodes* (LE, Shiitake) edible mushroom exert an anti-inflammatory effect in animal models of immune-mediated colitis [15]. Mushrooms are an abundant source of ergosterol, which is the precursor of vitamin D_2. Ergosterol converts into ergocalciferol (vitamin D_2) following the exposure to ultraviolet (UV) light. Then, after ingestion and absorption, it goes through hydroxylation into the active form 25-hydroxyvitamin D [25(OH)D]. Recently, the vitamin D_2-enriched mushrooms were studied, in order to verify the impact of both ingredients [16].

The aim of the present study is to determine the immunomodulatory effect of oral administration of vitamin D-enriched mushrooms extracts, and to assess its corresponding clinical effect on fatty liver disease and the related insulin resistance in the high-fat diet (HFD) animal model of non-alcoholic steatohepatitis (NASH).

Methods

Animals and experimental design

Experiments were carried out on animals according to the guidelines of the Hebrew University-Hadassah Institutional Committee for the Care and Use of Laboratory Animals with the committee's approval. 10 weeks old male C57BL/6 mice were obtained from Harlan Laboratories (Jerusalem, Israel) and maintained in the Animal Core Facility of the Hadassah-Hebrew University Medical School. The mice were weighted weekly and fed in a liberal, restriction-free, commercially available HFD (Harlan, TD88137; 42% of the calories are from fat). Four groups of mice ($n = 6$, each) were orally treated three times a week for 25 weeks with one of the following: Group A (Control), saline (0.9% NaCl); Group B (Vitamin D), 25 μL of commercially available, over-the-counter, vitamin D supplement, containing 400 IU per drop, diluted at commercially available, over-the-shelf, ready-to-use, locally-made olive oil, equal to 10 UI per mouse per feed; Group C (LE), 25 μL of LE mushrooms extract containing 8.3 mg of dried mushroom, suspended in double-distilled water (DDW), per mouse per feed; Group D (LE + Vitamin D), 25 μL of vitamin D-enriched LE mushrooms extract containing 8.3 mg of dried mushroom and 10 IU for vitamin D, suspended in DDW, per mouse per feed. Mice were sacrificed using anesthetics.

Preparation of vitamin D-enriched extract

Fruit bodies of LE at different development stages were picked. Immediately after picking the fruit bodies, they were exposed, post-harvest, to short pulses of UV-B irradiation in order to raise their vitamin D_2 content [16]. The highest vitamin content was found in the fruit bodies that were picked at the "flat" development stage, two days following the optimal marketing picking time. The mushrooms were frozen-dried, milled to powder, and their vitamin D_2 contents (on dry weight basis) were measured by high-performance liquid chromatography (HPLC) (MIGAL labs, Israel).

Effect of UV-B exposure on shiitake Ergosterol, vitamin D_2 and glucan content

As shown in Table 1, Shiitake mushroom's Ergosterol and α-Glucans concentrations were not significantly altered following radiation exposure. However, Vitamin D_2 content was increased significantly following UV-B exposure from a negligible concentration to 42.96 ± 7.21 μg/g DM (p value <0.05). Furthermore, in response to UV-B exposure Shiitake β-Glucan and total-Glucan concentrations were decreased significantly by 30% and 27.5%, respectively (p value <0.05).

Table 1 Active components in radiated (LE + D) and unirradiated (LE) *L. edodes* mushrooms

	LE (n = 3)		LE + D (n = 3)		
	M	SD	M	SD	p value
Ergosterol (mg/1 g DM)	1.98	0.84	1.24	0.70	0.327
Vit. D$_2$ (µg/1 g DM)	ND	ND	42.96	7.21	0.0005
β-Glucan (% w/w)	22.35	1.01	15.80	0.88	0.0023
α-Glucan (% w/w)	1.3	0.04	1.38	0.07	0.2019
total-Glucan (% w/w)	23.64	1	17.18	0.81	0.0021

Mushroom culture

Mushrooms were not exposed to UV-B along the growing process. LE mushrooms (S61 var., Fungisem) were grown on sterilized 3:2 mixture of eucalyptus sawdust and olive mill cake. Mixture was wetted to 60% water content and packed into Unicorn Type M filter polypropylene bags. Bags were autoclaved at 121 °C for 1 h, and cooled to 25 °C for inoculation with the spawn. Culture was incubated at 25 °C for 21 days. For fruiting, the temperature was reduced to 16 °C with a relative humidity of 90%, daily illumination for 12 h by fluorescent 500 lx "Daylight" and air CO$_2$ concentration of 600–800 ppm [17].

Irradiation procedure

A LH-840 (Xenon Corporation, Wilmington, MA) was used for pulsed UV light exposure. A 16″ linear B-type lamp was used (240 nm, No ozone generated). The LE mushrooms were exposed to 10 UV-B radiation pulses, at doses of 507 J/pulse at room temperature. The non-radiated and irradiated mushrooms were separately freeze-dried (Dr. Golik Co.), grind by mortar and pestle with liquid nitrogen, and then stored at −20 °C until analysis.

Analysis of the Ergosterol and vitamin D$_2$

The compounds of the vitamin D and Ergosterol fraction were extracted as described previously with minor modifications [17]. Their analysis was performed by UHPLC (Ultimate 3000, Thermo Scientific, MA, USA) coupled with diode array detector (DAD). The chromatographic separation was conducted on a C18 column (Aqua 3u C18 125A New Column 150 × 4.6 mm, Silicol). The sampler oven temperature was set to 4 °C, while the column oven temperature was set to 15 °C, with injection volume of 20 µL and flow rate at 1 mL/min. The separation was isocratic plan with 75% methanol: 25% acetonitrile. UV detection was performed in 210, 250, 265 and 280 nm. Ergosterol, vitamin D$_3$ (Internal Standard) and vitamin D$_2$ were determined by comparing the retention times of standards (ergosterol, cholecalciferol and ergocalciferol, Sigma Chemicals, Steinheim, Germany), and quantification was done by using a calibration curve.

Total glucans, β-glucans and α-glucans analysis

The glucan concentrations were evaluated by using a Glucan Assay Kit (Megazyme® International Ireland Ltd., Bray Co, Wicklow, Ireland), based on a colorimetric reaction, according to the manufacturer's instructions. Absorbance was measured at 510 nm using Ultrospec 2100 pro UV/Visible Spectrophotometer (Amersham Bioscience, Freiburg, Germany) against the GOPOD reagent blank and unknowns were compared to a glucose standard to calculate percent of glucan. Total Glucan (% w/w) and α-Glucan (% w/w) were measured and the difference between those two was calculated as the β-glucan (% w/w).

Isolation of splenocytes

Spleens were kept in RPMI-1640 supplemented with FCS 10%. Spleens were crushed through a 70 µm nylon cell strainer [18] and centrifuged (1250 rpm for 7 min) to remove debris. Red blood cells were lysed. Splenocytes were suspended in 1 mL of fluorescence-activated cell sorting (FACS) buffer. Viability was assessed using trypan blue staining and was above 90%.

FACS analysis

Flow cytometry was performed on splenocytes lymphocytes with antibodies for CD4, CD8, CD25 (eBioscience, San Diego, CA, USA) and NK1.1 (Biogem, Westlake village, CA, USA) epitopes using the LSR-II. Analysis was performed using FSC express software.

Cytokine measurement

Serum interleukin 1-α(IL-1$_\alpha$), IL-1$_\beta$, IL-4, IL-6, IL-10, IL-12, IL-13 IL-17, tumor necrosis factor alpha (TNF$_\alpha$) and interferon gamma (IFN$_\gamma$) levels were measured in each animal using Custom Q-plex-10plex ELISA-based Chemiluminescent assay (Quansys Biosciences, Logan, UT, USA). Transforming growth factor beta (TGF$_\beta$) levels were measured in each animal using Quantikine ELISA Mouse/Rat/Porcine/Canine TGF-b1 (R&D Systems, Minneapolis, MN, USA).

Biochemistry analysis

Blood was collected from individual mice at euthanasia and serum aspartate aminotransferase (AST), alanine aminotransferase (ALT) and gamma-glutamyl transferase (gGT) levels were determined using Reflotvet Plus (Roche). Serum triglyceride (TG), total cholesterol (T-chol) and high-density lipoprotein (HDL) levels were measured using the Cobas®C 111 analyzer (Roche, Switzerland). Tail-end venous blood glucose levels were measured bi-weekly using Accu-Check Performa Tests (Roche). Low-density lipoproteins (LDL-c, was calculated by (0.9xT-Chol)-(0.9xTG/5)-28) at the end of the study [19].

Body and liver fat content

The total in vivo body and ex vivo liver fat contents were evaluated by using the EchoMRI™-100H (EchoMRI, TX) at weeks 7 and 25 and after sacrifice, respectively.

Liver histology

4–5 μm paraffin-embedded liver sections were prepared from each mouse and stained with hematoxylin-eosin (H&E). An unsighted pathologist examined the tissues using a light microscopy to score for morphological and histopathological changes that are characteristic of NAFLD Activity Score (NAS). The maximal score for steatosis (=3) was assigned for greater than 66%. The maximal score for lobular inflammation (=3) was assigned for >4 foci/200×, and hepatocyte ballooning (=2) was assigned for many cells/prominent ballooning. The maximal NAS score is a simple arithmetic combination of all three features (min. 0, max. 8) [20]. In addition, fibrosis was evaluated and semi-quantified (score 0–4).

Hepatic triglyceride (hTG) content

Accumulation of intracellular TGs within the liver was quantified using a modification of the Folch method [21]. hTGs were extracted from aliquots of snap-frozen livers and then assayed using a GPO-Trinder kit (Sigma, Israel), and the levels were normalized to per gram of liver tissue in the homogenate.

Statistical analysis

Statistical analysis was performed using Kruskal-Wallis test and Mann-Whitney (only if the former showed statistical significance, p value <0.05) (Using GraphPad Prism 6.01). Standard Error (SE) is indicated by error bars at all figures.

Results

Effect of treatment on metabolic parameters

The aim of the study was to determine the immunomodulatory effect of oral administration of vitamin D-enriched mushrooms extracts, and to assess its corresponding clinical effect on fatty liver disease and the related insulin resistance in the HFD model of NASH. Treatment with LE + vitamin D significantly attenuated the rate of body fat accumulation as calculated by the trend-lines and their slope [Fig. 1a].

As noted, the slope decreases from 4.31, 4.39 and 4.66 at Control, Vitamin D and LE groups to 2.10 at the LE + vitamin D group. At week 25, there was a decrease in the percentage of total body fat between the control group and all three treatment groups [Fig. 1b].

The TG levels, T-Chol and LDL-c were decreased in all treatment groups, compared to the control group [Fig. 2a-d], while the ratio between serum HDL and LDL-c was increased at all treatment group [Fig. 2e].

Starting from week 3 (data not shown), and throughout all of the experiment, the three treatment groups showed a statistically significant decrease in the average serum glucose levels, compared to the control group. No significant differences were noted between the average serum glucose levels for three treatment groups, except at anecdotal point - week 11 (data not shown), [Fig. 2f].

Treatment was also associated with a significant decrease in body weight. For example, at week 25, the average weight of the control group was 47.4 g, compared with 40.6 g, 40.2 g and 40.5 g at the vitamin D, LE and LE + vitamin D treated groups, respectively (all p values <0.05. Data not shown).

The effect of treatment on liver damage

A significant alleviation of the liver damage as manifested by a marked decrease in serum ALT, AST and GGT levels in all three treated groups at week 25, compared with the control group [Fig. 3a].

The hTG content did not change between the three treated groups and the control group.

A statistically significant decrease in the hepatic fat content (by Post-mortem Liver EchoMRI) was noted following treatment with mushrooms extracts compared to the control group. This effect was not achieved when treating with vitamin D alone [Fig. 3b].

Upon histological examination, a reduction was noted for hepatocytes ballooning score, and in the NAS score, in the Vitamin D group [Fig. 3c-f].

Representative photographs of liver sections (H&E, ×10) from all groups are shown in Fig. 3g. A reduction in the ballooning is noted in Vitamin D and LE groups, and a reduction in the inflammation was noted in Vitamin D and LE + Vitamin D treated groups. Photos courtesy of Dr. Areej A. S. Khatib, M.D., Bethlehem University.

Effect of treatment on the immune system

A significant reduction was noted in pro-inflammatory cytokines serum levels in all three treated groups - TNF$_\alpha$, IL-1$_\alpha$ and IL-1$_\beta$. TGF$_\beta$1 serum levels increased in all three treated groups, compared to the control group. A trend for an increase IL-10 was noted, following treatment with Vitamin D and LE + Vitamin D. The IL-10/TNF$_\alpha$ ratio and IL-4/TNF$_\alpha$ ratio were increased in all the treated groups, compared to control group (data not shown) [Fig. 4a-f].

The oral administration of vitamin D-enriched mushrooms exerted a systemic immune modulatory effect as noted by a trend for alteration of splenic lymphocytes sub-populations. A change in the CD4/CD8 lymphocyte ratio was noted with an increased ratio in all three treated groups, compared with the control group. No other significant changes were noted in other studied subsets of lymphocytes [Fig. 4g].

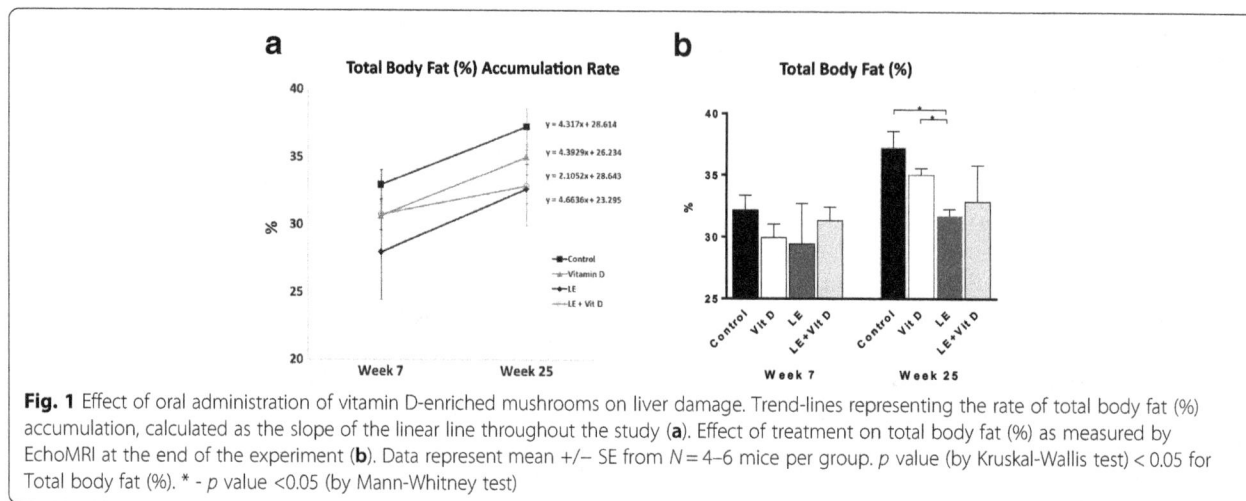

Fig. 1 Effect of oral administration of vitamin D-enriched mushrooms on liver damage. Trend-lines representing the rate of total body fat (%) accumulation, calculated as the slope of the linear line throughout the study (**a**). Effect of treatment on total body fat (%) as measured by EchoMRI at the end of the experiment (**b**). Data represent mean +/− SE from N = 4–6 mice per group. p value (by Kruskal-Wallis test) < 0.05 for Total body fat (%). * - p value <0.05 (by Mann-Whitney test)

Discussion

Much progress in the understanding of the pathophysiology of NASH has been made. However, there is still no approved therapy for this epidemic [1]. Several of the drugs being developed for NASH target fibrosis, and/or carry side effects. These may prohibit their long term use in patients with mild to moderate disease, when inflammation (and not fibrosis) underlines the liver damage [1]. The results of the present study show that vitamin-D enriched mushrooms extract exerts a beneficial immunomodulatory effect alleviating the liver damage and the metabolic parameters in the HFD model of NASH. Each of the compounds

exerted a beneficial effect on their own. However, a synergistic effect was noted on body fat accumulation.

A pro-inflammatory status underlines the development of NASH. Immune modulatory treatments are being evaluated for NASH [3, 22–28]. A correlation between TNF_α and degree of severity of the liver disease were described [29, 30]. Adaptive immune responses triggered by TNF_α-mediated oxidative stress contribute to hepatic inflammation in NASH [31]. Similarly, activation of kupffer cells enhances IL-1 production, contributing to hepatocyte dysfunction, necrosis, apoptosis, and generation of extracellular matrix proteins leading to fibrosis.

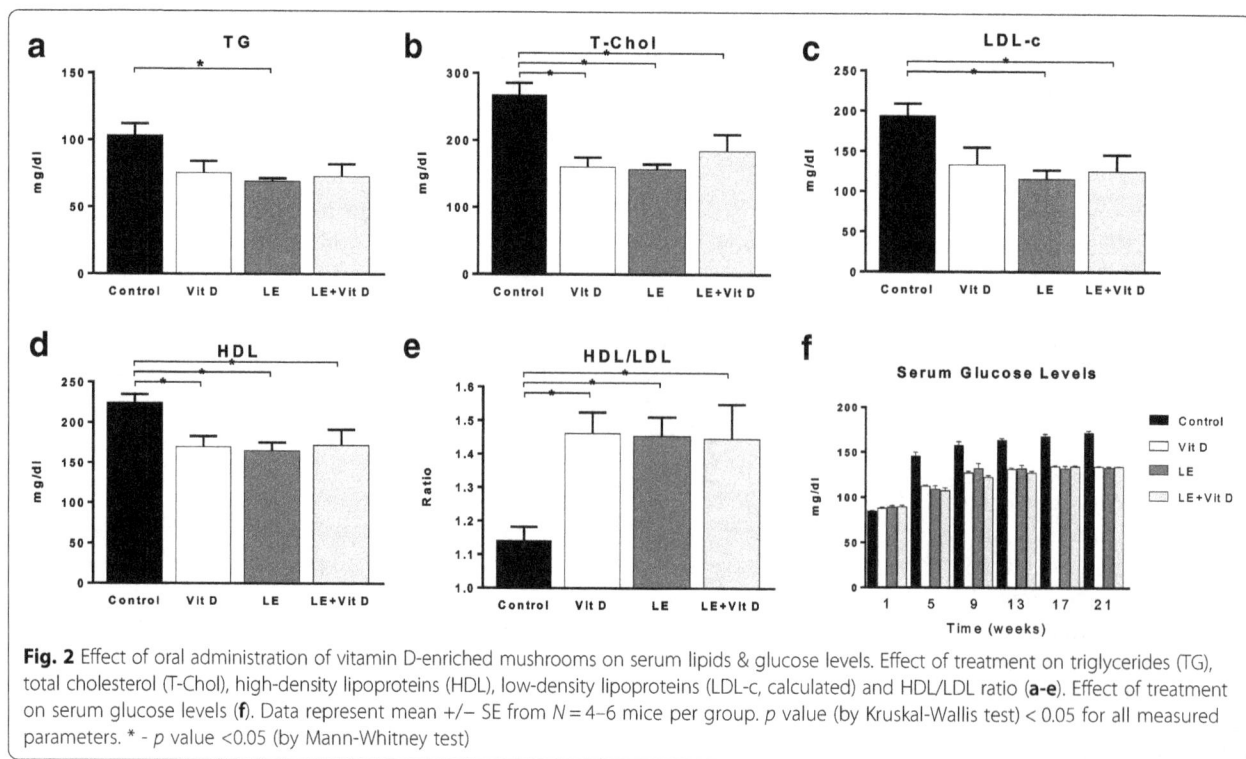

Fig. 2 Effect of oral administration of vitamin D-enriched mushrooms on serum lipids & glucose levels. Effect of treatment on triglycerides (TG), total cholesterol (T-Chol), high-density lipoproteins (HDL), low-density lipoproteins (LDL-c, calculated) and HDL/LDL ratio (**a-e**). Effect of treatment on serum glucose levels (**f**). Data represent mean +/− SE from N = 4–6 mice per group. p value (by Kruskal-Wallis test) < 0.05 for all measured parameters. * - p value <0.05 (by Mann-Whitney test)

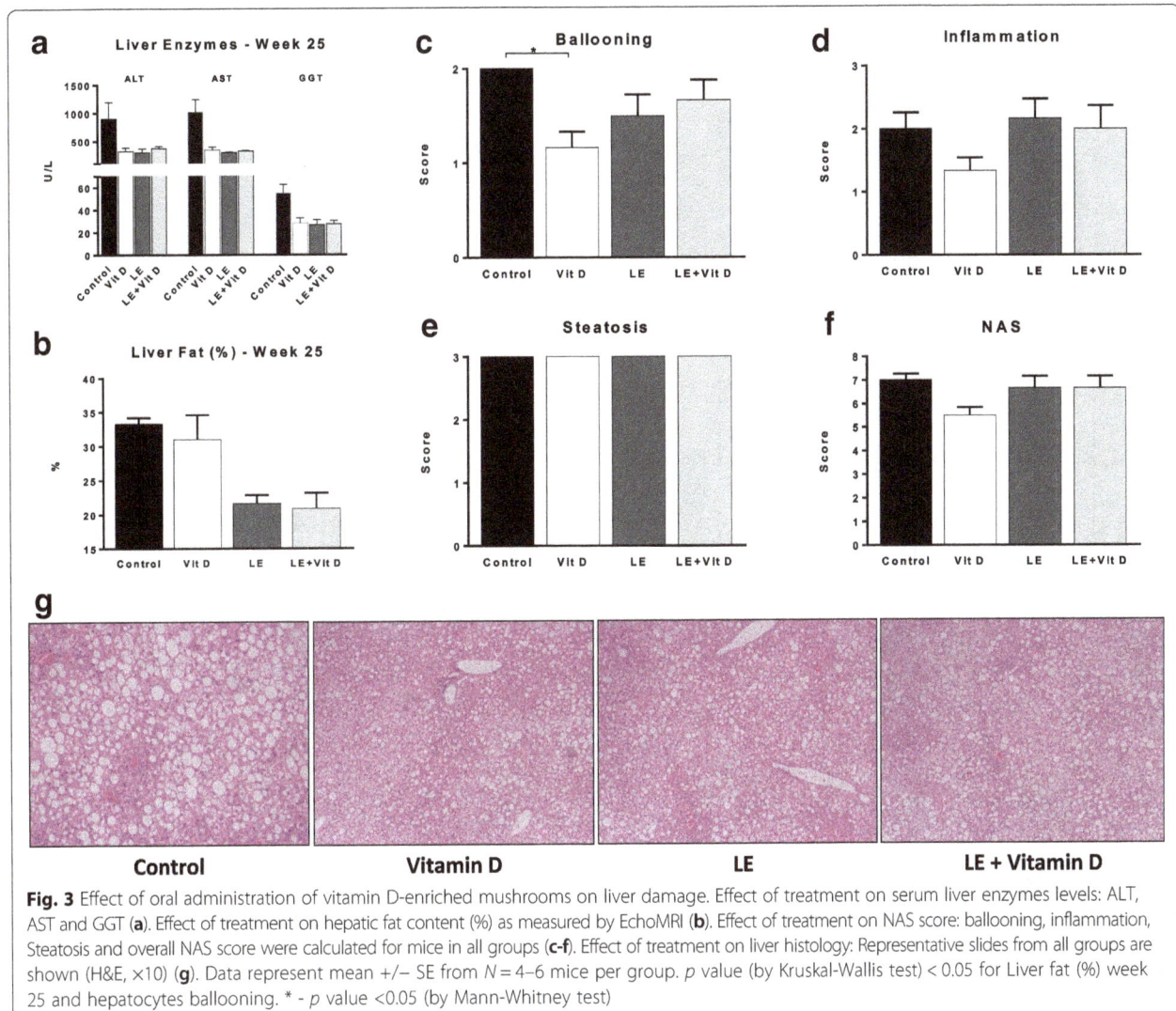

Fig. 3 Effect of oral administration of vitamin D-enriched mushrooms on liver damage. Effect of treatment on serum liver enzymes levels: ALT, AST and GGT (**a**). Effect of treatment on hepatic fat content (%) as measured by EchoMRI (**b**). Effect of treatment on NAS score: ballooning, inflammation, Steatosis and overall NAS score were calculated for mice in all groups (**c-f**). Effect of treatment on liver histology: Representative slides from all groups are shown (H&E, ×10) (**g**). Data represent mean +/− SE from N = 4–6 mice per group. p value (by Kruskal-Wallis test) < 0.05 for Liver fat (%) week 25 and hepatocytes ballooning. * - p value <0.05 (by Mann-Whitney test)

IL-1 is also known to regulate hepatic steatosis [32]. Increased pro-IL-1$_\beta$ levels correlate with disease severity [33]. Neutralization of IL-1 by IL-1 receptor antagonist (IL-1Ra) prevents liver injury [32]. Serum IL-1 receptor antagonist (IL-1RA) and liver mRNA expression of IL-1RN are associated with NASH and with the degree of lobular inflammation in liver [34]. In the present study, oral administration of vitamin D-enriched LE extracts exerted a systemic immune modulatory effect as noted by the alteration of splenic lymphocytes sub-populations. Treatment was also associated with a significant decrease in the serum levels TNF$_\alpha$, IL-1$_\alpha$, and IL-1$_\beta$.

The role of TGF$_\beta$ serum levels in the pathogenesis of NASH is somewhat controversial. Some studies showed lack of correlation with degree of severity of disease [35], while other suggested that TGF$_\beta$ signaling pathway in hepatocytes contributes to hepatocyte death and lipid accumulation through *Smad* signaling and reactive oxygen species production that promote the development of NASH [36, 37]. In some clinical trials using immune modulatory agents in patients with NASH, an increase in TGF$_\beta$ serum levels correlated with the beneficial effect of the drug [26]. In the present study, an increase in TGF$_\beta$ serum levels was noted in all treated groups. Being a multifactorial disease, NASH is also multiple cytokine-mediated disorder [38, 39].

The immune modulatory effects were associated with a significant alleviation of the liver damage manifested by a marked decrease in ALT, AST, and GGT serum levels in all three treatment groups. A corresponding decrease in hepatic fat content and attenuation of body fat accumulation is established. A significant decrease in serum TGs, T-Chol, along with an increase in the HDL/LDL ratio, and improved glucose levels, were noted in all treated groups.

The vitamin D-enriched LE extract described in the present study was previously shown to have a potent anti-inflammatory effect. Oral administration of LE extracts is

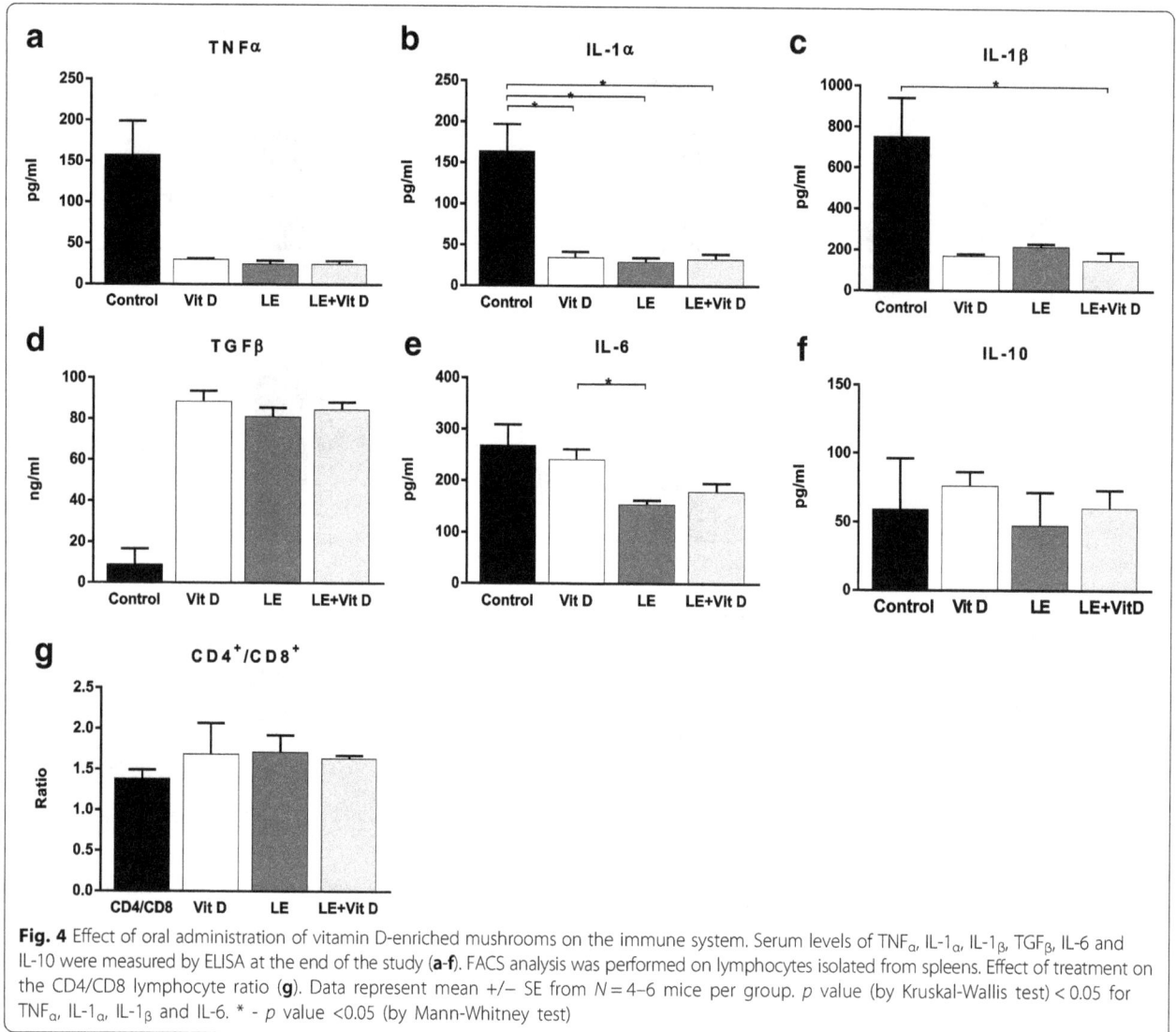

Fig. 4 Effect of oral administration of vitamin D-enriched mushrooms on the immune system. Serum levels of TNF_α, $IL-1_\alpha$, $IL-1_\beta$, TGF_β, IL-6 and IL-10 were measured by ELISA at the end of the study (**a-f**). FACS analysis was performed on lymphocytes isolated from spleens. Effect of treatment on the CD4/CD8 lymphocyte ratio (**g**). Data represent mean +/− SE from $N = 4$–6 mice per group. p value (by Kruskal-Wallis test) < 0.05 for TNF_α, $IL-1_\alpha$, $IL-1_\beta$ and IL-6. * - p value <0.05 (by Mann-Whitney test)

known to alleviate immune-mediated colitis [15]. The effect is associated with altered NKT regulatory lymphocyte distribution and increased intrahepatic CD8+ T lymphocyte trapping.

Treatment with vitamin D_2-enriched mushrooms extracts alleviates Concanavalin A- immune-mediated liver injury [16]. Following feeding of the vitamin D-enriched mushrooms extracts to immune-mediated hepatitis harboring mice, ALT serum levels are decreased and proportion of severe liver injury is declined. A corresponding histological improvement of the immune mediated liver injury is also noted in treated mice. The data showed a synergistic effect between the anti-inflammatory effect of the mushroom extracts and that of the vitamin D [16]. In the present study, oral administration of vitamin D-enriched LE extracts had a beneficial effect on all tested immune, liver, and metabolic parameters, while the administration of non-vitamin

enriched extracts or vitamin D alone exerted an effect only on some of these endpoints. A synergistic effect for the vitamin D-enriched LE extract was noted for the rate of body fat accumulation.

Mushrooms-associated immunomodulatory polysaccharides, such as Glucans (α-Glucans and β-Glucans) contribute to their anti-inflammatory effect [40]. Innate immune cells express pattern recognition receptors (PRRs) including dectin-1, Toll-like receptors, and mannose receptors on their cell surfaces. These PRRs recognize pathogens by binding to highly conserved pathogen-associated molecular patterns (PAMPS) such as beta-glucan, mannan, and lipopolysaccharide. Binding of β-glucans to dectin-1 expressed by macrophages or dendritic cells leads to innate cells activation of adaptive immune cells via secretion of interleukins (IL-4, IL-6) and TNF_α [40]. In vitro, the immune effect of β-glucans was dependent of their structure, molecular weight and compositional characteristics [41]. β-D-glucan manifested an immunomodulatory activity on THP-1 macrophages, inhibited the inflammatory phase of nociception, and reduced the number of total leukocytes and myeloperoxidase levels induced by LPS, supporting their anti-inflammatory activity [42].

Hypovitaminosis D is associated with NAFLD, increased insulin resistance, impaired insulin secretion, and is related to type 2 diabetes mellitus (T2DM) [43]. Local vitamin D signaling regulates hepatic and pancreatic islet functions contributing to both hepatic insulin sensitivity and islet insulin secretion [43]. Studies have suggested the benefits for vitamin D maintenance, or dietary manipulation, for prevention and treatment of obesity-induced T2DM and NAFLD. A recent cross-sectional study evaluated the correlation between NAFLD and vitamin D in 5000 men and women [44]. Decreased vitamin D levels were associated with an increased risk of NAFLD. Vitamin D was found to be an independent factor for NAFLD prevalence, implying that vitamin D interventional treatment may control the disease [44]. In a NASH animal model of choline-deficient diet, 1,25-vitamin D3 supplement slowed the development and progression of NASH [45]. Administration of 1,25-vitamin D3 decreased free fatty acids, triglycerides, thiobarbituric acid-reactive substances, number of apoptotic cells, expression of tissue inhibitor of metalloproteinase-1,and CK18-M30 in the liver, and improved liver histology. No change was noted in total antioxidant capacity of the liver [45, 46].

A recent 239 patient's trial showed that plasma vitamin D levels are not associated with insulin resistance, amount of liver fat accumulation, or the severity of NASH [47]. A 398 patient's trial showed that low levels of 25-OH vitamin D were not independently associated with liver damage in morbidly obese patients with NAFLD [48]. However, 25-OH vitamin D levels were inversely correlated to NAS biopsy score and steatosis. Vitamin D levels were lower in patients with significant fibrosis [47]. This discrepancy may be explained by population differences, and other confounding factors which were not accounted for. In addition, the beneficial effect of vitamin D-enriched mushrooms in NASH, as noted in the present study, may be due to a direct synergistic effect of the mushrooms extract and vitamin D, independent of baseline vitamin D serum levels.

The exact mechanism in which either vitamin D or LE mushrooms extracts exert all the above beneficial effects is still unknown. The fact that some beneficial effects were achieved by the Vitamin D and other effects were achieved by the LE might suggest a different biochemical mechanism, with a synergistic effect of both pathways. Another study, in an attempt to decipher these mechanisms and isolate the active ingredient (or ingredients) of LE, is underway.

Conclusions

In summary, the data of the present study supports a beneficial effect of oral administration of LE extracts enriched with vitamin D in alleviating the liver damage, and insulin resistance in a mouse model of NAFLD. A synergistic effect was noted on body fat accumulation. Considering the high safety profile of these extracts, the data supports their potential use in patients with early-stage NASH.

Abbreviations
(U)HPLC: (Ultra-) High-Performance Liquid Chromatography; ALT: Alanine aminotransferase; AST: Aspartate aminotransferase; DDW: Double-Distilled Water; DM: Dried Mushroom; GGT: Gamma-Glutamyl Transferase (gGT); HDL: High Density Lipoprotein; HFD: High-Fat Diet; IFN$_\gamma$: Interferon gamma; IL: Interleukin; IL-1Ra: IL-1 receptor antagonist; IL-1RA: Interleukin 1 receptor antagonist; LE: Shiitake: *Lentinula edodes*; NAFLD: Nonalcoholic Fatty Liver Disease; NAS: NAFLD Activity Score; NASH: Nonalcoholic Steatohepatitis; PAMPS: Pathogen-associated Molecular Patterns; PRRs: Pattern Recognition Receptors; TG: Triglycerides; TGF$_\beta$: Transforming Growth Factor beta; TNF$_\alpha$: Tumor Necrosis Factor alpha; Tregs: T-regulatory T cells; VDR: Vitamin D receptor

Acknowledgements
Not applicable

Funding
This work was supported in part by a grant from Kamin, Israel Ministry of the Economy, and the Roaman-Epstein Liver Research Foundation (to Y.I.), and the Israel Science Foundation (ISF) grant (#1471/14 to J.T.).

Authors' contributions
AD, DR, AS, DA, ZL performed the studies and prepared the data. AD, DA, DO, LD, TJ, YI designed the studies, analyzed the results, and took part in writing the manuscript. All authors read and approved the final manuscript.

Competing interests
The authors declare that they have no competing interests.

Author details
[1]Gastroenterology and Liver Units, Department of Medicine, Hadassah-Hebrew University Medical Center, P.O.B 12000, -91120 Jerusalem, IL, Israel. [2]Migal, Galilee Research Institute, Kiryat Shmona, Israel. [3]Obesity and Metabolism Laboratory, The Institute for Drug Research, School of Pharmacy, Faculty of Medicine, The Hebrew University of Jerusalem, Jerusalem, Israel.

References

1. Ratziu V, Goodman Z, Sanyal A. Current efforts and trends in the treatment of NASH. J Hepatol. 2015;62(1 Suppl):S65–75.

2. Meli R, Mattace Raso G, Calignano A. Role of innate immune response in non-alcoholic fatty liver disease: metabolic complications and therapeutic tools. Front Immunol. 2014;5:177.

3. Ilan Y. Immune therapy for nonalcoholic steatohepatitis: are we there yet? J Clin Gastroenterol. 2013;47(4):298–307.

4. Mehal WZ. The Gordian knot of dysbiosis, obesity and NAFLD. Nat Rev Gastroenterol Hepatol. 2013;10(11):637–44.

5. Wree A, Broderick L, Canbay A, Hoffman HM, Feldstein AE. From NAFLD to NASH to cirrhosis-new insights into disease mechanisms. Nat Rev Gastroenterol Hepatol. 2013;10(11):627–36.

6. Lee SM, Jun DW, Cho YK, Jang KS, Vitamin D. Deficiency in non-alcoholic fatty liver disease: the chicken or the egg? Clin Nutr. 2015;

7. Eliades M, Spyrou E, Vitamin D. A new player in non-alcoholic fatty liver disease? World J Gastroenterol. 2015;21(6):1718–27.

8. Strange RC, Shipman KE, Ramachandran S. Metabolic syndrome: a review of the role of vitamin D in mediating susceptibility and outcome. World J Diabetes. 2015;6(7):896–911.

9. Lu Z, Pan X, Hu Y, Hao Y, Luo Y, Hu X, Ma X, Bao Y, Jia W. Serum vitamin D levels are inversely related with non-alcoholic fatty liver disease independent of visceral obesity in Chinese postmenopausal women. Clin Exp Pharmacol Physiol. 2015;42(2):139–45.

10. Beilfuss A, Sowa JP, Sydor S, Beste M, Bechmann LP, Schlattjan M, Syn WK, Wedemeyer I, Mathe Z, Jochum C, et al. Vitamin D counteracts fibrogenic TGF-beta signalling in human hepatic stellate cells both receptor-dependently and independently. Gut. 2015;64(5):791–9.

11. Suzuki H, Kunisawa J. Vitamin-mediated immune regulation in the development of inflammatory diseases. Endocr Metab Immune Disord Drug Targets. 2015;15(3):212–5.

12. van Etten E, Stoffels K, Gysemans C, Mathieu C, Overbergh L. Regulation of vitamin D homeostasis: implications for the immune system. Nutr Rev. 2008;66(10 Suppl 2):S125–34.

13. Han YP, Kong M, Zheng S, Ren Y, Zhu L, Shi H, Duan Z, Vitamin D. In liver diseases: from mechanisms to clinical trials. J Gastroenterol Hepatol. 2013;28(Suppl 1):49–55.

14. Mallard SR, Howe AS, Houghton LA, Vitamin D. Status and weight loss: a systematic review and meta-analysis of randomized and nonrandomized controlled weight-loss trials. Am J Clin Nutr. 2016;104(4):1151–9.

15. Shuvy M, Hershcovici T, Lull-Noguera C, Wichers H, Danay O, Levanon D, Zolotarov L, Ilan Y. Intrahepatic CD8(+) lymphocyte trapping during tolerance induction using mushroom derived formulations: a possible role for liver in tolerance induction. World J Gastroenterol. 2008;14(24):3872–8.

16. Drori A, Shabat Y, Ben Ya'acov A, Danay O, Levanon D, Zolotarov L, Ilan Y. Extracts from Lentinula edodes (shiitake) edible mushrooms enriched with vitamin D exert an anti-inflammatory Hepatoprotective effect. J Med Food. 2016;19(4):383–9.

17. Wittig M, Krings U, Berger RG. Single-run analysis of vitamin D photoproducts in oyster mushroom (Pleurotus ostreatus) after UV-B treatment. J Food Compos Anal. 2013;31(2):266–74.

18. Falcone M, Facciotti F, Ghidoli N, Monti P, Olivieri S, Zaccagnino L, Bonifacio E, Casorati G, Sanvito F, Sarvetnick N. Up-regulation of CD1d expression restores the immunoregulatory function of NKT cells and prevents autoimmune diabetes in nonobese diabetic mice. J Immunol. 2004;172(10):5908–16.

19. Kapoor R, Chakraborty M, Singh N, Leap A. Above Friedewald formula for calculation of low-density lipoprotein-cholesterol. J Lab Physicians. 2015;7(1):11–6.

20. Kleiner DE, Brunt EM, Van Natta M, Behling C, Contos MJ, Cummings OW, Ferrell LD, Liu YC, Torbenson MS, Unalp-Arida A, et al. Design and validation of a histological scoring system for nonalcoholic fatty liver disease. Hepatology. 2005;41(6):1313–21.

21. Folch J, Lees M, Sloane Stanley GH. A simple method for the isolation and purification of total lipides from animal tissues. J Biol Chem. 1957;226(1):497–509.

22. Adar T, Ben Ya'acov A, Lalazar G, Lichtenstein Y, Nahman D, Mizrahi M, Wong V, Muller B, Rawlin G, Ilan Y. Oral administration of immunoglobulin G-enhanced colostrum alleviates insulin resistance and liver injury and is associated with alterations in natural killer T cells. Clin Exp Immunol. 2012;167(2):252–60.

23. Shabat Y, Lichtenstein Y, Zolotarov L, Ben Ya'acov A, Ilan Y. Hepatoprotective effect of DT56a is associated with changes in natural killer T cells and regulatory T cells. J Dig Dis. 2013;14(2):84–92.

24. Zigmond E, Tayer-Shifman O, Lalazar G, Ben Ya'acov A, Weksler-Zangen S, Shasha D, Sklair-levy M, Zolotarov L, Shalev Z, Kalman R, et al. Beta-glycosphingolipids ameliorated non-alcoholic steatohepatitis in the Psammomys Obesus model. J Inflamm Res. 2014;7:151–8.

25. Khoury T, Ben Ya'acov A, Shabat Y, Zolotarovya L, Snir R, Ilan Y. Altered distribution of regulatory lymphocytes by oral administration of soy-extracts exerts a hepatoprotective effect alleviating immune mediated liver injury, non-alcoholic steatohepatitis and insulin resistance. World J Gastroenterol. 2015;21(24):7443–56.

26. Lalazar G, Mizrahi M, Turgeman I, Adar T, Ben Ya'acov A, Shabat Y, Nimer A, Hemed N, Zolotarovya L, Lichtenstein Y, et al. Oral administration of OKT3 MAb to patients with NASH, promotes regulatory T-cell induction, and alleviates insulin resistance: results of a phase IIa blinded placebo-controlled trial. J Clin Immunol. 2015;35(4):399–407.

27. Mizrahi M, Shabat Y, Ben Ya'acov A, Lalazar G, Adar T, Wong V, Muller B, Rawlin G, Ilan Y. Alleviation of insulin resistance and liver damage by oral administration of Imm124-E is mediated by increased Tregs and associated with increased serum GLP-1 and adiponectin: results of a phase I/II clinical trial in NASH. J Inflamm Res. 2012;5:141–50.

28. Elinav E, Pappo O, Sklair-Levy M, Margalit M, Shibolet O, Gomori M, Alper R, Thalenfeld B, Engelhardt D, Rabbani E, et al. Amelioration of non-alcoholic steatohepatitis and glucose intolerance in ob/ob mice by oral immune regulation towards liver-extracted proteins is associated with elevated intrahepatic NKT lymphocytes and serum IL-10 levels. J Pathol. 2006;208(1):74–81.

29. Basaranoglu M, Basaranoglu G, Senturk H. From fatty liver to fibrosis: a tale of "second hit". World J Gastroenterol. 2013;19(8):1158–65.

30. Zhang X, Shen J, Man K, Chu ES, Yau TO, Sung JC, Go MY, Deng J, Lu L, Wong VW, et al. CXCL10 plays a key role as an inflammatory mediator and a non-invasive biomarker of non-alcoholic steatohepatitis. J Hepatol. 2014;61(6):1365–75.

31. Sutti S, Jindal A, Locatelli I, Vacchiano M, Gigliotti L, Bozzola C, Albano E. Adaptive immune responses triggered by oxidative stress contribute to hepatic inflammation in NASH. Hepatology. 2014;59(3):886–97.

32. Tilg H, Moschen AR, Szabo G. Interleukin-1 and inflammasomes in ALD/AAH and NAFLD/NASH. Hepatology. 2016;

33. Wree A, McGeough MD, Pena CA, Schlattjan M, Li H, Inzaugarat ME, Messer K, Canbay A, Hoffman HM, Feldstein AE. NLRP3 inflammasome activation is required for fibrosis development in NAFLD. J Mol Med. 2014;92(10):1069–82.

34. Pihlajamaki J, Kuulasmaa T, Kaminska D, Simonen M, Karja V, Gronlund S, Kakela P, Paakkonen M, Kainulainen S, Punnonen K, et al. Serum interleukin 1 receptor antagonist as an independent marker of non-alcoholic steatohepatitis in humans. J Hepatol. 2012;56(3):663–70.

35. Sepulveda-Flores RN, Vera-Cabrera L, Flores-Gutierrez JP, Maldonado-Garza H, Salinas-Garza R, Zorrilla-Blanco P, Bosques-Padilla FJ. Obesity-related non-alcoholic steatohepatitis and TGF-beta1 serum levels in relation to morbid obesity. Ann Hepatol. 2002;1(1):36–9.

36. Yang L, Roh YS, Song J, Zhang B, Liu C, Loomba R, Seki E. Transforming growth factor beta signaling in hepatocytes participates in steatohepatitis through regulation of cell death and lipid metabolism in mice. Hepatology. 2014;59(2):483–95.

37. Schwartz JJ, Emerson L, Hillas E, Phan A, Thiesset H, Firpo M, Sorensen J, Kennedy T, Rinella M. Amelioration of hepatic inflammation in a mouse model of NASH using a dithiocarbamate derivative. Hepatol Int. 2013;7(2):600–9.

38. Szabo G, Petrasek J. Inflammasome activation and function in liver disease. Nat Rev Gastroenterol Hepatol. 2015;12(7):387–400.

39. Marra F, Tacke F. Roles for chemokines in liver disease. Gastroenterology. 2014;147(3):577–94. e571

40. Lee DH, Kim HW. Innate immunity induced by fungal beta-glucans via dectin-1 signaling pathway. Int J Med Mushrooms. 2014;16(1):1–16.

41. Chanput W, Reitsma M, Kleinjans L, Mes JJ, Savelkoul HF, Wichers HJ. Beta-glucans are involved in immune-modulation of THP-1 macrophages. Mol Nutr Food Res. 2012;56(5):822–33.

42. Silveira ML, Smiderle FR, Moraes CP, Borato DG, Baggio CH, Ruthes AC, Wisbeck E, Sassaki GL, Cipriani TR, Furlan SA, et al. Structural characterization and anti-inflammatory activity of a linear beta-D-glucan isolated from Pleurotus sajor-caju. Carbohydr Polym. 2014;113:588–96.

43. Leung PS. The potential protective action of vitamin D in hepatic insulin resistance and pancreatic islet dysfunction in type 2 diabetes mellitus. Nutrients. 2016;8(3)

44. Zhai HL, Wang NJ, Han B, Li Q, Chen Y, Zhu CF, Chen YC, Xia FZ, Cang Z, Zhu CX, et al. Low vitamin D levels and non-alcoholic fatty liver disease, evidence for their independent association in men in East China: a cross-sectional study (survey on prevalence in East China for metabolic diseases and risk factors (SPECT-China)). Br J Nutr. 2016:1–8.

45. Han H, Cui M, You X, Chen M, Piao X, Jin G. A role of 1,25(OH)2D3 supplementation in rats with nonalcoholic steatohepatitis induced by choline-deficient diet. Nutr Metab Cardiovasc Dis. 2015;25(6):556–61.

46. Aad G, Abbott B, Abdallah J, Abdelalim AA, Abdesselam A, Abdinov O, Abi B, Abolins M, Abramowicz H, Abreu H, et al. Observation of a centrality-dependent dijet asymmetry in lead-lead collisions at sqrt[S(NN)] =2.76 TeV with the ATLAS detector at the LHC. Phys Rev Lett. 2010;105(25):252303.

47. Bril F, Maximos M, Portillo-Sanchez P, Biernacki D, Lomonaco R, Subbarayan S, Correa M, Lo M, Suman A, Cusi K. Relationship of vitamin D with insulin resistance and disease severity in non-alcoholic steatohepatitis. J Hepatol. 2015;62(2):405–11.

48. Anty R, Hastier A, Canivet CM, Patouraux S, Schneck AS, Ferrari-Panaia P, Ben-amor I, Saint-Paul MC, Gugenheim J, Gual P, et al. Severe vitamin D deficiency is not associated with liver damage in morbidly obese patients. Obes Surg. 2016;

15

CCL4 is the only predictor for non-responder in GT-1 CHC patients with favorable IL28B genotype when treated with PegIFN/RBV

Chia-Chen Lin[1], Shih-Huan Su[1], Wen-Juei Jeng[2], Chien-Hao Huang[2], Wei Teng[2], Wei-Ting Chen[2], Yi-Cheng Chen[1,2], Chun-Yen Lin[1,2*] (iD) and I-Shyan Sheen[1,2]

Abstract

Background: Chemokines/cytokines play important roles in the pathogenesis of chronic hepatitis C (CHC). However, their clinical characteristics and implications in treatment responses to pegylated interferon plus ribavirin treatment (PegIFN/RBV) have not been fully illustrated yet. In this study, we intended to investigate the possible predictability of serum chemokines/cytokines on the treatment response in Taiwanese of CHC, genotype-1 (GT-1).

Methods: 60 Patients with GT-1 CHC infection who had been treated with PegIFN/RBV were enrolled, including 27 (45%) with sustained virological response (SVR), 11 (18%) with relapse after 48 weeks of treatment and 22 (37%) non-response (NR). Clinical parameters, seven chemokines/cytokines, CCL3, CCL4, CXCL9, CXCL10, CXCL11, IL-10 and IFN-γ, and genotypes of rs12979860, the single nucleotide polymorphisms (SNPs) of interleukin-28B (IL28B) were analyzed for their relationship to treatment response.

Results: Baseline serum levels of CXCL10, CXCL11, CCL3 and CCL4 were significantly higher in NR group while comparing with non-NR group. (CXCL10: $p = 0.001$; CXCL11: $p < 0.001$; CCL3: $p = 0.006$; CCL4: $p = 0.005$). However, only rs12979860 CC genotype was the independent factors for NR in GT-1 CHC infection (OR, 8.985; $p = 0.008$). In addition, baseline serum level of CCL4 was found to be the only independent factor for NR in GT-1 CHC patients with favorable IL28B genotype (OR, 1.134; $p = 0.039$).

Conclusions: IL28B genotype is the predictor for NR in GT-1 CHC patients treated with PegIFN/RBV, while baseline serum level of CCL4 is the only predictor for NR in GT-1 CHC patients with favorable IL28B genotype.

Keywords: Chemokines, Cytokines, Treatment response, Chronic hepatitis C, Genotype-1, Interleukin-28B polymorphism

Background

Chronic hepatitis C is currently one of the leading causes of cirrhosis and hepatocellular carcinoma (HCC) in the whole-wide world [1, 2]. Eradication of HCV virus infection could reduce the risk of cirrhosis, hepatocellular carcinoma and hepatic decompensation [3, 4]. Though the direct

antiviral agents (DAAs) are now the standard of care in Western countries [5], dual therapy of pegylated interferon-α/ribavirin (PegIFN/RBV) still is a popular and effective treatment in several countries where DAAs are not available or not affordable [6–8]. In the treatment with PegIFN/RBV, the patients with non-response (NR) are a troublesome group of patients [9]. Even in the era of DAAs, NR group also highlight a special group of patient that needs special attention [10]. Recently, in the present newer generation of DAAs, this group of patients has finally achieved satisfactory SVR rate. However, in the next

* Correspondence: chunyenlin@gmail.com
[1]School of Medicine, College of Medicine, Chang-Gung University, 5, Fu-Xin street, Quain San, TaoYuan 330, Taiwan
[2]Division of Hepatology, Department of HepatoGastroenterology, Chang-Gung Memorial Hospital, Linkou Medical Center, TaoYuan, Taiwan

development of chronic hepatitis C treatment, shorter duration of interferon-free DAAs will be a hot issue to be investigated [11]. In this possible new trend of treatment development, this potential NR group is worthy of re-revaluation.

Host immune response strongly correlates to the success of antiviral treatment. According to the previous studies, chemokines/cytokines do play important roles in the pathogenesis of chronic hepatitis C. Chemokines and chemokine receptors are crucial in T cell recruitment into infected sites and are involved in inflammation, infection and tissue damage [12, 13]. Type I interferons upregulate either directly or indirectly the expression of CCL3–5, which were potent ligands of the chemokine receptors CCR5 and CCR1. Similarly, Type II interferons are recognized as the most potent inducers of CXCL9–10, which bind to the chemokine receptor-CXCR3 [13]. A previous study revealed that the predominant liver infiltration by majorly CCR5 high/ CXCR3 high phenotype CD8+ lymphocytes in GT-1 CHC patients correlates to intrahepatic chemokine expression level and the inflammatory activity of chronic hepatitis C [14, 15]. However, the clinical implications in treatment responses to pegylated interferon plus ribavirin (PegIFN/RBV) treatment have not yet been fully illustrated. In the era of PegIFN/RBV treatment, the treatment would be terminated if HCV RNA still detectable by 24 weeks (so-called NR). The host immune reaction between non-responder and responder under Peg-IFN/RBV remained unclear. Here, we examined the impact of cytokine and chemokine (CXCL9, CXCL10, CXCL11, CCL3, CCL4, IFN-γ and IL10) from peripheral blood mononuclear cells between NR and non-NR to elucidate why host immune failed to response toward PegIFN/RBV treatment.

Methods

Patient recruitment

We retrospectively analyzed naive GT-1 CHC patients who had been treated with PegIFN/RBV at Chang Gung Memorial Hospital, Linkou Medical center with available stored serum between 2011 and 2013. There were 22 patients with treatment outcome of non-responder. Therefore, 38 age and gender matched non-NR patients with stored serum were recruited as well (Table 1). Patients with other concomitant liver diseases, such as hepatitis B virus, human immunodeficiency virus, alcoholic liver disease, and autoimmune hepatitis, were excluded. Liver cirrhosis was evaluated by liver biopsy or by FIB-4.

The treatment regimens of our patients were standard weight-based pegylated interferon plus ribavirin (PegIFN/RBV) treatment (peginterferon alfa-2a (180 mcg/week) or peginterferon alfa-2b (1.5 mcg/kg/week) subcutaneously plus weight-based ribavirin (1000 mg/d for weight < 75 kg and 1200 mg/d for weight > 75 kg)). Patients who did not fulfill the 80/80/80 adherence rule were excluded. Patients

Table 1 Baseline Characteristics of CHC, GT1 Patients

Variables	Overall	NR (22)[a]	non-NR (38)[a]	P value
Age (years)	58.23 ± 9.19	55.6 ± 9.2	59.8 ± 9.0	0.090
Male (%)	55.0	50.0	57.9	0.599
BMI (Kg/m²)	25.44 ± 3.22	25.5 ± 3.7	25.4 ± 2.9	0.865
AST (U/L)	80.85 ± 40.27	91 ± 48	75 ± 34	0.118
ALT (U/L)	105.63 ± 59.86	108 ± 53	104 ± 64	0.797
HCV RNA (log₁₀ IU/ ml)	3.38(5.17)[b]	2.48(4.74)[b]	3.72(5.66)[b]	0.591
Diabetes Mellitus (%)	25.0	13.6	31.6	0.215
IL28B (CC %)	75.0	50.0	89.5	**0.001**
Liver cirrhosis (%)	28.3	45.5	18.4	**0.038**

[a]number of patients shown in parentheses
[b]median (IQR) shown in parentheses
Data are shown as mean ± standard deviation. Statistic analysis was done by Mann-Whitney test for comparison. Significant P values are shown in bold. AST, aspartate aminotransferase; ALT, alanine aminotransferase; HCV, hepatitis C virus; IL28B, Interleukin-28B

with no rapid virological response (RVR) had received a 48-week treatment while 24-week treatment for patients with RVR and low baseline viral load (HCV-RNA <0.4 × 106 IU/ml). No early virological responses (EVR) as the stop rule was applied to the treatment regimen. Treatment was terminated if detectable HCV-RNA at week 24 weeks.

Definitions of the treatment responses by serum level of HCV-RNA, assessed according to international definitions, were undetectable HCV-RNA 24 weeks after the cessation of treatment as sustained virological response (SVR), positive HCV-RNA at the end of at least 24 weeks of treatment as NR, and positive HCV-RNA after 48 weeks of treatment as relapser.

Laboratory assay

The HCV-RNA levels were measured by commercial quantitative polymerase chain reaction (PCR) assay, either VERSANT HCV RNA 3.0. Assay (HCV 3.0 bDNA assay, Bayer Diagnostics, Berkeley, Calif., lower limit of detection: 5.2 × 102 IU/ml) or COBAS TaqMan HCV Test (TaqMan HCV; Roche Molecular Systems Inc., Branchburg, N.J., lower limit of detection: 15 IU/ml). Serum sample was tested further by COBAS® AMPLICOR HCV Test, v2.0 (CA V2.0, Roche Diagnostic Systems., lower limit of detection: 50 IU/ml) if non-detection of HCV-RNA by VERSANT HCV RNA 3.0. Assay. HCV genotype was determined by a genotype specific probe based assay in the 5′ untranslated region (LiPA; Innogenetics, Ghent, Belgium).

Seven chemokines and cytokines assessed in this study were CXCL9–11, CCL3–4, IL-10 and IFN-γ. Serum samples were analyzed by BD Cytometric Bead Array

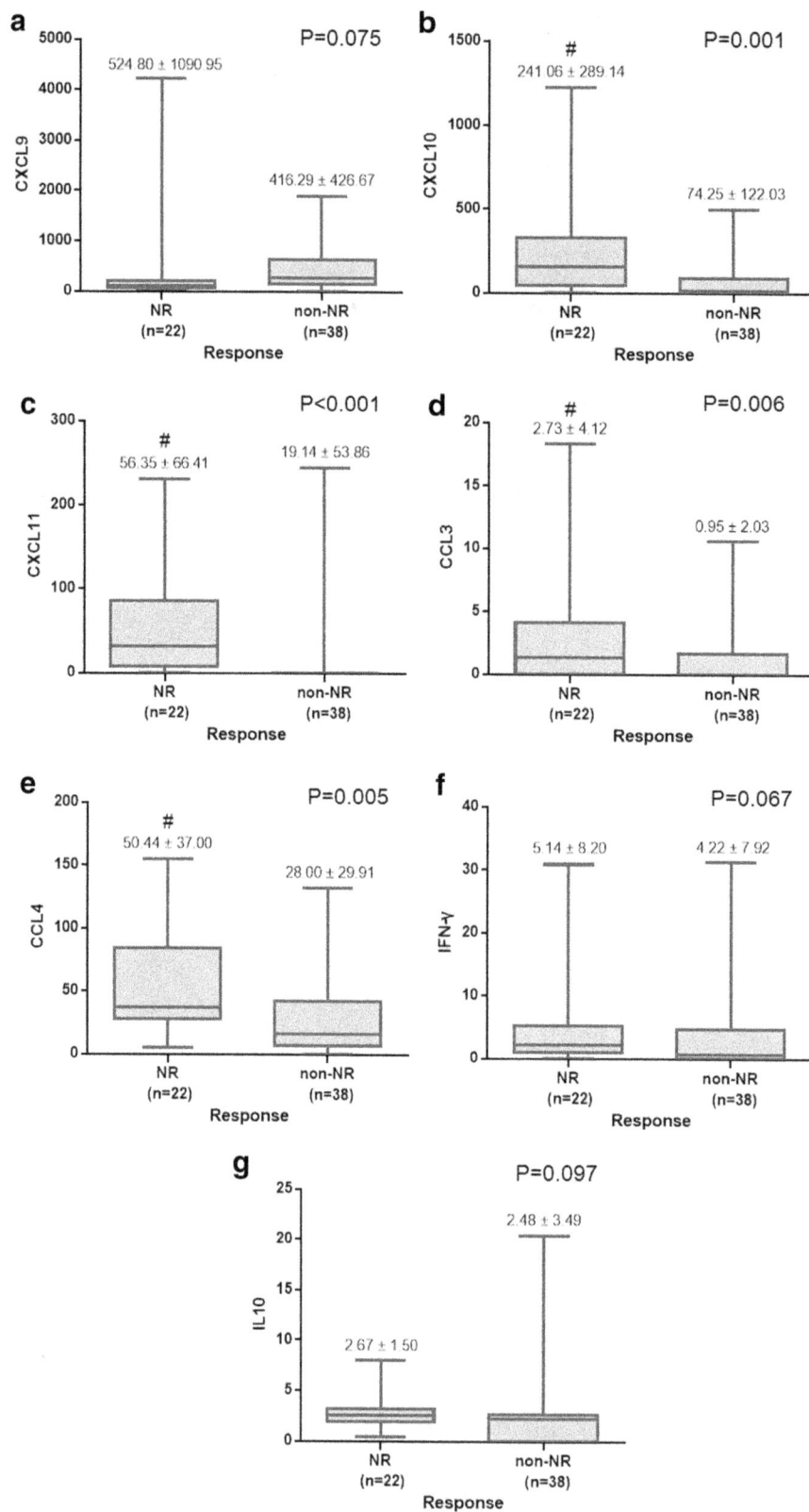

Fig. 1 (See legend on next page.)

Human Inflammatory Cytokines Kit, produced by Becton, Dickinson and Company BD Biosciences, U.S.

Genomic DNA extraction and IL28 B genotyping
Anti-coagulated peripheral blood was obtained from HCV patients. Genomic DNA was isolated from EDTA anti-coagulated peripheral blood using the Puregene DNA isolation kit (Gentra Systems, Minneapolis, MN) as previously described. The oligonucleotide sequences flanking ten IL28B polymorphisms were designed as primers for Taqman allelic discrimination. The allele specific primers for rs12979860 were labeled with a fluorescent dye (FAM and VIC) and used in the PCR reaction. Aliquots of the PCR product were genotyped with allele specific probe of SNPs using real-time PCR (ABI).

Ethics statements
All patients in this study provided written informed consent. The study protocol conformed to the ethical guidelines of the 1975 Declaration of Helsinki and was approved by the ethical committees of Chang Gung Memorial Hospital.

Statistical analysis
Chi-square test was used to compare the categorical variables of the groups. Continuous variables were compared with student's t test or Mann-Whitney U test. Logistic

regression analyses for predictors of treatment response were conducted using patients' demographic, clinical variables, IL28B SNPs and serum levels of chemokines/cytokines. The clinical variables included gender, age, viral load of HCV-RNA, grading of modified HAI and fibrosis stages, body mass index (BMI), Glycohemoglobin (HbA1c), aspartate aminotransferase (AST), alanine aminotransferase (ALT), and rs12979860 SNPs. The odds ratios (OR) and 95% confidence intervals (95% CI) were also calculated. All P values less than 0.05 by the two-tailed test were considered statistically significant. Variables that achieved a statistical significance less than 0.10 on univariate analysis were entered into multivariate logistic regression analysis to identify the significant independent predictive factors. All statistical analyses were performed with statistical software, SPSS for Windows (version 19, SPSS. Inc., Chicago, IL, USA).

Results
Patients' characteristics
A total of 60 patients with chronic hepatitis C genotype 1 infection were recruited into analysis. The majority of the patients are non-cirrhotic (71.7%) and more than half are male (55%). Twenty-two patients were NR and the other 38 are responders (non-NR) (including 27

Table 2 Predictors of NR in the patients of CHC GT1, Treated with P/R by univariate and multivariate Logistic regression analysis

Variables	UV			MV		
	OR	95%C.I	P value	OR	95%C.I	P value
IL28B	8.500	2.246–32.174	**0.002**	8.985	1.778–45.406	**0.008**
CXCL9	1.000	0.999–1.001	0.584			
CXCL10	1.005	1.001–1.009	**0.012**	1.004	0.997–1.011	0.292
CXCL11	1.011	1.001–1.021	**0.039**	0.999	0.985–1.013	0.839
CCL3	1.270	0.987–1.634	**0.064**	1.292	0.910–1.835	0.152
CCL4	1.021	1.003–1.039	**0.022**	1.011	0.980–1.042	0.500
IFN-γ	1.015	1.022–0.696	0.663			
IL10	1.023	0.845–0.397	0.800			
Liver cirrhosis	0.271	0.084–0.876	**0.029**	0.267	0.058–1.223	0.089

UV Univariate logistic regression analysis. *MV* Multivariate logistic regression analysis. *OR* Odds ratio, *CI* Confidence interval
Significant *P* values are shown in bold

Table 3 Baseline Characteristics of CHC, GT1 and IL28B-CC patients

Variables	Overall	NR (11)[a]	non-NR (34)[a]	P value
Age (years)	59.60 ± 8.62	60.00 ± 7.01	59.47 ± 9.17	0.862
Male (%)	60.0	63.6	58.8	0.725
BMI (Kg/m²)	25.24 ± 3.01	25.56 ± 3.39	25.14 ± 2.92	0.693
AST (U/L)	75.76 ± 35.93	85 ± 42	73 ± 34	0.313
ALT (U/L)	98.82 ± 55.79	104 ± 56	97 ± 56	0.741
HCV RNA (log$_{10}$ IU/ml)	2.39(6.22)[b]	4.09(12.27)[b]	3.97(5.56)[b]	0.927
Diabetes Mellitus (%)	26.7	13.6	32.3	0.072
Liver cirrhosis (%)	24.4	45.5	17.6	**0.039**

[a]number of patients shown in parentheses
[b]median (IQR) shown in parentheses
Data are shown as mean ± standard deviation. Statistic analysis was done by Mann-Whitney test for comparison. Significant *P* values are shown in bold.
AST, aspartate aminotransferase; ALT, alanine aminotransferase; HCV, hepatitis C virus; IL28B, Interleukin-28B

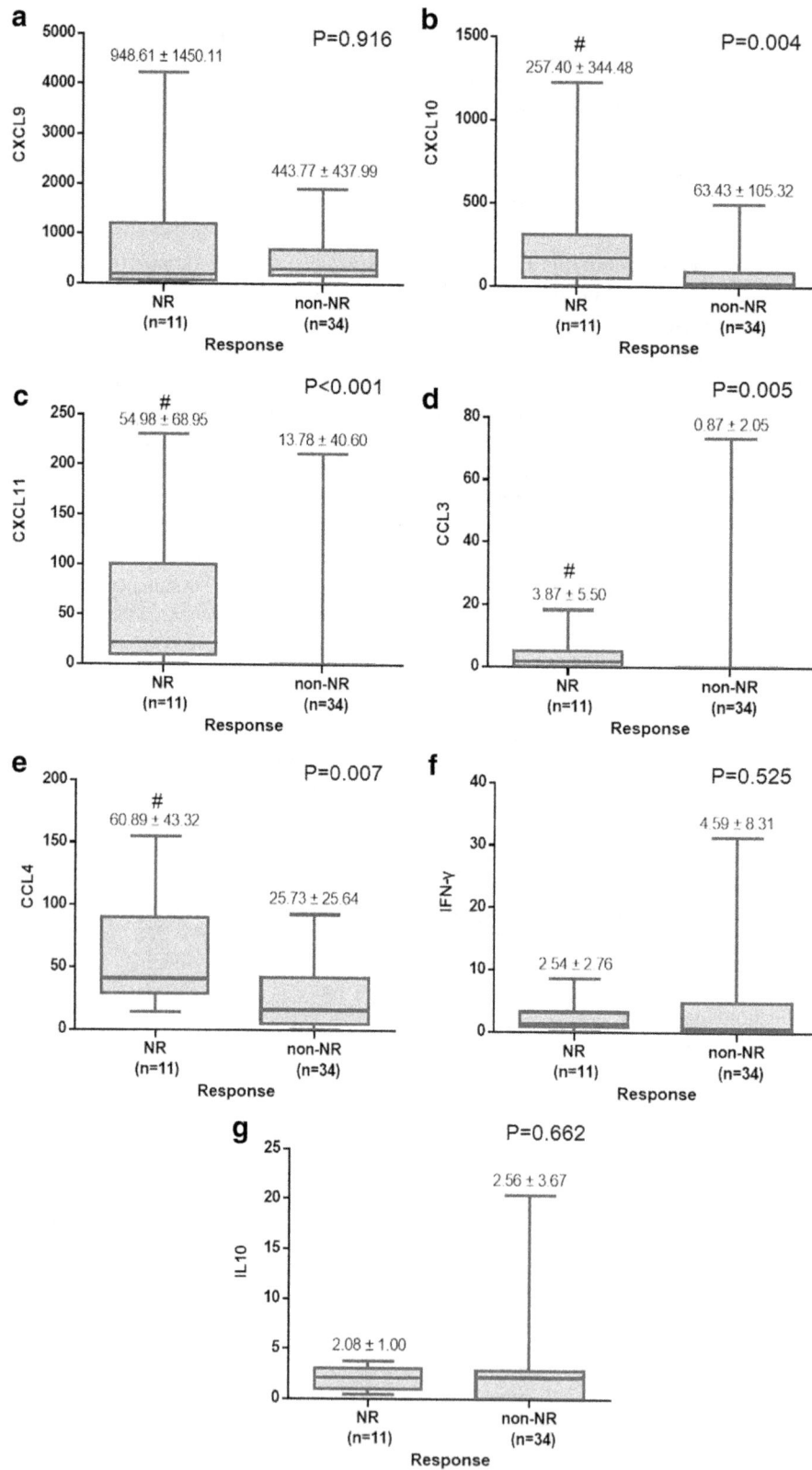

a CXCL9

948.61 ± 1450.11

443.77 ± 437.99

P=0.916

NR (n=11)   non-NR (n=34)

Response

b CXCL10

#
257.40 ± 344.48

63.43 ± 105.32

P=0.004

NR (n=11)   non-NR (n=34)

Response

c CXCL11

#
54.98 ± 68.95

13.78 ± 40.60

P<0.001

NR (n=11)   non-NR (n=34)

Response

d CCL3

0.87 ± 2.05

#
3.87 ± 5.50

P=0.005

NR (n=11)   non-NR (n=34)

Response

e CCL4

#
60.89 ± 43.32

25.73 ± 25.64

P=0.007

NR (n=11)   non-NR (n=34)

Response

f IFN-γ

2.54 ± 2.76

4.59 ± 8.31

P=0.525

NR (n=11)   non-NR (n=34)

Response

g IL10

2.08 ± 1.00

2.56 ± 3.67

P=0.662

NR (n=11)   non-NR (n=34)

Response

Fig. 2 (See legend on next page.)

patients with SVR and 11 patients with relapse after 48 weeks of treatment (relapser) (Table 1).

By comparison of baseline characteristics, there were no significant differences between NR and non-NR groups in terms of age, gender, BMI, baseline viral load, serum levels of liver enzymes and diabetes mellitus. However, the frequency of IL28B-related rs12979860 CC genotype in NR group was significantly lower than that in non-NR group (NR vs. Non-NR: 50.0% vs. 89.5%, *p* = 0.001). In addition, a significantly higher percentage of liver cirrhosis was associated in non-response group (NR vs. non-NR = 45.5% vs. 18.4%, *p* = 0.038) (Table 1).

IL28B genotype is the only predictor for NR
The baseline pre-treatment level of chemokines/cytokines, including CXCL9, CXCL10, CXCL11, CCL3, CCL4, IFN-γ and IL10 were measured between NR and non-NR. CXCL10, CXCL11, CCL3 and CCL 4 were significantly higher in NR group while comparing with non-NR group (CXCL10: NR vs. non-NR = 241.06 ± 289.14 vs. 74.25 ± 122.03, p = 0.001; CXCL11: NR vs. non-NR = 56.35 ± 66.41 vs. 19.14 ± 53.86, *p* < 0.001; CCL3: NR vs. non-NR = 2.73 ± 4.12 vs. 0.95 ± 2.03, *p* = 0.006; CCL4: NR vs. non-NR = 50.44 ± 37.00 vs. 28.00 ± 29.91, *p* = 0.005) (figure 1).

Furthermore, the impacts of these chemokines/cytokines were evaluated along with baseline clinical factors by logistic regression analysis. By univariate logistic regression analysis (Table 2), rs12979860 CC genotype, CXCL10, CXCL11, CCL3, CCL4 and liver cirrhosis were the factors for non-NR. However, rs12979860 CC genotype was the only independent factor for NR by multivariate logistic analysis. (Table 2).

CCL4 is the only predictor in CHC GT1 patients with advantageous IL28B genotype
The IL28B genotype polymorphism has significant impact on the treatment outcome with PegIFN/RBV but host immune factors for prediction of NR among the patients with advantageous rs12979860 CC allele were uncertained. Considering patients with rs12979860 CC allele, higher percentage of cirrhosis in the patients with NR was revealed (NR vs. non-NR = 45.5% vs. 17.6%, *p* = 0.039) (Table 3), and so were CXCL10, CXCL11, CCL3 and CCL 4 (CXCL10: NR vs. non-NR = 257.40 ± 344.48 vs. 63.43 ± 105.32, *p* = 0.004; CXCL11: NR vs. non-NR = 54.98 ± 68.95 vs. 13.78 ± 40.60, *p* < 0.001; CCL3: NR vs. non-NR = 3.87 ± 5.50 vs. 0.87 ±

2.05, *p* = 0.005; CCL4: NR vs. non-NR = 60.89 ± 43.32 vs. 25.73 ± 25.64, *p* = 0.007) (figure 2). CXCL10, CXCL11, CCL3, CCL4 and liver cirrhosis were the predictive factors for non-NR by univariate logistic analysis, but only the CCL4 was the independent predictor for non-NR by multivariate logistic analysis. (Table 4) Thus, our study indicated the advantageous genotype of IL28B is the only predictor for NR. As for patients with CC allele of rs12979860, higher baseline level of CCL4 is the only predictor for NR.

Discussion
In the present study, we focus on this group of patients with NR and found the rs12979860 non-CC genotype were strongly associated with treatment outcome of NR. Furthermore, in patients with advantageous rs12979860 CC genotype, higher baseline serum level of CCL4 was the only factor that is independently associated with non-response.

The role of IL28B genotype in predicting Peg/RBV treatment outcome like non-responder had been explored before like our previous studies [16, 17] and others [18–20]. Interesting, in the rapid advance of DAAs treatment, the role of IL28B on the SVR had gradually dwindled when treatment regimen are non- pegylated-IFN based [21].

Table 4 Predictors of NR in the patients of CHC GT1 and IL28B-CC, Treated with P/R by univariate and multivariate Logistic regression analysis

Variables	UV			MV		
	OR	95%C.I	P value	OR	95%C.I	P value
CXCL9	1.001	1.000–1.002	0.117			
CXCL10	1.006	1.000–1.012	**0.034**	0.985	0.965–1.005	0.150
CXCL11	1.014	1.000–1.029	**0.054**	1.020	0.995–1.046	0.118
CCL3	1.305	0.998–1.706	**0.052**	4.822	0.407–57.146	0.212
CCL4	1.032	1.007–1.057	**0.010**	1.134	1.006–1.277	**0.039**
IFN-γ	0.948	0.830–1.084	0.439			
IL10	0.943	0.720–1.236	0.673			
Liver cirrhosis	0.257	0.059–1.128	**0.072**	0.005	0.000–1.108	0.055

UV Univariate logistic regression analysis. *MV* Multivariate logistic regression analysis. *OR* Odds ratio, *CI* Confidence interval
Significant P values are shown in bold

However, in consideration of minor group with possible treatment failure by DAAs, the IL28B might still have impacts on the outcome [21].

The finding about chemokines be influential to the treatment outcome was compatible with another report that serum CXCL10 and CCL4 levels decreased significantly in GT-1 CHC patients with virological response [22]. Furthermore, CCL3, CCL4, CCL5, CXCL9, CXCL10 and CXCL11 were found to increase in both liver and peripheral blood during chronic hepatitis C in several studies [14, 22, 23]. The intra-hepatic levels of CXCL11 and CXCL10 were reported to correlate with HCV disease severity [13]. Patients with high CXCL10 at baseline were much less likely to achieve SVR, and the CXCL10 level was observed to be decreased following successful antiviral therapy [24, 25]. In HCV-infected livers, inflammation and fibrosis are mainly located in the portal areas, which may explain the up-regulation of CCL3–5 in the portal tracts [13]. However, the relationship existed between CCL3, CCL4 levels and the therapeutic responses were still controversial. A study showed that a low pretreatment CCL4 concentration was not only an independent predictor of early but also sustained virological response in CHC patients, while another study didn't found significant differences [26, 27]. Interestingly, patients of advantageous IL28B genotype predominated among all recruited patients in the former study. To the best of our knowledge, no study yet had analyzed baseline CCL4 level in patient groups of advantageous IL28B genotype.

There were some limitations for this study. First of all, it was a retrospective study. However, in the new era of DAAs treatment, it is difficult to conduct a large-scale study just focused on PegIFN/RBV treatment. In addition, it is a medium-size study with case number of 60. However, in this scale of study, the serum levels of CCL4 become the only predictor for NR in patients with advantageous IL28B genotype. Therefore, it has emphasized the importance of CCL4 among other serum chemokines, especially in considering the future shorter duration of treatment for chronic hepatitis C patients receiving shorter duration of interferon-free DAAs.

Conclusion

IL28B genotype is the predictor for non-responder in GT-1 CHC patients treated with PegIFN/RBV, while baseline serum level of CCL4 is the only predictor for non-responder in GT-1 CHC patients with favorable IL28B genotype.

Abbreviations

CHC: Chronic hepatitis C; DAAs: Direct antiviral agents; EVR: Early virological responses; GT-1: Genotype-1; HCC: Hepatocellular carcinoma; IL28B: Interleukin-28B; NR: Non-response; PegIFN/RBV: Pegylated interferon plus ribavirin treatment; RVR: Rapid virological response; SVR: Sustained virological response

Acknowledgements

All the authors have read this manuscript and approved the submission for publication. All authors fulfill the criteria given in the Authorship defined by your journal.

All authors concur with the submission and none of the data have been previously reported or are under consideration for publication elsewhere. No conflict of interest exists for any of the authors.

Funding

This work was supported by CMRPG3A1021, CMRPG3A1022, and CMRPG3A1023 from Medical Research Project Fund, Chang Gung Memorial Hospital, and 104–2815-C-182A-004-B from Ministry of Science and Technology, Taiwan.

Authors' contributions

C-C. L., C-Y. L. and I-S. S. designed the research studies; C-C. L., S-H. S. and C-H. H., performed the research; C-C. L., W-J. J., C-H. H., W.T., W-T. C., Y-C. C., C-Y. L. and I-S. S. analyzed the data; and C-C. L., W-J. C and C-Y. L. wrote the paper. All authors read and approved the final manuscript.

Competing interests

The authors declare that they have no competing interests.

References

1. Poynard T, Yuen MF, Ratziu V, Lai CL. Viral hepatitis C. Lancet. 2003; 362(9401):2095–100.
2. Lauer GM, Walker BD. Hepatitis C virus infection. N Engl J Med. 2001; 345(1):41–52.
3. Pockros PJ, et al. Histologic outcomes in hepatitis C–infected patients with varying degrees of virologic response to interferon-based treatments. Hepatology. 2010;52(4):1193–200.
4. Swain MG, et al. A sustained virologic response is durable in patients with chronic hepatitis C treated with peginterferon alfa-2a and ribavirin. J Gastro. 2010;139(5):1593–601.
5. Panel AIHG. Hepatitis C guidance: AASLD-IDSA recommendations for testing, managing, and treating adults infected with hepatitis C virus. Hepatology. 2015;62(3):932–54.
6. Asselah T, Marcellin P. New direct-acting antivirals' combination for the treatment of chronic hepatitis C. Liver Int. 2011;31:68–77.
7. Mangia A, Andriulli A. Tailoring the length of antiviral treatment for hepatitis C. Gut. 2010;59(1):1–5.
8. Yu M-L, Chuang W-L. Treatment of chronic hepatitis C in Asia: when east meets west. J Gastroenterol Hepatol. 2009;24(3):336–45.
9. Heathcote EJ. Antiviral therapy: chronic hepatitis C. J Viral Hepat. 2007;14:82–8.
10. Wendt A, Bourlière M. An update on the treatment of genotype-1 chronic hepatitis C infection: lessons from recent clinical trials. Ther Adv Infect Dis. 2013;1(6):191–208.
11. Asselah T, Boyer N, Saadoun D, Martinot-Peignoux M, Marcellin P. Direct-acting antivirals for the treatment of hepatitis C virus infection: optimizing current IFN-free treatment and future perspectives. Liver Int. 2016;36:45–57.
12. Charo IF, Ransohoff RM. The many roles of chemokines and chemokine receptors in inflammation. N Engl J Med. 2006;354:610–21.
13. Wald O, Weiss ID, Galun E, Peled A. Chemokines in hepatitis C virus infection: pathogenesis, prognosis and therapeutics. Cytokine. 2007; 39(1):50–62.
14. Apolinario A, et al. Increased expression of T cell chemokines and their receptors in chronic hepatitis C: relationship with the histological activity of liver disease. Am J Gastroenterol Suppl. 2002;97(11):2861–70.

15. Larrubia JR, et al. The role of CCR5/CXCR3 expressing CD8+ cells in liver damage and viral control during persistent hepatitis C virus infection. J Hepatol. 2007;47(5):632–41.

16. Lin C-Y, et al. IL28B SNP rs12979860 is a critical predictor for on-treatment and sustained virologic response in patients with hepatitis C virus genotype-1 infection. PLoS One. 2011;6(3):e18322.

17. Lin C-Y, Sheen I-S, Jeng W-J, Huang C-W, Huang C-H, Chen J-Y. Patients younger than forty years old with hepatitis C virus genotype-1 chronic infection had treatment responses similar to genotype-2 infection and not related to interleukin-28B polymorphism. Ann Gastroentol Hepatol. 2013; 12(1):62–9.

18. Dill MT, et al. Interferon-induced gene expression is a stronger predictor of treatment response than IL28B genotype in patients with hepatitis C. Gastroenterol. 2011;140(3):1021–31.

19. Ge D, et al. Genetic variation in IL28B predicts hepatitis C treatment-induced viral clearance. Nature. 2009;461(7262):399–401.

20. Tanaka Y, et al. Genome-wide association of IL28B with response to pegylated interferon-alpha and ribavirin therapy for chronic hepatitis C. Nat Genet. 2009;41(10):1105–9.

21. Matsuura K, Watanabe T, Tanaka Y. Role of IL28B for chronic hepatitis C treatment toward personalized medicine. J Gastroenterol Hepatol. 2014; 29(2):241–9.

22. Apolinario A, et al. Increased circulating and intrahepatic T-cell-specific chemokines in chronic hepatitis C: relationship with the type of virological response to peginterferon plus ribavirin combination therapy. Aliment Pharmacol Ther. 2004;19(5):551–62.

23. Larrubia JR, Benito-Martínez S, Calvino M, Sanz-de-Villalobos E, Parra-Cid T. Role of chemokines and their receptors in viral persistence and liver damage during chronic hepatitis C virus infection. World J Gastroenterol. 2008;14(47):7149–59.

24. Butera D, et al. Plasma chemokine levels correlate with the outcome of antiviral therapy in patients with hepatitis C. Blood. 2005;106(4):1175–82.

25. Diago M, et al. Association of pretreatment serum interferon gamma inducible protein 10 levels with sustained virological response to peginterferon plus ribavirin therapy in genotype 1 infected patients with chronic hepatitis C. Gut. 2006;55(3):374–9.

26. Florholmen J, et al. A rapid chemokine response of macrophage inflammatory protein (MIP)-1α, MIP-1β and the regulated on activation, normal T expressed and secreted chemokine is associated with a sustained virological response in the treatment of chronic hepatitis C. Clin Microbiol Infect. 2011;17(2):204–9.

27. Zhang S, et al. Pretreatment serum macrophage inflammatory protein (MIP)-1 levels predict sustained virological responses to re-treatment in patients with chronic hepatitis C virus infection. Int J Infect Dis. 2015; 33:15–21.

16

Gut microbiota-mediated generation of saturated fatty acids elicits inflammation in the liver in murine high-fat diet-induced steatohepatitis

Shoji Yamada[1], Nobuhiko Kamada[2], Takeru Amiya[3], Nobuhiro Nakamoto[3], Toshiaki Nakaoka[1], Masaki Kimura[1], Yoshimasa Saito[1,3], Chieko Ejima[4], Takanori Kanai[3] and Hidetsugu Saito[1,3*]

Abstract

Background: The gut microbiota plays crucial roles in the development of non-alcoholic steatohepatitis (NASH). However, the precise mechanisms by which alterations of the gut microbiota and its metabolism contributing to the pathogenesis of NASH are not yet fully elucidated.

Methods: Mice were fed with a recently reported new class of high-fat diet (HFD), steatohepatitis-inducing HFD (STHD)-01 for 9 weeks. The composition of the gut microbiota was analyzed by T-RFLP. Luminal metabolome was analyzed using capillary electrophoresis and liquid chromatography time-of-flight mass spectrometry (CE- and LC-TOFMS).

Results: Mice fed the STHD-01 developed NASH-like pathology within a short period. Treatment with antibiotics prevented the development of NASH by STHD-01. The composition of the gut microbiota and its metabolic activities were markedly perturbed in the STHD-01-fed mice, and antibiotic administration normalized these changes. We identified that long-chain saturated fatty acid and n-6 fatty acid metabolic pathways were significantly altered by STHD-01. Of note, the changes in gut lipidome caused by STHD-01 were mediated by gut microbiota, as the depletion of the gut microbiota could reverse the perturbation of these metabolic pathways. A saturated long-chain fatty acid, palmitic acid, which accumulated in the STHD-01 group, activated liver macrophages and promoted TNF-α expression.

Conclusions: Lipid metabolism by the gut microbiota, particularly the saturation of fatty acids, affects fat accumulation in the liver and subsequent liver inflammation in NASH.

Keywords: Gut microbiota, Non-alcoholic steatohepatitis, Long-chain saturated fatty acids, Fat accumulation, Fat transportation

Background

The number of patients with fatty liver disease (FLD) has been steadily increasing in recent years. FLD due to causes other than excessive alcohol intake is termed non-alcoholic FLD (NAFLD) [1]. In patients with NAFLD, dysregulation of adipokines, insulin resistance, and dyslipidemia lead to fat accumulation in the liver [2–4]. Activation of Kupffer cells and hepatic stellate cells and lipid peroxidation elicit liver inflammation, thereby leading to the development of non-alcoholic steatohepatitis (NASH). The numbers of patients with NAFLD and NASH in Japan are more than 10 million and 1 million, respectively. Thus, it is required to understand the precise mechanism of action and develop better therapeutic treatments for NAFLD and NASH.

Since many environmental and genetic factors are associated with the development and progression of NASH, the precise mechanisms by which NASH develops are still not completely understood [5]. Animal

* Correspondence: hsaito@a2.keio.jp
[1]Division of Pharmacotherapeutics, Faculty of Pharmacy, Keio University, 1-5-30 Shiba-Kohen, Minato-ku, Tokyo 105-8512, Japan
[3]Division of Gastroenterology and Hepatology, Department of Internal Medicine, Keio University, Shinjuku-ku, Tokyo 160-8582, Japan
Full list of author information is available at the end of the article

models are useful tools for understanding the pathogenesis of human diseases inducing NASH. Feeding of mice with a high-fat diet (HFD) leads to the development of NASH in mice [6]. A recent accumulating evidence has highlighted that the gut microbiota and its metabolites play pivotal roles in the development of NASH [7]. It has been reported that feeding of a HFD induces the alteration of gut microbial communities, referred to as dysbiosis [8, 9]. HFD-induced dysbiosis impairs the integrity of the intestinal epithelium, and thereby eliciting the systemic dissemination of the gut microbiota and/or microbial products, such as lipopolysaccharides (LPS) [10]. The microbial stimuli activate the production of pro-inflammatory cytokines in the liver, and liver inflammation elicits the development of NASH [10]. In addition to the direct stimulation by microbial components, metabolic alterations caused by dysbiosis are also known to cause NASH development. In db/db mice, gut dysbiosis with accompanied enrichment of the genus *Bacteroides* alters fatty acid metabolism [11]. Fatty acids are absorbed in the intestine and transported to the liver through the portal vein for energy utility. Although fatty acid metabolism is believed to be involved in the pathogenesis of NASH, the precise mechanisms by which high-fat diet-induced dysbiosis affects fatty acid metabolism in the gut and the consequent effect of this imbalance on liver inflammation have not been fully elucidated.

A recent study has reported a new class of HFD, known as steatohepatitis-inducing HFD (STHD)-01. The consumption of STHD-01 promotes the development of NASH-like pathology within a short period of time [12]. However, since STHD-01 is a recently developed diet, it remains unclear whether this diet impacts the gut microbiota and its metabolic activities, promoting NASH development, similar to that of the commonly used HFD. Hence, in the present study, we comprehensively analyzed the alteration of the gut microbiota composition and its metabolic activities as well as potential mechanisms associated with the STHD-01-induced development of NASH-like symptoms.

Methods
Animals
SPF C57BL/6J mice were fed a conventional CE-2 diet (CLEA Japan Inc., Tokyo, Japan) until 8 weeks of age. The gut microbiota was normalized by exchanging beddings between cages every 2–3 days for 2 weeks. From 8 weeks of age, the mice were fed the STHD-01 (11% kcal/protein, 72% kcal/fat, and 17% kcal/nitrogen-free extracts; EA Pharma Co. Ltd., Kawasaki, Kanagawa) [12] for 9 weeks. The control group was fed the Standard diet (SD) (AIN-93G) (19% kcal/protein, 12% kcal/fat, and 69% kcal/nitrogen-free extract). In the microbiota-depleted group, the mice fed with the

STHD-01 diet were treated with an antibiotic (Abx) cocktail (ceftazidime, Sigma-Aldrich, Tokyo, Japan; C3809-5G plus metronidazole; Sigma-Aldrich M3761-25G, both 1 g/L) from 7 weeks until 17 weeks. The mice were killed at week 17 with isoflurane (Mylan Inc., Nagoya, Japan) [13] and peripheral blood, intestinal tissues, and liver samples were harvested. Histological evaluation was performed in a blind manner by a hepatologist and two pathologists from Keio University Hospital as described previously [14].

Measurement of disease markers
The levels of aspartate aminotransferase (AST) and alanine aminotransferase (ALT) were measured using the Spotchem EZ (Sp-4430, Arkrey USA Inc., MN). The levels of triiodothyronine (T3), thyroxin (T4) and monocyte chemoattractant protein (MCP)-1 were measured with an enzyme-linked immunosorbent assay kit (T3 and T4, Alpha Diagnostic Intl. Inc., Antonio, TX. MCP-1, R&D System, Inc., Minneapolis, MN). For the measurement of triglyceride (TG) in the liver tissue, a Folch solution (2:1 chloroform: methanol; Wako Pure Chemical Industries Ltd., Tokyo, Japan; 4 mL) was added to each liver tissue sample (0.1 g), which was then homogenized. After adding and mixing with 0.5% NaCl (1 mL), the mixture was centrifuged at 180 g at 20 °C for 20 min. The lower layer was obtained and vacuum-dried, and then 1 mL of isopropanol (Wako Pure Chemical Industries Ltd.) was added to the precipitate. The levels of TG were measured using the Pureauto S TG-N (Sekisui Medical Co., Ltd., Tokyo, Japan). At week 15, mice were fasted 1 day before measuring the levels of fasting blood glucose. The levels of fasting blood glucose were measured with GT-1640 (Arkrey USA Inc.). The plasma levels of insulin were measured with mouse insulin enzyme-linked immunosorbent assay kit (Shibayagi Co.,Ltd., Gunma, Japan).

Microbiome analysis
At week 17, feces were obtained from the mice and resuspended in a phosphate-buffered saline solution (PBS) (0.1 g/mL). The fecal suspension was crushed using the Bug Crashar (Taitec GM-01, Saitama, Japan) at maximal rotation for 10 min. The sample was incubated on ice for 5 min and centrifuged at 2300 g at 4 °C for 1 min. The supernatant (500 μL) was placed in another tube and vortexed with 100 μL of 10% SDS and 500 μL of phenol/chloroform/isoamylalcohol. Then, the sample was centrifuged at 20,000 g at 20 °C for 3 min. The supernatant was treated with chloroform/isoamylalcohol and then isoamylalcohol alone, and the DNA pellet was resuspended in 100 μL Tris/ethylenediamine tetraacetic acid buffer (TE) (Sigma) and 0.5 μL RNase A (Qiagen, Hilden, Germany). The DNA was further purified using the Template Preparation Kit (Roche, Basel, Switzerland).

The obtained DNA was analyzed by a terminal restriction fragment length polymorphism analysis (TechnoSuruga Laboratory Co., Ltd., Shizuoka, Japan). The DNA was amplified with fluorescence-labeled primers, and the amplified DNA was then treated with the restriction enzyme BS/I (Takara Bio Inc., Tokyo, Japan) and analyzed using the ABI Prism 3130xl DNA Sequencer (Applied Biosystems, CA) and Gene Mapper (Applied Biosystems). Cluster analysis was performed using the Gene Maths (Applied Maths, Sint-Martens-Latem, Belgium).

To measure the total number of gut bacteria in the feces, a standard curve using *Escherichia coli* genome DNA (JCM1649T, kindly provided by RIKEN, Saitama, Japan) was drawn and inserted into the pGEM®-T EASY vector system (Promega Co., WI). The sample DNA was amplified with primers 8F (5′ AGAGTTTGATYMTGG CTCAG 3′) and 1510R (5′ TACGGYTACCTTGTTACG ACTT 3′). Quantitative polymerase chain reaction (qPCR) was performed using the SYBR Green PCR Master Mix (Applied Biosystems). Quantification was carried out using the CFX96Touch™ (Applied Biosystems). The cycle step was 50 °C × 2 min, 95 °C × 10 min, (95 °C × 30 s, 60 °C × 30 s, 72 °C × 1 min) × 50 cycles.

Quantitative RT-PCR

RNA extraction from the liver and intestinal tissues was carried out in accordance with a previously described method [15] using Isogen (Wako Pure Chemical Industries, Ltd.). The RNA was transcribed into cDNA using the High Capacity cDNA Reverse Transcription kit (Applied Biosystems), and qPCR was performed using the SYBR Green PCR Master Mix (Applied Biosystems). Quantification was carried out using the CFX96Touch™ (Applied Biosystems). The cycle step was 50 °C × 2 min, 95 °C × 10 min, (95 °C × 30 s, 60 °C × 30 s, 72 °C × 1 min) × 50 cycles. The primers used are summarized in Additional file 1.

Luminal metabolomic analysis

The metabolomic analysis was conducted using the Dual Scan package of Human Metabolome Technologies Inc. (HMT; Yamagata, Japan) using liquid chromatography time-of-flight mass spectrometry (LC-TOFMS) and capillary electrophoresis (CE)-TOFMS for ionic and non-ionic metabolites, respectively, on the basis of the methods described elsewhere [16, 17]. Briefly, for extracting ionic metabolites, approximately 50 mg of feces sample was dissolved in MilliQ water with ratio of 1:9 (*w/v*). After centrifugation, 20 µL of the supernatant was suspended with 20 µL of internal standard solution (HMT, Tsuruoka, Yamagata, Japan) and 80 µL of MilliQ water. The solution was then centrifugally filtered through a Millipore 5000-Da cutoff filter (UltrafreeMC-PLHCC, HMT) to

remove macromolecules (9100 × g, 4 °C, 60 min) for subsequent analysis with CE-TOFMS. For extracting non-ionic metabolites, approximately 50 mg of feces sample was dissolved in 1 mL of methanol containing internal standard (HMT). After centrifugation, 300 µL of the supernatant was moved into glass vial for evaporation under nitrogen gas and reconstituted with 300 µL of 50% isopropanol (*v/v*) for subsequent analysis with LC-TOFMS. CE-TOFMS analysis was performed using a CE capillary electrophoresis system with a 6210 time-of-flight mass spectrometer, 1100 isocratic high-performance liquid chromatography (HPLC) pump, G1603A CE-MS adapter kit, and G1607A CE-ESI-MS sprayer kit (Agilent Technologies, Waldbronn, Germany). The G2201AA ChemStation software version B.03.01 for CE (Agilent Technologies) was used to control the systems, which were connected by a fused silica capillary (50 µm i.d. × 80 cm total length) with a commercial electrophoresis buffer (H3301–1001 and H3302–1021 for cation and anion analyses, respectively; HMT) as the electrolyte. The spectrometer was scanned from m/z 50 to 1000. LC-TOFMS analysis was performed using an LC System (Agilent 1200 series RRLC system SL) equipped with a 6230 time-of-flight mass spectrometer (Agilent Technologies). The systems were controlled by the G2201AA ChemStation software version B.03.01 for CE equipped with an octadecylsilyl column (2 × 50 mm, 2 µm). Peaks were extracted using an automatic integration software, MasterHands (Keio University, Tsuruoka, Yamagata, Japan), to obtain peak information, including m/z, peak area, and migration time (MT) for CE-TOFMS and retention time (RT) for LC-TOFMS analyses. The following were excluded: signal peaks corresponding to isotopomers, adduct ions, and other product ions of known metabolites. The HMT metabolite database was used to annotate the remaining peaks on the basis of their m/z values with the MTs and RTs determined by TOFMS. Areas of the annotated peaks were then normalized based on internal standard levels and sample amounts to obtain relative levels of each metabolite. Hierarchical cluster analysis and principal component analysis were conducted using HMT's proprietary software, PeakStat and SampleStat, respectively. Detected metabolites were plotted on metabolic pathway maps using the VANTED software.

Liver cell preparation

The livers were perfused through the portal vein with fluorescence-activated cell sorting (FACS) buffer [1 g bovine serum albumin (BSA) in 500 mL PBS] and then minced well. The filtrate was centrifuged at 50 g for 1 min, and the supernatant was washed once. The cells were suspended in 25% Percoll and overlaid in 50% Percoll to distinguish resident macrophages from monocytes. After centrifugation at 2000 rpm for 20 min, the cells were collected from the middle layer and were washed and resuspended in an RPMI1640 medium. Flow cytometry was performed as described previously [18]. Briefly, the cells were collected from the upper phase of a Percoll gradient. After blocking with anti-FcR (CD16/32, BD bioscience, NJ) for 20 min, the cells were incubated with specific monoclonal antibodies at 4 °C for 30 min. The liver mononuclear cells were gated as 7-AAD negative CD45.2-FITC (BD bioscience) positive cells. Liver macrophages were stained with PE-conjugated anti-mouse F4/80 mAb and antigen-presenting cell (APC)-conjugated anti-mouse CD11b mAb (both from BD biosciences). Background fluorescence was assessed by staining with the relevant isotype control Abs. Stained cells were analyzed by flow cytometry (FACS Cant II, Becton Dickinson Co. Franklin Lakes, NJ), and data were analyzed using the FlowJo software (FlowJo, LLC, Ashland, OR).

Liver CD11b$^+$ mononuclear phagocytes ex vivo culture

Liver CD11b$^+$ mononuclear phagocytes were separated from all other mononuclear phagocytes using MicroBeads (Miltenyi Biotec K.K., Japan). Then, separated CD11b$^+$ cells were cultured in an RPMI1640 containing 0.1% penicillin/streptomycin (Sigma), supplemented with 10% fetal bovine serum (Biowest SAS, Nualle, France) with or without 200 μM palmitic acid (PA; Wako). After incubation for 20 h, mRNA was collected from the CD11b$^+$ cells using Isogen.

Statistical analysis

Results were shown as mean ± standard errors. A one-way ANOVA followed by the Tukey's post-hoc test was used for comparisons of multi groups. The Mann-Whitney U-test was used for comparisons of two groups. All comparisons were two-sided, and a P-value < 0.05 was considered significant. All statistical analyses were performed using the SPSS 22 for Windows (SPSS, IBM Japan, Tokyo, Japan).

Results

STHD-01 induced steatohepatitis through alteration of the gut microbiota

C57BL/6 J mice were fed a control diet (SD diet; CONT), HFD (STHD-01 diet; STHD-01), or STHD-01 plus Abx (STHD-01 + Abx) for 9 weeks (Fig. 1a). Total calorie intake and total water intake were not different between the three groups (Fig. 1b). The STHD-01 HFD-fed mice exhibited an increased liver mass without an increase in body weight (Fig. 1b). The levels of fasting blood glucose at the week 15 and the plasma levels of insulin were not different between the CONT and HFD group (Additional file 2). Plasma T4, thyroxine, was not altered by STHD-01 (Fig. 1b). In contrast, T3, a thyroid hormone metabolized from T4, was significantly

elevated in the STHD-01-fed mice (Fig. 1b). Administration of Abx significantly improved the increased liver weight and plasma T3 induced by STHD-01, suggesting that these changes are mediated by gut dysbiosis induced by STHD-01 (Fig. 1b). Likewise, the STHD-01 group showed significantly larger and more numerous fat droplets throughout the liver (Fig. 1c). Fat droplets were found in both the pericentral and periportal regions (Fig. 1c and Additional file 3). Significant numbers of ballooning and Mallory bodies were observed in the periportal region in the STHD-01 group (Additional file 3). Moreover, several fibrotic extensions were observed in the STHD-01 group (Fig. 1c and Additional file 3). Not only the lipid accumulation but also the STHD-01 induced the infiltration of inflammatory cells in the peripheral region in the liver (Fig. 1c). Notably, these pathological changes in the liver seen in the STHD-01-fed mice were not developed when the mice were administrated with Abx (Fig. 1c). Consistent with these histological changes, the STHD-01-fed mice exhibited increased levels of AST and ALT in the plasma and TG in the liver (Fig. 1d). Moreover, transcription of inflammatory markers tumor nuclear factor (TNF)-α and Interleukin (IL) -1β; and fibrosis markers α-smooth muscle antigen (α-SMA) and α1 type 1 collagen (Col 1α1) mRNAs in the liver were dramatically upregulated in the STHD-01-fed mice (Fig. 1d). These changes were not observed in mice that receive Abx, suggesting that STHD-01-induced alteration of the gut microbiota plays a critical role in the development of steatohepatitis.

Metabolic activities of the gut microbiota were dramatically altered in the STHD-01-fed mice

Next, we analyzed the composition of the gut microbiota in all three groups. The total number of bacteria in the feces was not affected by feeding of STHD-01 (Fig. 2a). In contrast, treatment with Abx dramatically reduced the number of gut microbes (Fig 2a). After feeding of STHD-01, an abundance of *Bifidobacterium*, *Enterococcus*, and *Bacteroides* genera decreased, while an abundance of *Clostridium* subclusters XIVa and XVIII increased (Fig. 2a). The treatment of Abx almost completely deleted these major genera of bacteria found in the STHD-01 group, and the genus of *Enterococcus* was dominated within the gut microbiota after the Abx administration. To address the influence of STHD-01-induced dysbiosis on the metabolic activities of the gut microbiota, we analyzed the gut metabolome. Lipid metabolites in the feces were analyzed by liquid LC-TOFMS and hydrophilic metabolites by CE-TOFMS. The detected peaks were categorized into glycolysis/gluconeogenesis, pentose-phosphate, tricarboxylic acid (TCA) cycle, urea cycle, purine-pyrimidine, coenzyme, amino acids, acyl-carnitine, and

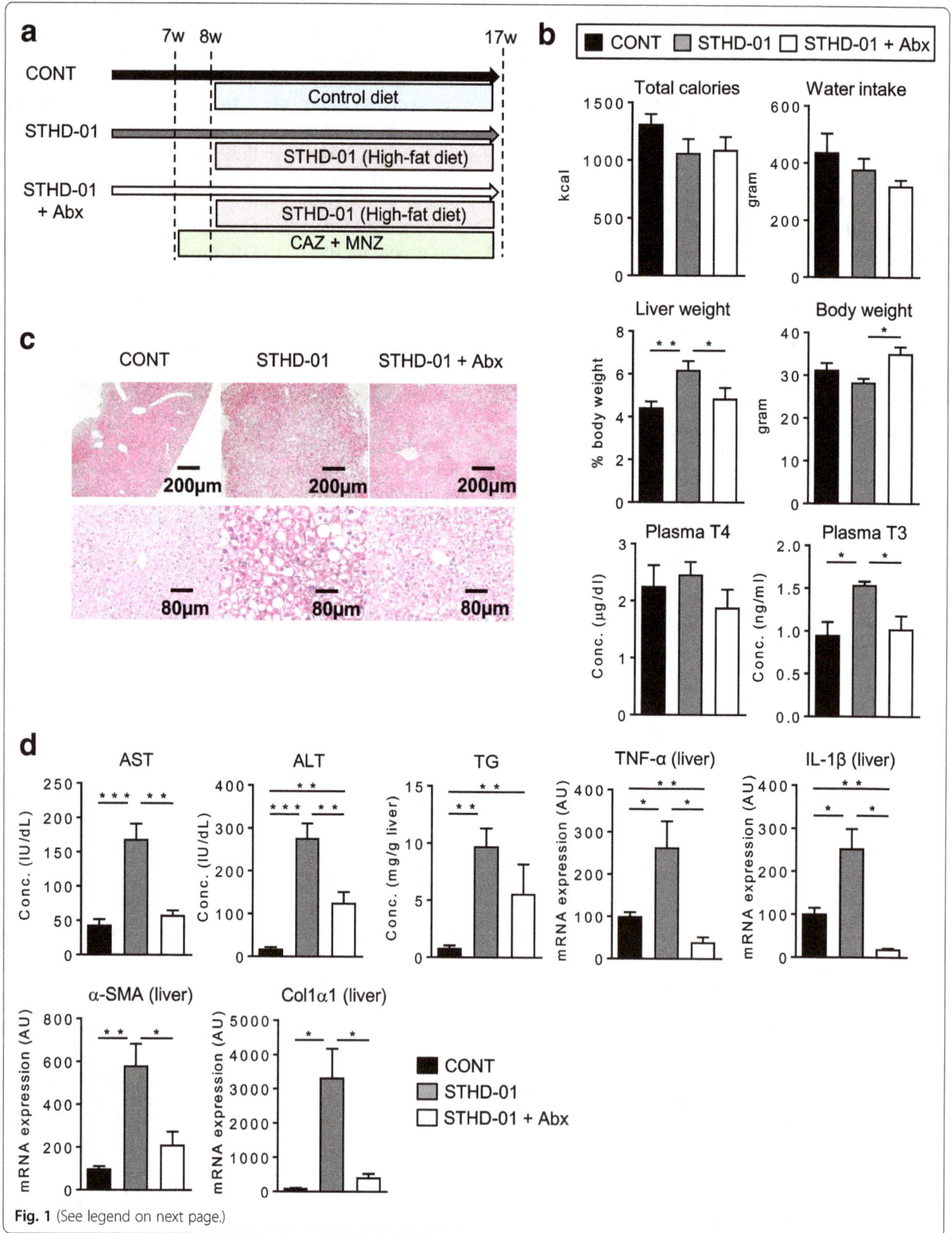

Fig. 1 (See legend on next page.)

(See figure on previous page.)
Fig. 1 The gut microbiota contributes to the development of NASH induced by STHD-01. **a** Experimental protocol. CAZ; Ceftazidime. MNZ; Metronidazole. **b** Total calorie intake, total water intake, liver/body weight ratios, body weight, and plasma triiodothyronine (T3) and thyroxin (T4) were measured at 17 weeks. **c** Representative histological image of the liver. **d** Plasma aspartate aminotransferase (AST) and alanine aminotransferase (ALT), liver triglyceride (TG), and transcription of TNF-α, IL-1β, α-SMA, and Col1α1 in the liver tissue were measured. **b, d** Data are presented as mean ± SEM ($N = 7$). *$P < 0.05$, ***$P < 0.001$ by the Tukey's test. The cut-off value of T3 was 0.16 ng/ml and T4 was 0.5 μg/dl. The cut-off value of AST and ALT were 9 IU/dl. The cut-off value of TG was 0.19 mg/g liver

fatty acid pathways and were included in a pathway map (Additional file 4 A). There were also many detected metabolite peaks that were not categorized into any aforementioned metabolic pathways (Additional file 4 B–C). The relative area ratios of the three experimental groups were compared and shown in a heatmap with hierarchical clustering. This cluster analysis revealed that the luminal metabolic profiles in all three experimental groups were completely different (Fig. 2b). Among the largely different metabolites found in the STHD-01 group, we attempted to identify metabolic pathways in which the metabolites were constantly elevated throughout the pathway. We found that the pathways of long-chain saturated fatty acids, fatty acids longer than C14, and n-6 unsaturated fatty acids were constantly elevated in the STHD-01 group compared with the control group. Strikingly, the elevation of these pathways was normalized to control levels after the treatment with Abx, suggesting that these metabolic pathways were up-regulated due to gut dysbiosis induced by STHD-01 (Figs. 2b and 3).

Saturated long-chain fatty acids promoted liver inflammation through activation of migratory macrophages in the liver

So far, we have found that STHD-01-induced gut dysbiosis altered microbial metabolic activities, and therefore resulted in an accumulation of saturated long-chain fatty acids and n-6 unsaturated fatty acids. However, it remains unclear whether these metabolic changes in the gut lead to liver inflammation. To investigate the detailed phenotype of liver inflammation induced by the STHD-01, we next analyzed the macrophage populations, which play central roles in the development of inflammation in the liver [19]. Macrophages in the liver can be subdivided into resident and migratory macrophages [20]. Although both macrophage subsets express F4/80 and CD11b, resident macrophages reveal F4/80high CD11blow phenotypes, and

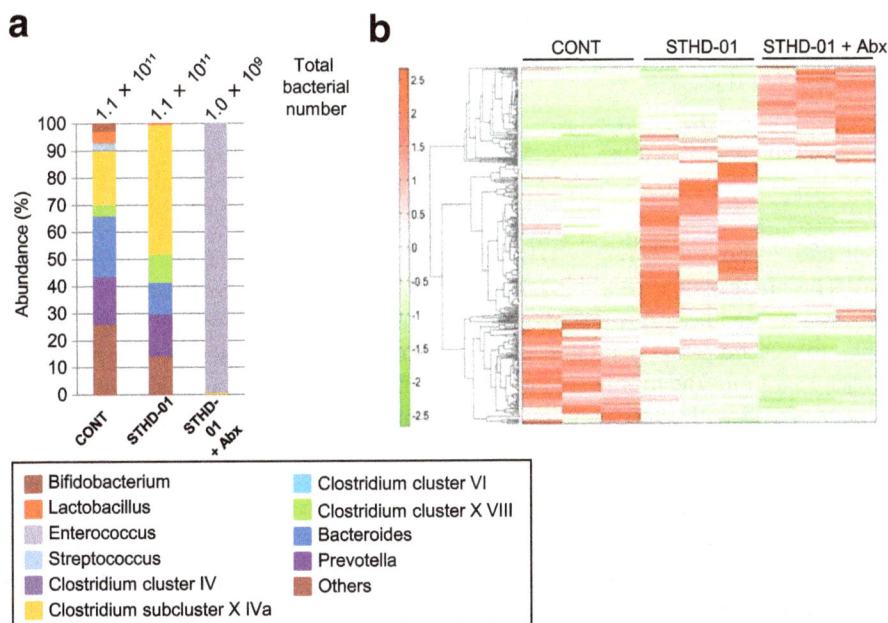

Fig. 2 Gut microbiome and luminal metabolomic analyses in NASH mice. **a** Fresh fecal samples were obtained from each group of mice ($N = 7$) on week 17. Microbial. DNA was extracted from feces and analyzed by T-RFLP. The abundance of bacterial genus is indicated. The total number of bacteria (/g feces) is shown at the top of each column. The cut-off value of total number of bacteria was 1.0×10^6 /g feces (**b**) Fresh fecal samples were obtained from each group of mice (3 individual mice) on week 17 and analyzed using capillary electrophoresis time-of-flight mass spectrometry (CE-TOFMS) and liquid chromatography TOFMS (LC-TOFMS). The hierarchical cluster analysis is shown with a heat map of the metabolite

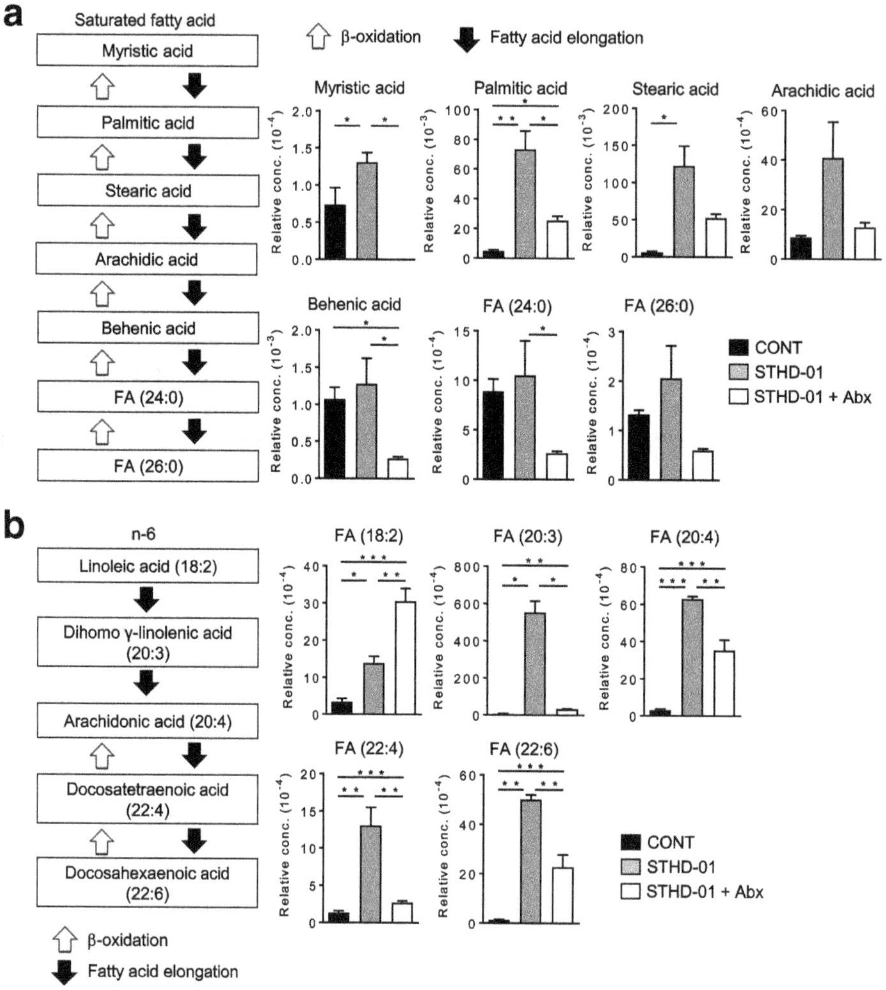

Fig. 3 Alteration of fatty acid metabolism induced by STHD-01. Changes in the luminal metabolites categorized into long-chain saturated fatty acids longer than C14 (**a**) and into n-6 unsaturated fatty acids (**b**) are shown. Data are presented as mean ± SEM ($N = 3$). *$P < 0.05$, **$P < 0.01$, ***$P < 0.001$ by the Tukey's test

migratory macrophages show F4/80^high^CD11b^high^ phenotypes (Fig. 4a). The number of F4/80^high^CD11b^high^ migratory macrophages was significantly elevated in the STHD-01 group (Fig. 4b). Of note, the migration of F4/80^high^CD11b^high^ macrophages into the liver, which is elicited by STHD-01, was significantly decreased by Abx treatment (Fig. 4b). Next, we examined the plasma level of MCP-1, a chemokine that is responsible for the recruitment of monocytes from the bone marrow to the blood, thereby leading to the migration of monocytes to inflammatory tissue sites. Consistent with the number of migratory macrophages in the liver, plasma MCP-1 level was significantly elevated in the STHD-01 group and it was suppressed by the administration of Abx (Fig. 4c). We next asked the impact of long-chain saturated fatty acids in the induction of liver inflammation. CD11b^+^ macrophages were isolated from the liver of the control (CONT), STHD-01-fed (STHD-01). Isolated CD11b^+^

macrophages were then stimulated with palmitic acids (PA), in which the level was correlated to liver inflammation induced by STHD-01 (Figs. 1c, 2, and 3). We measured the transcription of *Tnfa* mRNA as a marker of liver inflammation. In the CONT group, PA stimulation did not induce *Tnfa* expression in liver macrophages (Fig. 4d). In contrast, PA stimulation significantly induced the expression of *Tnfa* in liver macrophages isolated from STHD-01 (Fig. 4d). Since migratory macrophages were dominated within CD11b^+^ mononuclear cell (MNC)s in the STHD-01 fed mice (Fig. 4a-d), this result indicated that PA could activate migratory, but not the resident, macrophages in the liver. PA was able to induce *Tnfa* expression in liver CD11b^+^ macrophages isolated from this group of mice. This result suggests that STHD-01-induced liver inflammation leads to the increased F4/80^high^CD11b^high^ macrophage migration in the liver. Lipid mediators, which are generated by the gut microbiota,

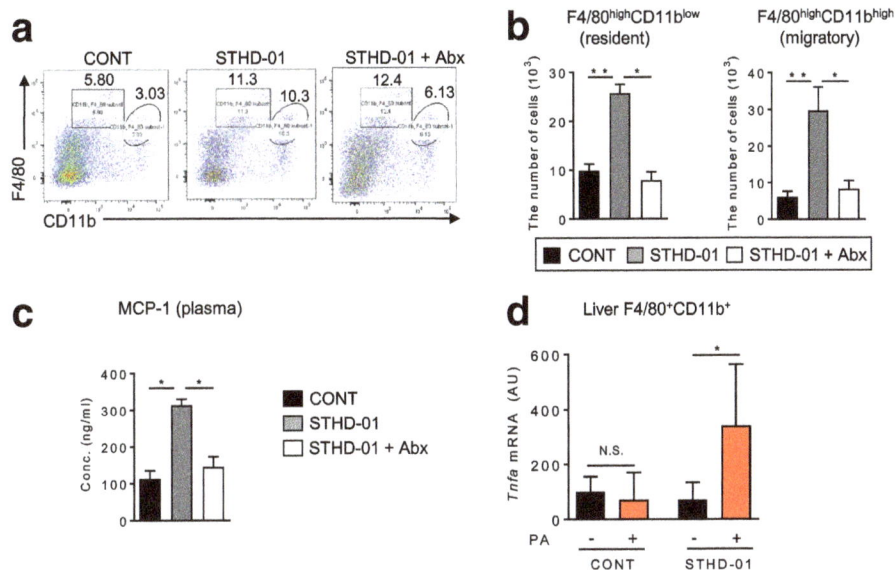

Fig. 4 Migratory macrophages in the liver produce TNF-α in response to palmitic acid. At week 17. All three groups of mice were sacrificed, and liver mononuclear cells were isolated. **a** Representative fluorescence-activated cell sorting (FACS) plot for liver macrophages. CD45.2$^+$7-AAD$^-$ liver mononuclear cells were further expanded by CD11b and F4/80. F4/80^{high}CD11b^{low} resident macrophages (square area) and F4/80^{high}CD11b^{high} migratory macrophages (circle area) are shown. **b** The absolute number of resident and migratory macrophages in the liver. Data are presented as mean ± SEM ($N = 7$). *$P < 0.05$ by the Tukey's test. **c** Monocyte chemoattractant protein (MCP)-1 level in plasma ($N = 3$). (D) Isolated liver CD11b$^+$ macrophages were stimulated with palmitic acid (PA) ($5.12*10^{-3}$ mg/mL) for 20 h. The transcription of Tnfa mRNA was measured by quantitative polymerase chain reaction (qPCR). The expression of Tnfa mRNA was normalized to that of GAPDH. Data are presented as mean ± SEM ($N = 3$). *$P < 0.05$ by the Mann-Whitney U-test

such as PA, promote the progression of liver inflammation by activating the migrated macrophages.

Discussion

The gut microbiota plays a critical role in the pathogenesis of NASH [21]. Here, we comprehensively analyzed the impact of feeding of a new class of HFD, STHD-01, on the gut microbiota and subsequent development of steatohepatitis. As reported previously in conventional HFDs, feeding of STHD-01 induced significant alterations in the gut microbial composition and subsequent luminal metabolic profiles. Depletion of the gut microbiota by treatment of Abx significantly improved the STHD-01-induced mal-metabolic profile in the gut and attenuated liver inflammation. Our present study highlighted a role of the long-chain saturated fatty acid, PA, which accumulated due to STHD-01-induced dysbiosis, in the induction of liver inflammation (Fig. 5).

It has been extensively reported that the intake of HFD causes NASH in experimental animal models [6]. In the present study, we used a recently developed novel steatohepatitis-inducing HFD, STHD-01 [12], to induce NASH. This novel HFD contains a high amount of cholesterol, which is not contained in conventionally used HFDs, and induces the development of severe NASH, while conventionally-used HFDs only induce mild to moderate NASH in a shorter period of time [22]. Another specific feature of STHD-01 is that STHD-01 does not affect

fasting blood glucose levels (Additional file 2). While certain type of diet, such as methionine- and choline-deficient diet (MCD), can also cause an advanced NASH [23], this diet decreases fasting blood glucose levels in experimental animals [24]. Since non-overweight human patients with NAFLD do not show decreased fasting blood glucose levels compared to non-fatty liver disease patients [25], STHD-01 is a better approximation of the clinical condition. One obvious difference in the phenotypes between the mice fed with the STHD-01 and the conventional HFD is body weight gain. Contrary to conventional HFD feeding, the STHD-01-fed mice did not gain body weight while experiencing liver weight gain and lipid accumulation (Fig. 1). These phenotypes may in part be explained by the increased plasma T3 levels, which increase energy expenditure in brown adipose tissues. It has been demonstrated that bile acids generated by the metabolism of dietary fat activate the G-protein-coupled receptor (TGR) 5, which in turn stimulates Iodothyronine Deiodinase (DIO) 2 activity. DIO2 metabolizes T4 and converts it into T3 [26]. In our model, the level of total bile acids in the plasma was significantly elevated in the STHD-01-fed mice (data not shown), suggesting that the increased bile acids subsequently increase T3-mediated energy expenditure in brown adipose tissues and therefore prevent body weight gain.

Consistent with previous observations [27–29], STHD-01-induced NASH pathology was mediated by an

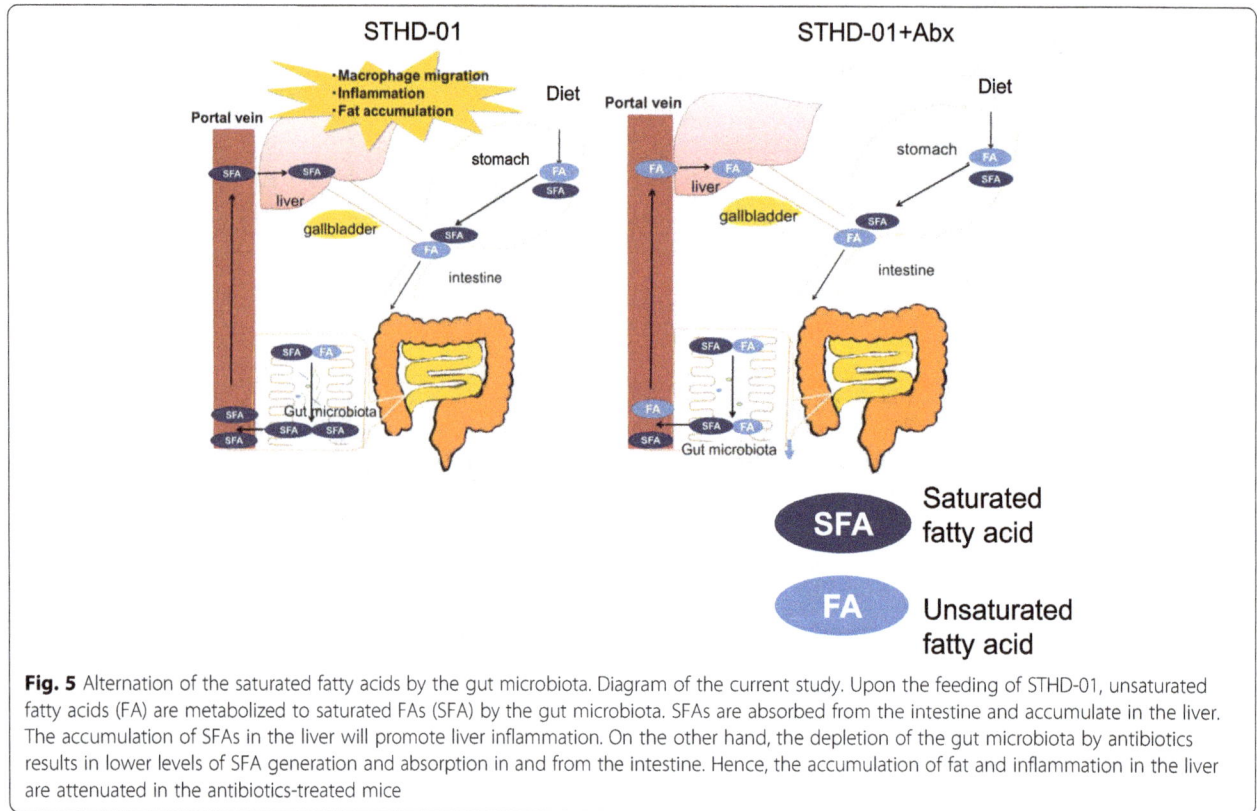

Fig. 5 Alternation of the saturated fatty acids by the gut microbiota. Diagram of the current study. Upon the feeding of STHD-01, unsaturated fatty acids (FA) are metabolized to saturated FAs (SFA) by the gut microbiota. SFAs are absorbed from the intestine and accumulate in the liver. The accumulation of SFAs in the liver will promote liver inflammation. On the other hand, the depletion of the gut microbiota by antibiotics results in lower levels of SFA generation and absorption in and from the intestine. Hence, the accumulation of fat and inflammation in the liver are attenuated in the antibiotics-treated mice

alteration of the gut microbiota and its metabolic activities. In our study, feeding STHD-01 decreased the occurrence of *Bifidobacterium, Lactobacillus, Enterococcus, Streptococcus* and *Bacteroides*, while increasing the presence of *Clostridium* subclusters XIVa and XVIII. The decline in *Bacteroides* in FLD has been reported previously in ob/ob obese mice [11], and a decrease in *Bacteroides* and an increase in *Streptococcus* were observed in patients with hepatitis compared with healthy subjects [30]. The luminal metabolomic analysis showed significant alterations of the luminal metabolic profiles of the mice when fed with the STHD-01. We identified two major pathways (saturated fatty acid and n-6 fatty acid pathways) as candidates of metabolic pathways overrepresented in the STHD-01 group. Although saturated and unsaturated fatty acids are contained in the diet, the overrepresentation of these lipid metabolism pathways was markedly normalized by the depletion of the gut microbiota. This fact indicates that the accumulation of fatty acids is not merely caused by the diet; rather, the generation of saturated fatty acid is enhanced by the gut microbiota. Consistent with this notion, it has been reported that certain types of gut bacteria can saturate fatty acids [31–33]. However, it is still possible that other bacteria metabolites beside fatty acids are involved in the development of NASH induced by STHD-01. Since the involvement of saturated fatty acids in fatty liver

disease has already been reported [34], this was not so unique feature caused by STHD-01. This suggests that different types of HFDs (e.g., different formulations of fatty acids) may bring about a similar microbial/metabolic shift. However, since STHD-01 causes more severe NASH, there might be yet to be determined differences in the abundance of specific microbes and/or metabolites between animals receiving STHD-01 compared to those on conventionally used HFDs. We found that migratory macrophages were significantly increased in the liver upon feeding of the STHD-01. The recruitment of migratory macrophages was significantly suppressed by antibiotics treatment, suggesting that the gut microbiota and their metabolites are indispensable for the macrophage recruitment to the liver. Not only the migration of macrophages, but also the gut microbiota is required for the activation of the migratory macrophages in the liver. Saturated fatty acids, such as PA, which are accumulated upon the feeding of STHD-01 in a gut microbiota dependent manner, can activate migratory macrophages in the liver.

Conclusions

The gut microbiota and its lipid metabolism play a central role in the pathogenesis of NASH induced by a novel steatohepatitis-inducing STHD-01. Comprehensive experiments that utilize multi-OMICS "dry" analyses (gut microbiome and metabolomic analysis) together with "wet" immunological approaches will allow us to understand the precise mechanisms of development of this disease. Targeting the gut microbiota to modify the metabolism of fatty acids might be a new preventive or therapeutic approach in NAFLD and NASH.

Additional files

Additional file 1: Primers used in this study. (PDF 32 kb)

Additional file 2: The levels of fasting blood glucose at week 15 and plasma levels of insulin. The levels of fasting blood glucose at week 15 and plasma level of insulin were shown CONT group and STHD-01 group. Data are presented as mean ± SEM (N = 4). The cut-off value of fasting blood glucose is 9 mg/dl. The cut-off value of plasma level of insulin is 3.12 ng/ml. (PDF 5 kb)

Additional file 3: Liver histology characteristic of non-alcoholic steatohepatitis (NASH). Upon feeding of steatohepatitis-inducing high-fat diet (STHD-01), ballooning, Mallory-Denk body, fibrosis, inflammatory cell infiltration in the periportal regions and fat accumulation both in the pericentral and periportal regions were observed in the liver. (PDF 72 kb)

Additional file 4: Schematic illustration of the substances detected in the metabolomic analysis of the metabolic pathways. (A) Global metabolomic profiling comparing the detectable molecules in the feces among the 3 experimental groups was performed (N = 3 in each group) to determine how different gut bacteria metabolize food. Lipid metabolites in the feces were analyzed using liquid chromatography time-of-flight mass spectrometry (LC-TOFMS), and hydrophilic metabolites were analyzed by capillary electrophoresis time-of-flight mass spectrometry (CE-TOFMS). We identified 225 peaks (158 cations and 67 anions) of hydrophobic metabolites by CE-TOFMS, 115 peaks (65 positives and 50 negatives) of hydrophilic metabolites by LC-TOFMS, and 340 candidate compounds (CE-TOFMS 225 and LC-TOFMS 115). These detected peaks were categorized into glycolysis/glyconeogenesis, pentose-phosphate, tricarboxylic acid (TCA) cycle, urea cycle, purine-pyrimidine, coenzyme, amino acids, acyl-carnitine, and fatty acid pathways and were included in a pathway map. Pathway mapping shows a quantitative comparison of the molecules in the 3 experimental groups. (B) The 38 selected metabolites that were increased specifically in antibiotics treated group compared to the control or STHD-01 groups. (N = 3 in each group) Among these metabolites, 6 metabolites were detected in STHD-01 + Abx group in high concentration, while these were undetectable in the STHD-01 group. The concentration of 32 metabolites were as >3-fold higher in STHD-01 + Abx group than that in the STHD-01 group. (C) The 78 selected metabolites that were increased specifically in the STHD-01 group compared to the STHD-01 + Abx group. (N = 3 in each group) Among these metabolites, 16 metabolites were detected in the STHD-01 group in high concentration, while these were undetectable in the STHD-01 + Abx group. The concentration of 62 metabolites were as >3-fold higher in the STHD-01 group than that in the STHD-01 + Abx group. (ZIP 552 kb)

Abbreviations

Abx: Antibiotics; ALT: Alanine aminotransferase; APC: Antigen-presenting cell; AST: Aspartate aminotransferase; BSA: Bovine serum albumin; CE: Capillary electrophoresis; Col 1α1: α1 type 1 collagen; CONT: Control diet; DIO: Iodothyronine deiodinase; FACS: Fluorescence-activated cell sorting; FLD: Fatty liver disease; HFD: High-fat diet; HPLC: High-performance liquid chromatography; IL: Interleukin; LC-TOFMS: Liquid chromatography time-of-flight mass spectrometry; LPS: Lipopolysaccharides; MCD: Methionine- and choline-deficient diet; MCP-1: Monocyte chemoattractant protein; MNC: Mononuclear cell; MT: Migration time; NAFLD: Non-alcoholic FLD; NASH: Non-alcoholic steatohepatitis; PA: Palmitic acid; PBS: Phosphate-buffered saline solution; qPCR: Quantitative polymerase chain reaction; RT: Retention time; SD: Standard diet; SFA: Saturated long-chain fatty acid; STHD: Steatohepatitis-inducing HFD; T3: Triiodothyronine; T4: Thyroxin; TCA: Tricarboxylic acid; TE: Tris/ethylenediamine tetraacetic acid buffer; TG: Triglyceride; TGR: The G-protein-coupled receptor; TNF: Tumor nuclear factor; α-SMA: α-smooth muscle antigen

Acknowledgements

The *Escherichia coli* JCM1649T genome DNA was provided by the RIKEN BRC through the Bio-Resource Project of the MEXT, Japan.
This research is supported in part by research assistantship of Grant-in-Aid to the Program for Leading Graduate School for "Science for Development of Super Mature Society" from the Ministry of Education, Culture, Sport, Science, and Technology in Japan.

Funding

This work was supported by a Keio University Fukuzawa Memorial Fund (to H.S.) and a Grant-in-Aid for Scientific Research C (15 K09021) from the Japan Society for Promotion of Science (to H.S.). The fund was used for obtaining materials.

Authors' contributions

SY conduced all experiments and analyzed the data with help from TA, NN and TN. MK and YS contributed interpretation of results. CE and NK contributed to the concept, design of the study, interpretation of results. TK contributed the design of the study. SY, NK, and HS wrote the manuscript. HS is responsible for the overall contents. All authors have read and approved the final manuscript.

Competing interests

The authors declare that they have no competing interests.

Author details

[1]Division of Pharmacotherapeutics, Faculty of Pharmacy, Keio University, 1-5-30 Shiba-Kohen, Minato-ku, Tokyo 105-8512, Japan. [2]Division of Gastroenterology, Department of Internal Medicine, The University of Michigan Medical School, Ann Arbor, MI 48109, USA. [3]Division of Gastroenterology and Hepatology, Department of Internal Medicine, Keio University, Shinjuku-ku, Tokyo 160-8582, Japan. [4]Research Institute, EA Pharma Co. Ltd, Kawasaki, Kanagawa 210-8681, Japan.

References

1. Bellentani S, Sacoccio G, Masutti F, Crocè LS, Brandi G, Sasso F, Cristanini G, Tiribelli C. Prevalence of and risk factors for hepatic steatosis in northern Italy. Ann Intern Med. 2000;18(132):112–7.
2. Arata M, Nakajima J, Nishimata S, Nagata T, Kawashima H. Nonalcoholic steatohepatitis and insulin resistance in children. World J Diabetes. 2014; 5(6):917–23.
3. Moraes Ados S, Pisani L, Corgosinho FC, Carvalho LO, Masquio DC, Jamar G, Sanches RB, Oyama LM, Dâmaso AR, Belote C, et al. The role of leptinemia state as a mediator of inflammation in obese adults. Horm Metab Res. 2013; 45(8):605–10.
4. Imajo K, Hyogo H, Yoneda M, Honda Y, Kessoku T, Tomeno W, Ogawa Y, Taguri M, Mawatari H, Nozaki Y, et al. LDL-migration index (LDL-MI), an indicator of small dense low-density lipoprotein (sdLDL), is higher in non-

    alcoholic steatohepatitis than in non-alcoholic fatty liver: a multicenter cross-sectional study. PLoS One. 2014;9(12):e115403.

5. Tilg H, Moschen AR. Evolution of inflammation in nonalcoholic fatty liver disease: the multiple parallel hits hypothesis. Hepatology. 2010;52(5):1836–46.

6. Ito M, Suzuki J, Tsujioka S, Sasaki M, Gomori A, Shirakura T, Hirose H, Ito M, Ishihara A, Iwaasa H. Longitudinal analysis of murine steatohepatitis model induced by chronic exposure to high-fat diet. Hepatol Res. 2007;37(1):50–7.

7. Yoshimoto S, Loo TM, Atarashi K, Kanda H, Sato S, Oyadomari S, Iwakura Y, Oshima K, Morita H, Hattori M, et al. Obesity-induced gut microbial metabolite promotes liver cancer through senescence secretome. Nature. 2013;499(7456):97–101.

8. De Minicis S, Rychlicki C, Agostinelli L, Saccomanno S, Candelaresi C, Trozzi L, Mingarelli E, Facinelli B, Magi G, Palmieri C, Marzioni M, et al. Dysbiosis contributes to fibrogenesis in the course of chronic liver injury in mice. Hepatology. 2014;59(5):1738–49.

9. Hildebrandt MA, Hoffmann C, Sherrill-Mix SA, Keilbaugh SA, Hamady M, Chen YY, Ahima RS, Bushman F, Wu GD. High-fat diet determines the composition of the murine gut microbiome independently of obesity. Gastroenterology. 2009;137:1716–24.

10. Imajo K, Fujita K, Yoneda M, Nozaki Y, Ogawa Y, Shinohara Y, Kato S, Mawatari H, Shibata W, Kitani H, et al. Hyperresponsivity to low-dose endotoxin during progression to nonalcoholic steatohepatitis is regulated by leptin-mediated signaling. Cell Metab. 2012;16(1):44–54.

11. Ridaura VK, Faith JJ, Rey FE, Cheng J, Duncan AE, Kau AL, Griffin NW, Lombard V, Henrissat B, Bain JR, et al. Gut microbiota from twins discordant for obesity modulate metabolism in mice. Science. 2013;341(6150):1241214.

12. Ejima C, Kuroda H, Ishizaki S. A novel diet-induced murine model of steatohepatitis with fibrosis for screening and evaluation of drug candidates for nonalcoholic steatohepatitis. Physiological Reports. 2016;4(21):e13016.

13. Roustan A, Perrin J, Berthelot-Ricou A, Lopez E, Botta A, Courbiere B. Evaluating methods of mouse euthanasia on the oocyte quality: cervical dislocation versus isoflurane inhalation. Lab Anim. 2012;46(2):167–9.

14. Takaki Y, Saito Y, Takasugi A, Toshimitsu K, Yamada S, Muramatsu T, Kimura M, Sugiyama K, Suzuki H, Arai E, et al. Silencing of microRNA-122 is an early event during hepatocarcinogenesis from non-alcoholic steatohepatitis. Cancer Sci. 2014;105(10):1254–60.

15. Hibino S, Saito Y, Muramatsu T, Otani A, Kasai Y, Kimura M, Saito H. Inhibitors of enhancer of zeste homolog 2 (EZH2) activate tumor-suppressor microRNAs in human cancer cells. Oncogene. 2014;3:e104.

16. Ooga T, Sato H, Nagashima A, Sasaki K, Tomita M, Soga T, Ohashi Y. Metabolomic anatomy of an animal model revealing homeostatic imbalances in dyslipidaemia. Mol BioSyst. 2011;7(4):1217–23.

17. Sugiyama K, Ebinuma H, Nakamoto N, Sakasegawa N, Murakami Y, Chu PS, Usui S, Ishibashi Y, Wakayama Y, Taniki N, et al. Prominent steatosis with hypermetabolism of the cell line permissive for years of infection with hepatitis C virus. PLoS One. 2014;9(4):e94460.

18. Chu PS, Nakamoto N, Ebinuma H, Usui S, Saeki K, Matsumoto A, Mikami Y, Sugiyama K, Tomita K, Kanai T, et al. C-C motif chemokine receptor 9 positive macrophages activate hepatic stellate cells and promote liver fibrosis in mice. Hepatology. 2013;58(1):337–50.

19. Nakamoto N, Ebinuma H, Kanai T, Chu PS, Ono Y, Mikami Y, Ojiro K, Lipp M, Love PE, Saito H, Hibi T. CCR9+ macrophages are required for acute liver inflammation in mouse models of hepatitis. Gastroenterology. 2012;142(2):366–76.

20. Hettinger J, Richards DM, Hansson J, Barra MM, Joschko AC, Krijgsveld J, Feuerer M. Origin of monocytes and macrophages in a committed progenitor. Nat Immunol. 2013;14(8):821–30.

21. Malaguarnera M, Vacante M, Antic T, Giordano M, Chisari G, Acquaviva R, Mastrojeni S, Malaguarnera G, Mistretta A, Li Volti G, et al. Bifidobacterium longum with fructo-oligosaccharides in patients with non alcoholic steatohepatitis. Dig Dis Sci. 2012;57(2):545–53.

22. Itoh M, Suganami T, Nakagawa N, Tanaka M, Yamamoto Y, Kamei Y, Terai S, Sakaida I, Ogawa Y. Melanocortin 4 receptor-deficient mice as a novel mouse model of nonalcoholic steatohepatitis. Am J Pathol. 2011;179(5):2454–63.

23. Machado MV, Michelotti G, Xie G, Almeida PT, Boursier J, Bohnic B, Guy CD, Diehl AM. Mouse models of diet-induced nonalcoholic steatohepatitis reproduce the heterogeneity of the human disease. PLoS One. 2015;10(5):e0127991.

24. Rinella ME, Green RM. The methionine-choline deficient dietary model of steatohepatitis does not exhibit insulin resistance. J Hepatol. 2004;40(1):47–51.

25. Omagari K, Kadokawa Y, Masuda J, Egawa I, Sawa T, Hazama H, Ohba K, Isomoto H, Mizuta Y, Hayashida K, et al. Fatty liver in non-alcoholic non-overweight Japanese adults: incidence and clinical characteristics. J Gastroenterol Hepatol. 2002;17(10):1098–105.

26. Watanabe M, Morikawa K, Houten SM, Kaneko-Iwasaki N, Sugizaki T, Horai T, Mataki C, Sato H, Murahashi K, Arita E, et al. Bile acid binding resin improves metabolic control through the induction of energy expenditure. PLoS One. 2012;7(8):e38286.

27. Jiang C, Xie C, Li F, Zhang L, Nichols RG, Krausz KW, Cai J, Qi Y, Fang ZZ, Takahashi S, et al. Intestinal farnesoid X receptor signaling promotes nonalcoholic fatty liver disease. J Clin Invest. 2015;125(1):386–402.

28. Vanderhoof JA, Tuma DJ, Antonson DL, Sorrell MF. Effect of antibiotics in the prevention of jejunoileal bypass-induced liver dysfunction. Digestion. 1982;23(1):9–15.

29. Bergheim I, Weber S, Vos M, Krämer S, Volynets V, Kaserouni S, McClain CJ, Bischoff SC. Antibiotics protect against fructose-induced hepatic lipid accumulation in mice: role of endotoxin. J Hepatol. 2008;48(6):983–92.

30. Qin N, Yang F, Li A, Prifti E, Chen Y, Shao L, Guo J, Le Chatelier E, Yao J, Wu L, et al. Alterations of the human gut microbiome in liver cirrhosis. Nature. 2014;513(7516):59–64.

31. Takeuchi M, Kishino S, Hirata A, Park SB, Kitamura N, Ogawa J. Characterization of the linoleic acid Δ9 hydratase catalyzing the first step of polyunsaturated fatty acid saturation metabolism in lactobacillus plantarum AKU 1009a. J Biosci Bioeng. 2015;119(6):636–41.

32. Kishino S, Takeuchi M, Park SB, Hirata A, Kitamura N, Kunisawa J, Kiyono H, Iwamoto R, Isobe Y, Arita M, et al. Polyunsaturated fatty acid saturation by gut lactic acid bacteria affecting host lipid composition. Proc Natl Acad Sci U S A. 2013;110(44):17808–13.

33. Hirata A, Kishino S, Park SB, Takeuchi M, Kitamura N, Ogawa J. A novel unsaturated fatty acid hydratase toward C16 to C22 fatty acids from lactobacillus acidophilus. J Lipid Res. 2015;56(7):1340–50.

34. Reichardt F, Chassaing B, Nezami BG, Li G, Tabatabavakili S, Mwangi S, Uppal K, Liang B, Vijay-Kumar M, Jones D, et al. Western diet induces colonic nitrergic myenteric neuropathy and dysmotility in mice via saturated fatty acid- and lipopolysaccharide-induced TLR4 signalling. J Physiol. 2017;595(5):1831–46.

17

A comparison of pyogenic liver abscess in patients with or without diabetes: a retrospective study of 246 cases

Wenfei Li[†], Hongjie Chen[†], Shuai Wu and Jie Peng[*] ⓘ

Abstract

Background: Pyogenic liver abscess(PLA) has become common in patients with diabetes mellitus (DM), but it is unclear whether differences exist between patients with and without DM. A retrospective study was performed to identify these differences, summarize the clinical experience, and improve the diagnosis and treatment of PLA.

Methods: The patients were enrolled in a teaching hospital from January 2012 to December 2016. The patients were separated into two groups based on comorbidity with diabetes mellitus (DM). The DM group was further separated into two subgroups according to the HbA1C concentration to investigate whether glycaemic control affected the clinical characteristics of PLA patients with DM. Chi-square, Fisher's exact test, and t-tests were used to analyse and evaluate differences between the two groups.

Results: Two hundred and forty-six PLA patients were identified and 90 (36.6%) had comorbid DM. Patients with DM were older, had higher levels of alkaline phosphatase and γ-glutamyl transferase, hypertension, a loss of body weight, a single abscess, and combined antibiotic therapy with the use of carbapenems and *Klebsiella pneumoniae* in their blood cultures but a less frequent history of abdominal surgery and *Escherichia coli* in their pus cultures. When DM patients were compared to non-DM patients, each of these differences was significant ($P < 0.05$). Diabetic PLA patients with poor glycaemic control had a significantly higher proportion of fever and both lobes abscess($P < 0.05$).

Conclusion: PLA patients with diabetes are older, have more serious complications, a higher prevalence of cardiovascular disease, an increased use of combined antibiotic therapy with carbapenem, and *K. pneumoniae* as the predominant pathogen, but these patients had fewer abdominal surgeries and fewer *E. coli* infections. In addition, poorly controlled glycaemia in diabetic PLA patients is associated with high incidence of fever and both lobes abscess.

Keywords: Pyogenic liver abscess, Diabetes, Diagnosis, Treatment

Background

Pyogenic liver abscess (PLA), which is a suppurating infection of the hepatic parenchyma, remains a condition associated with mortality and is reported in China and throughout the world, especially in Asia. The incidence rate of PLA is different worldwide and continues to increase annually [1]. In Taiwan, the annual all-age incidence of PLA has gradually increased from 10.83 to 15.45 cases per 100,000 individuals from 2000 to 2011 [2]. In northeast China, an incidence of 5.7 cases per 100,000 individuals was reported in a large population-based retrospective study [3]. In the United States, a large study described an incidence of 3.59 cases per 100,000 individuals [1]. PLA is concomitant with many diseases. These diseases are important risk factors and include diabetes mellitus (DM), malignancy, cholangitis, urinary tract disease, pneumonia, cardiovascular disease, autoimmune disease and malnutrition [1, 4–6]. In recent years, PLA patients with concomitant DM have become more common in this hospital, and previous case reports

* Correspondence: pjie138@163.com
†Wenfei Li and Hongjie Chen contributed equally to this work.
Department of Infectious Diseases, Nanfang Hospital of Southern Medical University, Guangzhou 510515, China

demonstrate that DM results in an increased risk of PLA [7]. Tian et al. provided a comprehensive perspective of PLA [8], but whether differences exist among PLA patients with and without concomitant DM is unknown, especially in South China. Furthermore, there is little information regarding the effects of glycaemic control on the characteristics of PLA in diabetic patients. In addition, it is unknown whether glycaemic control affects the clinical characteristics of PLA with DM. Therefore, the purpose of this investigation was to compare the clinical characteristics of PLA patients with and without concomitant DM, to investigate whether glycaemic control affects the clinical characteristics of PLA patients with DM and to improve the diagnosis and treatment of PLA.

Methods
Study population
All of the hospitalized patients diagnosed with PLA (International Classification of Disease, Clinical Modification 572.0) and treated at the Nanfang Hospital of Southern Medical University in Guangzhou, China, from January 2012 to December 2016 were enrolled. This hospital is a public-care, teaching-medical centre in Guangzhou that serves as a patient referral centre and accepts patient referrals from every part of Guangzhou. The diagnosis of PLA was based on the following criteria: 1) clinical features, such as fever, chills, abdominal fullness, and abdominal pain; 2)etiological tests of the blood and the abscess; and 3)imaging evidence of the abscess cavity in the liver as judged by abdominal ultrasonography (US), computerized tomography (CT), or magnetic resonance imaging (MRI). Patients were excluded who did not have clear records or did not complete the treatment. The included patients were divided into two groups: those with and those without DM. The criteria for type II DM were defined according to the 2017 standards [9]: 1)fasting plasma glucose (FPG) $\geq$ 126 mg/dL (7.0 mmol/L); 2)2-h plasma glucose (2-hPG) $\geq$ 200 mg/dL (11.1 mmol/L); 3) HbA1C $\geq$ 6.5% (48 mmol/mol); and 4) a random plasma glucose $\geq$200 mg/dL (11.1 mmol/L) in patients with classic symptoms of hyperglycaemia or hyperglycaemic crisis. To monitor glycaemic control, haemoglobin A1c (HbA1c) provides an estimate of average blood glucose during the preceding 3 months and is widely accepted as the primary indicator of the level of glycaemic control for the optimal management of diabetes [10]. The DM group was further categorised into two subgroups according to the HbA1C concentration: group 1, HbA1C < 7.0%, which indicated good glycaemic control, and group 2, HbA1C $\geq$ 7%, which indicated poor glycaemic control. The HbA1C cut-off value selection was based on previous studies [11].

Data collection
Data were collected by reviewing the medical records of each patient. The records included demographic characteristics (age and sex), length of stay, hospital stay, duration aetiology, underlying diseases, clinical parameters (signs and symptoms), HbA1C levels, laboratory values (hematologic, biochemical, and microbiological findings), imaging features, diagnoses, antimicrobial therapy, catheter drainage, and outcomes at discharge (i.e., recovered or died).

Statistical analysis
The statistical analysis was completed using the SPSS version 17.0 statistical software package(SPSS Inc., Chicago,Illinois, USA). All of the categorical variables were reported as percentages. The chi-square or Fisher's exact test was applied to evaluate the differences in the categorical variables. Continuous data were presented as the mean with the standard deviation (SD) and the Student's t-test was used to evaluate the differences in continuous variables. The statistical tests were performed with a two-tailed significance level of 0.05.

Results
Demographic characteristics
A total of 286 patients received hospital treatment for PLA during the study period. A total of 12 patients were excluded who did not fit the inclusion criteria, 18 were excluded whose medical treatment data were incomplete, and 10 were excluded who were transferred to another hospital before the completion of the treatment. Ultimately, 246 patients were included in this retrospective study. The demographic characteristics and clinical features of the PLA patients are shown in Table 1. We found that males were predominant (n = 160, 65%) and age ranged from 3 to 89 years with a mean age of 54.2 $\pm$ 14.2 years. The length of the hospital stay was 3 to 71 days with an average of 18.5 $\pm$ 11.4 days. Of the 246 patients, 90 (36.6%) had DM and 64 of these were men with a male-to-female ratio of 2.5:1.0. The mean age was 56.5 $\pm$ 10.9 years (26–84 years) for the DM group, which was higher than the 52.9 $\pm$ 15.6 years (3–89 years)for the non-DM group (P = 0.039). However, there was no difference in gender between the two groups (P = 0.129). Table 5 shows the clinical features in diabetic patients with good controlled or poorly controlled glycaemia. All of the diabetic patients had recorded HbA1C levels. Based on the HbA1C levels of the diabetic patients, 27 patients (30.0%) had good glycaemic control and 67 (70.0%) had poor glycaemic control. In our study, the age and gender were not identified between the controlled glycaemia groups (Table 5).

Table 1 Characteristics and clinical findings for patients with pyogenic liver abscess with diabetes mellitus (DM) or without DM (non-DM)

Characteristic	DM cases (%)	Non-DM cases (%)	P value (chi-square test)
Sex			
Male	64(71.1)	96(61.5)	0.129
Female	26(28.9)	60(38.5)	
Age (year) (mean ± SD)	56.5 ± 10.9	52.9 ± 15.6	0.039[a]
Underlying conditions			
Gallbladder diseases	42(53.3)	81(51.9)	0.427
Hypertension	24(26.7)	17(10.9)	0.001
Gastrointestinal surgery	3(3.3)	20(12.8)	0.025
Liver surgery	1(1.1)	14(9.0)	0.013
Pulmonary tuberculosis	3(3.3)	4(2.6)	1.000
Symptoms			
Fever	80(88.9)	138(88.5)	0.919
Chills	58(64.4)	93(59.6)	0.454
Abdominal pain	48(53.3)	90(57.7)	0.507
Frailty	33(36.7)	57(36.5)	0.984
Nausea or Vomiting	10(11.1)	23(14.7)	0.421
Cough	13(14.4)	17(10.9)	0.413
Weight loss	18(20.0)	13(8.3)	0.008

[a]Student's t-test

Underlying diseases

Although most patients in both groups had gallbladder diseases (n = 123, 50.0%) (i.e., gallstones, choledocholithiasis, chronic cholecystitis, pancreatitis, or postcholecystectomy), no significant differences were found between the groups. Hypertension (n = 41, 16.7%) was the second most common underlying disease and was more common in the DM group (26.7% vs. 10.9%, P = 0.001). This was followed by gastrointestinal surgery (n = 23, 9.3%), liver surgery (n = 15, 6.1%), pulmonary tuberculosis (n = 7, 2.5%), nephrotic syndrome (n = 1, 0.4%) and hyperthyroidism (n = 1, 0.4%). Patients with DM had a lower prevalence of gastrointestinal surgery (3.3% vs. 12.8%, P = 0.025) and liver surgery (1.1% vs. 9.0%, P = 0.027) (Table 1). However, the underlying disease did not differ between the good controlled and poorly controlled glycaemia groups (Table 5).

Clinical features

In both groups, the most common symptom was fever (n = 218, 88.6%) with 88.9% in the DM group and 88.5% in the non-DM group; this symptom was followed by chills (n = 151, 61.4%), abdominal pain (n = 138, 56.1%), frailty (n = 90, 36.6%), nausea or vomiting (n = 33, 13.4%), weight loss (n = 31, 12.6%), cough (n = 30, 12.2%), abdominal fullness (n = 8, 3.3%) and jaundice (n = 5, 2.0%) in decreasing order. The DM group had a higher prevalence of body weight loss (20.0% vs. 8.3%, P = 0.008) (Table 1), but there were no significant differences among the glycaemic control groups. However, patients with poorly controlled glycaemia had a higher rate of fever (77.8% vs. 93.7%, P = 0.028) (Table 5).

Laboratory examination

In both groups, inflammatory biomarkers were generally elevated and included C-reactive protein (CRP), procalcitonin (PCT), erythrocyte sedimentation rate (ESR), and leukocyte and neutrophil count. Remarkably, the sensitivity of the erythrocyte sedimentation rate was 100% positive in all of the PLA patients. In addition, C-reactive protein and procalcitonin were approximately 100% positive in all PLA patients. A higher incidence of elevated alanine aminotransferase (ALT), aspartate aminotransferase (AST), total bilirubin (T.Bil), alkaline phosphatase (ALP), γ-glutamyl transferase (GGT) and decreased albumin (ALB)levels were detected in both groups. Additionally, patients with DM had a higher prevalence of ALP (73.5% vs. 49.2%, P = 0.020) and GGT(91.2% vs. 46.2%, P = 0.001) (Table 2). However, no laboratory examination was identified in the group with controlled glycaemia (Table 5).

Imaging

All of the cases were imaged by ultrasonography, computerized tomography (CT), or magnetic resonance imaging (MRI), but no significant difference was found between the groups. According to these images, most of the lesions (n = 171, 69.5%) were located in the right lobe (70.0% in the DM group and 69.2% in the non-DM

Table 2 Laboratory and image findings for pyogenic liver abscess patients with diabetes mellitus (DM) or without DM (non-DM)

Characteristic	DM cases (%)	Non-DM cases (%)	P value (chi-square test)
Laboratory findings			
WBC > 9.5 (× 10^9/L)	64/90(71.1)	96/156(61.5)	0.129
WBC < 3.5 (× 10^9/L)	1/90(1.1)	4/156(2.6)	0.397[a]
NEUT> 75%	62/90(68.9)	101/156(64.7)	0.508
Anaemia[b]	71/90(78.9)	113/156(72.4)	0.262
PLT > 350(× 10^9/L)	28/90(31.1)	59/156(37.8)	0.289
PLT < 125(× 10^9/L)	12/90(13.3)	23/156(14.7)	0.760
↑ESR(mm/1 h)	27/27(100)	32/32(100)	1.000
CRP > 5(mg/L)	81/83(97.6)	131/137(95.6)	0.449
PCT > 0.05(ng/ml)	66/66(100)	90/92(97.8)	0.510[a]
T.Bil > 20.5(μmol/L)	29/89(32.6)	39/155(25.2)	0.468
ALT> 50(U/L)	32/90(35.6)	54/155(34.8)	0.910
AST > 40(U/L)	27/90(30.0)	57/154(37.0)	0.266
ALP > 125(μmol/L)	25/34(73.5)	32/65(49.2)	0.020
GGT > 60(U/L)	31/34(91.2)	30/65(46.2)	0.001
ALB< 40(g/L)	87/90(96.7)	142/155(91.6)	0.123
Abscess location			
Right lobe	63/90(70.0)	108/156(69.2)	0.232
Left lobe	16/90(17.8)	29/156(18.6)	
Both lobes	9/90(10.0)	19/156(12.2)	
Caudate lobe	2/90(2.2)	0(0)	
Abscess size (cm)			
< 5	21/90(23.3)	37/156(23.7)	0.907
5–10	49/90(54.5)	88/156(56.4)	
> 10	20/90(22.2)	31/156(19.9)	
Count of abscess			
Single	75/90(83.3)	110/156(70.5)	0.025
Multiple	15/90(16.7)	46/156(29.5)	

WBC white blood cell count, *NEUT* neutrophil count, *PLT* platelets, *ESR* erythrocyte sedimentation rate, *PCT* procalcitonin, *CRP* C-reactive protein, *ALT* alanine aminotransferase, *AST* aspartate aminotransferase, *T.Bil* total bilirubin, *ALP* alkaline phosphatase, *GGT* γ-glutamyl transferase, *ALB* albumin
[a]Fisher's exact test; [b] Haemoglobin < 130 g/l in men, < 115 g/l in women; ↑ESR > 15 mm/1 h in men, > 20 mm/1 h in women

group) and the diameters ranged from 0.8 × 0.6 cm to 19.0 × 17.7 cm. Patients with a single abscess (*n* = 185, 75.2%) were three-fold as common as patients with multiple abscesses (*n* = 61, 24.8%), and the DM group had a higher prevalence of a single abscess(83.3% vs. 70.5%, *P* = 0.025); however, the difference was not statistically significant for either abscess lesion number or size (Table 2). Remarkably, patients with poor glycaemic control had a higher prevalence in both lobes and the left lobe but less in the right lobe abscess(14.3% vs. 0, 23.8% vs. 3.7%, and 60.3% vs. 92.6%, respectively, *P* = 0.010) (Table 5).

Aetiology

Blood cultures were collected from 118 patients and 24.6% (29 cases) were positive. The DM group had a higher positive proportion(36% vs. 16.2%, *P* = 0.013). Only 6.9%(two cases)of the culture-positive patients had polymicrobial growth. Pus cultures were collected from 121 patients and the overall positive growth rate was 58.7% (71 cases). Only 4.2%(three cases)had polymicrobial growth. A total of 9 cases were positive for both blood and pus cultures. A total of 5 cases had monomicrobial infections and 4 cases had polymicrobial infections. Among the culture-positive patients, 105 strains were identified, which included 10 Gram-positive organisms (9.5%) and 95 Gram-negative organisms (90.5%). *Klebsiella pneumoniae* was the most common pathogen identified in both blood and pus cultures for both groups and had a higher prevalence in blood cultures(26% vs. 1.5%, *P* = 0.001). The second most common pathogen was *Escherichia coli*, which was less frequently isolated from pus cultures of the DM group(16% vs. 2.2%, $P = 0.037$). Other pathogens were isolated from < 5% of the patients (Table 3). However, *K. pneumoniae* infections and *E. coli* infections showed no significant differences between the glycaemic control groups in our study (Table 5).

Treatments and outcomes

Antibiotic therapy was the most common treatment for both groups ($n = 241$, 98.0%), which included 46 patients (19.1%) who received a single antibiotic and 195 patients (80.9%) who received a combination antibiotic therapy. The remaining five patients only accepted simple abscess drainage. In both groups, the most frequently used antibiotics were third generation cephalosporins (including ceftriaxone, ceftazidime, or cefoperazone) ($n = 167$, 69.3%), which were followed by fluoroquinolone (including levofloxacin, moxifloxacin, or ciprofloxacin) ($n = 72$, 29.9%), carbapenems (imipenem or meropenem)($n = 64$, 26.6%), or combined with metronidazole ($n = 109$, 45.2%). It is notable that compared to the non-DM group, the DM group had a significantly higher frequency of combined antibiotic therapy (86.7% vs. 75.0%, $P = 0.009$) with carbapenems (36.7% vs. 19.9%, $P = 0.004$). In addition, percutaneous drainage was performed in 134 (54.5%) patients and surgical drainage was performed in 22 patients (8.9%), but there were no differences between the groups. The total effective rate of the therapy was 96.3%(237/246) and the two groups had similar rates. A total of 6 cases were invalid and 3 cases died from septic shock or multiple

organ failure (MOF). No significant difference was noted in the ratio of the effective treatment and the mortality between the groups (Table 4). Furthermore, the treatment strategy, hospitalization days and mortality were not significantly different between the controlled glycaemia groups either (Table 5).

Discussion

The morbidity of patients with PLA and diabetes has recently increased. This may be due to reduced immunity, neutrophil chemotaxis, mononuclear phagocyte activation, and/or opsonization in diabetes patients. In addition, hyperglycaemia can promote bacterial growth in tissues, and metabolic disorders impact the liver, gut, pancreas, stomach, and intestine, which induces biliary disease. DM is a risk factor for PLA with a hazard risk rate of 3.6 to 9-fold [6, 7] and it is relatively common in PLA patients with reported co-existence rates of 30% in Hong Kong [12], 31% in Canada [13], 28.7% in a single centre in Xi'an, China [14], 23% in Italy [15], and 36.6% in this study.

The majority of the patients in this study were males with a mean of 54.2 ± 14.2 years old, which is comparable with other studies [16]. Patients with DM were approximately 4 years older than patients without DM, which was similar to previous reports [17] and may relate to the fact that most DM patients are older and immunocompromised. Notably, biliary tract diseases were the major underlying disease process, which indicated that biliary infections were the predominate cause of

Table 3 Microbiological isolates in blood and pus cultures from patients with diabetes mellitus (DM) or without DM (non-DM)

Characteristic	Blood culture			Pus culture			Strains
	DM ($n = 50$)	Non-DM ($n = 68$)	P value (chi-square)	DM ($n = 46$)	Non-DM ($n = 75$)	P value (chi-square)	
Positive growth	18	11	0.013	28	43	0.701	–
Polymicrobial growth	1	1	1.000	1	2	1.000	–
Gram-positive aerobes							10 (9.5)
Staphylococcus	2	0	0.177[a]	1	2	1.000	5(4.7)
Streptococcus	1	0	0.424[a]	0	2	0.525[a]	3 (2.9)
Enterococcus	0	2	0.507[a]	0	0	–	2 (1.9)
Gram-negative organisms							95 (90.5)
Klebsiella pneumonia	13	1	0.001	23	25	0.069	62 (59.0)
Escherichia coli	2	7	0.357	1	12	0.037	22 (21.0)
Pseudomonas	0	1	1.000[a]	0	1	1.000[a]	2 (1.9)
Aeroenterobacter	0	0	–	2	1	0.665	3(2.9)
Burkholderia cepacia	1	0	0.424[a]	1	0	0.380[a]	2 (1.9)
Acinetobacter baumannii	0	0	–	1	0	0.380[a]	1(0.95)
Enterobacter cloacae	0	0	–	0	1	1.000[a]	1(0.95)
Bacillus citrate	0	1	1.000[a]	0	0	–	1(0.95)
Shewanella putrefaciens	0	0	–	0	1	1.000[a]	1(0.95)

[a]Fisher's exact test

Table 4 Treatment and outcome in pyogenic liver abscess patients with diabetes mellitus (DM) or without DM (non-DM)

Characteristic	DM cases (%)	Non-DM cases (%)	P value (chi-square test)
Antibiotic option			
Combined	78(86.7)	117(75.0)	0.009
Single	9(0.1)	37(23.7)	
Antibiotic drugs			
The third generation of cephalosporin	63(70.0)	104(66.7)	0.590
Fluoroquinolone	33(36.7)	39(25.0)	0.053
Carbapenems	33(36.7)	31(19.9)	0.004
Metronidazole	43(47.8)	66(42.3)	0.405
Method of abscess drainage			
Percutaneous drainage	51(56.7)	83(53.2)	0.599
Surgical drainage	7(7.8)	15(9.6)	0.627
Clinical outcomes			
Cured	85(94.4)	152(97.4)	0.395
Death	1(1.1)	2(1.3)	1

PLA, and this is consistent with a previous study from east China [18]. In addition, patients with DM had a higher prevalence of hypertension, which suggests that PLA patients with DM were more likely to have cardiovascular disease. In this investigation, gastrointestinal operations included appendectomy ($n = 10$), enterectomy ($n = 7$), laparotomy ($n = 4$) and hemigastrectomy ($n = 2$), and were more common in the non-DM group, which indicated that the gastrointestinal operation history for PLA patients without diabetes was relevant, especially for appendectomy [19]. In our study, liver surgery included a partial hepatectomy ($n = 11$), transcatheter arterial chemoembolization (TACE) ($n = 3$) and splenectomy (n = 1). Although no significant difference was found between the groups, TACE and splenectomy have been linked with certain PLA, which were statistically significant independent risk factors [20, 21]. In addition, patients without DM have been reported to have a higher prevalence of biliary tract diseases [17], but this investigation failed to support that finding.

In our study, the main clinical findings for PLA patients were fever, chills, and abdominal pain, which is consistent with other studies [13, 16–18, 22]. Clinical features, such as cough, jaundice, frailty, and abdominal fullness are not typical and may relate to a delayed diagnosis of PLA. The loss of body weight was higher in the DM group and this may be because DM patients ineffectively use glucose, which results in increased consumption of body fat and protein, and this metabolic condition may enhance more infection. In addition, we found that poorly controlled glycaemia patients were prone to have a fever, which is different from previous studies [23] indicating that glycaemia control affects the severity of PLA.

The laboratory outcomes did not differ between the groups. Most patients had elevated white blood cell counts (WBC), neutrophil counts, C-reactive protein (CRP), procalcitonin (PCT), erythrocyte sedimentation rate (ESR) levels, and abnormal liver function tests, but there was no significant difference between the groups. The CRP, PCT and ESR levels appeared to be more sensitive than WBC. Collectively, the analysis of these biomarkers may reduce the misdiagnosis of PLA. Furthermore, the alkaline phosphatase and γ-glutamyl transferase levels of the DM group were higher, which suggests that liver injury in PLA patients with DM was more remarkable with more fatty liver and biliary cell damage. Nevertheless, our study showed that no laboratory examination was significantly identified between good and poorly controlled glycaemia.

We all know that imaging is crucial for the diagnosis of PLA. In this investigation, most liver abscess was singular and located in the right lobe with a diameter of 5–10 cm, which was in agreement with previous studies [14, 17]. This may be due to the large area of the right liver lobe and its propensity to receive the most portal blood flow [17]. Interestingly, unlike the non-DM group, the overwhelming majority of DM patients had a single abscess. This may be because patients with non-DM had a higher incidence of previous surgeries with possible abdominal infection involving other areas of the liver. It is also interesting to note that patients with poorly controlled glycaemia had a higher rate of both lobes. This may be because poorly controlled glycaemia can help bacteria grow, which makes the overall condition worse. Thus, it is important to control good glycaemia.

Gram-negative bacteria predominated in this investigation, which indicates that antibiotics against Gram-negative

Table 5 Baseline characteristics, clinical presentation, and outcome of diabetic patients with good or poorly controlled glycaemia

Characteristic	Good control of glycaemia (n = 27)(%)	Poor control of glycaemia (n = 63)(%)	P value (chi-square test)
Male	20 (74.1)	44 (69.4)	0.685
Age (year) (mean ± SD)	57.2 ± 2.0	56.1 ± 1.4	0.681
Underlying conditions			
Gallbladder diseases	15 (55.6)	27 (42.9)	0.268
Hypertension	7 (25.9)	17 (26.9)	0.917
Abdominal surgery	2 (7.4)	1 (1.6)	0.159
Liver surgery	0 (0)	1 (1.6)	0.510
Pulmonary tuberculosis	1 (3.7)	2 (3.2)	0.909
Symptoms			
Fever	21 (77.8)	59 (93.7)	0.028
Chills	14 (51.9)	44 (69.8)	0.102
Abdominal pain	14 (51.9)	34 (54.0)	0.854
Weight loss	5 (18.5)	13 (20.6)	0.818
Laboratory findings			
WBC > 9.5 (×10^9/L)	18/27 (66.7)	46/63 (73.0)	0.543
NEUT> 75%	16/27 (59.3)	46/63 (73.0)	0.196
Anaemia[b]	22/27 (81.5)	49/63 (77.8)	0.693
PLT > 350(×10^9/L)	3/27 (11.1)	9/63 (14.3)	0.946
PLT < 125(×10^9/L)	11/27 (40.7)	17/63 (27.0)	0.196
↑ESR(mm/1 h)	7/7 (100)	20/20 (100)	1.000
CRP > 5(mg/L)	25/25 (100)	56/58 (96.6)	1.000[a]
PCT > 0.05(ng/ml)	20/20 (100)	46/46 (100)	1.000
T.Bil > 20.5(μmol/L)	11/27 (40.7)	18/62 (29.0)	0.279
ALT> 50(U/L)	11/27 (40.7)	21/63 (33.3)	0.501
AST > 40(U/L)	9/27 (33.3)	18/63 (28.6)	0.919
ALP > 125(μmol/L)	6/10 (60)	19/24 (79.2)	0.467
GGT > 60(U/L)	9/10 (90)	22/24 (91.7)	1.000[a]
ALB< 40(g/L)	26/27 (96.3)	61/63 (96.8)	1.000[a]
Abscess locations			
Right lobe	25 (92.6%)	38 (60.3%)	0.010
Left lobe	1 (3.7%)	15 (23.8%)	
Both lobes	0 (0)	9 (14.3%)	
Caudate lobe	1 (3.7%)	1 (1.6%)	
Abscess size (cm)			
< 5	4 (14.8)	16 (25.4)	0.526
5–10	16 (59.3)	34 (54.0)	
> 10	7 (25.9)	13 (20.6)	
Multiple abscesses	4 (14.8)	11 (17.5)	0.758
K. Pneumonia infections	6/18 (33.3)	25/50 (50)	0.223
E.coli infections	1/18 (5.6)	2/50 (4)	1.000[a]

Table 5 Baseline characteristics, clinical presentation, and outcome of diabetic patients with good or poorly controlled glycaemia (Continued)

Characteristic	Good control of glycaemia (n = 27)(%)	Poor control of glycaemia (n = 63)(%)	P value (chi-square test)
Treatment			
Percutaneous drainage	15 (55.6)	36 (57.1)	0.889
Surgical drainage	2 (7.4)	5 (7.9)	0.932
Antibiotics only	10 (37.0)	22 (35.0)	0.848
Clinical outcomes			
Cured	27 (100)	58 (92.1)	0.132
Death	0 (0)	1 (1.6)	1.000[a]
Hospitalization days	22.3 ± 2.3	19.4 ± 1.3	0.252

WBC white blood cell count, NEUT neutrophil count, PLT platelets, ESR erythrocyte sedimentation rate, PCT procalcitonin, CRP C-reactive protein, ALT alanine aminotransferase, AST aspartate aminotransferase, T.Bil total bilirubin, ALP alkaline phosphatase, GGT γ-glutamyl transferase, ALB albumin
[a]Fisher's exact test; [b] Haemoglobin < 130 g/l in men, < 115 g/l in women; ↑ESR > 15 mm/1 h in men, > 20 mm/1 h in women

bacteria should be used for empiric therapy. In addition, we also found that *K. pneumoniae* was the dominant pathogen (accounting for 59.0% of the pathogens), which is consistent with previous studies from Asian countries where it accounted for 40–80% [16, 24–26]. Followed by *E. coli,Staphylococcus*, *E. aerogenes*, and *Streptococcus*. In this investigation, the prevalence of *K. pneumoniae* in blood cultures was higher in the DM group. These findings are consistent with previous studies and could be explained by possible intimal vascular defects in DM patients [17]. In contrast, PLA patients without DM had a higher prevalence of *E. coli* in pus cultures, which is similar to a previous study by Tian et al. [8], which may be correlated with a higher incidence of post-abdominal operation and resulting liver infection. Remarkably, the incidence of positive pus cultures was similar between the two groups. Positive pus cultures were significantly higher than blood cultures, which is similar to a previous report [8, 14]. These findings imply that bacteria were primarily confined to the liver. The administration of antibiotics and anti-fever drugs was significantly lower than the incidence of positive blood cultures. Positive blood cultures were higher in the DM group, which suggests that PLA patients with DM are more likely to develop blood infections or even sepsis. Previous studies have shown that diabetic PLA patients with poor glycaemic control had higher *K. pneumoniae* infection rates [23], but our study failed to support this finding. In our study, 98.0% of the patients underwent antibiotic therapy, 54.5% underwent percutaneous drainage, and 8.9% underwent surgical drainage, which resulted in an effective rate of 96.7% and a fatality rate of 1.2%, which was similar to recent international reports of 0.9–2.5% [5, 16, 18]. For treatment, third generation cephalosporin or fluoroquinolone combined with metronidazole was used. Carbapenems were used if the outcomes were not optimal or if patients were in a critical condition. Remarkably, 5 patients presented with severe sepsis and 4 patients required an ICU stay and they all

received combination antibiotic therapy including carbapenems for broad coverage. It is notable that the DM group had a higher proportion of antibiotic combined therapy and carbapenems and a higher likelihood of severe complications with difficult to control infections. These observations suggest that PLA patients with DM may need more aggressive combined therapy with carbapenems. However, there was not a significant difference between percutaneous drainage and surgical therapy for the two groups. Our study showed that the treatment strategy, hospitalization days and mortality were not significantly different between the controlled glycaemia groups. Based on this investigation, antibiotic therapy and catheter drainage are the appropriate treatments for PLA patients with or without DM.

There were notable limitations to this study. This was a retrospective study, it was performed in a single centre, and the results may not be generalizable. However, the results are based on a large number of cases and should be valuable to other investigators and clinicians.

Conclusions

In conclusion, PLA was mainly due to biliary tract disease with a single lesion located in the right lobe, and the predominant pathogen was *K. pneumonia*. PLA patients with and without DM had many differing clinical characteristics. PLA patients with DM were older and had more complications including a higher prevalence of cardiovascular disease, a loss of body weight, *K. pneumonia* infections, antibiotic combined therapy with carbapenem, and a greater likelihood of sepsis. In contrast, a history of gastrointestinal surgery and *E. coli* were less frequent. Furthermore, diabetic PLA patients with poor glycaemic control had a significantly higher proportion of fever and both lobes abscess. Additional large-scale studies and fundamental research can build upon this investigation and should provide further insight into PLA.

Abbreviations

2-hPG: 2-h plasma glucose; ALB: Albumin; ALP: Alkaline phosphatase; ALT: Alanine aminotransferase; AST: Aspartate aminotransferase; CRP: C-Reactive protein; CT: computerized tomography; DM: Diabetes mellitus; *E. coli*: *Escherichia coli*; ESR: Erythrocyte sedimentation rate; FPG: Fasting plasma glucose; GGT: γ-Glutamyl transferase; MRI: Magnetic resonance imaging; NEUT: Neutrophil count; PCT: Procalcitonin; PLA: Pyogenic liver abscess; PLT: Platelets; SD: Standard deviation; T.Bil: Total bilirubin; US: Ultrasonography; WBC: White blood cell count

Authors' contributions

Study conception and design: JP and WFL. Acquisition, analysis and/or interpretation of data: WFL and HJC. Drafting/revision of the work for intellectual content and context: WFL, HJC and SW. Final approval and overall responsibility for the published work: JP. All of the authors read and approved the final manuscript.

Competing interests

The authors declare that they have no competing interests.

References

1. Meddings L, Myers RP, Hubbard J, Shaheen AA, Laupland KB, Dixon E, Coffin C, Kaplan GG. A population-based study of pyogenic liver abscesses in the United States: incidence, mortality, and temporal trends. Am J Gastroenterol. 2010;105(1):117–24.
2. Chen Y, Lin C, Chang S, Shi Z. Epidemiology and clinical outcome of pyogenic liver abscess: an analysis from the National Health Insurance Research Database of Taiwan, 2000–2011. J Microbiol Immunol Infect. 2016; 49(5):646–53.
3. Finch RG, Blasi FB, Verheij TJ, Goossens H, Coenen S, Loens K, Rohde G, Saenz H, Akova M. GRACE and the development of an education and training curriculum. Clin Microbiol Infect. 2012;18(9):E308–13.
4. Gallagher MC, Andrews MM. Postdischarge outcomes of pyogenic liver abscesses: single-center experience 2007-2012. Open Forum Infect Dis. 2017; 4(3):x159.
5. Rahimian J, Wilson T, Oram V, Holzman RS. Pyogenic liver abscess: recent trends in etiology and mortality. Clin Infect Dis. 2004;39(11):1654–9.
6. Tsai FC, Huang YT, Chang LY, Wang JT. Pyogenic liver abscess as endemic disease, Taiwan. Emerg Infect Dis. 2008;14(10):1592–600.
7. Thomsen RW, Jepsen P, Sorensen HT. Diabetes mellitus and pyogenic liver abscess: risk and prognosis. Clin Infect Dis. 2007;44(9):1194–201.
8. Tian LT, Yao K, Zhang XY, Zhang ZD, Liang YJ, Yin DL, Lee L, Jiang HC, Liu LX. Liver abscesses in adult patients with and without diabetes mellitus: an analysis of the clinical characteristics, features of the causative pathogens, outcomes and predictors of fatality: a report based on a large population, retrospective study in China. Clin Microbiol Infect. 2012;18(9):E314–30.
9. American Diabetes Association. 2. Classification and Diagnosis of Diabetes: Standards of Medical in Diabetes 2018. Diabetes Care. 2018;41(Suppl 1):S13–27.
10. American Diabetes Association. Standards of medical care in diabetes--2014. Diabetes Care. 2014;37(Suppl 1):S114–80.
11. Lin YT, Wang FD, Wu PF, Fung CP. Klebsiella pneumoniae liver abscess in diabetic patients: association of glycemic control with the clinical characteristics. BMC Infect Dis. 2013;13:56.
12. Yu SC, Ho SS, Lau WY, Yeung DT, Yuen EH, Lee PS, Metreweli C. Treatment of pyogenic liver abscess: prospective randomized comparison of catheter drainage and needle aspiration. HEPATOLOGY. 2004;39(4):932–8.
13. Kaplan GG, Gregson DB, Laupland KB. Population-based study of the epidemiology of and the risk factors for pyogenic liver abscess. Clin Gastroenterol Hepatol. 2004;2(11):1032–8.
14. Du ZQ, Zhang LN, Lu Q, Ren YF, Lv Y, Liu XM, Zhang XF. Clinical Charateristics and outcome of pyogenic liver abscess with different size: 15-year experience from a single center. Sci Rep. 2016;6:35890.
15. Serraino C, Elia C, Bracco C, Rinaldi G, Pomero F, Silvestri A, Melchio R, Fenoglio LM. Characteristics and management of pyogenic liver abscess: a European experience. Medicine (Baltimore). 2018;97(19):e628.
16. Kong H, Yu F, Zhang W, Li X. Clinical and microbiological characteristics of pyogenic liver abscess in a tertiary hospital in East China. Medicine (Baltimore). 2017;96(37):e8050.
17. Foo NP, Chen KT, Lin HJ, Guo HR. Characteristics of pyogenic liver abscess patients with and without diabetes mellitus. Am J Gastroenterol. 2010; 105(2):328–35.
18. Liu L, Chen W, Lu X, Zhang K, Zhu C. Pyogenic liver abscess: a retrospective study of 105 cases in an emergency department from East China. J EMERG MED. 2017;52(4):409–16.
19. Liao KF, Lai SW, Lin CL, Chien SH. Appendectomy correlates with increased risk of pyogenic liver abscess: a population-based cohort study in Taiwan. Medicine (Baltimore). 2016;95(26):e4015.
20. Lai SW, Lai HC, Lin CL, Liao KF. Splenectomy correlates with increased risk of pyogenic liver abscess: a Nationwide cohort study in Taiwan. J EPIDEMIOL. 2015;25(9):561–6.
21. Oshima S, Tani N, Takaishi K, Hirano M, Makari Y, Hoshi M, Doi T, Matsuno H, Kobori Y. Kobayashi T et al: [clinical evaluation of the risk factors for liver abscess after TACE or RFA]. Gan To Kagaku Ryoho. 2014;41(12):2113–5.
22. Ali AH, Smalligan RD, Ahmed M, Khasawneh FA. Pyogenic liver abscess and the emergence of Klebsiella as an etiology: a retrospective study. Int J Gen Med. 2013;7:37–42.
23. Liao WI, Sheu WH, Chang WC, Hsu CW, Chen YL, Tsai SH. An elevated gap between admission and A1C-derived average glucose levels is associated with adverse outcomes in diabetic patients with pyogenic liver abscess. PLoS One. 2013;8(5):e64476.
24. Lok KH, Li KF, Li KK, Szeto ML. Pyogenic liver abscess: clinical profile, microbiological characteristics, and management in a Hong Kong hospital. J Microbiol Immunol Infect. 2008;41(6):483–90.
25. Cerwenka H. Pyogenic liver abscess: differences in etiology and treatment in Southeast Asia and Central Europe. World J Gastroenterol. 2010;16(20):2458–62.
26. Luo M, Yang XX, Tan B, Zhou XP, Xia HM, Xue J, Xu X, Qing Y, Li CR, Qiu JF, et al. Distribution of common pathogens in patients with pyogenic liver abscess in China: a meta-analysis. Eur J Clin Microbiol Infect Dis. 2016;35(10): 1557–65.

Macrocytic anemia is associated with the severity of liver impairment in patients with hepatitis B virus-related decompensated cirrhosis: a retrospective cross-sectional study

Jian Yang[1†] (ID), Bin Yan[1†], Lihong Yang[1], Huimin Li[2], Yajuan Fan[2], Feng Zhu[3], Jie Zheng[1] and Xiancang Ma[2*]

Abstract

Background: Macrocytic anemia is common in liver disease. However, its role in hepatitis B virus (HBV)-related decompensated cirrhosis remains unknown. The aim of the present study was to determine the association between macrocytic anemia and the severity of liver impairment in patients with HBV-related decompensated cirrhosis according to the Model for End Stage Liver Disease (MELD) score.

Methods: A total of 463 participants who fulfilled our criteria were enrolled in this cross-sectional study. Patients were classified into three groups according to anemia types, diagnosed based on their mean corpuscular volume level. Multivariate linear regression analyses were used to determine the association between macrocytic anemia and the MELD score for patients with HBV-related decompensated cirrhosis.

Results: Patients with macrocytic anemia had evidently higher MELD scores (10.8 ± 6.6) than those with normocytic anemia (8.0 ± 5.5) or microcytic anemia (6.3 ± 5.1). The association remained robust after adjusting for age, gender, smoking, drinking, and total cholesterol ($\beta = 1.94$, CI: 0.81–3.07, $P < 0.001$).

Conclusions: Macrocytic anemia was found to be associated with the severity of liver impairment and might be a predictor for short-term mortality in patients with HBV-related decompensated cirrhosis.

Keywords: Macrocytic anemia, HBV-related decompensated cirrhosis, MELD score, Severity of liver impairment

Background

Cirrhosis is an end-stage disease that invariably leads to death. It is the 14th most common cause of death in adults worldwide and results in 1.03 million deaths per year [1]. Chronic infection with hepatitis B virus (HBV) is one of the major causes of cirrhosis and 30% of deaths are attributable to HBV [2, 3]. China is a highly endemic area of HBV, where 78% of patients with cirrhosis are HBsAg positive [4]. In patients with cirrhosis, the 5-year probability of decompensation is 15–20%, while the

5-year survival rate decreases from 84 to 14–35% once clinical decompensating events occur [5–7].

Anemia is a common comorbidity in cirrhosis that is associated with poor prognosis [8]. Erythrocyte abnormalities were clinically important and frequent findings in patients with chronic disease. Mean corpuscular volume (MCV), a measurement of the average volume of red blood cells (RBCs), has been documented to be associated with an increase in many clinical conditions [9–12]. Typically, anemia can be classified into macrocytic anemia (> 100 fL), normocytic anemia (80–100 fL), and microcytic anemia (< 80 fL) based on the patient's MCV level. A recent study has reported that the elevated MCV level was associated with increased liver cancer mortality, especially in men who are hepatitis B surface antigen (HBsAg)

* Correspondence: maxiancang@163.com
†Jian Yang and Bin Yan contributed equally to this work.
²Department of Psychiatry, the First Affiliated Hospital, Xi'an Jiaotong University, No.277 Yanta West Road, Yanta District, Xi'an 710061, People's Republic of China
Full list of author information is available at the end of the article

positive [13]. Therefore, in this study, we hypothesized that a common association might exist between macrocytic anemia and the severity of liver impairment in patients with HBV-related decompensated cirrhosis.

We used the Model for End Stage Liver Disease (MELD) score for evaluating the severity of liver impairment of HBV-related decompensated cirrhosis. The MELD score was developed to predict the short-term mortality of end-stage liver disease because of the shortage of donated livers. It had been validated subsequently as an accurate predictor of survival among different populations of patients with advanced liver disease and was adopted for organ allocation for liver transplantation instead of the older Child-Pugh score in the USA since 2002 [14–16]. Liver transplantation is generally recommended for patients with MELD score of > 15, if possible [17].

The goal of the present study is to investigate whether the MELD score is higher in the macrocytic anemia group in patients with HBV-related decompensated cirrhosis.

Methods
Study population
From May 2013 to July 2016, data of 1445 patients diagnosed as having HBV-related decompensated cirrhosis were extracted from the HIS Database at the First Affiliated Hospital of Xi'an Jiaotong University. For patients to be diagnosed as having HBV-related decompensated cirrhosis, the following conditions must be present: HBsAg carrier for

≥6 months; pathological or clinical evidence of cirrhosis; and occurrence of complications, such as ascites, upper gastrointestinal bleeding, spontaneous bacterial peritonitis, or hepatic encephalopathy [6, 18–20]. Anemia was defined according to WHO's haemoglobin thresholds, which is haemoglobin level of < 130 g/L in male and < 120 g/L in female [8]. After strictly screening according to the inclusion criteria and exclusion criteria, 463 patients were enrolled in this hospital-based cross-sectional study (Fig. 1). The study was approved by the Ethics Committee of the First Affiliated Hospital, Xi'an Jiaotong University. Since this is a retrospective study, a written consent is waived by the Ethics Committee and is deemed unnecessary. All methods were carried out in accordance with appropriate clinical practice guidelines and national legal requirements.

Data collection
Demographic characteristics were obtained from an interview during the patients' admission to our hospital. Venous blood samples were collected from the participants after an overnight fasting for laboratory assessments. Smoking was defined as having ≥1 cigarette per day and drinking was defined as alcohol intaking > 20 g per day for at least a year [21, 22]. Estimated glomerular filtration rate (eGFR) was calculated using a formula adapted from the Modification of Diet in Renal Disease (MDRD) equation [23, 24]. Unfortunately, body mass index (BMI) and HBV DNA data were not included in the analysis due to excessive missing values.

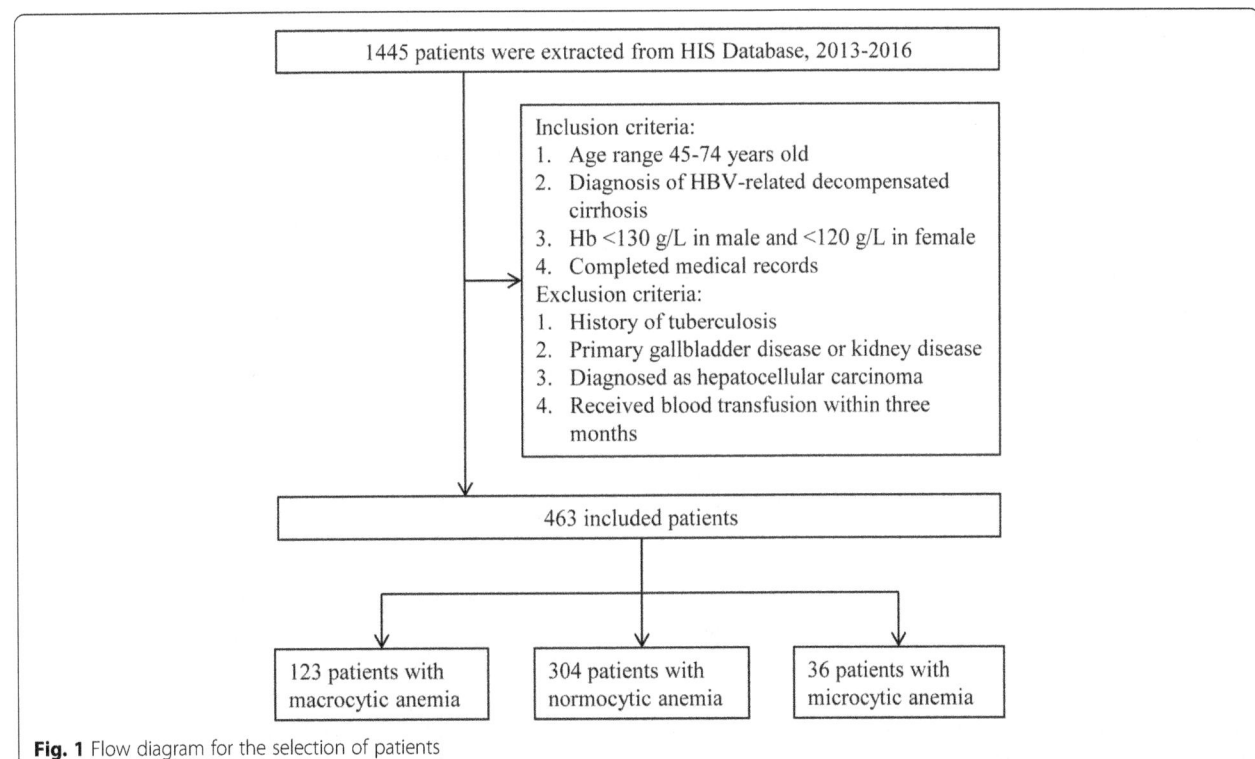

Fig. 1 Flow diagram for the selection of patients

MELD score

The MELD score was calculated using the following formula: $9.57 \times \log_e$ (creatinine mg/dl) $+ 3.78 \times \log_e$ (bilirubin mg/dl) $+ 11.2 \times \log_e$ (INR) $+ 6.43$, where INR is the international normalised ratio and 6.43 is the constant for liver disease aetiology [16].

Statistical analysis

Statistical analyses were conducted using R software (version 3.1.3). Continuous data were presented as mean $\pm$ SD, and categorical variables were presented as count and percentage. All participants were divided into three groups according to their anemia classification. We used one-way ANOVA to determine the differences among the three groups in terms of the continuous variables, because the variables were all normally distributed and homogeneous in variance. Simultaneously, the chi-square test was used for categorical variables. Univariate and multivariate linear regression analyses were used to examine the associations of the MELD score with macrocytic anemia. Variables with P value < 0.05 in univariate models were then included in the multivariate analyses. A two-tailed test was used to calculate the P value, and the results were considered statistically significant when the P value < 0.05.

Results

Characteristics of participants

Table 1 presents the baseline characteristics of the participants, which were divided into three groups according to anemia types. Among the 463 eligible participants, 304 had normocytic anemia, 123 had macrocytic anemia and 36 had microcytic anemia. The average age of participants was 54.3 (SD = 7.3) years and 63.5% of them were male. Our data showed that patients with macrocytic anemia were older and had higher levels of bilirubin, international normalized ratio (INR) and alkaline phosphatase (ALP) compared to patients with normocytic or microcytic anemia. MELD score was also observed to be higher in the macrocytic group. Oppositely, the total cholesterol and albumin were relatively low. There were no significant differences observed in terms of gender, smoking, drinking, hypertension, systolic blood pressure, diastolic blood pressure, creatinine, eGFR, aspartate aminotransferase (AST) and alanine aminotransferase (ALT). The haemoglobin level and prevalence of diabetes in the microcytic group were slightly different from that in the other two groups, but this difference was negligible.

Assessment of the association between MELD score and possible risk factors

We next assessed the correlation between the MELD score and possible risk factors using the univariate linear regression analyses (Table 2). Our results revealed a positive association between the MELD score and male, smoking and drinking. In addition, a negative association between the MELD score and the total cholesterol level was observed.

Association between macrocytic anemia and MELD score

Patients in the macrocytic group had evidently higher MELD scores than patients in the other two groups (Fig. 2). In univariate regression analysis, we found that there was a significant association between macrocytic anemia and the MELD score (estimated coefficient [β] = 2.80, 95% confidence interval [CI]: 1.59–4.01, P value [P] < 0.001), using the normocytic group as the reference. Furthermore, the association remained robust (β = 1.94, CI: 0.81–3.07, $P < 0.001$) after adjusting for age, gender, smoking, drinking and total cholesterol in multivariate analysis (Table 2).

Discussion

In this retrospective study, we demonstrated that macrocytic anemia, defined as anemia in which the RBCs are larger than their normal volume (100 fL), is associated with the severity of liver impairment in patients with HBV-related decompensated cirrhosis. This finding remains substantial even after adjusting for demographics and laboratory parameters, such as age, gender, smoking, drinking and total cholesterol.

An MCV level greater than 100 fL, which is also known as macrocytosis, may not always be associated with anemia. Moreover, it presents independently from anemia in most cases [10]. Nevertheless, we chose anemia as one of our inclusion criteria because 84.2% of the 1445 pre-screened patients have anemia. This result was consistent with the finding of another study, which reported that about 75% of patients with chronic liver disease have a diverse aetiology of anemia [25]. Furthermore, patients with cirrhosis may have anemia due to a lack of haematopoietic factors, shortened erythrocyte survival, reduced bone marrow function, or gastrointestinal bleeding. All these conditions indicate impaired liver function and a high risk of mortality. Therefore, patients without anemia were excluded from the data analysis to avoid potential bias in our present study.

The importance of macrocytic anemia or macrocytosis seems to be underestimated in the past. Only a few studies focused on its risk of adverse events or death [9–13]. Among these studies, Yoon et al. documented that the elevated MCV level was associated with increased liver cancer mortality in men [13]; this finding was consistent with the result of our study. A small-sample study also found a markedly higher MCV in patients with chronic liver failure than in healthy subjects [26]. These observations, though not directly, provided evidence for our conclusion that patients with HBV-related decompensated cirrhosis

Table 1 Demographic and biochemical characteristics of the study participants ($N = 463$)

Variable	Macrocytic anemia	Normocytic anemia	Microcytic anemia	P value
Number of subjects	123	304	36	
Mean corpuscular volume, fL	102.7 ± 2.6	91.2 ± 5.1[†]	74.2 ± 4.6[†¥]	< 0.001
Age, years	56.1 ± 7.6	53.9 ± 7.1[†]	51.8 ± 6.2[†]	0.002
Male, n(%)	78(63.4)	191(62.8)	25(69.4)	0.738
Drinking, n(%)	24(19.5)	74(24.3)	13(36.1)	0.118
Smoking, n(%)	48(39.0)	107(35.2)	15(41.7)	0.618
Diabetes, n(%)	10(8.1)	39(12.8)	9(25.0) [†]	0.026
Hypertension, n(%)	14(11.3)	36(11.8)	4(11.1)	0.985
Hemoglobin, g/L				
> 90	97(78.9)	230(75.7)	10(27.8)[†¥]	< 0.001
60–90	21(17.1)	63(20.7)	20(55.6)[†¥]	< 0.001
< 60	5(4.1)	11(3.6)	6(16.7)[†¥]	0.002
Total cholesterol, mmol/L	2.4 ± 0.7	2.7 ± 0.9[†]	2.7 ± 0.8	0.012
Systolic blood pressure, mmHg	117.9 ± 17.6	117.8 ± 15.2	113.8 ± 13.8	0.350
Diastolic blood pressure, mmHg	72.6 ± 11.7	73.4 ± 10.0	70.9 ± 8.6	0.354
Bilirubin, mg/dL	3.4 ± 3.4	2.6 ± 3.2[†]	1.8 ± 3.4[†]	0.011
Creatinine, mg/dL	0.8 ± 0.8	0.7 ± 0.4	0.7 ± 0.4	0.147
INR	1.5 ± 0.3	1.4 ± 0.4[†]	1.3 ± 0.1[†]	0.006
eGFR, mL/min/1.73m^2	123.6 ± 54.5	126.9 ± 43.4	130.3 ± 39.1	0.686
Albumin	27.0 ± 4.7	29.1 ± 4.7[†]	31.7 ± 4.8[†¥]	< 0.001
AST	78.3 ± 147.3	84.2 ± 196.6	41.7 ± 39.5	0.394
ALT	45.3 ± 42.4	59.4 ± 114.3	29.3 ± 31.8	0.113
ALP	122.9 ± 55.5	106.4 ± 61.1[†]	85.2 ± 32.7[†]	0.001
MELD score	10.8 ± 6.6	8.0 ± 5.5[†]	6.3 ± 5.1[†]	< 0.001
Complications, n(%)				
UGB	6(4.9)	34(11.2)	5(13.9)	0.093
SBP	36(29.3)	75(24.7)[†]	3(8.3)[†]	0.037
HE	14(11.4)	22(7.2)	3(8.3)	0.377

Values are presented as mean ± standard deviation or numbers (percentage)
INR international normalized ratio, *eGFR* estimated glomerular filtration rate, *AST* aspartate aminotransferase, *ALT* alanine aminotransferase, *ALP* alkaline phosphatase, *MELD* model for end stage liver disease, *UGB* upper gastrointestinal bleeding, *SBP* spontaneous bacterial peritonitis, *HE* hepatic encephalopathy
P indicates the difference among the three groups. [†]Indicates significance ($P < 0.05$) compared to macrocytic anemia; [¥]Indicates significance ($P < 0.05$) compared to normocytic anemia

who have macrocytic anemia were more likely to present worse liver condition.

There are several potential pathological mechanisms that explain why macrocytic anemia is associated with the severity of liver impairment. First, patients with advanced liver damage are more likely to have vitamin B_{12} or folate deficiencies [27], which directly result in macrocytic anemia. Vitamin B_{12} and folate coenzymes are required for thymidylate and purine synthesis, thus, their deficiencies result in retarded DNA synthesis and eventually will develop into macrocytic anemia [28–30]. Second, macrocytic anemia in liver disease may be due to an increased deposition of cholesterol on the membranes of circulating RBCs [31, 32]. This deposition effectively increases the surface area of the

erythrocyte. Third, hemolytic anemias are common in advanced liver failure. In this case, excessive destruction of RBCs and increased reticulocyte count can be observed. The immature erythrocytes are approximately 20% larger compared to the mature erythrocytes, which result in macrocytic anemia [25]. Moreover, erythrocyte morphology is affected by various factors in liver disease, such as causes, degree of liver damage, and drugs used. Complicated mechanisms, which allow the synchronized performance of their independent or collaborative functions, determine the shape of RBCs. Nevertheless, we firmly believe that there is a positive correlation between macrocytic anemia and the severity of liver impairment in patients with HBV-related decompensated cirrhosis.

Table 2 Univariate and multivariate linear regression analysis for MELD score

Variable	Univariate		Multivariate	
	β (CI 95%)	P value	β (CI 95%)	P value
Age	0.05(−0.02,0.13)	0.160	0.07(0.01,0.15)	0.028
Male	2.25(1.15,3.36)	< 0.001	1.49(0.29,2.70)	0.015
Smoking	1.93(0.82,3.03)	< 0.001	0.21(−1.03,1.44)	0.742
Drinking	1.59(0.34,2.85)	0.013	0.73(−0.56,2.01)	0.269
Diabetes	0.53(− 1.11,2.16)	0.527		
Hypertension	0.15(−1.53,1.84)	0.857		
Hemoglobin, g/L				
> 90	Ref	–		
60–90	1.09(−0.21,2.39)	0.100		
< 60	−1.35(−3.90,1.20)	0.298		
Total cholesterol	−2.77(−3.37,-2.16)	< 0.001	−2.53(− 3.14,-1.93)	< 0.001
Systolic blood pressure	−0.01(− 0.04,0.03)	0.863		
Diastolic blood pressure	−0.01(− 0.06,0.05)	0.900		
Anemia classification				
Normocytic anemia	Ref	–	Ref	–
Macrocytic anemia	2.80(1.59,4.01)	< 0.001	1.94(0.81,3.07)	< 0.001
Microcytic anemia	−1.73(−3.72,0.27)	0.089	− 1.77(− 3.59,0.05)	0.057

MELD model for end stage liver disease, *β* estimated coefficient, *95% CI* 95% confidence interval

In addition, we used the MELD score, which is a formula comprising creatinine, bilirubin, and INR values, to evaluate the severity of liver impairment and risk of death. In our study, patients with macrocytic anemia had higher levels of bilirubin and INR, but no significant difference was observed in creatinine levels and eGFR. Thus, macrocytic anemia might be unrelated to kidney damage in patients with HBV-related decompensated cirrhosis.

There were a few limitations in this study. First, we used the MELD score for evaluating the severity of liver impairment in patients with HBV-related decompensated cirrhosis. Although the MELD score could provide an accurate prediction of short-term mortality of patients with cirrhosis, a follow-up data might be better and more credible. Second, the analysis did not include data on serum vitamin B_{12}, folate, reticulocyte count, drugs, and measures of haemolysis, which could

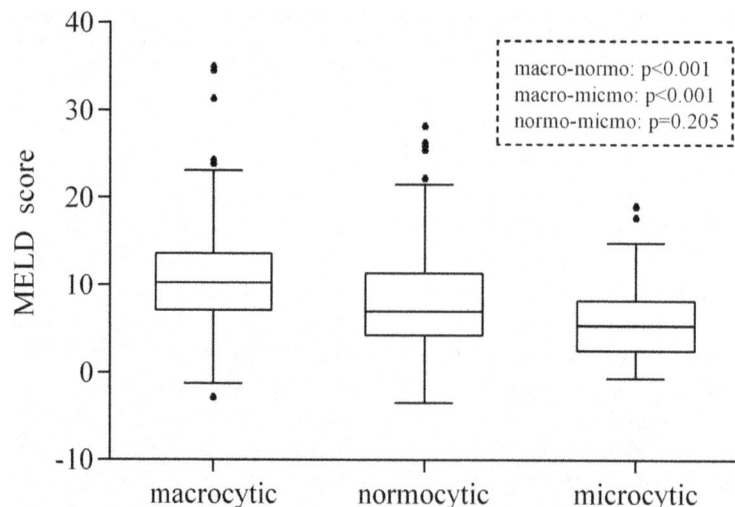

Fig. 2 Anemia types and MELD scores. Patients with macrocytic anemia had evidently higher MELD scores than those with normocytic anemia (*P* < 0.001) or microcytic anemia (*P* < 0.001)

contribute to better understand the mechanisms of macrocytic anemia in patients with cirrhosis.

Conclusions

Macrocytic anemia was found to be associated with the severity of liver impairment and might be a predictor for short-term mortality in patients with HBV-related decompensated cirrhosis. However, a large-scale cohort study is recommended to confirm the present results and to elucidate the mechanisms underlying the observed correlations between macrocytic anemia and the severity of liver impairment in patients with HBV-related decompensated cirrhosis.

Abbreviations

ALP: Alkaline phosphatase; ALT: Alanine aminotransferase; AST: Aspartate aminotransferase; BMI: Body mass index; eGFR: Estimated glomerular filtration rate; HBsAg: Hepatitis B surface antigen; HBV: Hepatitis B virus; HE: Hepatic encephalopathy; INR: International normalised ratio; MCV: Mean corpuscular volume; MDRD: Modification of diet in renal disease; MELD: Model for end stage liver disease; RBCs: Red blood cells; SBP: Spontaneous bacterial peritonitis; UGB: Upper gastrointestinal bleeding

Acknowledgements

We would like to acknowledge the participants in the study. We appreciated the Department of Epidemiology and Biostatistics, Xi'an Jiaotong University Health Science Center for statistical assistance.

Funding

There was no funding for this study.

Authors' contributions

XM, JY and BY designed the study. LY, HL and YF compiled the data and helped with the data interpretation. JY and BY analysed the data and drafted the manuscript. XM, JZ and FZ revised the manuscripts for important intellectual content helped with the data interpretation. All authors reviewed the manuscript.

Competing interests

The authors declare no competing financial interests.

Author details

[1]Clinical Research Center, the First Affiliated Hospital, Xi'an Jiaotong University, Xi'an 710061, People's Republic of China. [2]Department of Psychiatry, the First Affiliated Hospital, Xi'an Jiaotong University, No.277 Yanta West Road, Yanta District, Xi'an 710061, People's Republic of China. [3]Center for Translational Medicine, the First Affiliated Hospital, Xi'an Jiaotong University, Xi'an 710061, People's Republic of China.

References

1. Tsochatzis EA, Bosch J, Burroughs AK. Liver cirrhosis. Lancet. 2014;383(9930):1749–61.
2. Perz JF, Armstrong GL, Farrington LA, Hutin YJ, Bell BP. The contributions of hepatitis B virus and hepatitis C virus infections to cirrhosis and primary liver cancer worldwide. J Hepatol. 2006;45(4):529–38.
3. Lozano R, Naghavi M, Foreman K, Lim S, Shibuya K, Aboyans V, Abraham J, Adair T, Aggarwal R, Ahn SY, et al. Global and regional mortality from 235 causes of death for 20 age groups in 1990 and 2010: a systematic analysis for the global burden of disease study 2010. Lancet. 2012;380(9859):2095–128.
4. Merican I, Guan R, Amarapuka D, Alexander MJ, Chutaputti A, Chien RN, Hasnian SS, Leung N, Lesmana L, Phiet PH, et al. Chronic hepatitis B virus infection in Asian countries. J Gastroenterol Hepatol. 2000;15(12):1356–61.
5. Srivastava M, Rungta S, Dixit VK, Shukla SK, Singh TB, Jain AK. Predictors of survival in hepatitis B virus related decompensated cirrhosis on tenofovir therapy: an Indian perspective. Antivir Res. 2013;100(2):300–5.
6. Peng CY, Chien RN, Liaw YF. Hepatitis B virus-related decompensated liver cirrhosis: benefits of antiviral therapy. J Hepatol. 2012;57(2):442–50.
7. McMahon BJ. Epidemiology and natural history of hepatitis B. Semin Liver Dis. 2005;25(Suppl 1):3–8.
8. Benoist BD, Mclean E, Egll I, Cogswell M, Benoist BD, Mclean E, Egll I, Cogswell M. Worldwide prevalence of anaemia 1993–2005: WHO global database on anaemia. Geneva, World Health Organization. 2008 2(3):97-100.
9. Ueda T, Kawakami R, Horii M, Sugawara Y, Matsumoto T, Okada S, Nishida T, Soeda T, Okayama S, Somekawa S, et al. High mean corpuscular volume is a new Indicator of prognosis in acute decompensated heart failure. Circ J. 2013;77(11):2766–71.
10. Myojo M, Iwata H, Kohro T, Sato H, Kiyosue A, Ando J, Sawaki D, Takahashi M, Fujita H, Hirata Y, et al. Prognostic implication of macrocytosis on adverse outcomes after coronary intervention. Atherosclerosis. 2012;221(1):148–53.
11. Tennankore KK, Soroka SD, West KA, Kiberd BA. Macrocytosis may be associated with mortality in chronic hemodialysis patients: a prospective study. BMC Nephrol. 2011;12:19.
12. Kloth JS, Hamberg P, Mendelaar PA, Dulfer RR, van der Holt B, Eechoute K, Wiemer EA, Kruit WH, Sleijfer S, Mathijssen RH. Macrocytosis as a potential parameter associated with survival after tyrosine kinase inhibitor treatment. Eur J Cancer (Oxford, England : 1990). 2016;56:101–6.
13. Yoon HJ, Kim K, Nam YS, Yun JM, Park M. Mean corpuscular volume levels and all-cause and liver cancer mortality. Clin Chem Lab Med. 2016;54(7):1247–57.
14. Wiesner R, Edwards E, Freeman R, Harper A, Kim R, Kamath P, Kremers W, Lake J, Howard T, Merion RM, et al. Model for end-stage liver disease (MELD) and allocation of donor livers. Gastroenterology. 2003;124(1):91–6.
15. Bambha K, Kim WR, Kremers WK, Therneau TM, Kamath PS, Wiesner R, Rosen CB, Thostenson J, Benson JT, Dickson ER. Predicting survival among patients listed for liver transplantation: an assessment of serial MELD measurements. Am J Transplant Off J Am Soc Transplant Am Soc Transplant Surg. 2004;4(11):1798–804.
16. Kamath PS, Kim WR. Advanced liver disease study G: the model for end-stage liver disease (MELD). Hepatology (Baltimore, MD). 2007;45(3):797–805.
17. Murray KF, Carithers RL Jr. AASLD: AASLD practice guidelines: evaluation of the patient for liver transplantation. Hepatology (Baltimore, MD). 2005;41(6):1407–32.
18. Shim JH, Lee HC, Kim KM, Lim YS, Chung YH, Lee YS, Suh DJ. Efficacy of entecavir in treatment-naive patients with hepatitis B virus-related decompensated cirrhosis. J Hepatol. 2010;52(2):176–82.
19. Jang JW, Choi JY, Kim YS, Woo HY, Choi SK, Lee CH, Kim TY, Sohn JH, Tak WY, Han KH. Long-term effect of antiviral therapy on disease course after decompensation in patients with hepatitis B virus-related cirrhosis. Hepatology (Baltimore, MD). 2015;61(6):1809–20.
20. Wang FY, Li B, Li Y, Liu H, Qu WD, Xu HW, Qi JN, Qin CY. Entecavir for patients with hepatitis B decompensated cirrhosis in China: a meta-analysis. Sci Rep. 2016;6:32722.
21. Carter BD, Abnet CC, Feskanich D, Freedman ND, Hartge P, Lewis CE, Ockene JK, Prentice RL, Speizer FE, Thun MJ, et al. Smoking and mortality--beyond established causes. N Engl J Med. 2015;372(7):631–40.

22. Kim HM, Kim BS, Cho YK, Kim BI, Sohn CI, Jeon WK, Kim HJ, Park DI, Park JH, Joo KJ, et al. Elevated red cell distribution width is associated with advanced fibrosis in NAFLD. Clin Mol Hepatol. 2013;19(3):258–65.

23. National Kidney Foundation. K/DOQI clinical practice guidelines for chronic kidney disease: evaluation, classification, and stratification. Am J Kidney Dis. 2002;39(2 Suppl 1):S1–266.

24. Ma YC, Zuo L, Chen JH, Luo Q, Yu XQ, Li Y, Xu JS, Huang SM, Wang LN, Huang W, et al. Modified glomerular filtration rate estimating equation for Chinese patients with chronic kidney disease. J Am Soc Nephrol. 2006; 17(10):2937–44.

25. Gonzalez-Casas R. Spectrum of anemia associated with chronic liver disease. World J Gastroenterol. 2009;15(37):4653.

26. Remkova A, Remko M. Homocysteine and endothelial markers are increased in patients with chronic liver diseases. Eur J Intern Med. 2009;20(5):482–6.

27. Rocco A, Compare D, Coccoli P, Esposito C, Di Spirito A, Barbato A, Strazzullo P, Nardone G. Vitamin B12 supplementation improves rates of sustained viral response in patients chronically infected with hepatitis C virus. Gut. 2013;62(5):766–73.

28. Morris MS, Jacques PF, Rosenberg IH, Selhub J. Folate and vitamin B-12 status in relation to anemia, macrocytosis, and cognitive impairment in older Americans in the age of folic acid fortification. Am J Clin Nutr. 2007; 85(1):193–200.

29. Green R, Dwyre DM. Evaluation of macrocytic anemias. Semin Hematol. 2015;52(4):279–86.

30. Robinson AR, Mladenovic J. Lack of clinical utility of folate levels in the evaluation of macrocytosis or anemia. Am J Med. 2001;110(2):88–90.

31. Owen JS, Bruckdorfer KR, Day RC, McIntyre N. Decreased erythrocyte membrane fluidity and altered lipid composition in human liver disease. J Lipid Res. 1982;23(1):124–32.

32. Grattagliano I, Calamita G, Cocco T, Wang DQ, Portincasa P. Pathogenic role of oxidative and nitrosative stress in primary biliary cirrhosis. World J Gastroenterol. 2014;20(19):5746–59.

19

Symptom or faecal immunochemical test based referral criteria for colorectal cancer detection in symptomatic patients: a diagnostic tests study

Jesús-Miguel Herrero[1,2], Pablo Vega[1,2], María Salve[1,2], Luis Bujanda[3] and Joaquín Cubiella[1,2]*

Abstract

Background: Symptom based referral criteria for colorectal cancer (CRC) detection are the cornerstone of the strategy to improve prognosis in CRC. In 2017, the National Institute for Health and Care Excellence (NICE) updated their referral criteria (2017 NG12). Recently, several studies have evaluated the faecal haemoglobin (f-Hb) concentration in this setting. The aim of this study is to evaluate the diagnostic accuracy of the 2017 NG12 referral criteria and to compare them with the *CG27 referral criteria,* the f-Hb concentration and two f-Hb based prediction model: COLONPREDICT and FAST Score.

Methods: This is a post-hoc diagnostic test study performed within the COLONPREDICT study database (1572 patients, CRC prevalence 13.6%). We assessed symptoms, the 2017 NG12 and CG27 referral criteria and determined the f-Hb before performing a colonoscopy. We compared the discriminatory ability using the area under the curve (AUC) and the sensitivity and specificity at pre-stablished thresholds with the McNemar's test.

Results: The 2017 NG12 referral criteria discriminatory ability (AUC 0.53; 95% confidence interval- CI 0.49–0.57) was inferior to the CG27 version (AUC 0.59; 95% CI 0.55–0.63; $p = 0.01$), the f-Hb concentration (AUC 0.86; 95% CI 0.84–0-89; $p < 0.001$), the COLONPREDICT Score (AUC 0.92; 95% CI 0.91–0.94; $p < 0.001$) or the FAST Score (AUC 0.87; 95% CI 0.85–0.89; $p < 0.001$). The number of patients meeting each criteria were as follows: 2017 NG12 and CG27 = 94.1% and 52.2%; f-Hb ≥20 and ≥ 10 µg/g faeces = 38.6 and 44.3%; COLONPREDICT Score ≥ 5.6 and ≥ 3.2 = 29.4 and 63.2% and FAST Score ≥ 4.50 and ≥ 2.12 = 37.1 and 87.0%. The 2017 NG12 criteria were more sensitive (100%) than the CG27 criteria (68.2%), the f-Hb (≥20 µg/g) (91.2%), the f-Hb (≥10 µg/g) (93.5%), the COLONPREDICT Score (≥5.6) (90.1%) and the FAST Score (≥4.50) (89.8%) ($p ≤ 0.001$) and equivalent to the COLONPREDICT Score (≥3.5) (99.5%) or the FAST Score (≥2.12) (100.0%) ($p = 1$). However, their specificity (6.8%) was significantly lower than any of the evaluated criteria (50.3%, 69.6%, 63.4%, 78.7%, 45.8%, 71.3%, 13.9%; $p < 0.001$).

Conclusion: Referral criteria based on f-Hb measurement, either as a single test or within prediction models, are more accurate than symptom-based referral criteria for CRC detection in symptomatic patients.

Keywords: Colorectal cancer, Faecal immunochemical test, Diagnostic accuracy, Risk stratification

* Correspondence: joaquin.cubiella.fernandez@sergas.es
[1]Department of Gastroenterology, Complexo Hospitalario Universitario de Ourense, Ourense, Spain
[2]Instituto de Investigación Biomédica Galicia Sur, Centro de Investigación Biomédica en Red de Enfermedades Hepáticas y Digestivas (CIBERehd),, Ourense, Spain
Full list of author information is available at the end of the article

Background

Colorectal cancer (CRC) is the third most common cancer worldwide and the second leading cause of cancer-related death [1]. Two strategies are widely used to detect the disease at an early stage and, thus, improve the prognosis: CRC screening and early diagnosis strategies in symptomatic patients [2, 3]. Although screening programmes have been progressively implemented, most CRC are still detected when symptoms become apparent [4]. In addition, although gastrointestinal symptoms are extremely common in the population, the probability of CRC detection associated with any one symptom is low [5–7]. Thus, risk classification scores have been developed based on symptoms to determine which patients are most at risk of CRC with the aim of reducing this interval between the initial consultation and diagnostic colonoscopy [8, 9].

In this regard, one of the best known referral criteria for CRC detection are the National Institute for Health and Care Excellence (NICE) referral guideline for suspected cancer (CG27) [3]. This referral system has been extensively evaluated showing a low specificity and a variable sensitivity for CRC detection [6, 10–12]. In order to improve these results, the updated version of 2015 (NG12) introduced two significant changes. First, they recommended referral for those symptoms with a positive predictive value of 3% instead of previous 5%. Second, for the first time, testing for occult blood in faeces was recommended in several symptom scenarios with a positive predictive value below 3% [13]. However, the guideline did not recommend any particular method to determine occult blood in faeces.

Faecal immunochemical tests for haemoglobin (FIT) allow for quantitation of faecal haemoglobin concentration (f-Hb). FIT has proven to be the best currently available non-invasive test for CRC screening in asymptomatic individuals and an excellent test for rule-in of CRC and rule-out of significant colonic lesions (SCL) in patients presenting with lower gastrointestinal symptoms [14–21]. On the basis of the available evidence [22], the NICE diagnostic guidance (DG30) recommends the use of FIT with a 10 μg Hb/g faeces to guide referral for colorectal cancer in primary care [23]. However, the effect of the NG12 is not well understood and only one study has evaluated the diagnostic accuracy of this guidance [24]. In July 2017, NG 12 was amended and testing for occult blood in faeces was recommended in patients without rectal bleeding but with unexplained symptoms that do not meet the criteria for a suspected cancer pathway [13].

We have recently developed and validated two f-Hb based prediction models for CRC detection: COLON-PREDICT and FAST. The database of the COLONPRE-DICT Score derivation cohort [25, 26]. is an excellent platform to compare the most widely symptom based referral criteria with the f-Hb concentration based strategies. In this database, an extensive collection of information regarding symptoms as well as several blood and faecal determinations are included. This information allowed us to perform a post hoc analysis in order to evaluate the diagnostic accuracy of the 2017 NG12, compare these criteria with the CG27, the f-Hb concentration and two CRC prediction models based on the f-Hb concentration: COLONPREDICT and FAST Scores [25, 26].

Methods

Study design

The current study is a post hoc analysis performed within the COLONPREDICT study: a multicentre, cross-sectional, blinded study of diagnostic tests. The study aimed to create and validate a CRC prediction index based on available biomarkers, clinical and demographical data. We performed this post hoc analysis in the 1572 patients included in the derivation previously described [25].

Brief description of the COLONPREDICT study

The details of the study have been described extensively elsewhere and are summarized here [25, 26]. We used the Colonoscopy Research into Symptom Prediction questionnaire (CRISP) to record symptoms and demographic data [27]. Based on this questionnaire, they determined if patients met the CG27 referral criteria for CRC detection [3]. f-Hb concentration was assessed using the automated OC-SENSOR MICRO analyser (Eiken Chemical Co., Ltd., Tokyo, Japan). The faeces for the f-Hb determination were collected using the OC-Sensor probe. Moreover, we determined blood haemoglobin (b-Hb) and mean corpuscular volume with a Beckman Coulter Autoanalyzer (Beckman Coulter Inc., CA, USA). Colonoscopy was performed blind for the questionnaire and analytical results.

2017 NG12 referral criteria and the f-Hb based prediction models calculation

On the basis of the information obtained from the CRISP questionnaire and the analysis performed (f-Hb, b-Hb and mean corpuscular volume), we determined which of the 2017 NG12 criteria for CRC suspicion were met. Two researchers (JMH and JC) independently decided the equivalence between each NICE criteria and the information collected. Finally, they reached a consensus version. NG12 referral criteria are shown in Table 1 [13]. We considered a positive faecal occult blood test if the f-Hb concentration was ≥10 μg Hb/g faeces.

COLONPREDICT score is a CRC prediction model based on a multivariable logistic regression analysis [25]. The COLONPREDICT score is based in eleven variables and the mathematical formula is as follows: 0.789 x

Table 1 Criteria to refer people using a suspected cancer pathway referral for CRC according to the NG12 referral criteria. The number of patients meeting each of the referral criteria is shown

Criteria	Number of patients (n = 1572)
Patients ≥40 years with unexplained weight loss and abdominal pain	196 (12.5%)
Patients ≥50 years with unexplained rectal bleeding	811 (51.6%)
Patients ≥60 years with: iron–deficiency anaemia or changes in their bowel habit	890 (56.7%)
Patients with a rectal or abdominal mass	80 (5.1%)
Adults < 50 years with rectal bleeding and any of the following unexplained symptoms or findings: abdominal pain, change in bowel habit, weight loss or iron-deficiency anaemia.	124 (7.9%)
Offer testing for occult blood in faeces to assess for colorectal cancer in adults without rectal bleeding who but with unexplained symptoms that do not meet the criteria for a suspected cancer pathway referral A positive test for occult blood in faeces was considered if the haemoglobin concentration was ≥10 µg Hb/g faeces.	78 (4.9%)
Any of the referral criteria	1479 (94.1%)

rectal bleeding + 0.536 x change in bowel habit + 2.694 x rectal mass – 1.283 x benign anorectal lesions + 2.831 x f-Hb ≥20 µg Hb/g faeces + 1.561 x b-Hb (< 10 g/dL) + 0.588 x b-Hb (10–12 g/dL) + 1.511 x CEA ≥3 ng/mL + 0.040 x age (years) + 0.813 x sex (male) -2.073 x previous colonoscopy (last 10 years) -0.849 x continuous treatment with aspirin. It shows a high diagnostic accuracy for CRC detection. Two thresholds have been defined with 90% and 99% sensitivity for CRC: 5.6 and 3.5.

FAST Score is a CRC prediction model based on a multivariable logistic regression analysis [26]. The FAST score is based on three variables and the mathematical formula is as follows: 0 x f-Hb (0) µg Hb/g faeces 0.684 x f-Hb (1, 19) + 2.824 x f-Hb (20, 200) µg Hb/g faeces + 4.184 x f-Hb ≥200 µg Hb/g faeces + 0.031 x age (years) + 0.479 x sex (male). Two thresholds have been defined with 90% and 99% sensitivity for CRC: 4.50 and 2.12.

Outcomes

The main outcome was CRC detection. According to previous studies evaluating FIT in symptomatic patients, [14–21] we considered significant colonic lesion (SCL) detection as the secondary outcome. We defined SCL as CRC, advanced adenoma (≥10 mm, villous histology, high-grade dysplasia), polyposis (> 10 polyps of any histology, including serrated lesions), histologically confirmed colitis (any aetiology), polyps ≥10 mm, complicated diverticular disease (diverticulitis, bleeding), colonic ulcer and/or bleeding angiodysplasia.

Statistical analysis

First, we performed a descriptive analysis of the population included in the study. In order to determine differences in diagnostic accuracy between the NG12 referral criteria and the rest of diagnostic criteria, the CG27 referral criteria, the f-Hb concentration, the COLONPREDICT and the FAST score we performed two analysis. First, we determined the number of individuals with a positive result and the sensitivity and the specificity for CRC and SCL detection. We determined if the differences between the sensitivity and the specificity of the NG12 referral criteria and the rest of diagnostic criteria, CG27 referral criteria, the COLONPREDICT and the FAST scores at the pre-stablished thresholds and the f-Hb at a 10 and 20 µg Hb/g faeces concentration threshold, were statistically significant using the McNemar's test. Finally, we also calculated the positive and negative predictive value (PPV, NPV), the positive and negative likelihood ratios (LR) and the diagnostic Odds Ratio (OR) of all the diagnostic tests. Diagnostic OR is defined as the odds of positivity in subjects with disease relative to the odds in subjects without disease.

In a second step, we evaluated the discriminatory ability using receiver-operating characteristic (ROC) curves for CRC and SCL diagnosis, and we calculated the area under the curve (AUC). We determined whether there were statistically significant differences using the chi-square test of homogeneity of areas. Additionally, we determined if there were differences in the discriminatory ability of each of the diagnostic criteria according to the healthcare level referring the patient to colonoscopy. Primary healthcare referral was determined when a general practitioner was requesting the colonoscopy and secondary healthcare referral was determined when a specialist (gastroenterologist, surgeon..) was requesting the exploration.

We report differences with 95% confidence intervals (CI) and their significance. We consider a p-value < 0.05 statistically significant. We carried out the analyses using the IBM SPSS Statistics for Windows version 21.0 (IBM Corp, Armonk, USA) and EPIDAT 3.1 (Dirección Xeral de Saúde Pública, Santiago de Compostela, Spain).

Results

Description of the cohort

Among the 1572 patients included in the derivation cohort of the COLONPREDICT, a CRC was detected in 214 (13.6%) patients and a SCL in 463 (29.5%) patients: advanced adenomas in 251 (16.0%), a polyp ≥10 mm with non-adenoma histology in 6 (0.4%), colitis in 36 (2.3%) and other SCLs in 6 (0.4%) patients. Direct referrals from primary care to endoscopic evaluation accounted for 22.9% of the patients included.

As we show in the Table 1, 1,479 out of the 1572 (94.1%) met at least one of the 2017 NG12 referral criteria. In contrast, 52.2% of the patients met any of the CG27 referral criteria, 38.7% had a f-Hb concentration ≥ 20 μg Hb/g faeces, 44.4% had a f-Hb concentration ≥ 10 μg Hb/g faeces, 30.9% had a COLONPREDICT Score ≥ 5.6, 60.5% had a COLONPREDICT Score ≥ 3.5, 37.1% had a FAST Score ≥ 4.50 and 88.0% had a FAST Score ≥ 2.12.

Analysis of the diagnostic accuracy
The sensitivity of the 2017 NG12 referral criteria for CRC detection reaches 100% at the expense of a low specificity (6.8%). As we show in the Table 2, the sensitivity of the 2017 NG12 referral criteria is superior to the sensitivity of the CG27 referral criteria, the f-Hb (≥20 μg Hb/g and ≥ 10 μg Hb/g faeces), the COLONPREDICT Score at a 5.6 threshold ($p < 0.001$) and the FAST Score at a 4.50 threshold. In contrast, the sensitivity is similar to the COLONPREDICT Score at a 3.2 threshold and the FAST Score at a 2.12 threshold ($p = 1$) and the specificity is inferior to any of the other criteria ($p < 0.001$). The rest of the diagnostic accuracy analysis is displayed in Table 2.

On the other hand, 2017 NG12 referral criteria allows the diagnosis of 98.9% of SCL. As in the diagnostic accuracy for CRC detection, the specificity is extremely low (7.9%). As we show in the Table 3, the sensitivity of the 2017 NG12 referral criteria is similar to the FAST Score at a 2.12 threshold (p = 1) and superior the rest of the evaluated criteria. In contrast, the specificity of the 2017 NG12 criteria is inferior to any of the additional criteria evaluated (p < 0.001). We show the PPV, NPV, positive and negative LR and the diagnostic OR in Table 2.

Analysis of the discriminatory ability
The analysis of the discriminatory ability for CRC detection of the NICE referral criteria, the f-Hb concentration, the COLONPREDICT and the FAST Score is shown in Fig. 1. The discriminatory ability of the 2017 NG12 referral criteria is inferior to any of the evaluated criteria in the Chi-square homogeneity test comparison of AUC. Additionally, we found no differences in the performance of each diagnostic test in the evaluation of the discriminatory ability according to the healthcare referring the patient to colonoscopy: 2017 NG12 referral criteria (primary = 0.53, 95% CI 0.46–0.60; secondary = 0.53, 95% CI 0.48–0.58; p = 0.1), CG27 referral criteria (primary = 0.60, 95% CI 0.54–0.66; secondary = 0.59, 95% CI 0.55–0.63; p = 0.7), f-Hb concentration (primary = 0.85, 95% CI 0.80–0.89; secondary = 0.86, 95% CI 0.83–0.89; p = 0.5), COLONPREDICT Score (primary = 0.90, 95% CI 0.86–0.94; secondary = 0.93, 95% CI 0.91–0.95; p = 0.1), FAST Score (primary = 0.84, 95% CI 0.79–0.89;

secondary = 0.88, 95% CI 0.85–0.90; p = 0.1). Fig. 2 shows the discriminatory ability for SCL detection of the diagnostic tests evaluated. The discriminatory ability of the 2017 NG12 referral criteria is similar to the CG27 referral criteria and inferior to the rest of the evaluated criteria in the Chi-square homogeneity test comparison of AUC.

Discussion
Summary
We have evaluated the diagnostic accuracy of the 2017 NG12 referral criteria for suspected CRC. As we clearly show, these updated criteria are more sensitive than CG27 version. However, they produce a marked increase in the number of patients meeting them and a reduction in the specificity. Furthermore, we had the opportunity to compare them with the f-Hb concentration and two f-Hb based prediction model. As we clearly show, both diagnostic tools have a higher discriminatory ability than the NICE referral criteria.

Strengths and limitations
We have used a wide cohort of consecutive patients referred to colonoscopy due to gastrointestinal symptoms. Patients were evaluated homogenously using a symptom questionnaire and several analytics, including a FIT, were performed before colonoscopy. This questionnaire allowed us to gather all the details regarding type of symptoms, duration and evolution. Thus, we could evaluate the 2017 NG12 referral criteria for suspected CRC for the first time. Furthermore, we have been able to evaluate the use of FIT, with the 10 μg Hb/g faeces, as recommended in the DG30 [23]. On the other hand, our study has several limitations that must be taken in consideration. We cannot exclude a risk of bias of selection, as long as the symptomatic patients included in the study were previously selected for colonoscopy evaluation. However, we have included all consecutive patients referred both from primary and secondary healthcare to colonoscopy.

Comparison with existing literature
The update of the NICE referral criteria is based on reducing the PPV threshold required to refer patients from primary care using a suspected cancer pathway referral. The guideline development group agreed to use a threshold value of 3% PPV to underpin their recommendations [13]. So, those patients with symptoms (i.e ≥ 40 years with unexplained weight loss) with a PPV > 3% for CRC should be referred for further testing. Our results clearly demonstrate that this strategy increases the sensitivity for CRC detection in comparison with previous criteria. However, these criteria certainly introduce a risk of over investigation. In fact, what our analysis

Table 2 Evaluation of the diagnostic accuracy of the evaluated strategies for colorectal cancer detection

	Sensitivity[1]	P[2]	Specificity[1]	P[3]	Positive PV[1]	Negative PV[1]	Positive LR[4]	Negative LR[4]	Diagnostic OR[4]
2017 NG12 referral criteria (n = 1479)	100% (97.8–100.0)		6.8% (5.6–8.4)		14.5% (12.8–16.5)	100% (95.0–100.0)	1.07 (1.06–1.09)	NE	NE
CG27 referral criteria (n = 821)	68.2% (61.5–74.3)	p < 0.001	50.3% (47.6–53.0)	p < 0.001	17.8% (15.3–20.6)	91.0% (89.0–93.0)	1.4 (1.2–1.5)	0.6 (0.5–0.8)	2.2 (1.6–2.9)
f-Hb ≥ 20 μg Hb/g faeces (n = 607)	91.2% (86.3–94.4)	p < 0.001	69.6% (67.1–72.0)	p < 0.001	32.3% (28.6–36.2)	98.0% (96.9–98.8)	3.0 (2.7–3.3)	0.1 (0.08–0.2)	23.6 (14.5–38.3)
f-Hb ≥ 10 μg Hb/g faeces (n = 696)	93.5% (89.1–96.3)	p = 0.001	63.4% (60.7–66.0)	p < 0.001	28.9% (25.6–32.4)	98.4 (97.2–99.1)	2.6 (2.4–2.8)	0.1 (0.06–0.2)	24.8 (14.3–43.2)
COLONPREDICT Score ≥ 5.6 (n = 463)	90.1% (85.1–93.6)	p < 0.001	78.7% (76.4–80.9)	p < 0.001	40.7% (36.2–45.3)	98.0% (96.9–98.7)	4.2 (3.8–4.7)	0.1 (0.08–0.2)	33.8 (21.1–54.0)
COLONPREDICT Score ≥ 3.2 (n = 994)	99.5% (97.0–100.0)	1	45.8% (43.1–48.2)	p < 0.001	22.9% (20.3–25.8)	99.8% (98.9–100.0)	1.8 (1.7–1.9)	0.01 (0.0–0.07)	179 (25–1280)
FAST Score ≥ 4.50 (n = 583)	89.8% (84.7–93.3)	p < 0.001	71.3% (68.8–73.7)	p < 0.001	33.2% (29.4–37.2)	97.8% (96.6–98.6)	3.13 (2.84–3.44)	0.14 (0.10–0.21)	21.8 (13.8–34.4)
FAST Score ≥ 2.12 (n = 1383)	100.0% (97.8–100.0)	p = 1	13.9% (12.1–15.9)	p < 0.001	15.6% (13.7–17.6)	100% (97.5–100.0)	1.16 (1.14–1.19)	NE	NE

[1]Values are expressed as percentages and its 95% confidence interval

[2]Significance of the sensitivity differences when compared with the NG12 referral criteria in McNemar's test. Differences with p < 0.05 are considered statistically significant

[3]Significance of the specificity differences when compared with the NG12 referral criteria in McNemar's test. Differences with p < 0.05 are considered statistically significant

[4]Values are expressed as absolute numbers and its 95% confidence interval

PV, predictive value; LR, likelihood ratio; OR, odds ratio; f-Hb, faecal haemoglobin; NE, non evaluable

Table 3 Evaluation of the diagnostic accuracy of the evaluated strategies for significant colonic lesion detection

	Sensitivity[1]	P[2]	Specificity[1]	P[3]	Positive PV[1]	Negative PV[1]	Positive LR[4]	Negative LR[4]	Diagnostic OR[4]
2017 NG12 referral criteria (n = 1479)	98.9% (97.3–99.6)		7.9% (6.4–9.7)		30.9% (28.6–33.4)	94.6% (87.3–98.0)	1.07 (1.05–1.10)	0.14 (0.06–0.3)	7.9 (3.2–19.5)
CG27 referral criteria (n = 821)	58.3% (53.6–62.8)	p < 0.001	50.3% (47.3–53.3)	p < 0.001	32.9% (29.7–36.2)	74.3% (71.0–77.4)	1.17 (1.07–1.29)	0.83 (0.73–0.94)	1.4 (1.1–1.7)
f-Hb ≥ 20 µg Hb/g faeces (n = 607)	74.2% (70.0–78.1)	p < 0.001	76.1% (73.5–78.6)	p < 0.001	56.5% (52.4–60.5)	87.6% (85.3–89.6)	3.11 (2.76–3.50)	0.34 (0.29–0.40)	9.2 (7.1–11.8)
f-Hb ≥ 10 µg Hb/g faeces (n = 696)	79.4% (75.4–83.0)	p < 0.001	70.2% (67.4–72.9)	p < 0.001	52.7% (49.0–56.5)	89.1% (86.8–91.0)	2.67 (2.41–2.95)	0.29 (0.24–0.35)	9.1 (7.0–11.8)
COLONPREDICT Score ≥ 5.6 (n = 463)	64.2% (59.5–68.5)	p < 0.001	83.1% (80.7–85.2)	p < 0.001	61.4% (56.9–65.8)	84.7% (82.3–86.7)	3.79 (3.27–4.40)	0.43 (0.38–0.49)	8.8 (6.8–11.3)
COLONPREDICT Score ≥ 3.2 (n = 994)	88.7% (85.3–91.4)	p < 0.001	51.3% (48.3–54.3)	p < 0.001	43.3% (40.1–46.6)	91.5% (89.0–93.6)	1.82 (1.70–1.95)	0.22 (0.17–0.29)	8.3 (6.0–11.3)
FAST Score ≥ 4.50 (n = 583)	72.7% (68.4–76.7)	p < 0.001	77.8% (75.2–80.2)	p < 0.001	57.8% (53.7–61.9)	87.2% (84.9–89.2)	3.28 (2.90–3.71)	0.35 (0.30–0.41)	9.4 (7.3–12.0)
FAST Score ≥ 2.12 (n = 1383)	97.8% (95.9–98.9)	p = 1	16.1% (14.0–18.4)	p < 0.001	32.8% (30.3–35.3)	94.7% (90.2–97.3)	1.17 (1.13–1.2)	0.13 (0.07–0.25)	8.7 (4.5–16.5)

[1]Values are expressed as percentages and its 95% confidence interval
[2]Significance of the sensitivity differences when compared with the NG12 referral criteria in McNemar's test. Differences with p < 0.05 are considered statistically significant
[3]Significance of the specificity differences when compared with the NG12 referral criteria in McNemar's test. Differences with p < 0.05 are considered statistically significant
[4]Values are expressed as absolute numbers and its 95% confidence interval

PV, predictive value; LR, likelihood ratio; OR, odds ratio; f-Hb, faecal haemoglobin; NE, non evaluable

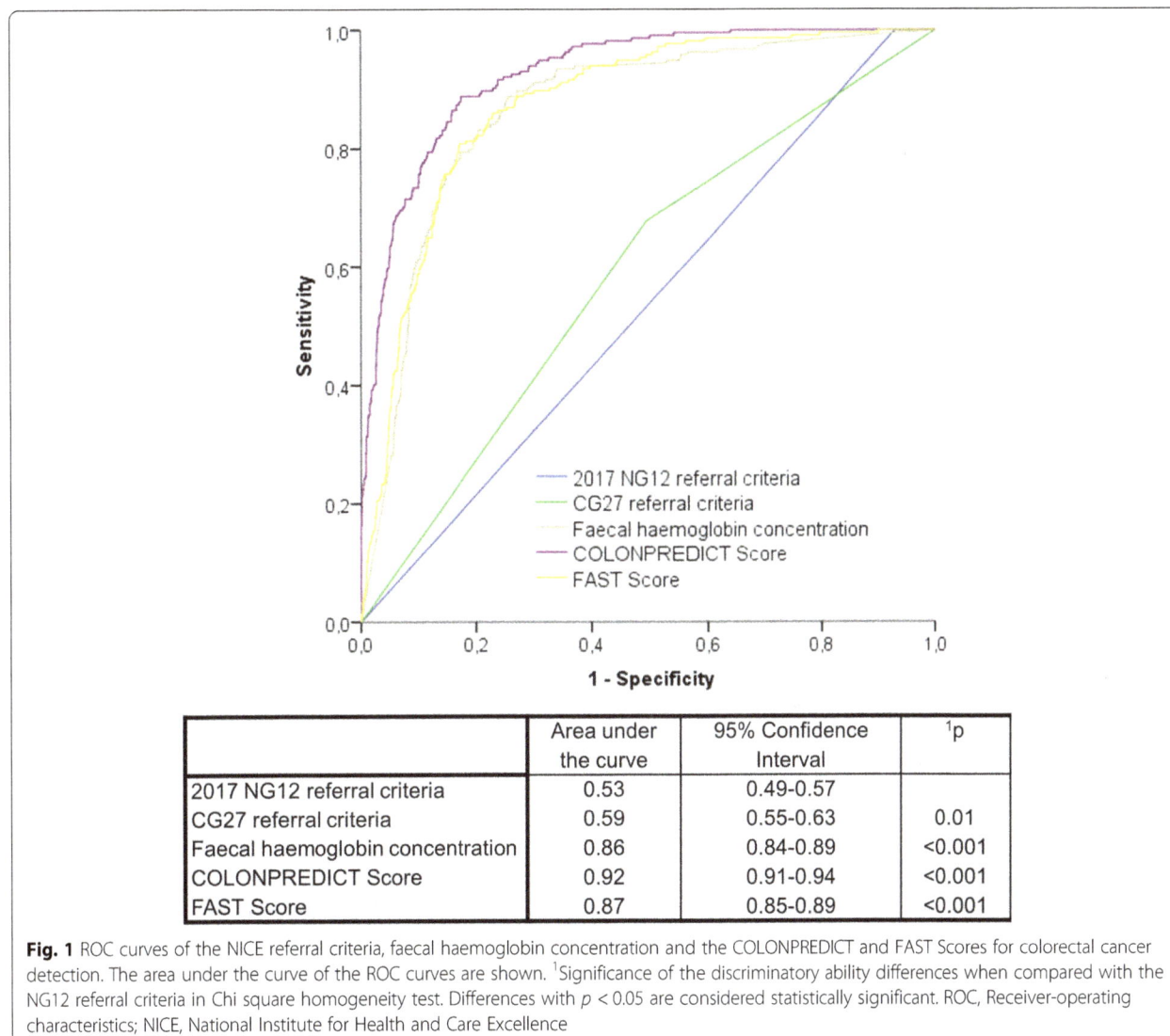

Fig. 1 ROC curves of the NICE referral criteria, faecal haemoglobin concentration and the COLONPREDICT and FAST Scores for colorectal cancer detection. The area under the curve of the ROC curves are shown. [1]Significance of the discriminatory ability differences when compared with the NG12 referral criteria in Chi square homogeneity test. Differences with $p < 0.05$ are considered statistically significant. ROC, Receiver-operating characteristics; NICE, National Institute for Health and Care Excellence

	Area under the curve	95% Confidence Interval	[1]p
2017 NG12 referral criteria	0.53	0.49-0.57	
CG27 referral criteria	0.59	0.55-0.63	0.01
Faecal haemoglobin concentration	0.86	0.84-0.89	<0.001
COLONPREDICT Score	0.92	0.91-0.94	<0.001
FAST Score	0.87	0.85-0.89	<0.001

confirms is that the discriminatory ability of any group of symptoms for CRC detection is suboptimal [6].

An additional innovation of the 2017 NG12 referral criteria is the inclusion of the faecal occult blood test in the evaluation of symptomatic patients. However, its use is only limited to patients without rectal bleeding and with unexplained symptoms that do not meet the criteria for a suspected cancer pathway referral [13]. Our results confirm the data previously published: the f-Hb concentration measured with a FIT shows a higher discriminatory ability for CRC detection than the NICE referral criteria [14–19]. So, probably, the strategy for the evaluation of the risk of CRC detection in symptomatic patients should be based on the f-Hb concentration irrespective of symptoms. Actually, in the COLONPREDICT Score, patients with a f-Hb concentration ≥ 20 μg Hb/g faeces have 17.0 times more risk of CRC detection. In contrast, patients with rectal bleeding or a change in

bowel habit have 2.2 and 1.7 times more risk of CRC detection, respectively [25].

Recently, an article has evaluated the diagnostic accuracy of the 2017 NG12 referral criteria for CRC and SCL detection and compared these criteria with the f-Hb concentration [24]. This study used the database of three diagnostic tests studies evaluating FIT in symptomatic patients [15, 17, 19]. and shows that the discriminatory ability of the 2017 NG12 referral criteria are inferior to the f-Hb concentration. This cohort has significant differences with ours: the prevalence of symptoms related to CRC diagnosis, rectal bleeding, changes in bowel habit, iron-deficiency anaemia or rectal mass, is inferior as well as the prevalence of CRC or SCL. Probably, these differences are responsible for the differences in the number of patients that meet 2017 NG12 referral criteria and in the inferior discriminatory ability documented in our study. However, are results are consistent

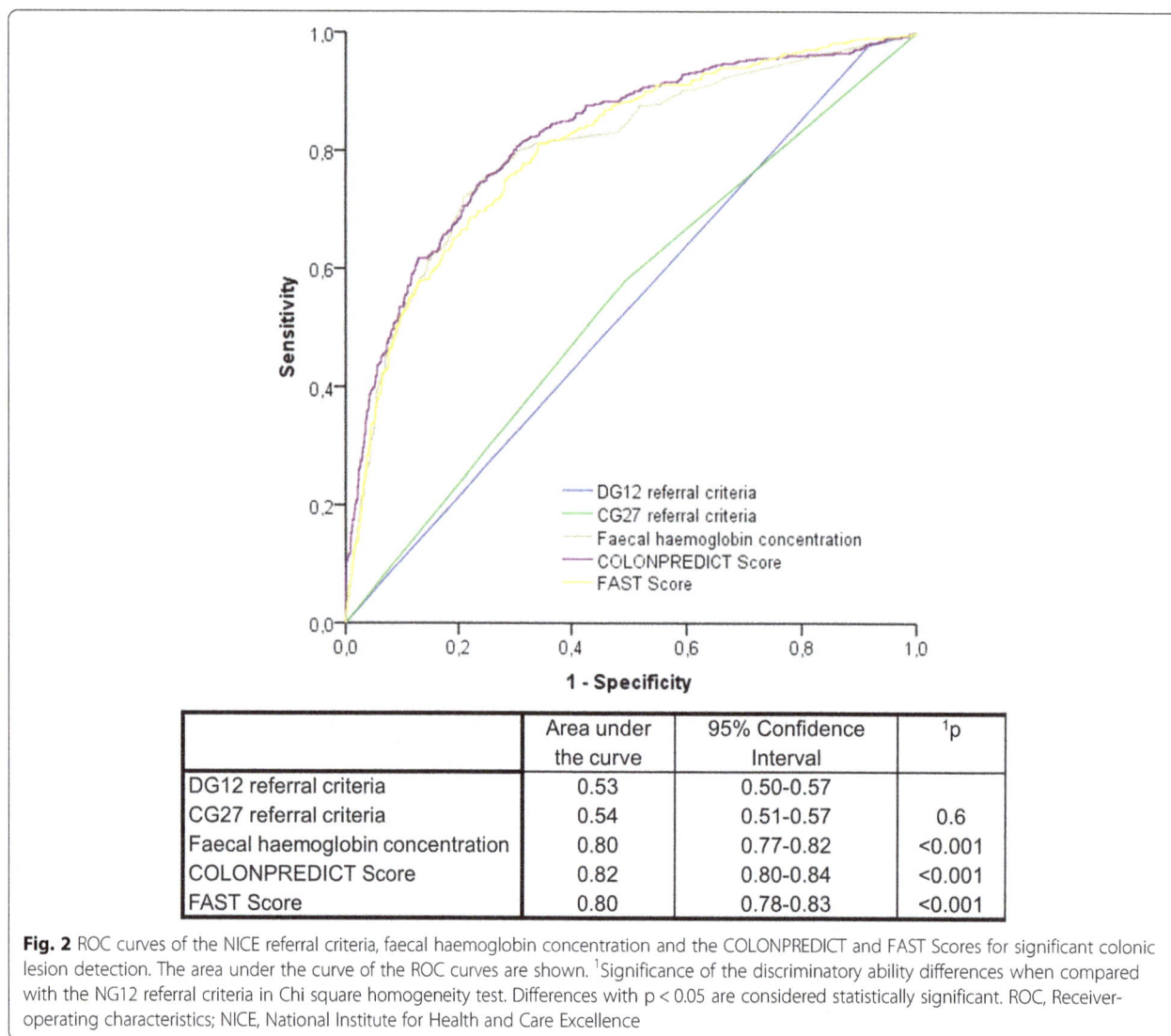

Fig. 2 ROC curves of the NICE referral criteria, faecal haemoglobin concentration and the COLONPREDICT and FAST Scores for significant colonic lesion detection. The area under the curve of the ROC curves are shown. [1]Significance of the discriminatory ability differences when compared with the NG12 referral criteria in Chi square homogeneity test. Differences with p < 0.05 are considered statistically significant. ROC, Receiver-operating characteristics; NICE, National Institute for Health and Care Excellence

in the comparison of the 2017 NG12 referral criteria with the f-Hb concentration.

Implications for research and/or practice

One of the main lessons learned in these years from the CRC screening programs is that lack of symptoms or the presence of non-specific symptoms do not exclude a CRC in adult population. Up to 20% of the incident CRC are detected in asymptomatic patients within a CRC screening program based in a guaiac faecal occult blood test [4]. So, the strategies for CRC detection in symptomatic patients should determine which patients require urgent referral, which require a normal referral and, finally, in what situations no additional evaluation is required. The NICE referral criteria only determine the scenarios where an urgent referral is required. Due to the increased discriminatory ability of the FIT for CRC, either the f-Hb concentration alone or a f-Hb

based prediction model can allow to establish these three risk groups with different diagnostic strategies. As we have recently proposed, at least 90% of CRC should be detected in a high-risk group, requiring a fast-track referral to colonoscopy. In contrast, in a low-risk group, where no additional explorations are required, the probability of a missing CRC should be well below 1%, so that the risk of CRC is balanced with the risk of colonoscopy complications, mainly perforation [28].

Conclusions

To conclude, the discriminatory ability of any symptom based criteria is limited when compared with a f-Hb concentration based strategy. An urgent evaluation of the diagnostic accuracy of FIT in symptomatic patients attending primary care is required.

Abbreviations

AUC: Area under the curve; CEA: Carcinoembryonic antigen; CI: Confidence interval; CRC: Colorectal cancer; CRISP: Colonoscopy Research into Symptom Prediction questionnaire; f-Hb: faecal haemoglobin; FIT: Faecal immunochemical test; LR: Likelihood ratio; NICE: National Institute for Health and Care Excellence; NPV: Negative predictive value; OR: Odds Ratio; PPV: Positive predictive value; ROC: Receiver-operating characteristic; SCL: Significant colonic lesion

Meeting presentations

This research was partially presented in the XIX Reunión Nacional de la Asociación Española de Gastroenterología held in Madrid 1-4th March, 2016.

Funding

This study was supported by a grant from Instituto de Salud Carlos III, Madrid, Spain (PI11/00094). Instituto de Salud Carlos III had no role in the study design; in the collection, analysis, and interpretation of data; in the writing of the report; or in the decision to submit the article for publication. JC has received an intensification grant through the European Commission funded "BIOCAPS" project (FP-7-REGPOT 2012–2013-1, Grant agreement no. FP7–316265).

Authors' contributions

The authors' contributions were as follows: JH and JC designed the analysis, PV, MS and LB collected the data, JH and JC performed the analysis and wrote the manuscript, and all the authors decided to submit the article for publication. All authors had full access to all of the data (including statistical reports and tables) in the study and can take responsibility for the integrity of the data and the accuracy of the data analysis. JC had full access to all of the data in the study and takes responsibility for the integrity of the data and the accuracy of the data analysis. All authors read and approved the final manuscript.

Competing interests

JC and MS had financial support from Instituto de Salud Carlos III for the submitted work but they had no financial relationships with any organisations that might have an interest in the submitted work in the previous five years, and no other relationships or activities that could appear to have influenced the submitted work. The remaining authors had no support from any organisation for the submitted work; no financial relationships with any organisations that might have an interest in the submitted work in the previous five years and no other relationships or activities that could appear to have influenced the submitted work.

Author details

[1]Department of Gastroenterology, Complexo Hospitalario Universitario de Ourense, Ourense, Spain. [2]Instituto de Investigación Biomédica Galicia Sur, Centro de Investigación Biomédica en Red de Enfermedades Hepáticas y Digestivas (CIBERehd),, Ourense, Spain. [3]Donostia Hospital, Biodonostia Institute, University of the Basque Country UPV/EHU, CIBERehd, San Sebastian, Spain.

References

1. Ferlay J, Shin HR, Bray F, Forman D, Mathers C, Parkin DM. Estimates of worldwide burden of cancer in 2008: GLOBOCAN 2008. Int J Cancer. 2010; 127:2893–917.
2. Zauber AG, Knudsen AB, Rutter CM, Lansdorp-Vogelaar I, Savarino JE, van Ballegooijen M, Kuntz KM. Cost-Effectiveness of CT Colonography to Screen for Colorectal Cancer. Technol. Assess. Rep. 2009:1–92. https://www.ncbi.nlm.nih.gov/pubmed/25834880.
3. NICE Clinical Guideline 27- Referral guidelines for suspected cancer. April 2011. www.nice.org.uk/CG027 [Internet]. 2011 [cited 2005 May 20]. Available from: www.nice.org.uk
4. Mansouri D, McMillan DC, Crearie C, Morrison DS, Crighton EM, Horgan PG. Temporal trends in mode, site and stage of presentation with the introduction of colorectal cancer screening: a decade of experience from the west of Scotland. Br J Cancer. 2015;113:556–61.
5. Ford AC. Veldhuyzen van Zanten SJO, Rodgers CC, Talley NJ, Vakil NB, Moayyedi P. diagnostic utility of alarm features for colorectal cancer: systematic review and meta-analysis. Gut. 2008;57:1545–53.
6. Jellema P, van der Windt DA, Bruinvels DJ, Mallen CD, van Weyenberg SJ, Mulder CJ, et al. Value of symptoms and additional diagnostic tests for colorectal cancer in primary care: systematic review and meta-analysis. BMJ. 2010;340:c1269.
7. Astin M, Griffin T, Neal RD, Rose P, Hamilton W. The diagnostic value of symptoms for colorectal cancer in primary care: a systematic review. Br J Gen Pract. 2011;61:e231–43.
8. Cotterchio M, Manno M, Klar N, McLaughlin J, Gallinger S. Colorectal screening is associated with reduced colorectal cancer risk: a case-control study within the population-based Ontario familial colorectal cancer registry. Cancer Causes Control. 2005;16:865–75.
9. Williams TGS, Cubiella J, Griffin SJ, Walter FM, Usher-Smith JA. Risk prediction models for colorectal cancer in people with symptoms: a systematic review. BMC Gastroenterol. 2016;16:63.
10. Zafar A, Mak T, Whinnie S, Chapman MA. The 2-week wait referral system does not improve 5-year colorectal cancer survival. Colorectal Dis. 2012;14: e177–80.
11. Rai S, Kelly MJ. Prioritization of colorectal referrals: a review of the 2-week wait referral system. Color Dis. 2007;9:195–202.
12. Thorne K, Hutchings HA, Elwyn G. The effects of the Two-Week Rule on NHS colorectal cancer diagnostic services: a systematic literature review. BMC Health Serv Res. 2006;6:43.
13. National Institute for Health and Clinical Excellence. Suspected cancer: recognitioin and referral [Internet]. NICE Guidel. 2017 [cited 2018 Mar 18]. Available from: https://www.nice.org.uk/guidance/ng12
14. Oono Y, Iriguchi Y, Doi Y, Tomino Y, Kishi D, Oda J, et al. A retrospective study of immunochemical fecal occult blood testing for colorectal cancer detection. Clin. Chim. Acta. 2010;411:802–5.
15. McDonald PJ, Digby J, Innes C, Strachan JA, Carey FA, Steele RJC, et al. Low faecal haemoglobin concentration potentially rules out significant colorectal disease. Colorectal Dis. [Internet]. 2013 [cited 2013 Jan 20];15:e151–e159.
16. Cubiella J, Salve M, Díaz-Ondina M, Vega P, Alves MT, Iglesias F, et al. Diagnostic accuracy of the faecal immunochemical test for colorectal cancer in symptomatic patients: comparison with NICE and SIGN referral criteria. Color Dis. 2014;16:O273–82.
17. Mowat C, Digby J, Strachan JA, Wilson R, Carey FA, Fraser CG, et al. Faecal haemoglobin and faecal calprotectin as indicators of bowel disease in patients presenting to primary care with bowel symptoms. Gut. 2016;65(9):1463–9.
18. Rodríguez-Alonso L, Rodríguez-Moranta F, Ruiz-Cerulla A, Lobatón T, Arajol C, Binefa G, et al. An urgent referral strategy for symptomatic patients with suspected colorectal cancer based on a quantitative immunochemical faecal occult blood test. Dig Liver Dis. 2015;47:797–804.
19. Godber IM, Todd LM, Fraser CG, MacDonald LR. Younes H ben. Use of a faecal immunochemical test for haemoglobin can aid in the investigation of patients with lower abdominal symptoms. Clin. Chem. Lab. Med. 2016;54:595–602.
20. Auge JM, Fraser CG, Rodriguez C, Lopez-Ceron M, Castells A, Roset A, et al. Clinical utility of one versus two faecal immunochemical test samples in the detection of advanced colorectal neoplasia in symptomatic patients. Clin Chem Lab Med. 2015;54:125–32.

21. Widlak MM, Thomas CL, Thomas MG, Tomkins C, Smith S, O'Connell N, et al. Diagnostic accuracy of faecal biomarkers in detecting colorectal cancer and adenoma in symptomatic patients. Aliment Pharmacol Ther. 2017;45:354–63.
22. Westwood M, Lang S, Armstrong N, van Turenhout S, Cubiella J, Stirk L, et al. Faecal immunochemical tests (FIT) can help to rule out colorectal cancer in patients presenting in primary care with lower abdominal symptoms: a systematic review conducted to inform new NICE DG30 diagnostic guidance. BMC Med. 2017;15:189.
23. Quantitative faecal immunochemical tests to guide referral for colorectal cancer in primary care [Internet]. [cited 2017 Mar 11]. Available from: https://www.nice.org.uk/guidance/dg30
24. Quyn AJ, Steele RJ, Digby J, Strachan JA, Mowat C, McDonald PJ, et al. Application of NICE guideline NG12 to the initial assessment of patients with lower gastrointestinal symptoms: not FIT for purpose? Ann Clin Biochem. 2017;0:4563217707981.
25. Cubiella J, Vega P, Salve M, Díaz-Ondina M, Alves MT, Quintero E, et al. Development and external validation of a faecal immunochemical test-based prediction model for colorectal cancer detection in symptomatic patients. BMC Med. 2016;14:128.
26. Cubiella J, Digby J, Rodríguez-Alonso L, Vega P, Salve M, Díaz-Ondina M, et al. The fecal hemoglobin concentration, age and sex test score: development and external validation of a simple prediction tool for colorectal cancer detection in symptomatic patients. Int. J. cancer [internet]. 2017;140:2201–2211.
27. Adelstein B-A, Irwig L, Macaskill P, Katelaris PH, Jones DB, Bokey L. A self administered reliable questionnaire to assess lower bowel symptoms. BMC Gastroenterol. 2008;8:8.
28. Rex DK, Schoenfeld PS, Cohen J, Pike IM, Adler DG, Fennerty MB, et al. Quality indicators for colonoscopy. Gastrointest Endosc. 2015;81:31–53.

20

A risk score system to timely manage treatment in Crohn's disease: a cohort study

Nadia Pallotta[1*], Giuseppina Vincoli[1], Patrizio Pezzotti[2], Maurizio Giovannone[3], Alessandro Gigliozzi[3], Danilo Badiali[1], Piero Vernia[1] and Enrico Stefano Corazziari[1]

Abstract

Background: Clinical severity and intestinal lesions of Crohn's disease (CD) usually progress over time and require a step up adjustment of the therapy either to prevent or to treat complications. The aim of the study was to develop a simple risk scoring system to assess in individual CD patients the risk of disease progression and the need for more intensive treatment and monitoring.

Methods: Prospective cohort study (January 2002–September 2014) including 160 CD patients (93 female, median age 31 years; disease behavior (B)1 25%, B2 55.6%, B3 19.4%; location (L)1 61%, L3 31.9%, L2 6%; L4 0.6%; perianal disease 28.8%) seen at 6–12-month interval. Median follow-up 7.9 years (IQR: 4.3–10.5 years). Poisson models were used to evaluate predictors, at each clinical assessment, of having the following outcomes at the subsequent clinical assessment a) use of steroids; b) start of azathioprine; c) start of anti-TNF-α drugs; d) need of surgery. For each outcome 32 variables, including demographic and clinical characteristics of patients and assessment of CD intestinal lesions and complications, were evaluated as potential predictors. The predictors included in the model were chosen by a backward selection. Risk scores were calculated taking for each predictor the integer part of the Poisson model parameter.

Results: Considering 1464 clinical assessments 12 independent risk factors were identified, CD lesions, age at diagnosis < 40 years, stricturing behavior (B2), specific intestinal symptoms, female gender, BMI < 21, CDAI> 50, presence of inflammatory markers, no previous surgery or presence of termino-terminal anastomosis, current use of corticosteroid, no corticosteroid at first flare-up. Six of these predicted steroids use (score 0–9), three to start azathioprine (score 0–4); three to start anti-TNF-α drugs (score 0–4); six need of surgery (score 0–11). The predicted percentage risk to be treated with surgery within one year since the referral assessment varied from 1 to 28%; with azathioprine from 3 to 13%; with anti-TNF-α drugs from 2 to 15%.

Conclusions: These scores may provide a useful clinical tool for clinicians in the prognostic assessment and treatment adjustment of Crohn's disease in any individual patient.

Keywords: Crohn's disease, Risk score system, Risk factors, small intestine contrast ultrasonography, Therapy, medical, surgical

* Correspondence: nadia.pallotta@uniroma1.it
[1]Dipartimento di Medicina Interna e Specialità Mediche, Università
"Sapienza", Policlinico "Umberto I", V.le del Policlinico, 155, 00161 Rome, Italy
Full list of author information is available at the end of the article

Background

Crohn's disease (CD) has a chronic course often characterized by progression toward increasing clinical severity. The outcome of treatments for Crohn's disease, including surgery, cannot be easily predicted since the available therapies achieve at best clinical and endoscopic remission (mucosal healing), without affecting the progressive course of the disease [1]. In addition, the course of CD varies considerably among patients making individual patient progression towards a complicated/disabling disease unpredictable. This has clinical management implications since complicated/disabling disease requires more intensive monitoring or treatment, including surgery.

Several independent predictors for complicated and severe CD have been so far identified across retrospective studies [2–4]. However, those predictors are diverse and not always consistent. Prospective studies assessing a risk prediction model are lacking. Although numerous techniques have been used to objectively describe disease activity and intestinal damage, no study has prospectively assessed the time-related change in severity of CD lesions nor the relative association of severity and progression of the disease. Small intestine contrast ultrasonography (SICUS) is a validated, standardized, radiation-free technique for assessment of small bowel CD lesions and associated complications [5–9]. The small amounts of oral contrast used and its simplicity make SICUS highly acceptable to patients, and well suited both for the follow-up of CD lesions and for the detection of complications.

Methods

Aim

The objective of this study was to develop a simple risk scoring system in order to quantify in individual patients the risk of disease progression and, among rapidly progressing CD patients, the indication for more intensive monitoring and for introducing changes in the treatment regimen in accordance with ECCO statements [10].

Study design

We prospectively monitored all CD patients referring to two tertiary GI centers (university hospital Policlinico Umberto I, Rome and San Camillo de Lellis's hospital, Rieti), from January 2002 to September 2014. Enrolled patients included both CD patients diagnosed prior to the study period and newly diagnosed patients in the participating hospitals during the study period.

The diagnosis of CD was based on Lennard-Jones criteria [9]. The disease characteristics at diagnosis were based on the Vienna and Montreal classifications [11]. Patients diagnosed and enrolled before 2005 were reclassified according to the Montreal classification.

All diagnosed patients then underwent complete clinical assessments at regular time intervals (6–12 months) that included both a physical examination and a clinical interview conducted by certified and experienced gastroenterologists (MG, AG, DB, PV, ESC) using a standardized clinical questionnaire. The following information was collected: symptoms, associated diseases, smoking status and load of cigarettes, family history, presence and number of surgical procedures, current treatment, BMI and Crohn's disease activity index (CDAI), endoscopic, radiological and imaging examinations. During each clinical assessment, laboratory exams and SICUS were also routinely performed. The following detailed records of aminosalicylate (sulphasalazine or mesalazine, 2–3 g daily), corticosteroid, and immunomodulatory therapies, were collected and included: timing of administration, dose, side-effects, end and/or change of prescription. Among patients who underwent intestinal resection, the type of anastomosis as well as the pathological findings of resection specimens and of section margins, were accurately reported.

Based on the results of the clinical assessments, the participating gastroenterologists modified the patients' treatments in accordance with the ECCO guidelines [10] using a step-up modality according to disease severity or complications. The need of additional investigations and the decision about surgery or start/change of a specific treatment class were independently decided by clinicians on clinical grounds.

Written informed consent was obtained from each subject and the study protocol was approved by the local committee of the Department of Clinical Science, University Hospital (Policlinico "Umberto I" viale del Policlinico 155, 00161 Roma, 6 December 2001).

Small intestine contrast US

SICUS was performed using Toshiba Tosbee (Tokyo, Japan) equipment with a 3.5 MHz convex and a 5 MHz linear array transducers. The apparatus can detect a bowel wall thickness variation of 0.1 mm. All SICUS examinations were performed by an experienced sonologist (NP), who had performed more than 10,000 SICUS examinations prior to the study. SICUS was performed after overnight fasting according to a previously published method [6] and CD lesions and complications were assessed in accordance with previously published studies [5–8, 12–14]. At the end of the US investigation, we reported on a standardized form: 1) the length of any intestinal lesion as the average of at least 3 measurements; the presence of, 2) stenoses, 3) fistulas, 4) abscesses, 5) mesenteric fat hypertrophy, 6) enlarged lymph nodes and spleen, 7) colonic-ileal reflux defined as the back flow of intestinal contents from colon to ileum through the ileo-cecal valve or the ileo-colonic anastomosis (ICA).

Statistical analysis

We developed a patient based model that considered all clinical assessments conducted and compared couples of consecutive clinical assessments on the basis of four outcomes: a) use of steroids; b) start of azathioprine; c) start of anti-TNF-α drugs; d) need of surgery. For each couple of clinical assessments, we defined the earlier visit as "referral visit".

Thirty-two baseline variables were evaluated as potential predictors for each of the aforementioned outcomes: gender, age at diagnosis (categorized as < 20 yrs., 20 yrs. to < 30 yrs., 30 yrs. to < 40 yrs., and ≥ 40 yrs), age at study enrollment, duration of the disease, location of the disease at diagnosis [small bowel only, i.e. ileal (L1) and isolated upper disease (L4), small bowel and colon (L3), colon only (L2)], disease behavior at diagnosis (B1 non-stricturing-non-penetrating, B2 stricturing, B3 penetrating), extraintestinal manifestations, presence/absence of perianal disease at diagnosis and at each clinical assessments, steroids required for the treatment of the first flare-up, smoking habits (at diagnosis and at each clinical assessments); family history for IBD, use of steroids, use of azathioprine, use of anti-TNF-α drugs, previous surgeries, extension of resected intestine, type of ileo-colonic anastomosis [i.e latero-lateral (L-L), termino-lateral (T-L), termino-terminal (T-T)], presence of specific intestinal symptoms, serological inflammatory markers (ESR, CRP), CDAI (< 50, 50–99, ≥ 100), body mass index (BMI) (< 22, 21–23, 23–25, > 25), and the following SICUS findings: site and extension of CD small bowel lesions, presence of stenosis, fistulas, abscesses, enlarged lymph nodes and spleen, mesenteric fat hypertrophy, presence of colon-ileal reflux.

The baseline variables "use of steroids", "use of azathioprine" and "use of anti-TNF-α drugs" were not assessed as potential predictors when "use of steroids", "start of azathioprine" and "start of anti-TNF-α drugs" were identified as outcomes. Descriptive analyses were initially performed to evaluate whether some of the aforementioned predictors needed to be grouped because of low frequency and/or because they consistently occurred together. Therefore, all patients that had undergone intestinal resection were classified combining type of ileo-colonic anastomosis and extension of intestine resected as follows: L-L/T-L and intestinal resection < 20 cm; T-T and intestinal resection < 20 cm; L-L/T-L and intestinal resection ≥ 20 cm; TT and intestinal resection ≥ 20 cm. Based on the presence/absence of CD lesions and CD complications at SICUS, the following five groups of patients were identified: 1) those without CD intestinal lesion or extending

≤ 0.5 cm and absence of CD complications; 2) those with CD intestinal lesion extension > 0.5 cm and < 20 cm and absence of CD complications; 3) those with CD intestinal lesion extension > 0.5 cm and < 20 cm and presence of at least one CD complication; 4) those with CD intestinal lesion extension ≥ 20 cm and absence of CD complications; 5) those with CD intestinal lesion extension ≥ 20 cm and presence of at least one CD complications.

Separate multiple Poisson models were used to evaluate the potential predictors of having, within the next clinical assessment, one of the previously described outcomes. For each couple of clinical assessments in the model, time between visits was considered as exposure time. For each outcome, the predictors included in the final model were selected using a backward selection excluding at each step the variable with the highest p-value > 0.15 (from log-likelihood ratio test) until only variables with an adjusted p-value < 0.15 remained. In each final model for the considered outcomes selected as described above, we further grouped some categories for the following predictors: age at diagnosis, CDAI (i.e., < 50, ≥ 50), BMI (i.e., < 21, 21–25, > 25), SICUS findings and surgical characteristics. This was done based on the similarities of the estimated parameters on the original categories. The standard errors of the multiple Poisson parameter models were adjusted for clinical assessment clustering within the same patient. Based on the final model for each outcome, risk scores were calculated taking for each predictor the integer part of each multiple Poisson model parameter [15] which is directly related to the probability of having the outcome within the next clinical assessment. The final score for each patient at each clinical assessment is the sum of each risk factor level. The probability of having any considered outcome was calculated for each month, and up to 12 months, after a referral visit for each score. We calculated this rate as follows: month rate = exp.(constant + score). A zero score therefore represents a patient at the lowest possible risk of having that outcome. For example, the 6-month risk of having an outcome was calculated as: [1 exp.(– 6*month rate)] and expressed as a percentage. Analogously, the 9-month risk was calculated as follows: [1 exp.(– 9*month rate)].

Model-predicted and observed outcomes (1 year after the referral visit) were then graphically compared.

Results

During a median follow-up period of 7.9 years (IQR: 4.3–10.5 years), 25 patients (female 11, median age 36 yrs.; disease behavior: 9 B1, 11 B2, 5 B3; disease location: 13 L1, 8 L3 2 L4, 2 L2) dropped out of study (nine moved to another town, 16 failed to present at follow-up); therefore 160 CD patients were included in the analysis for a total of 1464 assessments, being

10.5 months the minimum follow-up interval time. The main descriptive characteristics of patients at enrolment are shown in Table 1. At study enrolment, SICUS showed in 142 patients (88.8%) one or more small bowel CD lesions with a median extension of 25 cm (IQR 9–35 cm) and in 97 (60.6%) at least one CD complication. Nineteen patients (11.9%) developed complications during the follow-up period. The BMI and CDAI values measured during the study period are shown in Fig. 1. There were six deaths (two females) during the study period. Of those, three died due to renal failure and the remaining three, all on azathioprine therapy, died due to leukemia, multiple myeloma, and acute pancreatitis. After 7 years of azathioprine therapy, a female patient with terminal ileum CD, developed a Hodgkin lymphoma which was successfully treated, and subsequently a carcinoma on the ileal CD lesion.

Factors predictive of the need to use corticosteroids

Eighty nine patients (55.6%) (61 female, median age at diagnosis 30.1 years, IQR 21.2–38.1) required at least one cycle of corticosteroids. Six independent risk factors for the need of corticosteroid treatment within the next clinical assessment were identified (Table 2, section A), at SICUS evaluation the presence of 1) CD complications, 2) small bowel CD lesion > 20 cm in absence of CD complications, 3) the absence of colonic-ileal reflux; 4) age at diagnosis < 40 years; 5) stricturing (B2) behavior; 6) presence of specific intestinal symptoms. The integer risk score ranged from 0 to 9 points and observations were grouped according to the following scoring categories, 0–2, 3–4, 5–6 and 7–9. Figure 2a shows the predicted percentage risk of corticosteroids use up to 12 months after the referral visit for patients within different score groups. Figure 2b compares observed and model-predicted corticosteroid-use across the four risk groups according to the goodness-of-fit model.

Factors predictive of the need to start azathioprine

Sixty nine patients (43.1%) (45 female, median age at diagnosis 28.4 years, IQR 21.6–41.9) needed to start treatment with azathioprine. Three independent risk factors for the need to start azathioprine treatment within the next clinical assessment were identified (Table 2, section B), 1) female gender, 2) BMI value < 21, 3) CDAI > 50. The integer risk score ranged from 0 to 4 points and observations were grouped according to the following scoring categories, 0–1, 2 and 3–4, respectively. Figure 3a shows the predicted percentage risk to start azathioprine up to 12 months after the referral visit for patients within different score groups. Figure 3b compares observed and model-predicted start of azathioprine across the three risk groups according to the goodness-of-fit model.

Factors predictive of the need to start anti-TNF-α drugs

Fifty-seven patients (35.6%) (33 female, median age at diagnosis 29.4 years, IQR 22.5–40.3) needed to start anti-TNF-α drugs. Three independent factors for the need to start anti-TNF-α drugs treatment within the next clinical assessment were identified (Table 2 section C), at SICUS evaluation the presence of, 1) CD complications, and small bowel CD lesion > 20 cm in absence of CD complications, 2) presence of specific intestinal symptoms, and 3) positive inflammatory markers. The integer risk score ranged from 0 to 4 points and observations were grouped according to the following scoring categories: 0–1, 2 and 3–4, respectively. Figure 4a shows the predicted percentage risk to start anti-TNF-α drugs treatment up to 12 months after the referral visit for patients within different score groups. Figure 4b compares observed and model-predicted start of anti-TNF-α drugs across the three risk groups according to the goodness-of-fit model.

Factors predictive of the need of surgery

Fifty (31.2%) patients (28 female, median age at diagnosis 30 years, IQR 23.1–39.5), required surgical treatment on average 5 years from the diagnosis (IQR 1.6–9.9) and on average 16.1 months from the study enrolment (IQR 3.4–45.9). Six independent factors for the need of surgery within the next clinical assessment were identified (Table 2 section D): 1) the absence of previous surgery for CD or previous intestinal resection with termino-terminal ileo-colonic anastomosis; 2) the presence at SICUS evaluation of small bowel CD lesion length > 0.5 cm *plus* one or more complications; 3) the presence of specific intestinal symptoms; 4) no steroid requirement for treating the first flare-up of the disease; 5) the current use of corticosteroid; 6) positive inflammatory markers. The integer risk score ranged from 0 to 11 points and observations were grouped according to the following scoring categories: 0–6, 7–8 and 9–11, respectively. Figure 5a shows the predicted percentage risk of need of surgery up to 12 months after the referral visit for patients within different score groups. Figure 5b compares observed and model-predicted need of surgery across the three risk groups according to the goodness-of-fit model.

Discussion

Surgery, corticosteroids, immune-suppressants and anti-TNF-α drugs are often required in CD patients, but a significant proportion of them requires less aggressive, or no, treatment (4). Reliable predictors of short and long-term patient outcome would allow to individually

Table 1 Distribution of baseline characteristics of patients at diagnosis and at inclusion

		N	%	Median	IQR
Gender	Female	93	58.1		
Age at diagnosis				31	(22.8–42.6)
Age at study enrollment				40	(29.1–53.8)
Years from diagnosis to study enrollment				6.0	(1.3–11.3)
Smoker at diagnosis	Yes	91	56.9		
Smoker at study enrollment	Yes	74	46.2		
Family history	Yes	19	11.9		
Disease Behavior	B1	40	25.0		
	B2	89	55.6		
	B3	31	19.4		
Disease Location	L1	98	61.3		
	L2	10	6.3		
	L3	51	31.9		
	L4	1	0.6		
Steroids at first flare-up	Yes	50	31.2		
Perianal Disease at diagnosis	Yes	46	28.8		
Perianal Disease at study enrollment	Yes	15	9.4		
Previous surgery	Yes	53	33.1		
Number of surgery at study enrollment	1	34			
	≥ 2	19			
Extension of intestine resected [a] (cm)				30	(20–40)
Type of anastomosis[a]	L-L	28	52.8		
	T-L	11	20.8		
	T-T	10	18.9		
	Stoma	1	1.9		
Abdominal symptoms	Yes	71	44.4		
Serological inflammatory markers	Yes	94	58.8		
Extra-intestinal disease	Yes	27	16.9		
Use of azathioprine	Yes	29	18.1		
Use of corticosteroids at first flare-up	Yes	50	31.2		
Use of anti-TNF- α drugs	Yes	15	9.4		
SICUS FINDINGS					
• Site of CD lesion	No lesions	18	11.2		
	Ileal	142	88.8		
	ICA	0	0.0		
• Intestinal wall thickness (mm)				8	(5–10)
• Extension of CD lesion (cm)				25	(9–35)
• Presence of strictures	Yes	83	51.9		
• Presence of fistulas	Yes	29	18.1		
• Presence of abscesses	Yes	12	7.5		
• Presence of MFH	Yes	38	23.8		
• Presence of enlarged nodes	Yes	14	8.8		
• Presence of enlarged spleen	Yes	34	21.3		
BMI				22	(19.6–25.3)
CDAI				54	(24–96)

IQR: Interquartile range (i.e., the first value represents the 25th percentile and the 2nd one the 75th percentile of the distribution); [a]53 patients had a surgery before study enrollment and 50 among them had an intestinal resection

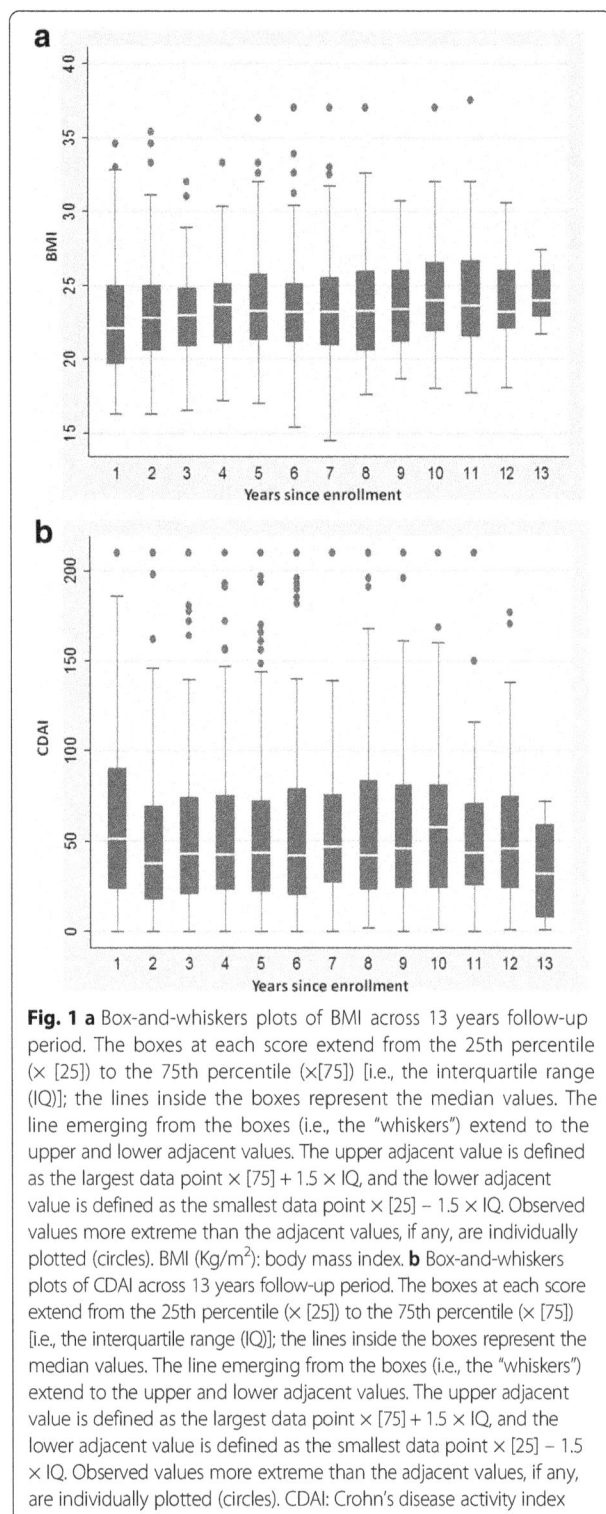

Fig. 1 a Box-and-whiskers plots of BMI across 13 years follow-up period. The boxes at each score extend from the 25th percentile (× [25]) to the 75th percentile (×[75]) [i.e., the interquartile range (IQ)]; the lines inside the boxes represent the median values. The line emerging from the boxes (i.e., the "whiskers") extend to the upper and lower adjacent values. The upper adjacent value is defined as the largest data point × [75] + 1.5 × IQ, and the lower adjacent value is defined as the smallest data point × [25] – 1.5 × IQ. Observed values more extreme than the adjacent values, if any, are individually plotted (circles). BMI (Kg/m²): body mass index. **b** Box-and-whiskers plots of CDAI across 13 years follow-up period. The boxes at each score extend from the 25th percentile (× [25]) to the 75th percentile (× [75]) [i.e., the interquartile range (IQ)]; the lines inside the boxes represent the median values. The line emerging from the boxes (i.e., the "whiskers") extend to the upper and lower adjacent values. The upper adjacent value is defined as the largest data point × [75] + 1.5 × IQ, and the lower adjacent value is defined as the smallest data point × [25] – 1.5 × IQ. Observed values more extreme than the adjacent values, if any, are individually plotted (circles). CDAI: Crohn's disease activity index

outcomes to assess the response to available treatments nor to quantify in a score model the predictive factors of severe disease. It is assumed that progressive bowel damage may, over time, result in the development of CD complications [1], nonetheless objective assessments of serial time-related disease modification and intestinal damage are lacking and it is not known whether the degree of bowel damage is an independent risk factor for disease progression. It has been recently shown that the Lémann index measures the cumulative bowel damage [16]. This index relies on high-quality abdominal MRI and radiology expertise, lacks, so far, of "gold standard" clinical references and is not applicable in clinical practice. To our knowledge, no prospectively estimated score indexes have been used to predict the CD clinical outcome, except the one proposed by Rutgeerts [17], based on endoscopic findings. In patients submitted to curative ileo-colon resection, SICUS is an accurate method for detecting early post-operative lesions and is comparable to the Rutgeerts score [12]. Differently from MRI, SICUS is based on a widely available technique not requiring costly and highly technological equipment and it has been proven to accurately assess CD small bowel intestinal lesions and complications both in adult and pediatric CD patients [6–9]. Of the 32 prospectively evaluated predictors, twelve independent predictors of the need of short-term treatment modification, including surgery, have been identified. In the present study, differently from previous studies assessing predictors of severe or disabling CD [2–4], the risk model has been converted into an integer score. This score can easily be translated in probability of the need of a short-term step-up therapeutic change. The most relevant result is that the predicted percentage of risk within 1 year was low across all the outcomes explored. In particular, the predicted risk of surgery varied from 1% (score 0–6) to 28% (score 9–11); that of starting azathioprine from 3% (score 0–1) to 13% (score 3–4); that of starting anti-TNF-α drugs from 2% (score 0–1) to 15% (score 3–4). These results are consistent with those reported by two studies, a large retrospective cohort [4] and a population-based study [18], showing that the probability of surgery and severity course of CD is overall low.

Bowel damage, as assessed by SICUS, is per se the most important predictor for any of the considered outcomes except for the need to start azathioprine. Age at diagnosis < 40 yrs is predictive for the use of corticosteroids and not for the other outcomes. A prior retrospective cohort study [2] found that younger age (< 40 yrs) at diagnosis was a predictive risk factor of disabling disease, alone or in association with steroids treatment for the first flare-up and presence at diagnosis of perianal disease. The different results

tailor therapy within a properly planned clinical follow-up. The outcome of any treatment of CD is determined by the clinical and pathological behavior and progression of the disease as well as by the response to treatment itself. However, in CD there are no unequivocal

Table 2 Adjusted incidence rate ratio (IRR) and score contribution of (A) use of corticosteroids, (B) start of azathioprine, (C) start of anti-TNF- α drugs, (D) need of surgery

	IRR	95% CI		p	score
A. Use of corticosteroids					
No or CD intestinal lesions < 20 cm and no complications (ref)	1				0
CD complications at SICUS	1.86	1.04	3.34	0.04	1
CD intestinal lesions > 20 cm and no complications at SICUS	3.38	1.80	6.35	< 0.01	3
Presence of colon-ileal reflux at SICUS (ref)	1				0
Absence of colon-ileal reflux at SICUS	1.54	1.00	2.37	0.05	1
Age at diagnosis ≥40 years (ref)	1				0
Age at diagnosis < 40 years	1.83	1.04	3.24	0.04	1
B1 or B3 disease behavior (ref)	1				0
B2 disease behavior	2.23	1.26	3.93	0.01	2
Absence of specific symptoms at clinical assessment (ref)	1				0
Presence of specific symptoms at clinical assessment	1.93	1.36	2.73	< 0.01	2
B. Start of azathioprine					
Male (ref)	1				0
Female	2.08	1.19	3.64	0.01	1
BMI > 25 (ref)	1				0
BMI < 21	4.10	1.95	8.61	< 0.01	2
BMI 21–25	2.13	1.04	4.33	0.04	1
CDAI < 50 (ref)	1				0
CDAI ≥50	1.82	1.13	2.90	0.013	1
C. Start of anti-TNF-α drugs					
Absence of CD intestinal lesions or complications at SICUS (ref)	1				0
CD intestinal lesions > 20 cm and no complications at SICUS	5.72	1.88	17.40	< 0.01	2
CD complications at SICUS	2.34	0.81	6.73	0.12	1
Negative markers of inflammation (ref)	1				0
Positive markers of inflammation	2.63	1.45	4.78	< 0.01	1
Absence of specific symptoms at clinical assessment (ref)	1				0
Presence of specific symptoms at clinical assessment	2.52	1.46	4.34	< 0.01	1
D. Need of surgery					
No previous surgery	6.40	2.01	20.31	< 0.01	2
Previous surgery and type of ileocolonic anastomosis (ICA)					
• latero-lateral ICA (ref)	1				0
• termino-terminal ICA	3.90	0.62	24.69	0.15	2
No or CD intestinal lesions and no complications (ref)	1				0
CD intestinal lesions > 0.5 cm and complications at SICUS	10.63	3.04	37.11	< 0.01	3
Corticosteroid at first flare (ref)	1				0
No corticosteroid at first flare	2.32	1.29	4.17	0.01	1
Absence of specific symptoms at clinical assessment (ref)	1				0
Presence of specific symptoms at clinical assessment	3.75	2.01	7.01	< 0.01	2
No current use of corticosteroid (ref)	1				0
Current use of corticosteroid	3.60	1.99	6.51	< 0.01	2
Negative markers of inflammation (ref)	1				0
Positive markers of inflammation	2.31	1.15	4.66	0.02	1

ICA: ileo-colonic anastomosis, IRR: incidence rate ratio
IRR and score estimates were obtained by Poisson models based on clinical assessment findings; models evaluated the occurrence of each specified outcome within the subsequent clinical assessment; 95% confidence intervals and p-values were calculated taking into account that clinical assessments were clustered within patient; selected predictors for each outcome were obtained starting from a multiple model including all the variables described in the method section and then excluding at each step that with the highest p-value > 0.15 (from log-likelihood ratio test). Final models include only predictors with a log-likelihood ratio test p < 0.15; IRR > 1 indicate an increased risk of having the specified outcome compared to the reference group

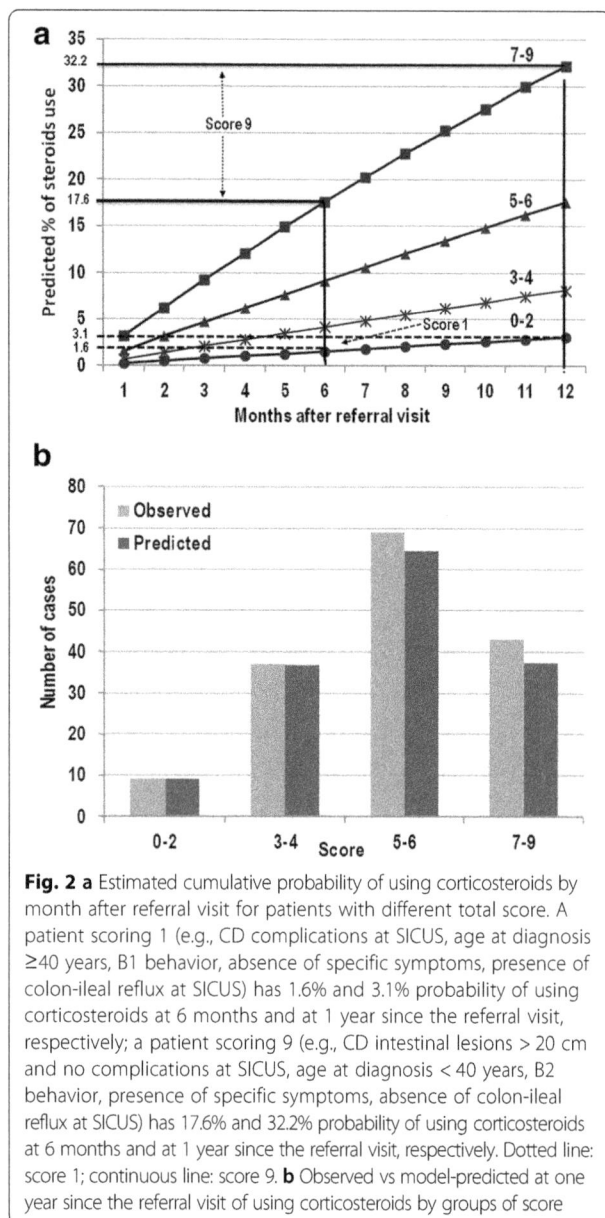

Fig. 2 a Estimated cumulative probability of using corticosteroids by month after referral visit for patients with different total score. A patient scoring 1 (e.g., CD complications at SICUS, age at diagnosis ≥40 years, B1 behavior, absence of specific symptoms, presence of colon-ileal reflux at SICUS) has 1.6% and 3.1% probability of using corticosteroids at 6 months and at 1 year since the referral visit, respectively; a patient scoring 9 (e.g., CD intestinal lesions > 20 cm and no complications at SICUS, age at diagnosis < 40 years, B2 behavior, presence of specific symptoms, absence of colon-ileal reflux at SICUS) has 17.6% and 32.2% probability of using corticosteroids at 6 months and at 1 year since the referral visit, respectively. Dotted line: score 1; continuous line: score 9. **b** Observed vs model-predicted at one year since the referral visit of using corticosteroids by groups of score

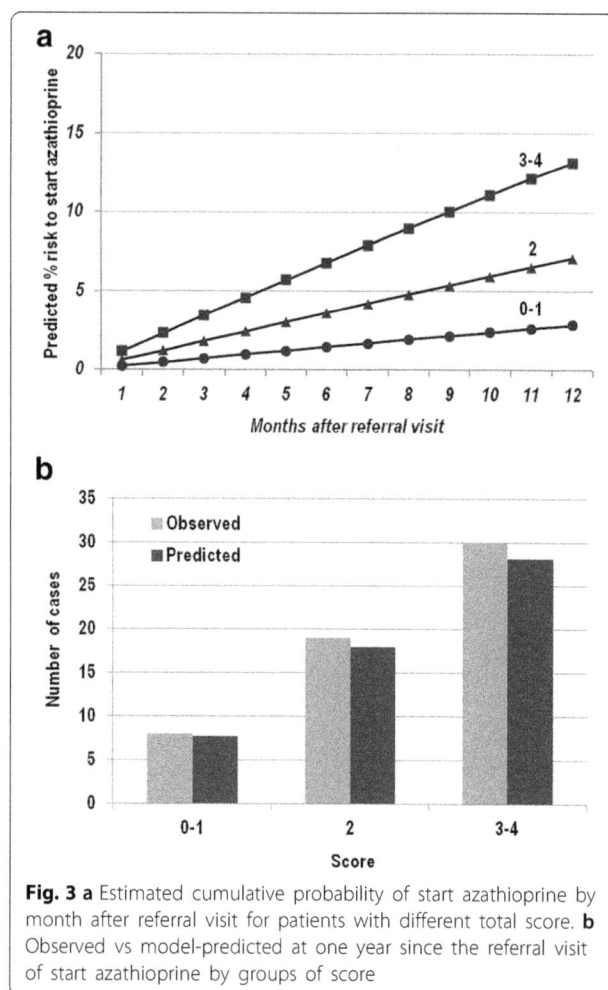

Fig. 3 a Estimated cumulative probability of start azathioprine by month after referral visit for patients with different total score. **b** Observed vs model-predicted at one year since the referral visit of start azathioprine by groups of score

of the present and Beaugerie et al. studies can be explained by the different short-term outcome (i.e., the need of therapeutic change or surgery within the next clinical assessment), the different number of predictors evaluated, 32 vs 9, and the exclusion in the present study of patients with childhood CD onset. Similarly to previous studies, we did not find an association between the short-term need of surgery and the use of azathioprine and anti-TNF-α drugs [19–23]. The association between the current use of corticosteroids and the need of surgery confirms the results of the Danish nationwide population-based cohort study [24]. The absence of previous surgery was associated with the need of surgery indicating that surgical removal of diseased bowel is followed by a favorable

short-term clinical outcome [25]. We did not find an association between the need of surgery and the early age of onset and long duration of the disease [26–28]. The analysis here performed was adjusted for the age at diagnosis and at enrollment, and for the duration of follow-up. At diagnosis more than two third of patients had stricturing and penetrating disease and one third perianal disease, ruling out an inclusion bias. Confirming a previous retrospective study [29], complicated disease at diagnosis had no predictive value for the need of surgery or step-up therapy except for the association of stricturing disease with the use of corticosteroids. The duration of the disease, the time interval between diagnosis and enrollment were not associated with the need to start azathioprine or anti-TFN-α drugs. The analyses were adjusted for the use of any other treatment. Female gender, CDAI > 50, and a low BMI concur in a score that predicts the start of azathioprine.

CD lesions of the upper gastrointestinal (GI) tract have been variably reported (28) to be associated with younger age at diagnosis, stricturing disease and two

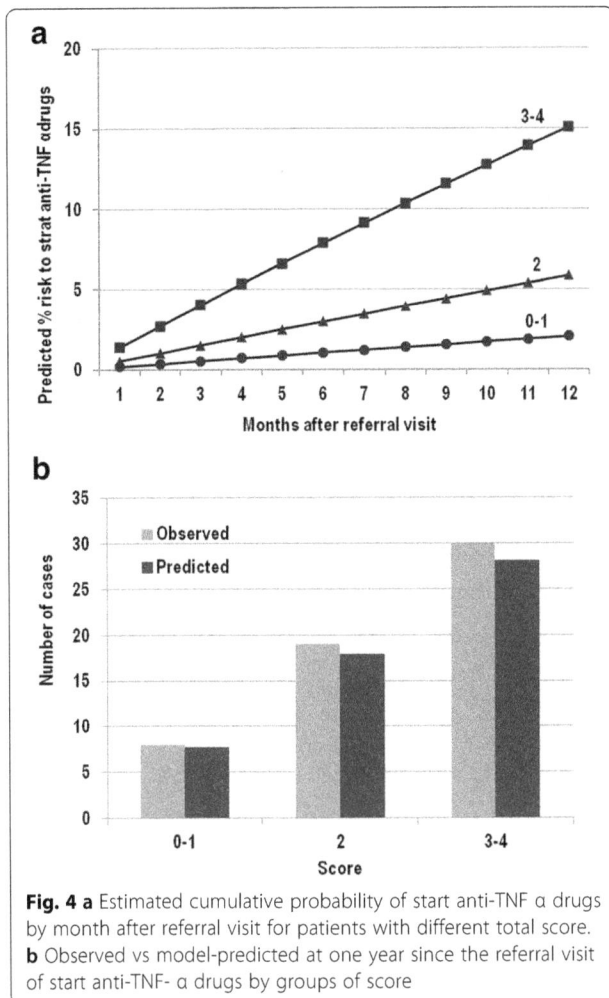

Fig. 4 a Estimated cumulative probability of start anti-TNF α drugs by month after referral visit for patients with different total score. **b** Observed vs model-predicted at one year since the referral visit of start anti-TNF- α drugs by groups of score

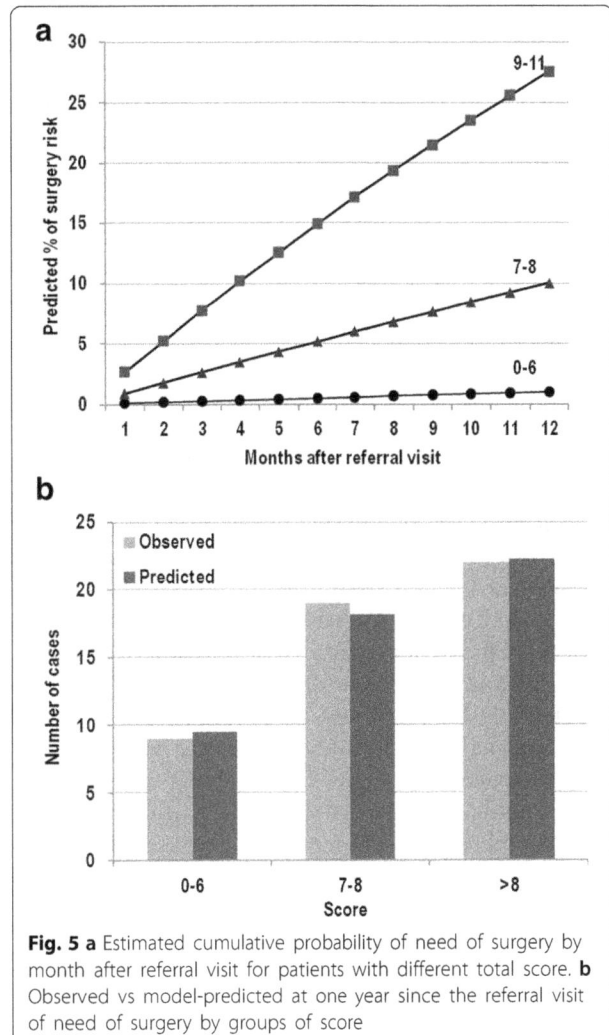

Fig. 5 a Estimated cumulative probability of need of surgery by month after referral visit for patients with different total score. **b** Observed vs model-predicted at one year since the referral visit of need of surgery by groups of score

or more abdominal surgeries. Due to the small number of patients with upper CD, as expected in adult CD patients, we did not evaluate separately the upper CD location as a predictive risk factor for any of the outcomes evaluated.

At multivariate analysis neither the extension of intestinal lesions at SICUS nor the length of intestine resected at surgery, adjusting for all potential confounding variables including immunosuppressive therapy and smoking habit, had an independent predictive effect on the need of surgical outcome. Conversely, the extension of the intestinal lesions evaluated at SICUS was independently associated with the short-term outcome to use steroids and to start anti-TNF-α drugs.

Similarly to population-based cohort and tertiary referral studies, we did not find an independent association between smoking status [29–32] and family history [33, 34] (defined on subject report) for IBD and the need of surgery or step-up treatment. The presence of family history for IBD was accurately assessed enquiring the patients repeatedly at each clinical assessment therefore

updating the new diagnoses occurring among relatives during the follow-up. The smoking behavior and the current number of cigarettes per day were assessed at each clinical assessment according to the threshold value previously published, avoiding recall bias [35].

Some drawbacks of the study need to be mentioned. This is a cohort study evaluating CD patients afferent to tertiary referral centers for IBD so they could not be representative of the patients population seen in a general gastroenterological setting. It is of note that, in our population at enrollment, one third of patients were previously submitted to one or more surgeries, one third had perianal disease and more than half had CD complications while patients with CD of the colon were a minority. The study was based on only 160 patients. As expressed by the 95% CIs estimated, for some predictors identified, the estimated effect on the evaluated outcomes presents a relatively large uncertainty even if the analysis was performed on 1464 assessments, thus increasing the statistical power [36]. Furthermore, due to the limited number of patients, we had to group some categories thus missing the possibility of detecting differences within those categories. Inflammatory markers (ESR and CRP) were considered as dichotomy variables not evaluating different cut-off value [37]. Lastly, we should consider that SICUS, as all ultrasound methods, is operator-dependent. It should be pointed out, however, that the score described in this study may be applied with any technique, including MRI, that allows to accurately assess the length of intestinal lesions and occurrence of CD complications.

The strength of the study is that patients were invited to outpatient clinic at regular time intervals, regardless of symptoms, thus minimizing the influence of follow-up duration in the development of severe course of CD and including in the analysis also asymptomatic patients. In addition, we enrolled in the study patients from 2002 when anti-TFN-α drugs became available and widely used in the hospitals of Lazio region, Italy. Thus the availability of drug treatments did not affect the proportion of patients that started azathioprine and anti-TNF-α drugs.

Differently from previous studies that rely mainly on data assessed retrospectively on clinical records or on mailed questionnaires, in this study at each clinical assessment all potential predictors of having, within the next clinical assessment, one of the considered outcomes were evaluated prospectively in a systematic way. Although the outcomes were arbitrarily chosen based on available therapeutic options and chosen on clinical grounds, it is of note that these choices were done by gastroenterologists with over 20 years experience in IBD in accordance with the diagnostic classification and treatment protocols of the ECCO consensus guidelines. The scores here proposed were based on the selection of some predictors by goodness of fit among 32 variables initially considered. Each predictor included contributes to the total score with a different weight based on the ability of that characteristic of predicting the outcome considered independently from all other predictors included. By assessing clinical factors, usually taken into consideration in the gastroenterological practice, this study has identified the main risk factors that make up four scores able to predict the four most relevant short-term clinical treatment strategy changes in the management of CD patients.

Conclusion

The four risk scores developed here, should be submitted to a future validation in a larger population and possibly in several centers. In conclusion, the identified scores provide a useful tool for clinicians allowing an objective prognostic assessment of individual patients with Crohn's disease, including an estimation of the need for treatment adjustment. Such timely awareness of the patient risk profile may be of value for physicians in determining the most appropriate management and treatment of patients with Crohn's disease.

Abbreviations
B1, B2, B3: Behavior 1,2,3; BMI: Body mass index; CD: Crohn's disease; CDAI: Crohn's disease activity index; CRP: C reactive protein; ESR: Erythrocyte sedimentation rate; IBD: Inflammatory bowel disease; ICA: Ileo-colonic anastomosis; IQR: Interquartile range; IRR: Incidence rate ratio; L1,L2,L3,L4: Location,1,2,3,4; MRI: Magnetic resonance imaging; PD: Perianal disease; SICUS: Small intestine contrast ultrasonography; TNF-α: Tumor necrosis factor-α

Acknowledgements
The authors wish to thank and acknowledge, Flavia Riccardo, MD PhD for editing the English and for her critical review.

Funding
Not applicable. No funding was received.

Public trial register
Not applicable.

Authors' contributions
NP and ESC contributed equally to this work; NP and ESC designed research; NP and GV acquired data and take the responsibility of the integrity of the data and the accuracy of the data analysis. ESC, NP, MG, AG, DB, PV recruited patients; PP, NP analyzed and interpreted the data. PP performed the statistical analysis; NP and ESC wrote the paper. All authors read and approved the final manuscript.

Competing interests
The authors declare that they have no competing interests.

Author details
[1]Dipartimento di Medicina Interna e Specialità Mediche, Università "Sapienza", Policlinico "Umberto I", V.le del Policlinico, 155, 00161 Rome, Italy. [2]Dipartimento di Malattie Infettive, Istituto Superiore di Sanità, Rome, Italy. [3]UOC di Gastroenterologia, Ospedale San Camillo De Lellis, Rieti, Italy.

References
1. Baumgart DC, Sandborn WJ. Crohn's disease. Lancet. 2012;380:1509–605.
2. Beaugerie L, Seksik P, Nion-Larmurier I, Gendre JP, Cosnes J. Predictors of Crohn's disease. Gastroenterology. 2006;130:650–6.
3. Loly C, Belaiche J, Louis E. Predictors of severe Crohn's disease. Scand J Gastroenterol. 2008;43:948–54.
4. Cosnes J, Bourrier A, Nion-Larmurier I, Sokol H, Beaugerie L, Seksik P. Factors affecting outcomes in Crohn's disease over 15 years. Gut. 2012;61:1140–5.
5. Pallotta N, Baccini F, Corazziari E. Ultrasonography of the small bowel after oral administration of anechoic contrast solution. Lancet. 1999;353:985–6.

6.   Pallotta N, Tomei E, Viscido A, Calabrese E, Marcheggiano A, Caprilli R, Corazziari E. Small intestine contrast ultrasonography: an alternative to radiology in the assessment of small bowel disease. Inflamm Bowel Dis. 2005;11:146–53.

7.   Parente F, Greco S, Molteni M, Cucino C, Maconi G, Sampietro GM, Danelli PG, Cristalli M, Bianco R, Gallus S, Bianchi Porro G. Role of the early ultrasound in detecting inflammatory intestinal disorders and identifying their anatomical location within the bowel. Aliment Pharmacol Ther. 2003; 18:1009–16.

8.   Pallotta N, Vincoli G, Montesani C, Chirletti P, Pronio A, Caronna R, Ciccantelli B, Romeo E, Marcheggiano A, Corazziari E. Small intestine contrast ultrasonography (SICUS) for the detection of small bowel complications in Crohn's disease: a prospective comparative study versus intraoperative findings. Inflamm Bowel Dis. 2012;18:74–84.

9.   Pallotta N, Civitelli F, Di Nardo G, Vincoli G, Aloi M, Viola F, Capocaccia P, Corazziari E, Cucchiara S. Small intestine contrast ultrasonography in pediatric Crohn's disease. J Pediatr. 2013;163:778–84.

10. Travis SPL, Stange EF, Lemann M, Oresland T, Chowers Y, Forbes A, D'Haens G, Kitis G, Cortot A, Prantera C, Marteau P, Colombel J-F, Gionchetti P, Bouhnik Y, Tiret E, Kroesen J, Starlinger M, Mortensen NJ, for the European Crohn's and Colitis Organisation (ECCO). European evidence based consensus on the diagnosis and management of Crohn's disease. Gut. 2006;55(Suppl I):i16–35.

11. Satsangi J, Silverberg MS, Vermeire S, Colombel JF. The Montreal classification of inflammatory bowel disease: controversies, consensus, and implications. Gut. 2006;55:749–53.

12. Pallotta N, Giovannone M, Pezzotti P, Gigliozzi A, Barberani F, Piacentino D, Hassan NA, Vincoli G, Tosoni M, Covotta A, Marcheggiano A, Di Camillo M, Corazziari E. Ultrasonographic detection and assessment of the severity of Crohn's disease recurrence after ileal resection. BMC Gastroenterol. 2010;10:69.

13. Maconi G, Bollani S, Bianchi Porro G. Ultrasonographic detection of intestinal complications in Crohn's disease. Dig Dis Sci. 1996;41:1643–8.

14. Maconi G, Greco S, Duca P, Ardizzone S, Massari A, Cassinotti A, Radice E, Porro GB. Prevalence and clinical significance of sonographic evidence of mesenteric fat alterations in Crohn's disease. Inflamm Bowel Dis. 2008;14: 1555–61.

15. Pocock SJ, Ariti CA, McMurray JJ, Maggioni A, Køber L, Squire IB, Swedberg K, Dobson J, Poppe KK, Whalley GA, Doughty RN, on behalf of the meta-analysis global Groupin chronic heart failure (MAGGIC). Predicting survival in heart failure: a risk score based on 39,372 patients from 30 studies. Eur Heart J. 2013;34:1404–13.

16. Pariente B, Mary JY, Danese S, Chowers Y, De Cruz P, D'Haens G, Loftus EV Jr, Louis E, Panés J, Schölmerich J, Schreiber S, Vecchi M, Branche J, Bruining D, Fiorino G, Herzog M, Kamm MA, Klein A, Lewin M, Meunier P, Ordas I, Strauch U, Tontini GE, Zagdanski AM, Bonifacio C, Rimola J, Nachury M, Leroy C, Sandborn W, Colombel JF, Cosnes J. Development of the Lémann index to assess digestive tract damage in patients with Crohn's disease. Gastroenterology. 2015;148:52–63.

17. Rutgeerts P, Geboes K, Vantrappen G, Beyls J, Kerremans R, Hiele M. Predictability of the postoperative course of Crohn's disease. Gastroenterology. 1990;99:956–63.

18. Solberg IC, Vatn MH, Høie O, Stray N, Sauar J, Jahnsen J, Moum B, Lygren I, the IBSEN study group. Clinical course in Crohn's disease: results of a Norwegian population-based ten year follow-up study. Clin Gastroenterol Hepatol. 2007;5:1430–8.

19. Cosnes J, Nion-Larmurier I, Beaugerie L, Afchain P, Tiret E, Gendre J-P. Impact of the increasing use of immunosuppressants in Crohn's disease on the need for intestinal surgery. Gut. 2005;54:237–41.

20. Nugent Z, Blanchard JF, Bernstein CN. A population-based study of health-care resource use among infliximab users. Am J Gastroenterol. 2010;105: 2009–16.

21. Cosnes J, Bourrier A, Laharie D, Nahon S, Bouhnik Y, Carbonnel F, Allez M, Dupas J-L, Reimund J-M, Savoye G, Jouet P, Moreau J, Mary J-Y, Colombel J-F, the Groupe d'Etude Therapeutique des Affectionns Inflammatories du Tube Digestif (GETAID). Early administration of azathioprine vs conventional management of Crohn's disease: a randomized controlled trial. Gastroenterology. 2013;145:758–65.

22. Chatu S, Subramanian V, Saxena S, Pollok RCG. The role of thiopurines in reducing the need for surgical resection in Crohn's disease:a systematic review and meta-analysis. Am J Gastroenterol. 2014;109:23–34.

23. Chatu S, Saxena S, Subramanian V, Curcin V, Yadegarfar G, Gunn L, Majeed A, Pollok RCG. The impact of timing and duration of thiopurine treatment on first intestinal resection in Crohn's disease: nation UK population-based study 1989-2010. Am J Gastroenterol. 2014;109:409–16.

24. Rungoe C, Langholz E, Andersson M, Basit S, Nielsen NM, Wohlfahrt J, Jess T. Changes in medical treatment and surgery rates in inflammatory bowel disease: a nationwide cohort study 1979-2011. Gut. 2014;63:1607–16.

25. Mekhjian HS, Switz DM, Melnyk CS, Rankin GB, Brooks RK. Clinical features and natural history of Crohn's disease. Gastroenterology. 1979;77:898–906.

26. Ramadas AV, Gunes S, Thomas GAO, Williams GT, Hawthorne AB. Natural history of Crohn's disease in a population-based cohort from Cardiff (1986-2003): a study of changes in medical treatment and surgical resection rates. Gut. 2010;59:1200–6.

27. Kruis W, Katalinic A, Klugmann T, Franke GR, Weismüller J, Leifeld L, Ceplis-Kastner S, Reimers B, Bokemeyer B. Predictive factors for an uncomplicated long-term course of Crohn's disease: a retrospective analysis. J Crohns Colitis. 2013;7:e263–76.

28. Lazarev M, Huang C, Bitton A, Cho JH, Duerr RH, McGovern DP, Proctor DD, Regueiro M, Rioux JD, Schumm PP, Tayolor KD, Silverberg MS, Steinhart AH, Huttfless S, Brant SR. Relatiosip between proximal Crohn's disease location and disease behavior and surgery: a cross sectional study of the IBD genetics consortium. Am J Gastroenterol. 2013;108:106–12.

29. Cosnes J, Cattan S, Blain A, Beaugerie L, Carbonnel F, Parc R, Gendre J-P. Long-term evolution of disease behavior of Crohn's disease. Inflamm Bowel Dis. 2002;8:244–50.

30. Moum B, Ekbom A, Vatn MH, Aadland E, Sauar J, Lygren I, Schulz T, Stray N, Fausa O. Clinical course during the 1st year after diagnosis in ulcerative colitis and Crohn's disease. Results of a large, prospective population-based study in southeastern Norway, 1990-93. Scand J Gastroenterol. 1997;32: 1005–12.

31. Aldhous MC, Hazel ED, Drummond HE, Anderson N, Smith LA, Arnott DR, Satsangi J. Does cigarette smoking influence the phenotype of Crohn's disease? Analysis using the Montreal classification. Am J Gastroenterol. 2007; 102:577–88.

32. Nunes T, Etchevers MJ, Merino O, Gallego S, García-Sánchez V, Marín-Jiménez I, Menchén L, Barreiro-de Acosta M, Bastida G, García S, Gento E, Ginard D, Gomollón F, Arroyo M, Monfort D, García-Planella E, Gonzalez B, Loras C, Agustí C, Figueroa C, Sans M, TABACROHN Study Group of GETECCU, Spanish Working Group in Crohn's Disease and Ulcerative Colitis. Does smoking influence Crohn's disease in the biologic era? The TABACROHN study. Inflamm Bowel Dis. 2013;8:244–50.

33. Carbonnel F, Macaigne G, Beaugerie L, Gendre JP, Cosnes J. Crohn's disease severity in familial and sporadic cases. Gut. 1999;44:91–5.

34. Henriksen M, Jahnsen J, Lygren I, Vatn MH, Moum B, the IBSEN Study Group. Are there any differences in phenotype or disease course between familial an sporadic cases of inflammatory bowel disease? Results of a population-based follow-up study. Am J Gastroenterol. 2007;102:1955–63.

35. Cosnes J, Carbonnel F, Carrat F, Beaugerie L, Cattan S, Gendre PJ. Effects of current and former cigarette smoking on the clinical course of Crohn's disease. Aliment Pharmacol Ther. 1999;13:1403–11.

36. Guo Y, Logan HL, Glueck DH, Muller KE. Selecting a sample size for studies with repeated measures. BMC Med Res Methodol. 2013;13:100.

37. Henriksen M, Jahnsen J, Lygren I, Stray N, Sauar J, Vatn MH, Moum B, the IBSEN Study Group. C-reactive protein: a predictive factor and marker of inflammation in inflammatory bowel disease. Results from a prospective population-based study. Gut. 2008;57:1518–23.

21

Predictors of distant metastasis on exploration in patients with potentially resectable pancreatic cancer

Xinchun Liu[1,2†] (iD), Yue Fu[1,3†], Qiuyang Chen[1,2], Junli Wu[1,2], Wentao Gao[1,2], Kuirong Jiang[1,2], Yi Miao[1,2*] and Jishu Wei[1,2*]

Abstract

Background: Patients with potentially resectable pancreatic ductal adenocarcinoma (PDAC) are frequently found to be unresectable on exploration due to small distant metastasis. This study was to investigate predictors of small distant metastasis in patients with potentially resectable PDAC.

Methods: Patients who underwent surgical exploration for potentially resectable PDAC from 2013 to 2014 were reviewed retrospectively and divided into two groups according to whether distant metastases were encountered on exploration. Then, univariate and multivariate logistic regression analyses were used to identify predictors of distant metastasis. A scoring system to predict distant metastasis of PDAC on exploration was constructed based on the regression coefficient of a multivariate logistic regression model.

Results: A total of 235 patients were included in this study. Mean age of the study population was 61.7 ± 10.4 years old. Upon exploration, distant metastases were found intraoperatively in 62 (26.4%) patients, while the remaining 173 were free of distant metastases. Multivariate logistic regression analysis identified that age ≤ 62 years old ($p < 0.001$), male sex ($p = 0.011$), tumor size ≥ 4.0 cm ($p < 0.001$), alanine aminotransferase level (ALT) < 125 U/L ($p < 0.001$), and carbohydrate antigen (CA19–9) level ≥ 385 U/mL ($p < 0.001$) were independent risk factors for occult distant metastasis of PDAC. A preoperative scoring system (0–8 points) for distant metastasis on exploration was constructed using these five factors. The receiver operating characteristic curves showed that the area under the curve of this score was 0.85. A score of 6 points was suggested to be the optimal cut-off value, and the sensitivity and specificity were 85% and 69%, respectively.

Conclusions: Distant metastasis is still frequently encountered on exploration for patients with potentially resectable PDAC. Younger age, male sex, larger tumor size, low ALT level and high CA19–9 level are independent predictors of unexpected distant metastasis on exploration.

Keywords: Distant metastasis, Pancreatic cancer, Predictive factor, Surgical exploration

Background

Pancreatic ductal adenocarcinoma (PDAC) is one of the most dismal malignancies with an overall 5-year survival rate of < 7% [1, 2]. Despite enormous efforts directed at the treatment of PDAC, radical resection remains the most effective treatment modality, and it increases the 5-year survival rate for PDAC patients to 10–25% [3–5]. However, due to a lack of presentations at early stages and the aggressive nature of this disease, the majority of PDAC patients present an unresectable disease at the time of diagnosis, and only around 20% of newly diagnosed PDAC patients were suitable candidates for curable surgical resection [6].

Multidetector computed tomography (MDCT) is currently the optimal imaging modality for preoperative diagnosis and staging of PDAC [7, 8]. However, this imaging modality has a poor sensitivity for identifying

---

* Correspondence: miaoyi@njmu.edu.cn; weijishu@njmu.edu.cn
†Xinchun Liu and Yue Fu contributed equally to this work.
[1]Pancreas Center, The First Affiliated Hospital of Nanjing Medical University, 300 Guangzhou Road, Nanjing, Jiangsu Province, China
Full list of author information is available at the end of the article

small liver or peritoneal metastasis [7, 9]. Among the patients subjected to surgical exploration, a significant proportion (40%) of them are found to be unresectable due to occult distant metastasis or infiltration of local structures [10–12]. The proportion of patients successfully resected during surgical exploration might be as low as 50% [12, 13].

For patients with distant occult metastasis, surgical resection is unnecessary as it does not prolong survival in the overwhelming majority of patients [14, 15]. Besides, unnecessary surgical exploration often delays administration of other treatments, for example systematic chemotherapy, which currently is the preferred treatment for metastatic PDAC patients [16]. Therefore, it is important to differentiate PDAC patients with distant metastasis from those with truly resectable cancers to avoid unnecessary surgery and offer these patients tailored treatments in a timely manners. The objective of this retrospective study was to analyze the predictive factors for distant occult metastasis in patients with resectable PDAC based on preoperative MDCT.

Methods
Study design and patients
This was a single institution, retrospective study, from a high-volume center, the Pancreas Center, The First Affiliated Hospital of Nanjing Medical University, China. All patients who underwent elective pancreatic surgery at our unit between January 2014 and December 2015 were reviewed retrospectively. Only patients with a final diagnosis of PDAC were included. Exclusion criteria were as follows: 1) patients underwent an operation with palliative intent, 2) patients without preoperative internal MDCT, and 3) patients with distant metastasis detected with preoperative MDCT. All patients underwent a triple-phase 16-row MDCT, consisting of unenhanced, early arterial, and venous phases.

Patients were included in the "with metastasis" (WM) group when distant metastasis, such as liver and peritoneal metastasis, was encountered during surgery. The remaining patients were included in the "no metastasis" (NM) group. During the surgery, distant metastasis was discovered through manual palpation by experienced surgeons and further confirmed with frozen resection. Intra-operative ultrasound was not used.

Data collected included age at diagnosis; sex; drinking and smoking history; comorbidities (Hypertension and Diabetes Mellitus); chief complaint (with pain or without pain); preoperative laboratory data, such as alanine aminotransferase (ALT), aspartate aminotransferase (AST), total bilirubin (TBil), direct bilirubin (DBil), albumin, alpha fetoprotein (AFP), carbohydrate antigen (CA19–9), and carcinoembryonic antigen (CEA); tumor size and location on MDCT; and time interval between MDCT

and operation. The possible risk factors for distant metastasis were then examined statistically. Data were obtained from the patients' medical records and the hospital electronic database. All the imaging results were reviewed by a dedicated radiologist. This study was approved by the institutional review board with a waiver of informed consent (No. 2016-SR-210).

Statistical analysis
Quantitative variables are presented as the mean ± standard deviation and qualitative variables are expressed as absolute and relative frequencies. Comparisons between the WM and NM groups are performed using the Student's t-test or Chi-square test accordingly. The association between the predictive factors and presence of distant metastasis was first evaluated by univariate logistic regression. Factors with a $p < 0.1$ in the univariate regression analysis were included in multivariate logistic regression analysis. Backward stepwise elimination was used to exclude variables with $p > 0.05$ from the model. Continuous variables were divided into two groups according to the mean value of each parameter. All statistical analyses were performed using Stata/SE version 10.0 for Windows (StataCorp, Texas, USA). All tests for significance were two-sided and a value of $p < 0.05$ was considered statistically significant.

Results
Demographic and clinicopathologic characteristics
In the study period, a consecutive series of 501 patients with PDAC underwent laparotomy in our center. Of these, 26 patients were excluded because they had unresectable disease detected radiologically and underwent an operation with palliative intent. Another 240 patients were excluded for having no internal MDCT: 218 didn't have any image studies in our hospital, and 22 had only Magnetic Resonance Imaging or magnetic resonance cholangiopancreatography or positron emission tomography/computed tomography other than MDCT. Ultimately, a total of 235 patients were included in the analysis (Fig. 1).

All the included 235 patients underwent upfront surgery, and received no neoadjuvant therapy. Distant metastasis was found in 62 (26.4%) patients, including 31 liver metastases and 31 peritoneal metastases. Of the 62 patients with metastases, three patients underwent pancreaticoduodenectomy for primary cancer and the remaining patients underwent different palliative procedures accordingly. Of the 173 NM patients, 164 patients underwent resection successfully and 9 patients underwent palliative operations because the tumor was locally advanced. Details of the procedures are shown in Table 1.

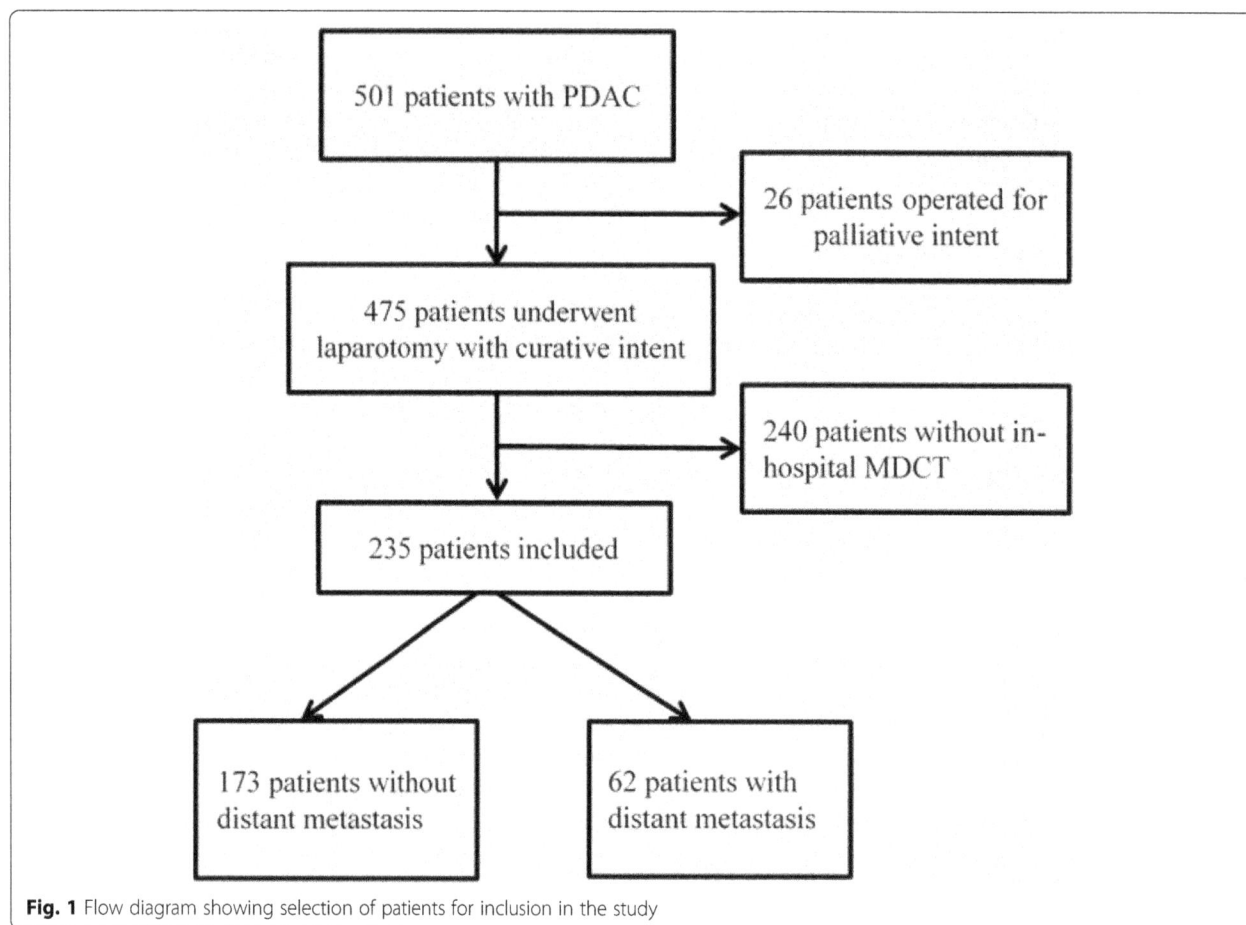

Fig. 1 Flow diagram showing selection of patients for inclusion in the study

Comparisons between the patients with metastasis (WM) and patients with no metastasis (NM)

Patients' demographics and laboratory values at the time of diagnosis are shown in Table 2. The mean age of all patients was 61.7 ± 10.4 years (median 62 years, range 29–87 years), and 64.3% ($n = 151$) were male. The metastasis

Table 1 Procedures performed for 235 patients

	Total ($n = 235$)	No Metastasis ($n = 173$)	With Metastasis ($n = 62$)
Resected	167	164	3
PD/PPPD	124	121	3
Distal pancreatectomy	39	39	0
Total pancreatectomy	1	1	0
Appleby Operation	3	3	0
Not Resected	68	9	59
Double Bypass	13	1	12
Biliary Bypass	9	4	5
Gastric Bypass	4	0	4
Celiac plexus neurolysis	16	0	16
Exploration alone	26	4	22

PD pancreaticoduodenectomy, PPPD
pylorus-preserving pancreaticoduodenectomy

group had a younger age (59.4 vs. 62.5 years, $p = 0.041$) and larger tumor size compared with the NM group (4.2 vs. 3.8 cm, $p < 0.001$). Additionally, patients in the NM group had a higher ALT level ($p = 0.010$) and a higher AST level ($p = 0.010$) when compared with patients in the WM group. Levels of TBil and DBil in the WM group were found to be lower than those in the NM group; however, these differences were not significant ($p = 0.057$ and 0.085, respectively).

Predictive factors for occult distant metastases on exploration
Table 3 summarizes the univariate and multivariate logistic regression analyses of the risk factor for distant metastasis using the significant univariate predictors. In univariate analyses, significant predictive factors for finding distant metastasis during surgery were younger age ($p = 0.003$), larger tumor size ($p < 0.001$), tumor location ($p = 0.048$), lower ALT level ($p < 0.001$), lower AST level ($p = 0.006$), lower TBil level ($p < 0.019$), higher CA199 level ($p = 0.007$), and higher CEA level ($p < 0.001$) (Table 3). In multivariate analysis, the following variables remained significantly associated with presence of distant metastasis: an age < 62 years old (Odds ratio (OR) = 3.97; 95% Confidence interval (CI): 1.87–8.42; $p < 0.001$), male sex (OR =

Table 2 Demographic and clinical characteristics of included patients

	Total (n = 235)	NM (n = 173)	WM (n = 62)	p
Age (years) (mean ± SD)	61.7 ± 10.4	62.5 ± 10.4	59.4 ± 10.0	0.041
Sex, male/female	151/84	105/68	46/16	0.057
Chief complaint				
Pain	150	106	44	0.173
Without pain	85	67	18	
Jaundice	73	61	12	0.200
Without jaundice	162	112	50	
Weight loss	100	70	30	0.279
Without weight loss	135	103	32	
Personal history				
Smoking, yes/no	48/187	34/139	14/48	0.624
Drinking, yes/no	38/197	32/141	6/56	0.106
Hypertension, yes/no	71/164	51/122	20/42	0.683
Diabetes, yes/no	36/199	25/148	11/51	0.537
Interval between imaging and surgery, days	6.3 ± 4.8	6.3 ± 4.6	6.2 ± 5.2	0.868
Tumor size on MDCT (cm)	4.2 ± 1.9	3.8 ± 1.6	5.5 ± 2.0	< 0.001
Tumor location				
Head	174	134	40	0.046
Body or tail	61	39	22	
Laboratory examinations				
ALT	124.6 ± 173.1	142.2 ± 179.1	75.9 ± 146.1	0.010
AST	84.3 ± 100.5	94.4 ± 105.0	56.3 ± 81.2	0.010
TBil	73.9 ± 103.8	81.6 ± 107.6	52.4 ± 89.5	0.057
DBil	50.3 ± 74.6	55.4 ± 77.2	36.3 ± 65.7	0.085
ALB	40.0 ± 5.4	40.1 ± 5.4	39.7 ± 5.2	0.686
AFP	2.9 ± 1.8	2.8 ± 1.4	3.1 ± 2.6	0.293
CA19-9	385.5 ± 378.8	335.7 ± 350.2	525.2 ± 422.0	< 0.001
CEA	8.9 ± 20.3	8.1 ± 21.9	11.1 ± 14.7	0.328

2.79, 95% CI: 1.26–6.19; $p = 0.011$), a tumor size ≥4.0 cm (OR = 16.02, 95% CI: 5.31–48.30; $p < 0.001$), ALT level < 125 U/L (OR = 6.19, 95% CI: 2.26–16.92, $p < 0.001$), and a CA19–9 level ≥ 385 U/ml (OR = 3.53, 95% CI: 1.87–6.67; $p < 0.001$) (Table 3).

The five independent risk factors found in the multivariate analysis were used to develop a score system based on the regression coefficient of the multivariate logistic regression model (Table 4). The score values for individual patient ranged from 0 to 8. The risk of patients with distant metastasis progressively increased as the score increased (Table 5, Fig. 2a). A receiver operating characteristic curve of the model showed that the area under curve of this score was 0.85 (95% CI: 0.80–0.89) (Fig. 2b). A score of 6 points was suggested to be the optimal cut-off value (Youden index = 0.548) to divide the risk strata with a sensitivity of 85% and a specificity of 69%.

Discussion

Currently, radical resection provides the only chance for long-term survival for patients with PDAC. As surgical skills and perioperative management developed, mortality after pancreatic surgery has dramatically decreased to less than 5% [17]. However, morbidity after pancreatic surgery is still very high. Non-curative exploratory laparotomy of pancreas can have a morbidity as high as 42.3% and does not increase survival [18]. Moreover, this unnecessary operation can postpone other more suitable therapies such as chemotherapy and can become the last straw to their debilitating state.

Unfortunately, not all patients with PDAC who undergo resection surgery can be resected successfully. Despite thorough pre-operative staging with advanced imaging techniques, incidental occult distant metastasis from PDAC is commonly encountered in during surgery

Table 3 Univariate and multivariate analyses of factors predicting distant metastases

		Total n = 235	NM n = 173	WM n = 62	Univariate analysis		Multivariate analysis[a]	
					p	OR (95% CI)	p	OR (95% CI)
Age	> 62	115	95	20	0.003	1	< 0.001	1
	≤62	120	78	42		2.55 (1.39, 4.71)		3.97 (1.87, 8.42)
Sex	Female	84	68	16	0.057	1	0.011	1
	Male	151	105	46		1.86 (0.98, 3.55)		2.79 (1.26, 6.19)
Pain	No	85	67	18	0.174	1		
	Yes	150	106	44		1.50 (0.82, 2.90)		
Jaundice	No	162	112	50	0.022	1		
	Yes	73	61	12		0.44 (0.22, 0.89)		
Weight loss	No	135	103	32	0.280	1		
	Yes	100	70	30		1.37 (0.77, 2.47)		
Smoking	No	187	139	48	0.624	1		
	Yes	48	34	14		1.19 (0.59, 2.41)		
Drinking	No	197	141	56	0.112	1		
	Yes	38	32	6		0.47 (0.19, 1.19)		
Hypertension	No	71	51	20	0.683	1		
	Yes	164	122	42		1.14 (0.61, 2.13)		
Diabetes	No	199	148	51	0.538	1		
	Yes	36	25	11		1.28 (0.59, 2.78)		
Interval between imaging and surgery	≤7	170	123	47		1		
	7–14	48	39	9	0.213	0.60 (0.27, 1.34)		
	≥14	17	11	6	0.461	1.49 (0.52, 4.31)		
Tumor size	< 4.0	96	92	4	< 0.001	1	< 0.001	1
	≥4.0	139	81	58		16.47 (5.73, 47.36)		16.02 (5.31, 48.30)
Tumor location	Head	174	134	40	0.048	1		
	Body/tail	61	39	22		1.88 (1.01, 3.55)		
ALT	≥125	71	64	7	< 0.001	1	< 0.001	1
	< 125	164	109	55		4.61 (1.98, 10.74)		6.19 (2.26, 16.92)
AST	≥ 85	75	64	11	0.006	1		
	< 85	160	109	51		2.72 (1.32, 5.60)		
TBil	≥75	78	65	13	0.019	1		
	< 75	157	108	49		2.27 (1.14, 4.50)		
DBil	≥50	75	61	14	0.069	1		
	< 50	160	112	48		1.87 (0.95, 3.66)		
ALB	≥40	124	89	35	0.498	1		
	< 40	111	84	27		0.82 (0.46, 1.47)		
AFP	< 3.0	153	111	42	0.612	1		
	≥3.0	82	62	20		0.85 (0.46, 1.57)		
CA19–9	< 385	144	115	29	0.007	1	0.015	1
	≥385	91	58	33		2.26 (1.25, 4.07)		2.49 (1.19, 5.21)
CEA	< 9	183	145	38	< 0.001	1		
	≥9	52	28	24		3.53 (1.87, 6.67)		

NM, No metastases; WM, with metastases
[a]A multivariable model was constructed by a backward stepwise method

Table 4 Predictive scoring system for pancreatic fistula

Preoperative factor	β coefficient	Points contributed
Age		
> 62 years old		0 point
≤ 62 years old	1.38	1 point
Sex		
Female		0 point
Male	1.02	1 point
Tumor size		
< 4.0 cm		0 point
≥ 4.0 cm	2.78	3 points
ALT		
≥ 125 U/L		0 point
< 125 U/L	1.89	2 points
CA19–9		
< 385 U/mL		0 point
≥ 385 U/mL	0.91	1 point

[19]. Previous studies revealed that up to 31% of patients with resectable PDAC staged by MDCT were found to have metastases in sbsequent laparotomy or staging laparoscopy [8, 20–22]. In patients with locally advanced PDAC, the likelihood of finding unresectable PDAC at operation is much higher [23].

Despite the emerging use of magnetic resonance imaging, endoscopic ultrasound, and positron emission tomography/computed tomography, MDCT remains the most commonly used imaging modality for the diagnosis and staging of PDAC [7, 24, 25]. However, small distant metastases, such as minimal peritoneal deposits and small liver metastases, can remain undetected even with modern computed tomography protocols [26]. Previous studies suggested that patients with PDAC should undergo the operation within 25 or 32 days of diagnostic imaging to reduce the risk of tumor progression to

unresectable disease [27, 28]. In the present study, we found that 26% of the patients selected for curative surgery for PDAC had distant metastasis. However, in our study, we found no affects attributable to the time interval between MDCT study and surgery on the accuracy of MDCT in determining the presence or absence of metastatic disease.

Due to the limitation of imaging, other techniques were reported in literature for determining the resectability of PDAC. One such technique is peritoneal lavage cytology (PLC), which is a routinely applied in the diagnosis and staging of several cancers. However, in PDAC, although a positive PLC represents an early recurrence and a worse prognosis, a positive PLC is not regarded as equal to a macrometastasis in patients with PDAC and it does not exclude a curative resection in patients without other distant metastasis [29–31]. Another technique is staging laparoscopy, which has been used to diagnose occult metastasis to decrease the number of unnecessary laparotomies in PDAC [32–34]. Patients who were found to harbor distant metastasis by laparoscopy staging received palliative chemotherapy earlier and lived longer than patients who underwent only laparotomy [33]. Moreover, a cost analysis indicated that use of laparoscopy in pancreatic cancer did not significantly increase the overall expense of treatment [34]. A recent review of 1146 patients found that diagnostic laparoscopy prior to laparotomy could decrease the rate of unnecessary laparotomy from 40 to 20% in patients with periampullary cancer [10]. As a minimally invasive modality, staging laparoscopy was suggested to be routinely used to identify radiographically occult metastases and prevent rewardless laparotomies [20, 21, 35, 36]. However, as the proportion of patients found to have metastases at laparoscopy is decreasing, its routine use is challenged, and some studies have investigated the indications for selective use of staging laparoscopy in pancreatic cancer [37]. Identifying patients at an increased risk of distant

Table 5 Risk of distant metastasis for patients with each score

Score	No. of patients		%				
	Total	WM		Sensitivity (%)	Specificity (%)	Accuracy (%)	Youden Index (%)
0	5	0	0	100	0	26.38	0
1	17	0	0	100	2.89	28.51	2.89
2	20	0	0	100	12.72	35.74	12.72
3	26	1	3.85	100	24.28	44.26	24.28
4	38	4	10.53	98.39	38.73	54.47	37.12
5	23	4	17.39	91.94	58.38	67.23	50.32
6	51	16	31.37	85.48	69.36	73.62	54.84
7	41	26	63.41	59.68	89.60	81.70	49.28
8	14	11	78.57	17.74	98.27	77.02	16.01

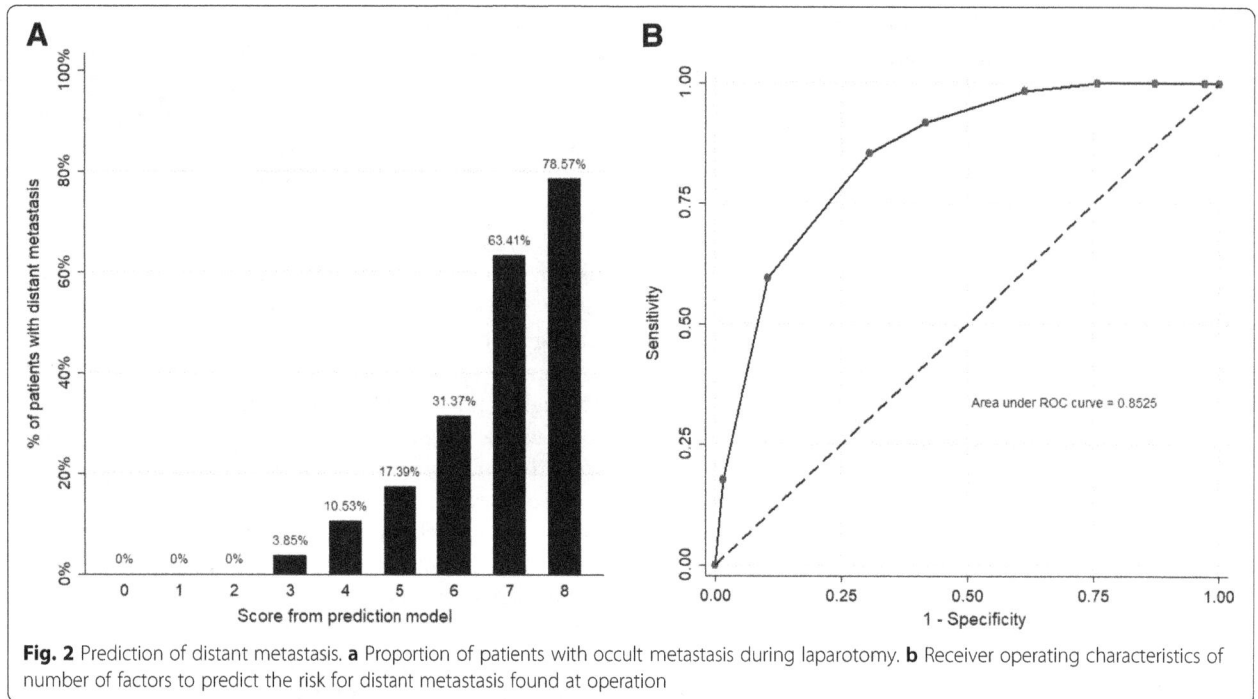

Fig. 2 Prediction of distant metastasis. **a** Proportion of patients with occult metastasis during laparotomy. **b** Receiver operating characteristics of number of factors to predict the risk for distant metastasis found at operation

metastasis seems to be a more reasonable approach, that can increase the diagnostic accuracy of staging laparoscopy and deliver optimal disease management.

By comparing a number of preoperative factors, this study identified that young age, male sex, low ALT level, large tumor size, and high CA 19–9 level were independent predictors of distant metastases in patients with resectable PDAC. Previous studies found that tumors in the pancreas body and tail, tumor size as determined by MDCT, serum CA 19–9 level, CEA, and weight loss were risk factors for unresectability in patients with potentially resectable PDAC [20, 38–41]. Our study confirmed that tumor in the body and tail, and high CEA were associated with distant metastasis in univariate analysis, but not in multivariate analysis. Weight loss was not associated with distant metastasis. In line with previous studies, CA19–9 and tumor size were independent predictive factors for distant metastasis [37]. Ong et al. found that age < =65 was a predictive factor of resectable disease [42]. On the contrary, our study found that age < =62 was an independent risk factor of distant metastasis. Also, we found that patients with distant metastatic PDAC had significantly lower levels of ALT and AST than patients without distant metastatic PDAC, which might be explained by the following reasons. First, this might be relevant to the population characteristics in our study. For example, all our patients underwent upfront surgery without neoadjuvant chemotherapy, which has liver toxicity and results in elevated levels of ALT and AST. Second, we found that patients with lower ALT levels are more likely to be without jaundice,

which, on the one hand is beneficial for liver function, but on the other hand may lead to late diagnosis of PDAC due to lack of symptoms. Third, we found that patients with peritoneal metastases had a slightly lower ALT level than patients with liver metastasis (52.7 ± 139.1 vs 99.2 ± 151.3 U/L, $p = 0.212$). This implies that liver metastasis could only slightly raise the level of ALT when there are no other contributing factors.

After identifying the risk factors associated with distant metastasis, this study developed a model for predicting occult distant metastasis in patients undergoing non-curative laparotomy for potentially resectable PDAC. When a score of 6 points was taken as the cut-off value, this score system had a sensitivity of 85% and a specificity of 69%. However, it is necessary to point out that the reliability and effectiveness of this score system still needs validation by further studies. Also, because successful resection is the only cure for PDAC, these preoperative predictors alone are not contraindications for pancreatic exploration. The predictive factors identified in this study only indicated that additional preoperative staging modalities, such as selective staging laparoscopy, may be needed before laparotomy is indicated.

This study has several limitations. First, due to the nature of its retrospective design, there was a potential for several biases. For example, small intrahepatic lesions may be missed by palpation. Second, the sample size of the present study is relatively small. Therefore, a well-designed, prospective study with more data will be needed to validate the results of this study. Third, though staging laparoscopy was discussed and suggested in this study, we had limited experience in using it. Lastly, although neoadjuvant therapy has become increasingly common in the practice, our findings may not apply to this group of patients.

Conclusions

In conclusion, we showed that for patients with potentially resectable PDAC based on MDCT, distant metastasis is still frequently encountered during surgery. Younger age, male sex, large tumor size, lower ALT and higher CA19–9 are independent predictive factors for finding distant metastasis during exploration.

Abbreviations

ALT: Alanine aminotransferase; AST: Aspartate aminotransferase; CA19–9: Carbohydrate antigen; CEA: Carcinoembryonic antigen; DBil: Direct bilirubin; MDCT: Multidetector computed tomography; NM: No metastasis; PDAC: Pancreatic ductal adenocarcinoma; PLC: Periton eal lavage cytology; TBil: Total bilirubin; WM: With metastasis

Acknowledgements

Not applicable

Funding

This work was supported by the Natural Science Foundation of China (81672449); Natural Science Foundation of Jiangsu Province (BK20161590); and the International Exchange and Cooperation Projects of Nanjing Medical University (C046). The founding resources had no role in study design, data collection and analysis, preparation of the manuscript, or decision to publish.

Authors' contributions

Study conception and design of the study: XL, JuW, WG, KJ, YM, and JiW. Acquisition of data: YF, and QC. Statistical analysis and interpretation of data: XL and YF. Drafting of the manuscript: XL, and JiW. Critical revision: YF, QC, JuW, WG, KJ, and YM. Approval of the final version: all authors.

Competing interests

The authors declare that they have no competing interests.

Author details

[1]Pancreas Center, The First Affiliated Hospital of Nanjing Medical University, 300 Guangzhou Road, Nanjing, Jiangsu Province, China. [2]Pancreas Institute, Nanjing Medical University, Nanjing, China. [3]Department of Gastrointestinal Surgery, The Affiliated Changzhou No.2 People's Hospital of Nanjing Medical University, Changzhou, China.

References

1. Waddell N, Pajic M, Patch AM, Chang DK, Kassahn KS, Bailey P, Johns AL, Miller D, Nones K, Quek K, et al. Whole genomes redefine the mutational landscape of pancreatic cancer. Nature. 2015;518(7540):495–501.
2. Siegel RL, Miller KD, Jemal A. Cancer statistics, 2016. CA Cancer J Clin. 2016; 66(1):7–30.
3. Perysinakis I, Avlonitis S, Georgiadou D, Tsipras H, Margaris I. Five-year actual survival after pancreatoduodenectomy for pancreatic head cancer. ANZ J Surg. 2015;85(3):183–6.
4. Schnelldorfer T, Ware AL, Sarr MG, Smyrk TC, Zhang L, Qin R, Gullerud RE, Donohue JH, Nagorney DM, Farnell MB. Long-term survival after pancreatoduodenectomy for pancreatic adenocarcinoma: is cure possible? Ann Surg. 2008;247(3):456–62.
5. Sener SF, Fremgen A, Menck HR, Winchester DP. Pancreatic cancer: a report of treatment and survival trends for 100,313 patients diagnosed from 1985-1995, using the National Cancer Database. J Am Coll Surg. 1999;189(1):1–7.
6. Speer AG, Thursfield VJ, Torn-Broers Y, Jefford M. Pancreatic cancer: surgical management and outcomes after 6 years of follow-up. Med J Aust. 2012; 196(8):511–5.
7. Pietryga JA, Morgan DE. Imaging preoperatively for pancreatic adenocarcinoma. J Gastrointest Oncol. 2015;6(4):343–57.
8. Loizou L, Albiin N, Leidner B, Axelsson E, Fischer MA, Grigoriadis A, Del Chiaro M, Segersvärd R, Verbeke C, Sundin A, Kartalis N. Multidetector CT of pancreatic ductal adenocarcinoma: Effect of tube voltage and iodine load on tumour conspicuity and image quality. Eur Radiol. 2016;26(11):4021-4029.
9. Vargas R, Nino-Murcia M, Trueblood W, Jeffrey RB Jr. MDCT in pancreatic adenocarcinoma: prediction of vascular invasion and resectability using a multiphasic technique with curved planar reformations. AJR Am J Roentgenol. 2004;182(2):419–25.
10. Allen VB, Gurusamy KS, Takwoingi Y, Kalia A, Davidson BR. Diagnostic accuracy of laparoscopy following computed tomography (CT) scanning for assessing the resectability with curative intent in pancreatic and periampullary cancer. Cochrane Database Syst Rev. 2016;7:CD009323.
11. Durczynski A, Kumor A, Hogendorf P, Szymanski D, Grzelak P, Strzelczyk J. Preoperative high level of D-dimers predicts unresectability of pancreatic head cancer. World J Gastroenterol. 2014;20(36):13167–71.
12. Schlieman MG, Ho HS, Bold RJ. Utility of tumor markers in determining resectability of pancreatic cancer. Arch Surg. 2003;138(9):951–5 discussion 955-956.
13. Ellsmere J, Mortele K, Sahani D, Maher M, Cantisani V, Wells W, Brooks D, Rattner D. Does multidetector-row CT eliminate the role of diagnostic laparoscopy in assessing the resectability of pancreatic head adenocarcinoma? Surg Endosc. 2005;19(3):369–73.
14. Gleisner AL, Assumpcao L, Cameron JL, Wolfgang CL, Choti MA, Herman JM, Schulick RD, Pawlik TM. Is resection of periampullary or pancreatic adenocarcinoma with synchronous hepatic metastasis justified? Cancer. 2007;110(11):2484–92.
15. Hackert T, Niesen W, Hinz U, Tjaden C, Strobel O, Ulrich A, Michalski CW, Buchler MW. Radical surgery of oligometastatic pancreatic cancer. Eur J Surg Oncol. 2016;43(2):358–363.
16. Merkow RP, Bilimoria KY, Tomlinson JS, Paruch JL, Fleming JB, Talamonti MS, Ko CY, Bentrem DJ. Postoperative complications reduce adjuvant chemotherapy use in resectable pancreatic cancer. Ann Surg. 2014;260(2): 372–7.
17. Gastinger I, Meyer F, Shardin A, Ptok H, Lippert H, Dralle H. Investigations on in-hospital mortality in pancreatic surgery: results of a multicenter observational study. Chirurg. 2018. https://doi.org/10.1007/s00104-018-0654-x.
18. Insulander J, Sanjeevi S, Haghighi M, Ivanics T, Analatos A, Lundell L, Del Chiaro M, Andren-Sandberg A, Ansorge C. Prognosis following surgical bypass compared with laparotomy alone in unresectable pancreatic adenocarcinoma. Br J Surg. 2016;103(9):1200–8.
19. Stefanidis D, Grove KD, Schwesinger WH, Thomas CR Jr. The current role of staging laparoscopy for adenocarcinoma of the pancreas: a review. Ann Oncol. 2006;17(2):189–99.
20. Contreras CM, Stanelle EJ, Mansour J, Hinshaw JL, Rikkers LF, Rettammel R, Mahvi DM, Cho CS, Weber SM. Staging laparoscopy enhances the detection of occult metastases in patients with pancreatic adenocarcinoma. J Surg Oncol. 2009;100(8):663–9.

21. Jimenez RE, Warshaw AL, Rattner DW, Willett CG, McGrath D, Fernandez-del Castillo C. Impact of laparoscopic staging in the treatment of pancreatic cancer. Arch Surg. 2000;135(4):409–14 discussion 414-405.

22. Glant JA, Waters JA, House MG, Zyromski NJ, Nakeeb A, Pitt HA, Lillemoe KD, Schmidt CM. Does the interval from imaging to operation affect the rate of unanticipated metastasis encountered during operation for pancreatic adenocarcinoma? Surgery. 2011;150(4):607–14.

23. Karabicak I, Satoi S, Yanagimoto H, Yamamoto T, Hirooka S, Yamaki S, Kosaka H, Inoue K, Matsui Y, Kon M. Risk factors for latent distant organ metastasis detected by staging laparoscopy in patients with radiologically defined locally advanced pancreatic ductal adenocarcinoma. J Hepatobiliary Pancreat Sci. 2016;23(12):750–755.

24. Feldman MK, Gandhi NS. Imaging evaluation of pancreatic Cancer. Surg Clin North Am. 2016;96(6):1235–56.

25. Tamburrino D, Riviere D, Yaghoobi M, Davidson BR, Gurusamy KS. Diagnostic accuracy of different imaging modalities following computed tomography (CT) scanning for assessing the resectability with curative intent in pancreatic and periampullary cancer. The Cochrane database of systematic reviews. 2016;9:CD011515.

26. Lavy R, Gatot I, Markon I, Shapira Z, Chikman B, Copel L, Halevy A. The role of diagnostic laparoscopy in detecting minimal peritoneal metastatic deposits in patients with pancreatic cancer scheduled for curative resection. Surgical laparoscopy, endoscopy & percutaneous techniques. 2012;22(4): 358–60.

27. Sanjeevi S, Ivanics T, Lundell L, Kartalis N, Andren-Sandberg A, Blomberg J, Del Chiaro M, Ansorge C. Impact of delay between imaging and treatment in patients with potentially curable pancreatic cancer. Br J Surg. 2016;103(3): 267–75.

28. Raman SP, Reddy S, Weiss MJ, Manos LL, Cameron JL, Zheng L, Herman JM, Hruban RH, Fishman EK, Wolfgang CL. Impact of the time interval between MDCT imaging and surgery on the accuracy of identifying metastatic disease in patients with pancreatic cancer. AJR Am J Roentgenol. 2015; 204(1):W37–42.

29. Steen W, Blom R, Busch O, Gerhards M, Besselink M, Dijk F, Festen S. Prognostic value of occult tumor cells obtained by peritoneal lavage in patients with resectable pancreatic cancer and no ascites: a systematic review. J Surg Oncol. 2016;114(6):743–51.

30. Yamada S, Fujii T, Kanda M, Sugimoto H, Nomoto S, Takeda S, Nakao A, Kodera Y. Value of peritoneal cytology in potentially resectable pancreatic cancer. Br J Surg. 2013;100(13):1791–6.

31. Yoshioka R, Saiura A, Koga R, Arita J, Takemura N, Ono Y, Yamamoto J, Yamaguchi T. The implications of positive peritoneal lavage cytology in potentially resectable pancreatic cancer. World J Surg. 2012;36(9):2187–91.

32. Ta R, O'Connor DB, Sulistijo A, Chung B, Conlon KC. The role of staging laparoscopy in Resectable and borderline Resectable pancreatic Cancer: a systematic review and meta-analysis. Dig Surg. 2018. https://doi.org/10. 1159/000488372.

33. Sell NM, Fong ZV, Del Castillo CF, Qadan M, Warshaw AL, Chang D, Lillemoe KD, Ferrone CR. Staging laparoscopy not only saves patients an incision, but may also help them live longer. Ann Surg Oncol. 2018;25(4):1009–16.

34. Enestvedt CK, Mayo SC, Diggs BS, Mori M, Austin DA, Shipley DK, Sheppard BC, Billingsley KG. Diagnostic laparoscopy for patients with potentially resectable pancreatic adenocarcinoma: is it cost-effective in the current era? J Gastrointest Surg. 2008;12(7):1177–84.

35. Hennig R, Tempia-Caliera AA, Hartel M, Buchler MW, Friess H. Staging laparoscopy and its indications in pancreatic cancer patients. Dig Surg. 2002;19(6):484–8.

36. Warshaw AL, Tepper JE, Shipley WU. Laparoscopy in the staging and planning of therapy for pancreatic cancer. Am J Surg. 1986;151(1):76–80.

37. De Rosa A, Cameron IC, Gomez D. Indications for staging laparoscopy in pancreatic cancer. HPB. 2016;18(1):13–20.

38. Maithel SK, Maloney S, Winston C, Gonen M, D'Angelica MI, Dematteo RP, Jarnagin WR, Brennan MF, Allen PJ. Preoperative CA 19-9 and the yield of staging laparoscopy in patients with radiographically resectable pancreatic adenocarcinoma. Ann Surg Oncol. 2008;15(12):3512–20.

39. Slaar A, Eshuis WJ, van der Gaag NA, Nio CY, Busch OR, van Gulik TM, Reitsma JB, Gouma DJ. Predicting distant metastasis in patients with suspected pancreatic and periampullary tumors for selective use of staging laparoscopy. World J Surg. 2011;35(11):2528–34.

40. Okada K, Kawai M, Tani M, Hirono S, Miyazawa M, Shimizu A, Kitahata Y, Yamaue H. Predicting factors for unresectability in patients with pancreatic ductal adenocarcinoma. J Hepatobiliary Pancreatic Sci. 2014;21(9):648–53.

41. Kim YC, Kim HJ, Park JH, Park DI, Cho YK, Sohn CI, Jeon WK, Kim BI, Shin JH. Can preoperative CA19-9 and CEA levels predict the resectability of patients with pancreatic adenocarcinoma? J Gastroenterol Hepatol. 2009;24(12): 1869–75.

42. Ong SL, Garcea G, Thomasset SC, Mann CD, Neal CP, Abu Amara M, Dennison AR, Berry DP. Surrogate markers of resectability in patients undergoing exploration of potentially resectable pancreatic adenocarcinoma. J Gastrointest Surg. 2008;12(6):1068–73.

22

Metabolic status and lifestyle factors associated with gallbladder polyps: a covariance structure analysis

Song Leng[1,2], Ai Zhao[3], Qiang Li[1], Leilei Pei[1], Wei Zheng[4], Rui Liang[2] and Hong Yan[1*]

Abstract

Background: Gallbladder Polyps (GBP) are highly prevalent in China; however, the etiology of GBP has not been clearly defined. This study explored the associations between lifestyle factors and GBP and whether it mediated by metabolic factors or not.

Methods: A total of 487 newly diagnosed GBP cases and 502 healthy controls were involved in this study. A questionnaire was used to investigate the socio-demographic characteristics and lifestyle factors. Food Intake Frequencies Questionnaire was used to obtain the food intake frequencies of seven food categories. Blood was tested for lipid profiles, fasting blood glucose and blood urine acid. A Covariance Structure Analysis was used in the analysis to explore the possible pathways between socio-demographic characteristics, lifestyle factors, metabolic factor and GBP.

Results: The Covariance Structure Analysis showed that a higher BMI and elevated triglyceride level mediated the association between age and GBP. Lifestyle factors (smoking and drinking) and higher intake frequencies of fatty food (meat and viscera) also linked to higher BMI and higher triglyceride level, respectively, which were associated with GBP.

Conclusion: In conclusion, age and lifestyle factors might be indirectly related with GBP through BMI and the triglyceride pathway.

Keywords: Gallbladder polyps, Blood lipid, Dietary intake, Body mass index, Metabolic status, Lifestyle factors

Background

Gallbladder Polyps (GBP) are defined as lesions protruding from the gallbladder mucosa and are one of the leading causes of hospital admissions related to gastrointestinal problems [1]. The presenting symptoms of GBP are non-specific and vague, and in many cases, asymptomatic, which leads to a late diagnosis [2]. Although the reported rate of malignancy GBP is only 3–8% [2], it is a common public health issue in many countries, affecting millions of people and the prevalence is continuing to increase [3]. The prevalence of GBP is reported in the range 0.3% to 9.5% worldwide, depending on the studied population and the study design [4]. Previous studies reported that compared to western populations, Asian populations (mainly Japanese, Korean and Chinese) have a higher GBP

prevalence and appear to be at a higher risk of gallbladder cancer [4–7]. Recently, the prevalence of GBP is estimated from 4 to 7% in different areas of China [4, 8].

To date, the etiology of GBP has not yet been clearly defined. Identifying risk factors for GBP will increase its understanding, diagnosis, and prevention. In China, HBV infection is highly prevalent, which is a strong risk factor for the development of GBP [4, 9]. The other reported risk factors associated with GBP mainly include unmodified socio-demographic factors such as age, gender, race, and family histories and modified lifestyle aspects, such as smoking, alcohol drinking, dietary habit and physical activity [4, 10]. According to previous studies, metabolic status such as obesity, hyperlipidemia, impaired glucose tolerance/diabetes and metabolic syndrome was strongly associated with GBP, however, there was paucity of the studies about the linkage between lifestyle factors and GBP [8, 10–12]. Therefore, it is important to explore whether these modifiable factors

* Correspondence: xjtu_yh.paper@aliyun.com
[1]Department of Epidemiology and Health Statistics, School of Public Health, Xi'an Jiaotong University Health Science Center, Xi'an, China
Full list of author information is available at the end of the article

independently contribute to GBP or through metabolic disorder pathways.

In this study, both intermediate factors and lifestyle factors including dietary habit, smoking, alcohol use, and physical activities were investigated. The aims of this study are to determine the association between lifestyle factors and GBP and additionally to examine whether these associations were mediated by BMI or metabolic factors, using path analysis.

Methods
Participants
Study participants were enrolled at Second hospital of Dalian Medical University, China, from January 2016 to November 2016. In this period, a total of 806 patients were diagnosed as GBP with B mode ultrasound based on the ICD-10: K82.808. We excluded those 1) with previously diagnosed or self-reported GBP and other gallbladder and hepatic disease (includes different types of hepatitis), 2) with cancer, infectious disease or other severe disease(such as autoimmune disease), 3) with physical disability and 4) with mental disease and impaired memory. There were 501 patients who were eligible, with 487volunteering to participate in this study, and who completed the questionnaire and blood test.

The control group was taken from 600 healthy volunteers who underwent annual routine physical examination during the same period as the case group and determined without GBP according to B mode ultrasound results and medical records. Total of 580 of them were eligible for this study according to the same exclusion criteria as the case group. Finally, 502 of them volunteered to participant in this study and completed the questionnaire. The results of blood test were obtained from the participants' routine physical examination with consent.

Data collection
Data were collected from cases and controls by trained registered nurses using an interviewer-administered questionnaire with regard to socio-demographic characteristics and lifestyle factors. The preliminary questionnaire tests were completed prior to data collection.

Regular patterns of food consumption were assessed using Food Frequency Questionnaire; seven different kinds of food groups were investigated: 1) meat, 2) viscera, 3) fried food,4) vegetable, 5) fruits, 6) alcoholic drinks and 7)tea. Smoking was defined as daily smoking one or more cigarettes (or any other types of tobacco equals to 1 cigarette) and lasting for at least one year. The previous smoking was defined as who successfully quitted smoking over 1 year. Physical activity of participants attending in the past months was asked for the types (categorized as light, moderate, or vigorous physical activities), frequencies and duration.

Anthropometric measurements (height, weight and blood pressure) were performed for each participant. Fasting serum blood samples(fasting over 8 h) were collected by trained nurse in the morning and tested for lipid profiles (total cholesterol (TC), total triglyceride (TG), high density lipoprotein cholesterol (HDL-C) and low density lipoprotein cholesterol (LDL-C), fasting blood glucose(FBG) and blood uric acid (BUA)).

Statistical analyses
SAS version 9.3 (SAS Institute, Inc., Cary, NC,USA) was used for statistical analysis. Data were presented as mean ± SD or percentage. Univariate analysis was performed to compare characteristics between case and control groups with Chi-square analysis or Independent T Test. Then, the crude associations were obtained by the method of logistic regression.

Covariance Structure Analysis was constructed to examine the pathways between predictors and GBP in AMOS 7.0(SPSS, Inc., Chicago, IL, USA). The outcome variable was GBP (binary variable). The independent variables were determined according to the univariate analysis (variables for which $P < 0.1$) which included age, lifestyle factors (smoking) and several dietary factors. The predictors which were highly relevant to smoking and meat intake (including drinking and viscera intake) were also involved in the model. The mediators were BMI and lipids profiles. The associations between the independent variables and the pathways that linked the independent variables to the GBP were determined by Structural Equation Model.

Results
Socio-demographic characteristics of participants
A total of 487 cases (292 men and 195 women) and 502 controls (275 men and 227 women) participated in this study. The majority ethnic group is Han(93.7%). The comparisons of socio-demographic characteristics were shown in Table 1. The case group had a higher age. There were no significant associations between gender, GBP and education level or family income.

Univariate analysis of lifestyle and dietary factors
According to the results of the univariate analysis, the current smokers and the ones with a higher intake frequencies of meat were significantly associated with GBP (Table 2). Physical activities, other types of food, alcoholic drinks and tea were not associated with GBP.

Univariate analysis of health indicators
Comparing health indicators between case and control groups, the case group had a significantly higher TG level. The BMI, blood pressure level, other lipid profiles, FBG and BUA were not associated with GBP(Table 3).

Table 1 Comparisons of socio-demographic characteristics between case and control

Variables	Case	Control	P	Crud OR (95%CI)
Age(years)	50.6 ± 14.0	46.1 ± 12.7	< 0.001	1.03 (1.02,1.04)
Gender				
Male	292 (51.5)	275 (48.5)	0.100	Ref.
Female	195 (46.2)	227 (53.8)		0.81 (0.63,1.04)
Education level				
Senior high school or under	88 (47.6)	97 (52.4)	0.603	Ref.
Bachelor degree or above	399 (49.7)	408 (50.3)		1.09 (0.79,1.50)
Family average Monthly income (RMB: yuan)				
< 2000	23 (5.4)	27 (6.6)	0.207	Ref.
2000~ 3999	121 (28.3)	95 (23.2)		1.50 (0.81,2.72)
≥4000	283 (66.3)	288 (70.2)		1.15 (0.65,2.06)

Ref. The reference group
Binary logistic regression was used to obtain the crud odds ratios OR and its 95% CI

Pathway analysis

The Structural Equation Model fit in the pathway analyses was adequate (The goodness of fit index (AGFI) was 0.96, comparative fit index (CFI) was 0.93, and the root mean square error of approximation was 0.04). The pathways determined in this study are depicted in Fig. 1. According to the Covariance Structure Analysis, elder and higher intake frequencies of meat are associated with the higher BMI; higher BMI linked to increased TG level; then the TG level is positively associated with GBP. In addition, age is also related to TG level. Meanwhile, the intake frequency of meat was highly correlated with the intake frequency of viscera, and these two predictors contribute to BMI. Smoking and drinking were also relevant, and were associated with TG.

Discussion

This study was focused on exploring the risk factors for GBP in the population of China, especially focused on the modifiable lifestyle factors. The current study has supported and extended previous findings by demonstrating that dyslipidemia is associated with GBP. In addition, through pathway analysis, lifestyle factors might indirectly contribute to GBP through increasing BMI and the TG level pathway.

Metabolic status with GBP

The etiology of GBP has not been clearly defined, the risk factors might be different among different types of GBP. In this study, we did not identify types of GBP; however, based on the previous study, the cholesterol polyps are the most common type (> 70%) [2]. Plenty of studies found that the abnormal metabolic status was associated with GBP. In Khairy's study of 74 patients with gallbladder cholesterol polyps, 85.1% had dyslipidemia [13]. Considering different lipid profiles, several studies found that HDL-C level was negatively associated with GBP, while LDL-C level was positively related with GBP; however, the study results were inconsistent [2, 4, 14–16]. The roles of TG and TC on GBP were not clear. In this study, we found that TG level in the case group was significantly higher than in the controls. One Korean study also found similar results, where the elevated TG level was significantly associated with GBP [3]. In addition, abnormal TG level was reported to be associated with other gallbladder diseases, such as gallstones and gallbladder cancer, which might share a similar pathogenesis with GBP [17, 18]. In the hypothesis, some researchers suggested that the direct deposition of bile or blood cholesterol might contribute to the formation of cholesterol polyps; others inferred the alterations in hepatic cholesterol metabolism and altered mucosal esterification of free sterols from bile could contribute to the development of cholesterolemia [19].

There are conflicting results about the relationship between GBP and obesity; some studies found that increasing BMI or obesity status is associated with GBP, while Cantürk et al. Conducted a study on 432 patients and found that patients with GBP were not severely obese(BMI > 30) [8, 20, 21]. However, it seems that most studies agree with the formation of GBP being associated with fat metabolism [21–23]. In this study, in univariate analysis, no strong and direct association was found between BMI and GBP ($P = 0.10$); however, based on pathway analysis, high BMI is one of the important predictors which contribute to GBP through increasing the TG level pathway. This result indicated that abnormal fat metabolism is a risk factor of GBP. In addition, a higher age was reported as a risk factor of GBP in many previous studies [4, 8]. Based on the current results, there might be a possibility that BMI and TG increase with age and contribute to GBP.

In the current study, the impaired blood glucose and abnormal blood pressures were not related to GBP; these

Table 2 Lifestyle and dietary factors between case and control groups

Variables		Case	Control	P	Crud OR (95%CI)
Smoking	Non-smoker	349 (71.7)	382 (76.1)	0.006	Ref.
	Current smoker	120 (24.6)	88 (17.5)		1.49 (1.09,2.04)
Physical activities	Previous smoker	18 (3.7)	32 (6.4)		0.62 (0.34,1.11)
	< 120 min/week	323 (90.5)	301 (93.2)	0.353	Ref.
	120~ 180 min/week	30 (8.4)	18 (5.6)		1.55 (0.85,2.84)
	> 180 min/week	4 (1.1)	4 (1.2)		0.93 (0.23,3.76)
Food intake frequencies(times/week)					
Meat	Never	159 (32.6)	229 (45.6)	< 0.001	Ref.
	1~ 2	215 (44.1)	209 (41.6)		1.48 (1.12,1.96)
	3~ 4	81 (16.6)	51 (10.2)		2.29 (1.53,3.43)
	≥5	32 (6.6)	13 (2.6)		3.55 (1.80,6.97)
Viscera	Never	225 (46.2)	273 (54.4)	0.207	Ref.
	1~ 2	223 (47.8)	206 (41.0)		1.37 (1.06,1.78)
	3~ 4	22 (4.9)	16 (3.2)		1.82 (0.94,3.51)
	≥5	5 (1.0)	7 (1.4)		0.87 (0.27,2.77)
Fried food	Never	143 (29.4)	184 (36.7)	0.109	Ref.
	1~ 2	265 (54.4)	247 (49.2)		1.38 (1.04,1.83)
	3~ 4	66 (13.6)	58 (11.6)		1.46 (0.97,2.22)
	≥5	13 (2.7)	13 (2.6)		1.29 (0.58,2.86)
Vegetables	Never	13 (2.7)	12 (2.4)	0.550	Ref.
	1~ 2	53 (10.9)	48 (9.6)		1.08 (0.49,2.41)
	3~ 4	97 (19.9)	118 (23.5)		1.10 (0.73,1.68)
	≥5	324 (66.5)	324 (64.5)		0.82 (0.60,1.12)
Fruits	Never	42 (8.6)	35 (7.0)	0.601	Ref.
	1~ 2	122 (25.1)	121 (24.1)		0.84 (0.50,1.41)
	3~ 4	108 (22.2)	147 (29.3)		0.61 (0.37,1.02)
	≥5	215 (44.1)	199 (39.6)		0.90 (0.55,1.47)
Alcohol drink	< 1	434 (89.0)	447 (89.0)	0.971	Ref.
	≥1	53 (10.9)	55 (11.0)		0.97 (0.67,1.48)
Tea	< 1	326 (66.9)	340 (67.7)	0.791	Ref.
	≥1	161 (33.1)	162 (32.3)		1.04 (0.80,1.35)

Ref. The reference group

Binary logistic regression was used to obtain the crud odds ratios *OR* and its 95% CI

findings have been reported in some studies [24], but not in others [4, 9].Further prospective investigations are still needed to clarify the roles of metabolic disorders on GBP. In addition, recent studies showed that the abnormal metabolism not only contribute to the formation of GBP, but are also related to the polyps' malignant transformation [25, 26]. Studies on exploring the metabolism effects of polyp transformation are also expected.

Lifestyle factors with GBP

With regard to smoking, several previous studies found that this was inversely related to GB polyps; however, a Chinese study failed to find any association [1, 27, 28].

In our study, we found that current smoking was positively associated with GBP in univariate analysis. Another Chinese study also found smoking to be positively associated with GBP in univariate analysis; however, it was ruled out from multivariate logistic regression model [4]. We could not clarify the mechanism of smoking involved in GBP formation; however, according to the results of pathway analysis, smoking might contribute to GBP by elevating the TG level pathway. Drinking was found to be highly relevant to smoking in this study, and might combine with smoking, contributing to increase TG to GBP pathway. On the contrary, one animal experimental study reported that

Table 3 Metabolic indicators between case and control groups

Variables	Case	Control	P	Crud OR (95%CI)
BMI (kg/m^2)	24.6 ± 3.3	24.5 ± 3.8	0.763	1.01(0.97,1.04)
Blood pressure				
Diastolic pressure	127.1 ± 16.1	126.2 ± 17.4	0.404	1.00(1.00,1.01)
Systolic pressure	78.0 ± 11.6	77.7 ± 11.9	0.651	1.00(0.99,1.01)
Lipid profiles				
TC(mmol/L)	4.84 ± 0.94	4.89 ± 0.92	0.385	0.94(0.82,1.08)
TG(mmol/L)	1.51 ± 1.10	1.37 ± 0.81	0.028	1.16(1.02,1.33)
HDL-C(mmol/L)	1.27 ± 0.33	1.31 ± 0.31	0.063	0.69(0.47,1.02)
LDL-C(mmol/L)	2.62 ± 0.72	2.58 ± 0.66	0.360	1.09(0.91,1.31)
FBG (mmol/L)	5.7 ± 1.4	5.7 ± 2.4	0.820	0.99(0.93,1.06)
BUA (μmol/L)	339.0 ± 92.5	341.9 ± 96.5	0.633	1.00(1.00,1.00)

Binary logistic regression was used to obtain the crud odds ratios *OR* and its 95% CI

alcohol reduces biliary cholesterol saturation and increases the serum levels of high-density lipoprotein [29]. Similarly, one population-based study found a protective effect of alcohol use on GBP [27]; however, other study results failed to find this relationship [4]. The inconsistent results might be due to the different study design and different types of alcoholic drink. As symbols of lifestyle, there are many factors between smoking/drinking and GBP; further studies including etiological studies are necessary to clarify the roles of smoking and drinking in GBP.

Lots of studies have focused on dietary effects of gallbladder stones or gallbladder cancer, but not GBP. High fat intake seems to contribute to many gallbladder diseases [30]. For GBP, one Korean study reported GBP tended to be less common in vegetarians than in controls; however, the difference was statistically insignificant [31]. In this study, we found a higher frequency of meat intake associated with GBP in univariate analysis, and through pathway analysis, fatty food was related to a higher BMI and resulted in a high TG level associated with GBP. We inferred that excessive fatty food intake might result in the imbalances and increased plasma cholesterol concentration and/or induced hepatic hypersecretion of biliary cholesterol which causes GBP. More studies on the dietary effects of GBP are needed to fill in the gaps regarding dietary recommendations to prevent gallbladder disease.

Limitation
With a case-control design, inherent limitations of this study were unavoidable and the results should be treated with caution. The causality between risk factors and GBP in this study could not been observed. Although the cases were all newly diagnosed, recall bias might exist and residual confounding by imprecisely measured or unmeasured factors remains possible for our findings.

In this study, we did not identify types of GBP, the risk factors and pathological pathways might be different for different types of GBP.

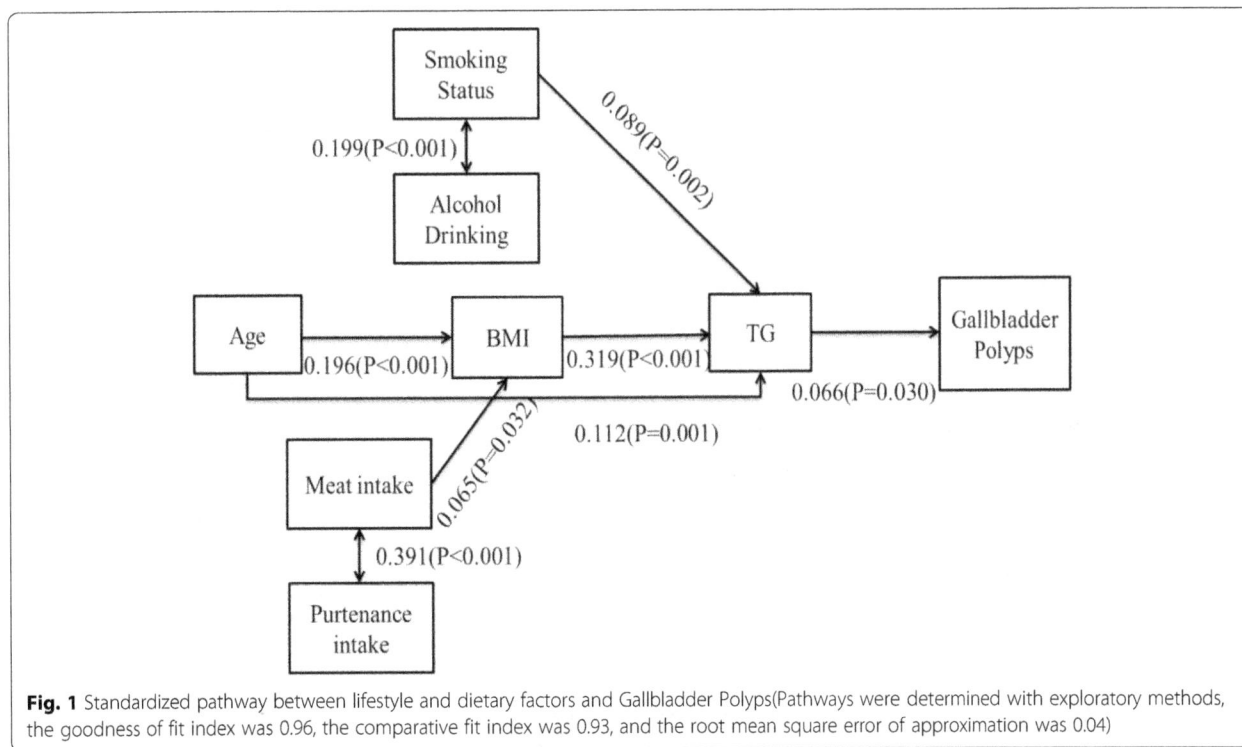

Fig. 1 Standardized pathway between lifestyle and dietary factors and Gallbladder Polyps(Pathways were determined with exploratory methods, the goodness of fit index was 0.96, the comparative fit index was 0.93, and the root mean square error of approximation was 0.04)

Conclusion

This study first use the Covariance Structure Analysis to explore the pathway among lifestyle factors, metabolic status and GBP. The current findings demonstrated that dyslipidemia is highly associated with GBP. More importantly, several modifiable factors such as smoking and high intake frequencies of meat or viscera might be the initial risk factors for GBP formation through increasing BMI and TG level pathways. More studies exploring modifiable factors with GBP are needed to build a strategy to prevent GBP.

Abbreviations

BUA: Blood uric acid; FBG: Fasting blood glucose; GBP: Gallbladder polyps; HDL-C: High density lipoprotein cholesterol; LDL-C: Low density lipoprotein cholesterol; TC: Total cholesterol; TG: Total triglyceride cholesterol

Acknowledgements
We sincerely acknowledged the volunteer participants involved in this study.

Funding
This study founded by National Natural Science Foundation of Liaoning Province (NO.:20170540239). The foundation not involved in the design of the study and collection, analysis, and interpretation of data and in writing the manuscript.

Authors' contributions
LS and YH conceived and designed the study; LS and PLL collected the data; AZ and ZW analyzed the data and draft the paper; LR, AZ and YH revised the manuscript and participated in the study supervision. All authors have read and approved the final manuscript.

Competing interests
The authors declare that they have no competing interests.

Author details
[1]Department of Epidemiology and Health Statistics, School of Public Health, Xi'an Jiaotong University Health Science Center, Xi'an, China. [2]Health Management Center, The Second Hospital of Dalian Medical University, Dalian, China. [3]School of Public Health, Peking University Health Science Center, Beijing, China. [4]Division of Endocrinology and Metabolism, Department of obstetrics, Beijing Obstetrics and Gynecology Hospital, Capital Medical University, Beijing, China.

References
1. Chen CY, Lu CL, Chang FY, Lee SD. Risk factors for gallbladder polyps in the Chinese population. Am J Gastroenterol. 1997;92:2066-8.
2. Lee KF, Wong J, Li JC, Lai PB. Polypoid lesions of the gallbladder. Am J Surg. 2004;188:186-90. https://doi.org/10.1016/j.amjsurg.2003.11.043.
3. Lee YJ, Park KS, Cho KB, Kim ES, Jang BK, Chung WJ, Hwang JS. Shifting prevalence of gallbladder polyps in Korea. J Korean Med Sci. 2014;29:1247-52. https://doi.org/10.3346/jkms.2014.29.9.1247.
4. Mao YS, Mai YF, Li FJ, Zhang YM, Hu KM, Hong ZL, Zhu ZW. Prevalence and risk factors of gallbladder polypoid lesions in Chinese petrochemical employees. World J Gastroenterol. 2013;19:4393-9. https://doi.org/10.3748/wjg.v19.i27.4393.
5. Aldouri AQ, Malik HZ, Waytt J, Khan S, Ranganathan K, Kummaraganti S, Hamilton W, Dexter S, Menon K, Lodge JP, Prasad KR, Toogood GJ. The risk of gallbladder cancer from polyps in a large multiethnic series. Eur J Surg Oncol. 2009;35:48-51. https://doi.org/10.1016/j.ejso.2008.01.036.
6. Park JK, Yoon YB, Kim YT, Ryu JK, Yoon WJ, Lee SH, Yu SJ, Kang HY, Lee JY, Park MJ. Management strategies for gallbladder polyps: is it possible to predict malignant gallbladder polyps? Gut Liver. 2008;2:88-94. https://doi.org/10.5009/gnl.2008.2.2.88.
7. Wiles R, Thoeni RF, Barbu ST, Vashist YK, Rafaelsen SR, Dewhurst C, Arvanitakis M, Lahaye M, Soltes M, Perinel J, Roberts SA. Management and follow-up of gallbladder polyps : Joint guidelines between the European Society of Gastrointestinal and Abdominal Radiology (ESGAR), European Association for Endoscopic Surgery and other Interventional Techniques (EAES), International Society of Digestive Surgery - European Federation (EFISDS) and European Society of Gastrointestinal Endoscopy (ESGE). Eur Radiol. 2017;27(9):3856-66. https://doi.org/10.1007/s00330-017-4742-y.
8. Xu Q, Tao LY, Wu Q, Gao F, Zhang FL, Yuan L, He XD. Prevalences of and risk factors for biliary stones and gallbladder polyps in a large Chinese population. HPB (Oxford). 2012;14:373-81. https://doi.org/10.1111/j.1477-2574.2012.00457.x.
9. Lin WR, Lin DY, Tai DI, Hsieh SY, Lin CY, Sheen IS, Chiu CT. Prevalence of and risk factors for gallbladder polyps detected by ultrasonography among healthy Chinese: analysis of 34 669 cases. J Gastroenterol Hepatol. 2008;23:965-9. https://doi.org/10.1111/j.1440-1746.2007.05071.x.
10. Unisa S, Jagannath P, Dhir V, Khandelwal C, Sarangi L, Roy TK. Population-based study to estimate prevalence and determine risk factors of gallbladder diseases in the rural Gangetic basin of North India. HPB (Oxford). 2011;13:117-25. https://doi.org/10.1111/j.1477-2574.2010.00255.x.
11. Lim SH, Kim DH, Park MJ, Kim YS, Kim CH, Yim JY, Cho KR, Kim SS, Choi SH, Kim N, Cho SH, Oh BH. Is metabolic syndrome one of the risk factors for gallbladder polyps found by ultrasonography during health screening? Gut Liver. 2007;1:138-44. https://doi.org/10.5009/gnl.2007.1.2.138.
12. Park EJ, Lee HS, Lee SH, Chun HJ, Kim SY, Choi YK, Ryu HJ, Shim KW. Association between metabolic syndrome and gallbladder polyps in healthy Korean adults. J Korean Med Sci. 2013;28:876-80. https://doi.org/10.3346/jkms.2013.28.6.876.
13. Khairy GA, Guraya SY, Murshid KR. Cholesterolosis. Incidence, correlation with serum cholesterol level and the role of laparoscopic cholecystectomy. Saudi Med J. 2004;25:1226-8.
14. Ivanchenkova RA, Sviridov AV, Ozerova IN, Perova NV, Grachev SV. High-density lipoproteins in cholesterosis of the gall bladder. Klin Med (Mosk). 2000;78:27-31.
15. Zak A, Zeman M, Hrubant K, Vecka M, Tvrzicka E. Effect of hypolipidemic treatment on the composition of bile and the risk or cholesterol gallstone disease. Cas Lek Cesk. 2007;146:24-34.
16. Yang HL, Kong L, Hou LL, Shen HF, Wang Y, Gu XG, Qin JM, Yin PH, Li Q. Analysis of risk factors for polypoid lesions of gallbladder among health examinees. World J Gastroenterol. 2012;18:3015-9. https://doi.org/10.3748/wjg.v18.i23.3015.
17. Goodloe R, Brown-Gentry K, Gillani NB, Jin H, Mayo P, Allen M, McClellan BJ, Boston J, Sutcliffe C, Schnetz-Boutaud N, Dilks HH, Crawford DC. Lipid trait-associated genetic variation is associated with gallstone disease in the diverse third National Health and nutrition examination survey (NHANES III). BMC Med Genet. 2013;14:120. https://doi.org/10.1186/1471-2350-14-120.
18. Jacyna MR, Bouchier IA. Cholesterolosis: A physical cause of "functional" disorder. Br Med J (Clin Res Ed). 1987;295:619-20.
19. Sandri L, Colecchia A, Larocca A, Vestito A, Capodicasa S, Azzaroli F, Mazzella G, Mwangemi C, Roda E, Festi D. Gallbladder cholesterol polyps and cholesterolosis. Minerva Gastroenterol Dietol. 2003;49:217-24.
20. Segawa K, Arisawa T, Niwa Y, Suzuki T, Tsukamoto Y, Goto H, Hamajima E, Shimodaira M, Ohmiya N. Prevalence of gallbladder polyps among apparently healthy Japanese: ultrasonographic study. Am J Gastroenterol. 1992;87:630-3.

21. Canturk Z, Senturk O, Canturk NZ, Anik YA. Prevalence and risk factors for gall bladder polyps. East Afr Med J. 2007;84:336–41.

22. Lee JK, Hahn SJ, Kang HW, Jung JG, Choi HS, Lee JH, Han IW, Jung JH, Kwon JH. Visceral obesity is associated with gallbladder polyps. Gut Liver. 2016;10:133–9. https://doi.org/10.5009/gnl14506.

23. Lim SH, Kim D, Kang JH, Song JH, Yang SY, Yim JY, Chung SJ, Kim JS, Cho SH. Hepatic fat, not visceral fat, is associated with gallbladder polyps: a study of 2643 healthy subjects. J Gastroenterol Hepatol. 2015;30:767–74. https://doi.org/10.1111/jgh.12841.

24. Kim SY, Lee HS, Lee YS, Chung KW, Jang BK, Chung WJ, Park KS, Cho KB, Hwang JS. Prevalence and risk factors of gallbladder polyp in adults living in Daegu and Gyeongbuk provinces. Korean J Gastroenterol. 2006;48:344–50.

25. Xue K, Li FF, Chen YW, Zhou YH, He J. Body mass index and the risk of cancer in women compared with men: a meta-analysis of prospective cohort studies. Eur J Cancer Prev. 2017;26:94–105. https://doi.org/10.1097/CEJ.0000000000000231.

26. John BJ, Irukulla S, Abulafi AM, Kumar D, Mendall MA. Systematic review: adipose tissue, obesity and gastrointestinal diseases. Aliment Pharmacol Ther. 2006;23:1511–23. https://doi.org/10.1111/j.1365-2036.2006.02915.x.

27. Okamoto M, Yamagata Z, Takeda Y, Yoda Y, Kobayashi K, Fujino MA. The relationship between gallbladder disease and smoking and drinking habits in middle-aged Japanese. J Gastroenterol. 2002;37:455–62. https://doi.org/10.1007/s005350200066.

28. Shinchi K, Kono S, Honjo S, Imanishi K, Hirohata T. Epidemiology of gallbladder polyps: an ultrasonographic study of male self-defense officials in Japan. Scand J Gastroenterol. 1994;29:7–10.

29. Schwesinger WH, Kurtin WE, Johnson R. Alcohol protects against cholesterol gallstone formation. Ann Surg. 1988;207:641–7.

30. Di Ciaula A, Garruti G, Fruhbeck G, De Angelis M, De Bari O, Q-H WD, Lammert F, Portincasa P. The role of diet in the pathogenesis of cholesterol gallstones. Curr Med Chem. 2017. https://doi.org/10.2174/0929867324666170530080636.

31. Jo HB, Lee JK, Choi MY, Han IW, Choi HS, Kang HW, Kim JH, Lim YJ, Koh MS, Lee JH. Is the prevalence of gallbladder polyp different between vegetarians and general population? Korean J Gastroenterol. 2015;66:268–73. https://doi.org/10.4166/kjg.2015.66.5.268.

23

Hepatocellular carcinoma is the most common liver-related complication in patients with histopathologically-confirmed NAFLD in Japan

Norio Akuta[1*], Yusuke Kawamura[1], Yasuji Arase[1], Satoshi Saitoh[1], Shunichiro Fujiyama[1,1], Hitomi Sezaki[1], Tetsuya Hosaka[1], Masahiro Kobayashi[1], Mariko Kobayashi[2], Yoshiyuki Suzuki[1], Fumitaka Suzuki[1], Kenji Ikeda[1] and Hiromitsu Kumada[1]

Abstract

Background: The incidence of liver-related events, cardiovascular events and type 2 diabetes mellitus in patients with histopathologically confirmed NAFLD remains unclear.

Methods: We retrospectively investigated the incidence of liver events, cardiovascular events, malignancy, and type 2 diabetes mellitus in 402 Japanese patients with histopathologically confirmed NAFLD for a median follow-up of 4. 2 years. We also investigated predictors of the development of hepatocellular carcinoma and type 2 diabetes mellitus in these patients.

Results: The rate of liver-related events per 1000 person years was 4.17 (hepatocellular carcinoma, 3.67; hepatic encephalopathy, 1.60; esophago-gastric varices, 2.43; ascites, 0.80; and jaundice, 0.40). The rate of cardiovascular events and type 2 diabetes mellitus was 5.73 and 9.95, respectively. Overall mortality was 3.33 (liver-related events, 1.25; cardiovascular events, 0.42; and malignancies other than hepatocellular carcinoma, 0.83), in patients free of previous or current malignancies. Multivariate analyses identified old age (≥70 years) and advanced fibrosis stage 4 as significant determinants of hepatocellular carcinoma development, and hepatocyte steatosis (> 33%), female sex, and serum ferritin (≤80 μg/l) as significant determinants of type 2 diabetes mellitus development in these patients.

Conclusions: Our results highlighted the importance of cardiovascular and liver-related events in Japanese patients with histopathologically-confirmed NAFLD. Hepatocellular carcinoma was the most common liver-related event, and the incidence of hepatocellular carcinoma was more than half of that of cardiovascular events.

Keywords: Nonalcoholic fatty liver disease, Nonalcoholic steatohepatitis, Hepatocellular carcinoma, Liver-related events, Cardiovascular events, Type 2 diabetes mellitus, Malignancy, Mortality, Fibrosis stage, Hepatocyte steatosis

Background

The most common liver disease worldwide is non-alcoholic fatty liver disease (NAFLD) [1–6]. Liver pathology ranges from the typically benign non-alcoholic fatty liver to non-alcoholic steatohepatitis (NASH), which may progress to liver cirrhosis, hepatocellular carcinoma (HCC), and liver failure [7].

The incidence of liver events, cardiovascular events, malignancy, and type 2 diabetes mellitus (T2DM) in patients with histopathologically confirmed NAFLD remains unclear. T2DM and fibrosis stage are significant and independent risk factors for HCC in patients with NAFLD [5]. Results of recent prospective studies have shown that antidiabetic drugs may improve histological features, including fibrosis stage [8–10]. Thus, it may be important to identify predictors of the development of

* Correspondence: akuta-gi@umin.ac.jp; norioakuta@toranomon.gr.jp
[1]Department of Hepatology, Toranomon Hospital and Okinaka Memorial Institute for Medical Research, 2-2-2 Toranomon, Minato-ku, Tokyo 105-0001, Japan
Full list of author information is available at the end of the article

HCC and T2DM to improve the prognosis of patients with NAFLD.

It has been suggested that fibrosis stage may be more reliable than the NAFLD activity score (NAS) for the prediction of liver-specific mortality [11]. Fibrosis stage, but not other histopathological features of steatohepatitis, was reported to be an independent and significant predictor of overall mortality, liver transplantation, and liver-related events [12].

The purpose of the present study was to determine the incidence of liver-related events, cardiovascular events, and T2DM, and the predictors of development of HCC and T2DM in patients with NAFLD by retrospectively analyzing the outcome of 402 Japanese patients with histopathologically confirmed NAFLD.

Methods

Patients

This is a retrospective cohort study of patients with histopathologically-confirmed NAFLD. Between 1976 and 2017, liver biopsy was performed at our hospital for patients with liver dysfunction and/or fatty liver diagnosed by abdominal ultrasonography. Of those, the diagnosis of NAFLD was confirmed in 402 patients by histopathology. The median duration of follow-up, from diagnosis to death or last visit, was 4.2 years (range, 0.0–41.4 years), and the total sum of person-years was 2625 years. The characteristics of the patients at the time of histopathological diagnosis of NAFLD are summarized in Table 1. Patients with histopathological changes of steatosis in at least 5% of hepatocytes and alcohol intake < 20 g/day were included in the analysis. We excluded patients with 1) underlying liver disease (e.g., viral hepatitis, autoimmune hepatitis, drug-induced liver disease, or primary biliary cirrhosis); 2) systemic autoimmune diseases (e.g., systemic lupus erythematosus and rheumatoid arthritis); and 3) metabolic diseases (e.g., hemochromatosis, α-1-antitrypsin deficiency, or Wilson disease).

The study was conducted in compliance with the International Conference on Harmonisation guidelines for Good Clinical Practice (E6) and the 2013 Declaration of Helsinki. The protocol was approved by the institutional review board at Toranomon Hospital (number 953). Written informed consent was provided by all patients prior to liver biopsy.

Diagnosis and follow-up

Liver-related events included HCC, hepatic encephalopathy, esophago-gastric varices with bleeding, ascites, and jaundice. Cardiovascular events included coronary artery disease, heart valve disease, arrhythmia, heart failure, hypertension, orthostatic hypotension, shock, endocarditis, diseases of the aorta and its branches, disorders of

Table 1 Patient characteristics at the time of histological diagnosis of NAFLD

Demographic data	
Numbers of patients	402
Gender, Male / Female, n	245 / 157
Age, y[a]	51 (20–87)
Body mass index, kg/m²[a]	26.1 (18.1–42.4)
Presence of previous and current malignancy	
None / Hepatocellular carcinoma / Other malignancy, n	351 / 26 / 30
Type 2 diabetes mellitus, Absence / Presence, n	276 / 126
Hypertension, Absence / Presence, n	230 / 172
Hyperlipidemia, Absence / Presence, n	274 / 128
Histological findings	
Steatosis, 5–33% / > 33–66% / > 66%, n	152 / 149 / 98
Lobular inflammation	
No foci / < 2 foci / 2–4 foci / > 4 foci per 200× field, n	28 / 242 / 116 / 13
Ballooning, None / Few cells / Many cells, n	39 / 252 / 108
Stage, 0 / 1 / 2 / 3 / 4, n	48 / 165 / 63 / 98 / 28
NAFLD activity score, ≤2 / 3, 4 / ≥5, n	34 / 181 / 184
Diagnosis according to FLIP algorithm, NASH / non-NASH, n	349 / 50
Laboratory data[a]	
Serum aspartate aminotransferase, IU/l	44 (3–378)
Serum alanine aminotransferase, IU/l	69 (15–783)
Gamma-glutamyl transpeptidase, IU/l	72 (11–990)
Platelet count, ×10³/mm³	213 (40–471)
Fasting plasma glucose, mg/dl	101 (65–287)
HbA1c, %	5.9 (4.4–12.6)
Uric acid, mg/dl	5.9 (1.9–11.1)
Total cholesterol, mg/dl	204 (101–370)
Triglycerides, mg/dl	140 (31–1088)
High-density lipoprotein cholesterol, mg/dl	45 (14–85)
Low-density lipoprotein cholesterol, mg/dl	120 (27–243)
Serum ferritin, µg/l	227 (< 10–2067)
High sensitive C-reactive protein, mg/dl	0.095 (0.006–2.240)
Alpha-fetoprotein, µg/l	4 (1–10,930)
PIVKA-II, AU/l	18 (1–157,050)

Data are number of patients, except those denoted by [a], which represent the median (range) values

the peripheral vascular system, and stroke. Furthermore, the incidence of T2DM and other malignancies, apart from HCCs, were also evaluated. The incidence of T2DM was assessed at least twice a year after baseline examination. T2DM was diagnosed as the presence of elevated fasting plasma glucose (≥126 mg/dl), elevated

HbA1c (≥6.5%) or self-reported history of clinical diagnosis.

Hematological and biochemical data were collected at least twice yearly after the diagnosis of NAFLD. Ultrasonography, computed tomography, or magnetic resonance imaging studies were performed at least once annually.

The clinical details of the events of 3 patients were missing. The rate of cancer development was evaluated only in patients confirmed to have no previous or existing HCC at the time of diagnosis of NAFLD, and no previous or current other malignancies apart from HCCs. The rates of development of hepatic encephalopathy, esophago-gastric varices, ascites, and jaundice were evaluated in patients confirmed to have no previous or current hepatic encephalopathy, esophago-gastric varices, ascites, jaundice or HCC at the time of NAFLD

diagnosis, respectively. Mortality was evaluated in patients, who had no previous or present malignancies at the time of NAFLD diagnosis. Details of patient enrolment are shown in Fig. 1.

Liver histopathology

Liver specimens were obtained with a 14-gauge modified Vim Silverman needle (Tohoku University style, Kakinuma Factory, Tokyo, Japan), a 16-gauge core tissue biopsy needle (Bard Peripheral Vascular Inc., Tempe, AZ) or surgical resection. Specimen was fixed in 10% formalin, and the prepared sections were stained with hematoxylin-eosin, Masson trichrome, silver impregnation, or periodic acid-Schiff after diastase digestion. Four pathologists (K.K., F.K., T.F., and T.F.), who were blinded to the clinical findings, evaluated each specimen, and the final assessment was reported by consensus. An

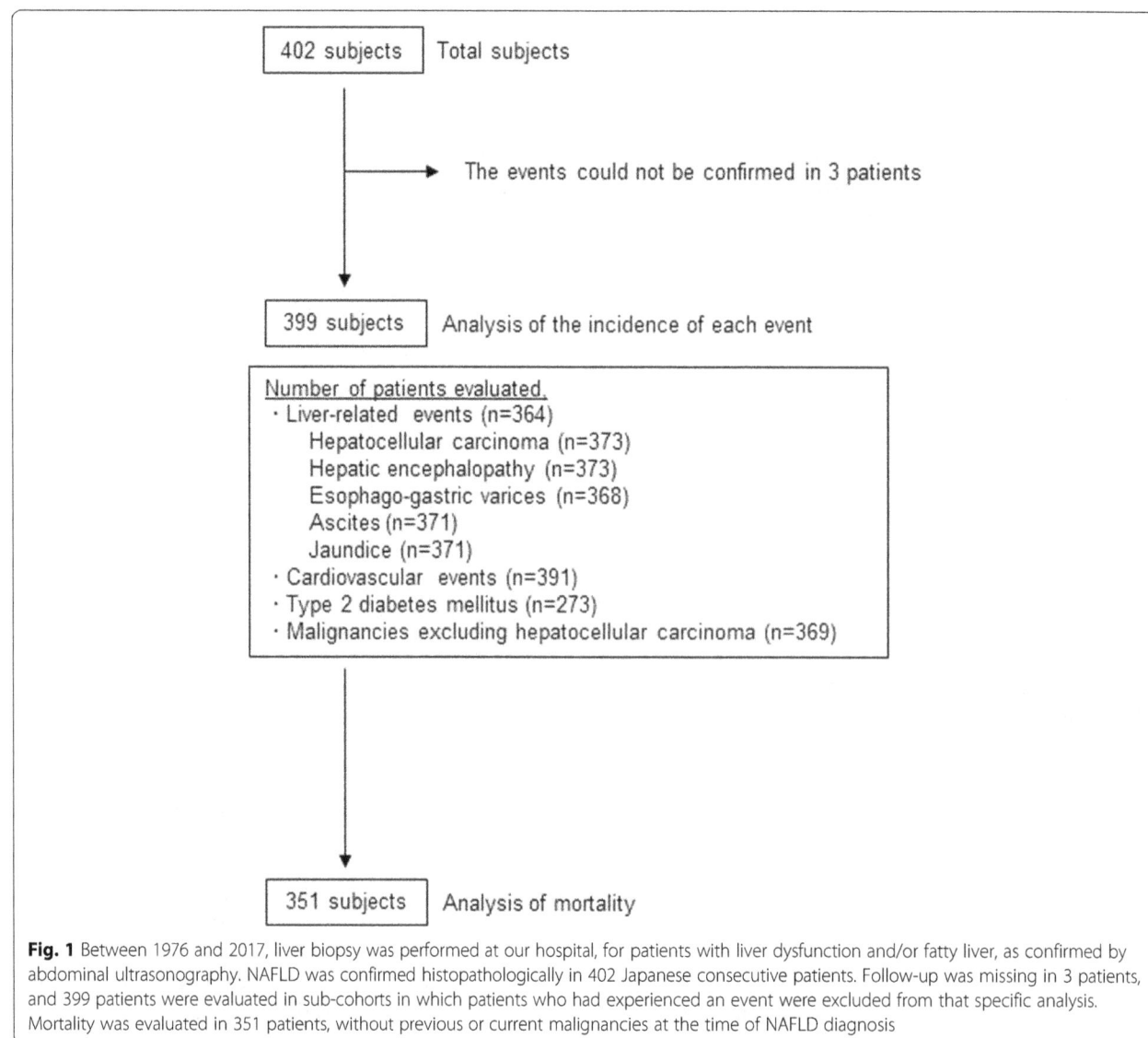

Fig. 1 Between 1976 and 2017, liver biopsy was performed at our hospital, for patients with liver dysfunction and/or fatty liver, as confirmed by abdominal ultrasonography. NAFLD was confirmed histopathologically in 402 Japanese consecutive patients. Follow-up was missing in 3 patients, and 399 patients were evaluated in sub-cohorts in which patients who had experienced an event were excluded from that specific analysis. Mortality was evaluated in 351 patients, without previous or current malignancies at the time of NAFLD diagnosis

adequate liver biopsy sample was defined as a specimen longer than 1.5 cm and/or containing more than 11 portal tracts.

Steatosis grade 0, 1, 2, and 3 corresponded to steatosis of < 5%, ≥5 to < 33%, ≥33 to < 66%, and ≥ 66% of hepatocytes, respectively. Lobular inflammation with no foci, < 2 foci, 2–4 foci, and ≥ 4 foci per 200× field was scored as 0, 1, 2, and 3, respectively. Hepatocyte ballooning of none, few, and many cells was scored as 0, 1, and 2, respectively. The sum of the steatosis, lobular inflammation, and hepatocyte ballooning scores (range, 0–8 points) was the NAS [13]. Fibrosis stage was defined as 0, 1, 2, 3, and 4 [13, 14]. NASH was defined according to the Fatty Liver Inhibition of Progression (FLIP) algorithm [15].

Clinical parameters
We analyzed clinicopathological parameters that could affect NAFLD prognosis. At our hospital, the normal range of aspartate aminotransferase (AST) was 13–33 IU/l, and the normal range of alanine aminotransferase (ALT) was 8–42 IU/l for males and 6–27 IU/l for females. Obesity was defined as body mass index of > 25.0 kg/m^2.

Statistical analysis
The incidence of each event was analyzed during the period from the time of histopathological diagnosis of NAFLD until the last visit or occurrence of event. Stepwise Cox regression analysis was used to determine independent predictive factors associated with the development of HCC and T2DM. The hazard ratio (HR) and 95% confidence interval (95% CI) were also calculated. Variables that were statistically significant on univariate analysis were tested by multivariate analysis to identify significant independent factors. Significance was set at p value < 0.05 by the two-tailed test. Statistical comparisons were performed with the SPSS software (SPSS Inc., Chicago, IL, USA).

Results
Incidence of liver-related events in NAFLD
During the follow-up, 9/373 (2.4%) patients developed HCC (rate per 1000 person years, 3.67), and 21/369 (5.7%) patients developed malignancies other than HCC (rate per 1000 person years, 8.93).

4/373 (1.1%) patients developed hepatic encephalopathy (rate per 1000 person years, 1.60). 6/368 (1.6%) patients developed esophago-gastric varices (rate per 1000 person years, 2.43). 2/371 (0.5%) patients developed ascites (rate per 1000 person years, 0.80). 1/371 (0.3%) patient developed jaundice (rate per 1000 person years, 0.40).

Hence, 10 of 364 patients (2.8%) confirmed to have no previous or current liver-related events at NAFLD diagnosis developed liver-related events (rate per 1000 person years, 4.17) (Table 2).

Predictors of development of HCC in patients with NAFLD
The characteristics of the 373 patients confirmed to have no previous or current HCC at the time of NAFLD diagnosis were evaluated for prediction of HCC development. Twenty-seven potential predictive factors of the clinicopathological parameters were analyzed (Table 3). Univariate analysis identified the following five parameters that correlated significantly with HCC development: age, fibrosis stage, platelet count, total cholesterol, and α-fetoprotein. These factors were entered into multivariate analysis, which identified two factors that significantly and independently influenced HCC development: advanced age (≥70 years; HR 9.54, 95% CI = 1.63–55.9, P = 0.012) and advanced fibrosis stage (stage 4; HR 7.14, 95% CI = 1.29–39.5, P = 0.024) (Table 3).

Rate of development of cardiovascular events in NAFLD
The characteristics of the 391 patients confirmed to have no previous or current cardiovascular events at NAFLD diagnosis were evaluated for the rate of development of cardiovascular events. During the follow-up, 14 patients (3.6%) developed cardiovascular events, and the development rate per 1000 person years was 5.73 (Table 2).

Rate and predictors of development of T2DM in NAFLD
The incidence of type 2 diabetes mellitus was evaluated in patients confirmed to have no previous or current T2DM (n = 273) at the time of NAFLD diagnosis. During the follow-up, 19 (7.0%) patients developed T2DM (rate per 1000 person years, 9.95) (Table 2).

The characteristics of the 273 patients confirmed to have no previous or current T2DM at the time of

Table 2 Incidence of liver events, cardiovascular events and type 2 diabetes mellitus in patients with NAFLD

Events	n/N (%)[a]	1000 person years
Liver-related events[b]	10/364 (2.8%)	4.17
Hepatocellular carcinoma	9/373 (2.4%)	3.67
Hepatic encephalopathy	4/373 (1.1%)	1.60
Esophago-gastric varices	6/368 (1.6%)	2.43
Ascites	2/371 (0.5%)	0.80
Jaundice	1/371 (0.3%)	0.40
Cardiovascular events	14/391 (3.6%)	5.73
Type 2 diabetes mellitus	19/273 (7.0%)	9.95
Malignancies except for hepatocellular carcinoma	21/369 (5.7%)	8.93

[a]n; number of events. N; number of patients, not having, or having had, the respective event simultaneously or previously to the time of NAFLD diagnosis
[b]Liver-related events were evaluated in patients, without previous or current hepatocellular carcinoma at the time of NAFLD diagnosis

Table 3 Predictors of development of hepatocellular carcinoma in patients with NAFLD

Factor	Category	Univariate Hazard ratio	(95% CI)	P value*	Multivariate Hazard ratio	(95% CI)	P value*
Demographic data							
Gender	Male	1					
	Female	0.24	(0.03–1.97)	0.186			
Age	< 70 y	1			1		
	≥70 y	18.6	(3.74–92.6)	< 0.001	9.54	(1.63–55.9)	0.012
Body mass index	< 25.0 kg/m^2	1					
	≥25.0 kg/m^2	0.46	(0.11–1.88)	0.276			
Type 2 diabetes mellitus	Absence	1					
	Presence	3.64	(0.95–14.0)	0.060			
Hypertension	Absence	1					
	Presence	1.06	(0.28–3.95)	0.932			
Hyperlipidemia	Absence	1					
	Presence	0.36	(0.05–2.91)	0.339			
Histological findings							
Steatosis	5–33%	1					
	> 33%	0.40	(0.10–1.63)	0.201			
Lobular inflammation	< 2 foci per 200× field	1					
	≥2 foci per 200× field	0.31	(0.04–2.50)	0.272			
Ballooning	None / Few cells	1					
	Many cells	0.47	(0.05–3.84)	0.482			
Stage	0–3	1			1		
	4	33.9	(7.14–161)	< 0.001	7.14	(1.29–39.5)	0.024
NAFLD activity score	< 5	1					
	≥5	0.19	(0.02–1.50)	0.114			
Diagnosis according to FLIP algorithm	non-NASH	1					
	NASH	1.34	(0.17–10.8)	0.784			
Laboratory data							
Serum aspartate aminotransferase	< 2 × ULN IU/l	1					
	≥2 × ULN IU/l	2.74	(0.73–10.2)	0.134			
Serum alanine aminotransferase	< 2 × ULN IU/l	1					
	≥2 × ULN IU/l	0.85	(0.22–3.22)	0.810			
Gamma-glutamyl transpeptidase	< 110 IU/l	1					
	≥110 IU/l	1.29	(0.34–4.86)	0.706			
Platelet count	< 200 × 10^3/mm^3	1			1		
	≥200 × 10^3/mm^3	0.06	(0.01–0.50)	0.009	0.14	(0.01–1.33)	0.086
Fasting plasma glucose	< 110 mg/dl	1					
	≥110 mg/dl	3.61	(0.85–15.3)	0.081			
HbA1c	< 5.8%	1					
	≥5.8%	56.2	(0.01–634,349)	0.397			
Uric acid	< 7.1 mg/dl	1					
	≥7.1 mg/dl	0.03	(0.00–21.0)	0.298			
Total cholesterol	< 200 mg/dl	1					
	≥200 mg/dl	0.18	(0.04–0.87)	0.033			

Table 3 Predictors of development of hepatocellular carcinoma in patients with NAFLD (Continued)

Factor	Category	Univariate Hazard ratio	(95% CI)	P value*	Multivariate Hazard ratio	(95% CI)	P value*
Triglycerides	< 150 mg/dl	1					
	≥150 mg/dl	0.46	(0.09–2.28)	0.342			
High-density lipoprotein cholesterol	< 41 mg/dl	1					
	≥41 mg/dl	0.58	(0.15–2.25)	0.428			
Low-density lipoprotein cholesterol	< 136 mg/dl	1					
	≥136 mg/dl	0.24	(0.03–2.06)	0.191			
Serum ferritin	< 81 μg/l	1					
	≥81 μg/l	0.71	(0.14–3.61)	0.674			
High sensitive C-reactive protein	< 0.2 mg/dl	1					
	≥0.2 mg/dl	1.02	(0.11–10.0)	0.984			
Alpha-fetoprotein	< 5 μg/l	1			1		
	≥5 μg/l	7.15	(1.44–35.6)	0.016	4.44	(0.84–23.4)	0.079
PIVKA-II	< 21 AU/l	1					
	≥21 AU/l	0.47	(0.06–4.05)	0.495			

*Significance was determined using a Cox proportional hazard model. CI confidence interval, ULN upper limit of normal

histopathological diagnosis of NAFLD were evaluated for prediction of T2DM development. Twenty-six potential predictive factors of the clinicopathological parameters were analyzed (Table 4). Univariate analysis identified the following five parameters that correlated significantly with T2DM development: gender, hepatocyte steatosis, γ-glutamyl transpeptidase, low-density lipoprotein cholesterol, and serum ferritin. These factors were entered into multivariate analysis, which identified three factors that significantly and independently influenced T2DM development: gender (female; HR 5.83, 95% CI = 1.47–23.1, P = 0.012), hepatocyte steatosis (> 33%; HR 9.52, 95% CI = 1.57–57.6, P = 0.014), and serum ferritin (≥81 μg/l; HR 0.18, 95% CI = 0.06–0.56, P = 0.003) (Table 4).

Mortality in NAFLD, without previous or current malignancies

In patients without previous or present malignancies at the time of NAFLD diagnosis, the overall mortality per 1000 person years was 3.33. The rate was 1.25 for those who died of liver-related events, 0.42 for those who died of cardiovascular events, and 0.83 for those who died of malignancies events other than HCC (Table 5). In the 3 patients who died from liver-related events, 2 of 3 patients and 1 of 3 patients had HCC and liver failure, respectively.

Discussion

The incidence of liver-related and cardiovascular events in patients with histopathologically confirmed NAFLD remains unclear. Furthermore, it is important to identify the predictors of development of HCC and T2DM to improve the prognosis of patients with NAFLD. There is limited information on the long-term development rate of these events in patients with histopathologically confirmed NAFLD [16, 17].

We found that patients with NAFLD were at increased risk of HCC (HR 6.55, P = 0.001) and cardiovascular diseases (HR 1.55, P = 0.01) [18]. In the present study, cardiovascular events had the highest incidence (5.73 per 1000 person years), with liver-related events the second highest incidence (4.17 per 1000 person years). Interestingly, among liver-related events, HCC was the event with the highest incidence (3.67 per 1000 person years). The incidence of HCC was more than half of that of cardiovascular events (3.67 vs. 5.73 per 1000 person years). In the present study, the mortality of liver-related events per 1000 person years (1.25) was not lower than that of cardiovascular events (0.42) and malignancies other than HCC (0.83). Hence, liver-related events accounted for about one-third of mortality in NAFLD patients who presented with no previous or present malignancies at the time of NAFLD diagnosis.

The present study has certain limitations. First, only a small number of deaths (8 patients) were recorded during the study period. Further studies of larger number of patients with NAFLD and longer follow-up period should be performed to investigate the impact of each event on mortality.

In another study, the incidence of HCC among all malignancies reported in 1600 patients with NAFLD diagnosed based on the presence of fatty liver by ultrasonography, was 6.0%, and the rate per 1000 person

Table 4 Predictors of development of type 2 diabetes mellitus in patients with NAFLD

Factor	Category	Univariate Hazard ratio	(95% CI)	P value*	Multivariate Hazard ratio	(95% CI)	P value*
Demographic data							
Gender	Male	1			1		
	Female	5.59	(2.07–15.1)	0.001	5.83	(1.47–23.1)	0.012
Age	< 70 y	1					
	≥70 y	0.05	(0.00–5618)	0.606			
Body mass index	< 25.0 kg/m^2	1					
	≥25.0 kg/m^2	1.41	(0.56–3.57)	0.472			
Hypertension	Absence	1					
	Presence	1.53	(0.62–3.77)	0.357			
Hyperlipidemia	Absence	1					
	Presence	1.20	(0.43–3.56)	0.732			
Histological findings							
Steatosis	5–33%	1			1		
	> 33%	3.30	(1.09–10.0)	0.035	9.52	(1.57–57.6)	0.014
Lobular inflammation	< 2 foci per 200× field	1					
	≥2 foci per 200× field	1.70	(0.63–4.57)	0.296			
Ballooning	None / Few cells	1					
	Many cells	0.57	(0.13–2.49)	0.452			
Stage	0–3	1					
	4	1.47	(0.20–11.0)	0.711			
NAFLD activity score	< 5	1					
	≥5	1.30	(0.51–3.26)	0.583			
Diagnosis according to FLIP algorithm	non-NASH	1					
	NASH	1.42	(0.41–4.90)	0.579			
Laboratory data							
Serum aspartate aminotransferase	< 2 × ULN IU/l	1					
	≥2 × ULN IU/l	1.19	(0.45–3.13)	0.730			
Serum alanine aminotransferase	< 2 × ULN IU/l	1					
	≥2 × ULN IU/l	1.47	(0.59–3.64)	0.408			
Gamma-glutamyl transpeptidase	< 110 IU/l	1					
	≥110 IU/l	0.28	(0.08–0.96)	0.043			
Platelet count	< 200 × 10^3/mm^3	1					
	≥200 × 10^3/mm^3	1.94	(0.64–5.87)	0.239			
Fasting plasma glucose	< 110 mg/dl	1					
	≥110 mg/dl	1.31	(0.37–4.62)	0.672			
HbA1c	< 5.8%	1					
	≥5.8%	2.33	(0.32–16.9)	0.404			
Uric acid	< 7.1 mg/dl	1					
	≥7.1 mg/dl	1.28	(0.49–3.38)	0.615			
Total cholesterol	< 200 mg/dl	1					
	≥200 mg/dl	2.43	(0.80–7.34)	0.116			
Triglycerides	< 150 mg/dl	1					
	≥150 mg/dl	0.78	(0.31–1.97)	0.594			

Table 4 Predictors of development of type 2 diabetes mellitus in patients with NAFLD *(Continued)*

Factor	Category	Univariate Hazard ratio	(95% CI)	P value*	Multivariate Hazard ratio	(95% CI)	P value*
High-density lipoprotein cholesterol	< 41 mg/dl	1					
	≥41 mg/dl	0.49	(0.20–1.20)	0.117			
Low-density lipoprotein cholesterol	< 136 mg/dl	1					
	≥136 mg/dl	3.20	(1.06–9.69)	0.040			
Serum ferritin	< 81 μg/l	1			1		
	≥81 μg/l	0.26	(0.10–0.70)	0.008	0.18	(0.06–0.56)	0.003
High sensitive C-reactive protein	< 0.2 mg/dl	1					
	≥0.2 mg/dl	1.84	(0.57–5.97)	0.312			
Alpha-fetoprotein	< 5 μg/l	1					
	≥5 μg/l	1.08	(0.38–3.04)	0.887			
PIVKA-II	< 21 AU/l	1					
	≥21 AU/l	0.23	(0.03–1.79)	0.160			

*Significance was determined using a Cox proportional hazard model. *CI* confidence interval, *ULN* upper limit of normal

years was 0.78, [19]. However, the results of our study indicated that the rate per 1000 person years was 3.67, and rate of HCC was higher compared to the above studies. The discrepant results could reflect patient selection bias, as all patients had histopathologically confirmed NAFLD, with elevated aminotransferases (indicators of high activity) and/or low levels of platelet counts (indicator of advanced fibrosis stage). Furthermore, patients treated with anti-platelet agents and anticoagulants for the prevention of cardiovascular events, did not undergo liver biopsy, and were thus not included. Also, patients who visit the hospital regularly tend to receive treatments for hypertension, hyperlipidemia, and diabetes mellitus, which are as risk factors of cardiovascular events. As previously reported [5], multivariate analysis identified advanced fibrosis stage and old age as significant and independent determinants of HCC development.

Seko and colleagues [20] reported that 13 of 89 (14.6%) patients with biopsy-confirmed NAFLD developed T2DM, and multivariate analysis identified the presence of insulin resistance as an independent risk factor for the development of T2DM. The present study showed that 19 of 273 (6.96%) patients developed T2DM, which is a lower rate compared to the above study. The discrepant results could be due to differences in the diagnostic methods for T2DM; patients in the previous study were diagnosed with a 75-g oral glucose tolerance test. The other reasons for the low frequency of T2DM development is probably that many patients had diabetes at the time of liver biopsy and the follow-up time was short, i.e. selection bias and short follow-up. Interestingly, multivariate analysis in the present study identified higher frequencies of hepatocyte steatosis, lower levels of serum ferritin, and female sex as significant and independent determinants of the incidence of T2DM. Previous reports showed that the incidence of T2DM is higher in postmenopausal female patients with hepatocyte steatosis [17, 21]. However, at this stage, we do not known why lower levels of serum ferritin influence the incidence of T2DM. This finding must be further explored and validated in a larger independent cohort.

Other limitations of the present study included the retrospective study design and the fact that the patients in our study were inpatients. We could not investigate whether factors during the course of observation, such as weight loss and exercise, might affect the development of HCC and T2DM. Furthermore, all participants were Japanese, and thus the results might not be applicable to patients of other races or ethnic groups. Also, the study did not address the epidemiological burden and complexity of the natural history of NAFLD [22, 23]. Identification of predictors of development of HCC and T2DM in patients with NAFLD is a clinical priority due to the currently available suboptimal surveillance criteria [5, 24].

Table 5 Mortality in patients with NAFLD, without previous and current malignancies

Cause of death	n/N (%)[a]	1000 person years
Overall	8/351 (2.3%)	3.33
Liver-related events	3/351 (0.9%)	1.25
Cardiovascular events	1/351 (0.3%)	0.42
Malignancies events except for hepatocellular carcinoma	2/351 (0.6%)	0.83
Other events	2/351 (0.6%)	0.83

[a]n; number of events. N; number of patients, not having, or having had, the respective event simultaneously or previously to the time of NAFLD diagnosis

In conclusion, the results of the present study suggest that cardiovascular and liver-related events are important in Japanese patients with histopathologically-confirmed NAFLD. Especially, HCC was the most common liver-related event, and the incidence of HCC was more than half of that of cardiovascular events. It may be important to identify fibrosis stage and hepatocyte steatosis as determinants of HCC and T2DM, respectively. Further large-scale prospective studies should be performed to identify the predictors of development of HCC and T2DM to improve the prognosis of patients with NAFLD.

Conclusions
Hepatocellular carcinoma was the most common liver-related event in Japanese patients with histopathologically-confirmed NAFLD.

Abbreviations
ALT: alanine aminotransferase; AST: aspartate aminotransferase; CI: confidence interval; FLIP: Fatty Liver Inhibition of Progression; HbA1c: Glycated hemoglobin type A1c; HCC: hepatocellular carcinoma; HR: hazard ratio; NAFLD: non-alcoholic fatty liver disease; NAS: NAFLD activity score; NASH: non-alcoholic steatohepatitis; T2DM: type 2 diabetes mellitus

Acknowledgments
The authors thank Drs. Keiichi Kinowaki and Takeshi Fujii (Department of Pathology, Toranomon Hospital) and also Drs. Fukuo Kondo and Toshio Fukusato (Department of Pathology, Teikyo University School of Medicine) for assistance in histopathological diagnosis.

Disclaimers
This paper has not been published or presented elsewhere in part or in entirety, and is not under consideration by another journal.

Funding
This study was supported in part by Grant-in-Aid from Japan Agency for Medical Research and Development (17fk0210304h0003).

Authors' contributions
N.A., Y.K., Y.A., S.S., S.F., H.S., T.H., M.K. (Masahiro Kobayashi), M.K. (Mariko Kobayashi), Y.S., F.S., K.I., and H.K. contributed to this work. N.A., Y.K., and Y.A. analyzed the data. N.A. wrote the manuscript. All authors read and approved the final manuscript.

Competing interests
(1) Hiromitsu Kumada has received honoraria from MSD K.K., Bristol-Myers Squibb, Gilead Sciences, AbbVie Inc., and Dainippon Sumitomo Pharma. (2) Norio Akuta has received an honorarium from Bristol-Myers Squibb and AbbVie Inc. (3) Yoshiyuki Suzuki has received an honorarium from Bristol-Myers Squibb and AbbVie Inc. All other authors declare no conflict of interest.

Author details
[1]Department of Hepatology, Toranomon Hospital and Okinaka Memorial Institute for Medical Research, 2-2-2 Toranomon, Minato-ku, Tokyo 105-0001, Japan. [2]Liver Research Laboratory, Toranomon Hospital, Tokyo, Japan.

References
1. Angulo P. Nonalcoholic fatty liver disease. N Engl J Med. 2002;346:1221–31.
2. Williams R. Global changes in liver disease. Hepatology. 2006;44:521–6.
3. Torres DM, Harrison SA. Diagnosis and therapy of nonalcoholic steatohepatitis. Gastroenterology. 2008;134:1682–98.
4. Vuppalanchi R, Chalasani N. Nonalcoholic fatty liver disease and nonalcoholic steatohepatitis: selected practical issues in their evaluation and management. Hepatology. 2009;49:306–17.
5. Kawamura Y, Arase Y, Ikeda K, Seko Y, Imai N, Hosaka T, et al. Large-scale long-term follow-up study of Japanese patients with non-alcoholic fatty liver disease for the onset of hepatocellular carcinoma. Am J Gastroenterol. 2012;107:253–61.
6. Sumida Y, Nakajima A, Itoh Y. Limitations of liver biopsy and non-invasive diagnostic tests for the diagnosis of nonalcoholic fatty liver disease/nonalcoholic steatohepatitis. World J Gastroenterol. 2014;20:475–85.
7. Kleiner DE, Brunt EM. Nonalcoholic fatty liver disease: pathologic patterns and biopsy evaluation in clinical research. Semin Liver Dis. 2012;32:3–13.
8. Sanyal AJ, Chalasani N, Kowdley KV, McCullough A, Diehl AM, Bass NM, et al. Pioglitazone, vitamin E, or placebo for nonalcoholic steatohepatitis. N Engl J Med. 2010;362:1675–85.
9. Armstrong MJ, Gaunt P, Aithal GP, Barton D, Hull D, Parker R, et al. Liraglutide safety and efficacy in patients with non-alcoholic steatohepatitis (LEAN): a multicentre, double-blind, randomised, placebo-controlled phase 2 study. Lancet. 2016;387:679–90.
10. Akuta N, Watanabe C, Kawamura Y, Arase Y, Saitoh S, Fujiyama S, et al. Effects of a sodium - glucose cotransporter 2 inhibitor in nonalcoholic fatty liver disease complicated by diabetes mellitus: preliminary prospective study based on serial liver biopsies. Hepatol Commun. 2017;1:46–52.
11. Younossi ZM, Stepanova M, Rafiq N, Makhlouf H, Younoszai Z, Agrawal R, et al. Pathologic criteria for nonalcoholic steatohepatitis: Interprotocol agreement and ability to predict liver-related mortality. Hepatology. 2011;53:1874–82.
12. Angulo P, Kleiner DE, Dam-Larsen S, Adams LA, Bjornsson ES, Charatcharoenwitthaya P, et al. Liver fibrosis, but no other histologic features, is associated with long-term outcomes of patients with nonalcoholic fatty liver disease. Gastroenterology. 2015;149:389–97.
13. Kleiner DE, Brunt EM, Van Natta M, Behling C, Contos MJ, Cummings OW, et al. Design and validation of a histological scoring system for nonalcoholic fatty liver disease. Hepatology. 2005;41:1313–21.
14. Brunt EM, Janney CG, Di Bisceglie AM, Neuschwander-Tetri BA, Bacon BR. Nonalcoholic steatohepatitis: a proposal for grading and staging the histological lesions. Am J Gastroenterol. 1999;94:2467–74.
15. Bedossa P. Utility and appropriateness of the fatty liver inhibition of progression (FLIP) algorithm and steatosis, activity, and fibrosis (SAF) score in the evaluation of biopsies of nonalcoholic fatty liver disease. Hepatology. 2014;60:565–75.
16. Hagström H, Nasr P, Ekstedt M, Hammar U, Stål P, Hultcrantz R, et al. Fibrosis stage but not NASH predicts mortality and time to development of severe liver disease in biopsy-proven NAFLD. J Hepatol. 2017;67:1265–73.
17. Björkström K, Stål P, Hultcrantz R, Hagström H. Histologic scores for fat and fibrosis associate with development of type 2 diabetes in patients with nonalcoholic fatty liver disease. Clin Gastroenterol Hepatol. 2017;15:1461–8.
18. Ekstedt M, Hagström H, Nasr P, Fredrikson M, Stål P, Kechagias S, et al. Fibrosis stage is the strongest predictor for disease-specific mortality in NAFLD after up to 33 years of follow-up. Hepatology. 2015;61:1547–54.
19. Arase Y, Kobayashi M, Suzuki F, Suzuki Y, Kawamura Y, Akuta N, et al. Difference in malignancies of chronic liver disease due to non-alcoholic fatty liver disease or hepatitis C in Japanese elderly patients. Hepatol Res. 2012;42:264–72.

20. Seko Y, Sumida Y, Tanaka S, Mori K, Taketani H, Ishiba H, et al. Insulin resistance increases the risk of incident type 2 diabetes mellitus in patients with non-alcoholic fatty liver disease. Hepatol Res. 2017 Jun 19. [Epub ahead of print].

21. Gaspard U. Hyperinsulinaemia, a key factor of the metabolic syndrome in postmenopausal women. Maturitas. 2009;62:362–5.

22. Lonardo A, Bellentani S, Argo CK, Ballestri S, Byrne CD, Caldwell SH, et al. Epidemiological modifiers of non-alcoholic fatty liver disease: focus on high-risk groups. Dig Liver Dis. 2015;47:997–1006.

23. Lonardo A, Sookoian S, Chonchol M, Loria P, Targher G. Cardiovascular and systemic risk in nonalcoholic fatty liver disease - atherosclerosis as a major player in the natural course of NAFLD. Curr Pharm Des. 2013;19:5177–92.

24. Della Corte C, Colombo M. Surveillance for hepatocellular carcinoma. Semin Oncol. 2012;39:384–98.

CT Enterography score: a potential predictor for severity assessment of active ulcerative colitis

Yingmei Jia[1†], Chang Li[1†], Xiaoyan Yang[2†], Zhi Dong[1], Kun Huang[1], Yanji Luo[1], Xuehua Li[1], Canhui Sun[1*], Shi-Ting Feng[1*] and Zi-Ping Li[1*]

Abstract

Background: Evaluate the possibility of CT enterography (CTE) score system as a predictor in assessing active ulcerative colitis (UC) severity.

Methods: Forty-six patients with active UC with CTE and colonoscopy were enrolled. Based on modified Mayo score, patients were divided into three groups: mild ($n = 10$), moderate ($n = 17$) and severe ($n = 19$). A cumulative CTE score was calculated in each patient and its correlation with modified Mayo score was analyzed. The optimal cutoff values of CTE score were determined by receiver operating characteristic (ROC) curves analysis.

Results: Significant between-group differences were observed in CTE spectrums of mucosal bubbles, mural stratification, loss of haustration, enlarged mesenteric lymph nodes and engorged mesenteric vessels ($P < 0.05$). The cumulative CTE scores were significant difference between three groups (CTE score:4.9 ± 2.3, 7.6 ± 2.6, and 10.9 ± 2.0, respectively, $P < 0.01$). The cumulative CTE score showed a positive correlation with modified Mayo score ($r = 0.835$, $P < 0.05$). The optimal cut-off value for CTE score predicting moderate and severe UC was 9.5 (area under the curve [AUC]:0.847, sensitivity:78.9%, specificity:82.4%).

Conclusion: Disease severity assessment by CTE score demonstrates strong positive correlation with severity established modified Mayo score. CTE score system maybe a potential predictor for active UC severity assessment.

Keywords: Ulcerative colitis, Disease activity, Multi-slice computed tomography, Computed tomography enterography, Modified Mayo score

Background

Ulcerative colitis (UC) is a chronic non-specific inflammatory bowel disease (IBD) characterized by diffuse inflammation of bowel mucosa and a relapsing disease course. UC mainly affects the rectum and sigmoid colon, but may involve the entire colon and terminal ileum [1–3]. As UC is a chronic condition, management of these patients requires prolonged treatment and regular follow-up throughout the course of the disease. Accurate evaluation of UC is a crucial component of therapeutic decision-making [4, 5].

However, owing to the non-specific symptoms, assessment of UC typically requires a combination of colonoscopic, histological and radiological examinations in addition to clinical examination [6].

Modified Mayo score is used frequently for assessment of UC activity [7], mainly depending on patient's symptoms and colonoscopy. Colonoscopy affords direct visualization of the colonic mucosa and has been the preferred method for defining the extent and site of inflammation, and to obtain biopsy specimen [8]. However, colonoscopy does not provide information on extra-intestinal manifestations and complications of UC. Moreover, in severe cases of UC, colonoscopy is contraindicated due to the risk of perforation or exacerbation of disease activity [9]. At present, computed tomography enterography (CTE), with its high contrast resolution

* Correspondence: canhuisun@sina.com; fengsht@mail.sysu.edu.cn; liziping163@163.com

†Yingmei Jia, Chang Li and Xiaoyan Yang contributed equally to this work.

[1]Department of Radiology, The First Affiliated Hospital, Sun Yat-Sen University, 58th, The Second Zhongshan Road, Guangzhou 510080, Guangdong, China

Full list of author information is available at the end of the article

and rapid images capability, allows evaluation of intra-mural and extra-intestinal involvement of UC and complications such as fistula, abdominal abscess or cellulitis. CTE is now widely used to diagnose and monitor inflammatory bowel disease (IBD), including UC [10, 11].

Establishment of a quick and accurate method to predict the severity of UC is an important goal for improving management of patients in future. Depending on the symptom, endoscopy and histology findings to predict the severity of UC is quite complex and time-consuming. Several studies have suggested the utility of CTE for assessment of severity of UC and a positive association of CTE findings with clinical and colonoscopic findings has been demonstrated [11]. Thus, identification of a CTE score system to assess and predict the severity of active UC is possible. However, to the best of our knowledge, no previous studies have investigated the utility of CTE score in predicting the severity of UC.

In this retrospective study, we assessed the individual CTE features in different severity of active UC, established a new CTE score system for UC, and analyzed the correlation between cumulative CTE score and modified Mayo score, so as to investigate the possibility of CTE score system as a predictor in assessing the severity of active UC.

Materials and methods

Patients

This is a retrospective study conducted in accordance with ethical guidelines for human research and was compliant with the Health Insurance Portability and Accountability Act (HIPAA). The study received ethical committee approval. The requirement for informed consent was waived off.

This study included 46 consecutive patients (29 men and 17 women) with a mean age (±SD) of 40.9 ± 17.2 years (age range: 19–77) at the First Affiliated Hospital, Sun Yat-Sen University between January 2010 and December 2015. The diagnosis of active UC was based on colonoscopic, clinical and histopathological examination. All patients had undergone CTE within 7 days of colonoscopy with biopsy.

The main symptoms included abdominal pain, fever, nausea and vomiting, intestinal bleeding and diarrhea. The duration of the disease course ranged from 1 month to 18 years.

Modified Mayo score

Reference the European consensus on diagnosis and management of UC reported by Dignass [7], classification of active UC was evaluated by modified Mayo scoring system (Table 1).

Table 1 Components of the modified Mayo score [20]

Stool frequency

0: Normal

1: 1–2 stools/day more than normal

2: 3–4 stools/day more than normal

3: > 4 stools/day more than normal

Rectal bleeding[a]

0: None

1: Visible blood with stool less than half the time

2: Visible blood with stool half of the time or more

3: Passing of blood alone

Mucosal appearance at endoscopy[b]

0: Normal or inactive disease

1: Mild disease (erythema, decreased vascular pattern, mild mucosal friability

2: Moderate disease (marked erythema, absent vascular pattern, friability, erosions)

3: Severe disease (spontaneous bleeding, ulceration)

Physician rating of disease activity

0: Normal

1: Mild

2: Moderate

3: Severe

[a]A score of 3 for bleeding required patients to have at least 50% of bowel motions accompanied by visible blood, and at least one bowel motion with blood alone
[b]Mucosal appearance at endoscopy is not included in the Partial Mayo Score
< 2, remission; 3–5, mild active; 6–10, moderately active; 11–12, severe active

CTE technique

Patients were asked to fast for more than 12 h before the CT scan. Cleaning enema was performed on the night before the examination. Prior to scan, patients ingested a total of 1600~ 2000 mL of 2.5% mannitol solution in 400–500 mL aliquots every 15 min, and administered 20 mg of anisodamine intramuscularly. For achievement of adequate entire colon distension, colon retention enema with 300~ 500 mL of 2.5% mannitol was performed before CT scan [12, 13]. Patients were scanned using Toshiba Aquilion 64-detector row CT from diaphragmatic top to ischial tuberosity. Three-phases were obtained; before injection of contrast (non-contrast), and 23–25 s, and 50–60 s after intravenous administration of 1.5 mL/Kg iopromide (ultravist 300, Schering, Berlin, Germany) injected at a rate of 3–4 mL/s using a power injector. CT scan parameters were 120 kv, 200–250 mAs, collimation 64 × 0.5 mm, section thickness and interval of 2 mm.

CTE image analysis

All data were reviewed on the workstation (Vitrea version 3.7). Each CTE study was evaluated by two trained abdominal radiologists who were blinded to the clinical and colonoscopic findings. Discrepancy, if any, was resolved by consensus.

With bowel well distended, bowel wall thickening was defined as > 4 mm [5]. Based on the Montreal classification [14], the extent of the disease was classified as E1, E2 and E3. E1 defined a proctitis with limited lesions until rectosigmoid junction, E2 defined a left-sided colitis with lesions under the splenic flexure and E3 defined an extensive colitis above the splenic flexure. Mural stratification was defined as circular intestinal wall and submucosal widening with decreased attenuation. Compared with the adjacent normal bowel, the features of mural hyperenhancement and mesenteric hyperemia were presented as increased mural density and engorgement of mesenteric vessels after enhancement. Perirectal stranding was depicted as a slightly increased attenuation (10-20HU) compared with normal fat as result of edema and inflammatory cell infiltrates [15]. Mesenteric lymph nodes with short axis > 5 mm were defined as enlarged. Mucosal bubbles present as round small bubbles in interrupted mucosal layer of intestinal wall. Intestinal pseudopolyp formed by colonic mucosal hyperplasia were shown as hummocky or nodules sample protrusions swelled to lumen. Luminal narrowing was defined by lack of full expansion of the bowel. Loss of haustration was also a feature of CTE images.

Once one of the active UC CTE features in any segment, a point was added. A cumulative CTE severity score (0–15 points) was calculated as the sum of all individual criteria scores. The cumulative CTE scores are shown in Table 2.

Statistical analysis

All data were analyzed by SPSS 17.0 software. Numerical data were expressed as mean ± SD and analyzed using R*C table method of Chi-squared test. After the difference is considered statistically significant among groups, partitions method of chi-square test were used to analyze. One-way Analysis of Variance (ANOVA) was performed for analysis of cumulative CTE score in 3 groups with the two-two comparisons. Correlation of cumulative CTE scores with the Mayo score was assessed using Spearman correlation (r). A P value of < 0.05 was considered statistically significant. Receiver-operating characteristic (ROC) curves were used to determine the optimal cut-off points of the CTE score for predicting severity of active UC.

Results
Modified Mayo score
According to the modified Mayo score, 46 patients were graded as mild (10), moderate (17) and severe (19) groups.

Table 2 Cumulative CT scores

CTE images	Scores
Extended range of UC	
Normal	0
E1	1
E2	2
E3	3
Bowel wall thickening	
< 3 mm	0
4–6 mm	1
7–9 mm	2
> 10 mm	3
Mural stratification	1
Mural hyperenhancement	1
Mesenteric hyperemia	1
Perirectal stranding	1
Lymph node enlargement	1
Mucosal bubbles	1
Luminal narrowing	1
loss of haustration	1
Intestinal pseudopolyp	1

CTE

According to the standard of study of Wold PB et al. [16], adequate luminal distention was defined as separation of the colon lumen by enteric contrast material without collapse. All patients ($n = 46$) had adequate distension of the entire colon.

In the total of 46 patients, involvement of the rectum was 2 cases (E1), involvement of a proportion of the colorectum distal to the splenic flexure was 23 cases (E2), and involvement extends proximal to the splenic flexure was 21 cases (E3). Overall, the consistency of CTE in assessment the extent of UC with endoscopy was 80.4% (80.0%, 82.3% and 79.0% for mild, moderate and severe group, respectively).

Of the total 46 cases, bowel wall thickening was seen in 43 cases (Figs. 1, 2, 3, 4). Mural hyperenhancement was observed in 45 cases (Figs. 1, 2, 3, 4). Mural stratification was present in 21 cases (Figs. 1, 2, 4). Mucosal bubbles were present in 30 cases (Fig. 1). Loss of haustration was identified in 28 cases (Fig. 3). Mesenteric hyperemia was present in 23 cases (Figs. 2, 3, 4). Perirectal stranding was seen in 14 cases (Fig. 2). Lymph node enlargement was present in 19 cases. Intestinal pseudopolyps were identified in five patients (Fig. 4). Luminal narrowing was seen in 12 cases (Fig. 3).

Statistical result

Among the individual CTE features, a significant difference in the spectrum of mucosal bubbles was observed

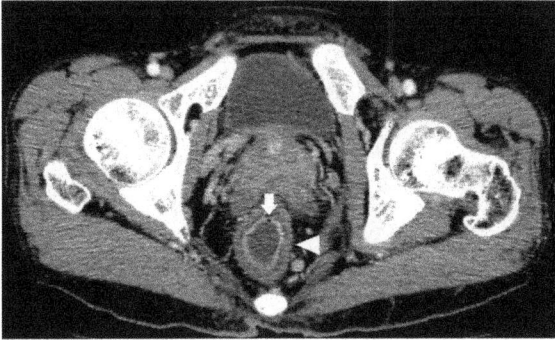

Fig. 1 Axial CTE of UC showed uniform mural thickening and stratification in rectum (arrowheads). Mucosal hyperenhancement and mucosal bubbles (arrows) sign were detected

between the mild and moderate groups ($P = 0.003$). A significant difference with respect to mural stratification, loss of haustration and enlarged mesenteric lymph nodes was observed between the moderate and severe groups ($P = 0.019$, $P < 0.001$, $P = 0.003$). Further, as significant difference was observed with respect to mucosal bubbles, loss of haustration, engorged mesenteric vessels and enlarged mesenteric lymph nodes between the mild and severe groups ($P = 0.016$, $P < 0.001$, $P = 0.002$, $P = 0.002$). There was no significant difference in the spectrum of bowel wall thickening, mural hyperenhancement, luminal narrowing and perirectal stranding between the 3 groups ($P > 0.05$). The spectrum of CTE features in 3 groups is shown in Tables 3 and 4.

The cumulative CTE scores for mild, moderate and severe groups were 4.9 ± 2.3, 7.6 ± 2.6, and 10.9 ± 2.0 (Fig. 5) with a statistically significant difference among the three groups ($P < 0.01$). On correlation analysis, a positive linear correlation between the cumulative CTE score and modified Mayo score was observed ($P < 0.05$, $r = 0.835$) (Fig. 6).

The optimal CTE score cut-off value for predicting moderate and severe UC was 9.5 with an area under the

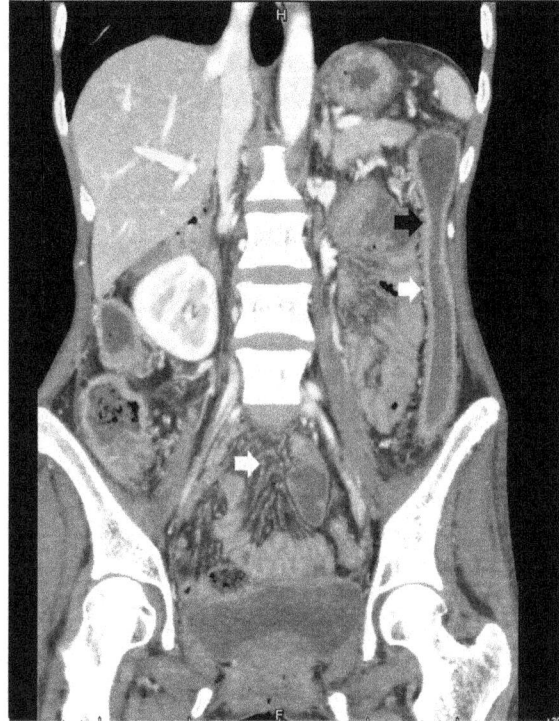

Fig. 3 Coronal CTE of UC showed loss of haustration, lumenal narrowing, mucosal hyperenhancement (black arrows) and engorgement of mesenteric vessels (white arrows)

ROC curve of 0.847 (Fig. 7). The sensitivity and specificity were 78.9% and 82.4%, respectively. There was no optimal cut-off value for predicting mild and moderate UC due to the low AUC (0.280).

Discussion

The symptoms of active UC include persistent or recurrent episodes of diarrhea, intestinal bleeding with abdominal pain, tenesmus and different levels of systemic symptoms [2]. Repeated bouts of inflammation lead to chronic active UC, and increase the grade of activity [11]. Based on the extent of involvement and degree of inflammatory activity, the active inflammatory severity of UC was divided into mild, moderate and severe disease.

In patients with UC, an exhaustive evaluation of disease extent and activity is crucial for therapeutic decision-making [17–19]. Therapeutic planning and follow-up is related to disease severity [10]. Modified Mayo score comprised of four categories (stool frequency, rectal bleeding, endoscopic appearance and physician assessment) is common used to evaluate severity of active UC [2, 20]. Nevertheless, these are indirect indices, mainly relying on self-assessment of symptoms by the patient [21]. Moreover, endoscopy can not provide information on bowel wall, extraintestinal manifestations and complications of UC [22].

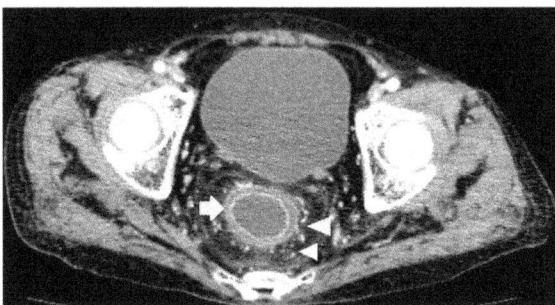

Fig. 2 Axial CTE of UC revealed bowel wall thickening, mural stratification and mural hyperenhancement (arrows) in rectum. Perirectal stranding was observed (arrowheads) displaying increased attenuation in perirectal fat

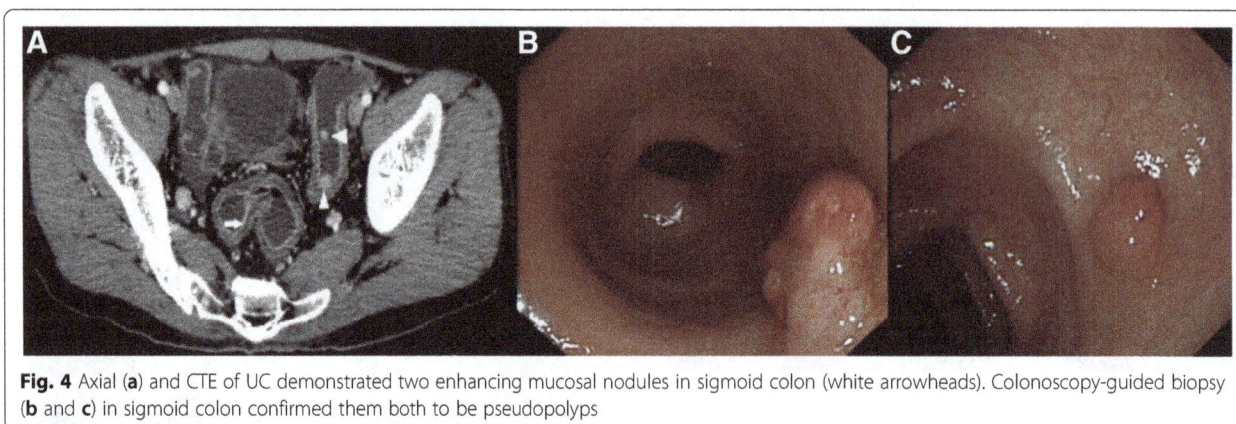

Fig. 4 Axial (**a**) and CTE of UC demonstrated two enhancing mucosal nodules in sigmoid colon (white arrowheads). Colonoscopy-guided biopsy (**b** and **c**) in sigmoid colon confirmed them both to be pseudopolyps

CTE with increased speed and resolution, allows for comprehensive assessment of the bowel wall and extra-intestinal manifestations and becomes a useful compliment to endoscopy [23–25]. A few studies have focused on the accuracy of CTE for the detection of UC. Johnson et al. [26] reported that an overall sensitivity of 74% for the detection of IBD (either Crohn or UC), and sensitivity was 93% for the detection of moderate and severe disease in well-distended colons and specificity was 91%. Andersen et al. [27] reported a moderate correlation of the loss of haustration, rigid bowel wall, and bowel thickness with severity of UC. Our study and previous studies showed that CTE was highly correlated with colonoscopic findings in assessment the extent of UC. Consequently, CTE is an ideal method and has great potential in evaluation for UC even at earlier occasion.

CTE spectrum are correlated closely with pathological findings and has the ability to reflect the pathological changes of UC. Pathologically, the early stages of UC are characterized by mucosal hyperplasia, increased mucosal vascularity, congestion and edema, which present as mucosal hyperenhancement and bowel wall thickening on CTE. With progression of disease course, the disease is characterized by multiple mucosal erosions or ulcers, which may manifest as mucosal bubbles in interrupted mucous. With further development of UC, the disease is characterized by edema, congestion, and inflammatory cells infiltration of submucosa, and hyperplasia and chronic fatty deposits of muscular layer. On CT, these changes appear as mural stratification and loss of haustration. In addition, luminal narrowing due to hyperplasia and fibrosis of muscularis mucosa occurs along with enlarged mesenteric lymph nodes and engorged mesenteric vessels due to chronic inflammation. Also, perirectal stranding is hallmark of chronic disease [11, 27, 28]. These pathological characteristics allow an objective assessment which reflects the severity of UC.

Table 3 Spectrum of CTE features in 3 groups

CTE features	Groups			P
	Mild (n = 10)	Moderate (n = 17)	Severe (n = 19)	
Extended range				0.309
E1	1	1	0	
E2	7	8	8	
E3	2	8	11	
Bowel wall thickening	9	15	19	0.318
Mural hyperenhancement	8	15	19	0.164
Mural stratification	3	5	13	0.034
Mucosal bubbles	2	14	14	0.003
loss of haustration	2	7	19	< 0.001
Mesenteric hyperemia	1	8	14	0.005
perirectal standing	1	6	7	0.282
Lymph nodes enlargement	1	4	14	0.001
Intestinal pseudopolyp	0	2	3	0.426
Luminal narrowing	1	4	7	> 0.05

Table 4 *P* values for between-group differences on ANOVA

| groups | CTE features | | | | |
	Mural stratification	Mucosal bubbles	loss of haustration	Mesenteric hyperemia	Lymph node enlargement
Mild-Moderate	1.000	0.003	0.406	0.091	0.621
Moderate-Severe	0.019	0.695	< 0.001	0.102	0.003
Mild-Severe	0.064	0.016	< 0.001	0.002	0.002

In our study, the spectrum of CTE findings in the three groups was difference. Bowel wall thickening and mucosal hyperenhancement were the essential characters and almost observed in all the cases. However, mucosal bubbles were more frequently observed in the moderate group as compared to that in the mild group. Mural stratification, loss of haustration and enlarged mesenteric lymph nodes in the severe group were significantly higher than that in the moderate group. Compared with the mild group, patients in the severe group were more likely to show mucosal bubbles, loss of haustration, engorged mesenteric vessels and enlarged mesenteric lymph nodes. Thus, increasing severity of UC demonstrated various CTE findings, reflecting the corresponding severity of intestinal inflammation. In mild UC, the intestinal inflammatory was mainly located in the mucosa and submucosa. In more severe disease, the inflammation spread from mucosa and submucosa to the whole intestinal wall, including ulceration and edema [27]. Small and tiny ulcerations are hard to detect by CTE. Mucosal bubbles represents obvious ulcer indicating more serious inflammatory activity. Mural stratification and loss of haustration indicated the UC involving the whole intestinal wall suggesting the severe disease. However, no statistically significant difference was found between the three groups with respect to luminal narrowing, perirectal stranding and pseudopolyp. Because these three signs may be more related to disease duration and individual differences rather than the disease severity [29].

Due to the correlation between the extent of UC and the clinical manifestations, the wider the extent of UC is, the worse are the symptoms. Due to this, the extent of UC was added to the CTE score system. A synthesis of all CTE features provides for a quantitative score system to evaluate the severity of UC. Our results showed a statistically significant difference in the CTE scores between the three groups. Moreover, the CTE score strongly correlated with modified Mayo score ($r = 0.835$). With aggravation of the disease course, CTE score increased significantly. Patel et al... [11], reported a weak correlation between the composite CT severity score and clinical assessment ($r = 0.45$), while bowel thickening, mucosal hyperenhancement, and mural stratification each individually showed a moderately positive association with clinical severity ($r = 0.58$; 0.57; 0.68). One possible reason is that our sample size is relatively large, and the modified Mayo scoring system (including colonoscopy) was used to evaluate active UC. Moreover, compared with the study of Patel et al [11], we developed a more comprehensive CTE score system in which CTE features correlated with disease severity as reflected in the extent of UC, mucosal bubbles, luminal narrowing and loss of haustration. Finally, we used plenty of low-density contrast media to expand the colon and the

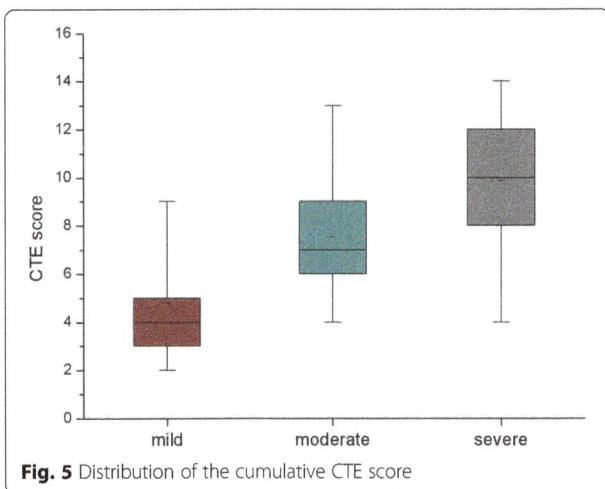

Fig. 5 Distribution of the cumulative CTE score

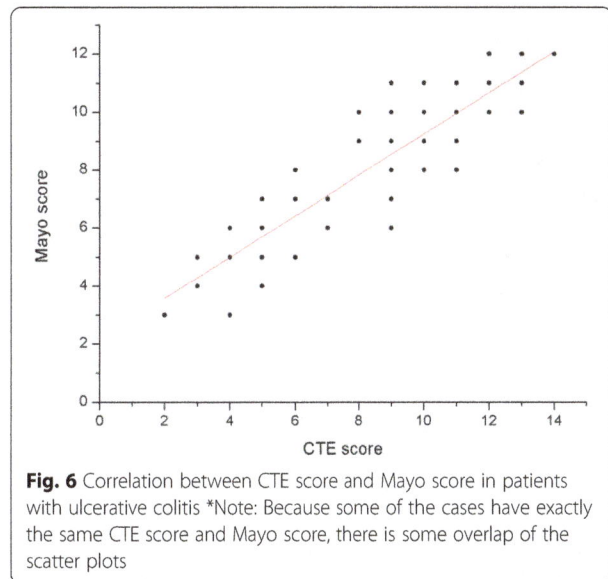

Fig. 6 Correlation between CTE score and Mayo score in patients with ulcerative colitis *Note: Because some of the cases have exactly the same CTE score and Mayo score, there is some overlap of the scatter plots

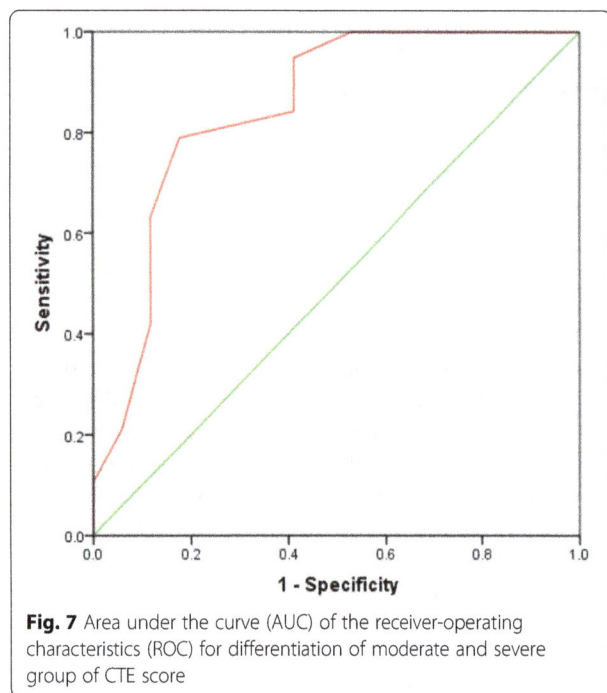

Fig. 7 Area under the curve (AUC) of the receiver-operating characteristics (ROC) for differentiation of moderate and severe group of CTE score

small intestine. The intraintestinal CT characteristics of UC such as mucosal bubbles, mural stratification, mural hyperenhancement may be displayed clearly with use of such agents, as opposed to high-density contrast media.

Accurate prediction of severity of active UC using a convenient method is necessary for management. Current methods (depending on the symptom, endoscopy and histology findings) to predict the severity of UC have some limitations. CTE provides more valuable information for judgment of active UC severity and maybe predict the severity. To our best knowledge, there are few studies using CTE score to predict severity of UC. In our study, based on ROC analysis, the CTE score system has the potential ability of predicting severity of UC. Our study showed CTE score was better for predicting moderate and severe disease of active UC with a CTE score cut-off value of 9.5 with high specificity. But there was no optimal cut-off value for predicting mild and moderate UC. This is probably due to the selection bias for the relative small number of mild UC. Another possible reason is there are more overlapping CTE findings between mild and moderate UC. Moreover, the CTE features are easier to identify with increasing inflammation degree. Even so, patients with UC whose CTE score more than 9.5 should be considered as having moderate or severe inflammatory severity. It is strongly recommended that such patients should be hospitalized.

Consequently, CTE enabled a comprehensively assessment of UC, helped determine the optimal treatment strategy and, to some extent, made up for the limitations of the conventional CT, as development of new signs on

CTE, such as mucosal bubbles and loss of haustration showed a correlation with pathological changes of UC. These advantages are of clinic relevance in the diagnosis and classification of UC. Thus, CTE can be a reliable examination method that helps in systematic evaluation of the severity of UC.

There are some limitations in our study. Firstly, the score given to each characteristic should ideally be derived based on regression analysis. However, for our study, the sample size is relative small. Most of the cases are severe groups (41.3%, 19/46) and selection bias can not be avoided. Thus, we did not use regression analysis in building CTE score system. Secondly, this CTE score system cannot be reliably used as a predictor of the outcomes of UC; however, it remains a very interesting subject to investigate. These need a further study enrolling a larger number of patients from multiple centers.

Conclusions
CTE enables assessment of extraintestinal manifestations and complications of UC. And, CTE score system provides a quantitative basis for accurate assessment of the severity of UC. Thus, CTE is a valuable supplement to the traditional methods such as colonoscopy and clinical assessment. It can be used as a potential predictor of severity assessment of active UC, help determine therapeutic strategy, and predict prognosis.

Acknowledgements
Not applicable.

Funding
This work was funded by National Natural Science Foundation of China (81771908,81571750, 81770654), The National Key Research and Development Program of China (2017YFC0113402). The Grants-in-Aid supported this study just financially, and had no role in the design of the study and collection, analysis, and interpretation of data and in writing the manuscript.

Authors' contributions
STF, CS and ZPL designed and carried out this study. XY, KH and XL collected patient data; YJ, CL and ZD analyzed and interpreted the data. All authors participated in writing the final manuscript. YL and STF revised manuscript critically for important intellectual content. All authors have read and approved the manuscript.

Competing interests
The authors declare that they have no competing interests.

Author details

[1]Department of Radiology, The First Affiliated Hospital, Sun Yat-Sen University, 58th, The Second Zhongshan Road, Guangzhou 510080, Guangdong, China. [2]Department of Radiology, Shenzhen Traditional Chinese Medicine Hospital, Shenzhen 518000, China.

References

1. Ouyang Q, Tandon R, Goh KL, et al. Management consensus of inflammatory bowel disease for the Asia-Pacific region. J Gastroenterol Hepatol. 2006;21(12):1772–82.
2. Chinese Society Of Gastroenterology. The consensus on diagnosis and management of inflammatory bowel disease(Guangzhou, 2012). Gastroenterol. 2012;17(12):763–81.
3. Ooi CJ, Fock KM, Makharia GK. The Asia-Pacific consensus on ulcerative colitis. J Gastroenterol Hepatol. 2010;25:453–68.
4. Deepak P, Bruining DH. Radiographical evaluation of ulcerative colitis. Gastroenterology report. 2014;2(3):169–77.
5. Panes J, Bouhnik Y, Reinisch W, et al. Imaging techniques for assessment of inflammatory bowel disease: joint ECCO and ESGAR evidence-based consensus guidelines. J Crohns Colitis. 2013;7(7):556–85.
6. Lee SD, Cohen RD. Endoscopy in inflammatory bowel disease. Gastroenterol Clin N Am. 2002;31:119–32.
7. Dignass A, Eliakim R, Magro F, et al. Second European evidence-based consensus on the dignosis and management of ulcerative colitis. J Crohns Colitis. 2012;6:965–90.
8. British Society of Gastroenterology. Guidelines for the management of inflammatory bowel disease in adults [J]. Gut. 2004;53(Suppl V):v1–v16.
9. Makkar R, Bo S. Colonoscopic perforation in inflammatory bowel disease. Gastroenterol Hepatol (N Y). 2013;9(9):573–83.
10. Patel NS, Pola S, Muralimohan R, et al. Outcomes of computed tomography and magnetic resonance enterography in clinical practice of inflammatory bowel disease. Dig Dis Sci. 2014;59(4):838–49.
11. Patel B, Mottola J, Sahni VA, et al. MDCT assessment of ulcerative colitis: radiologic analysis with clinical, endoscopic, and pathologic correlation. Abdom Imaging. 2012;37(1):61–9.
12. Raptopoulos V, Schwarta RK, McNicholas MM, et al. Multiplanar helical CT enterography in patients wih Crohn's disease. Am J Roentgenol. 1997; 169(6):1545–50.
13. Zhao J, Cui M-Y, Chan T, et al. Evaluation of intestinal tuberculosis by multi-slice computed tomography enterography. BMC Infect Dis. 2015;15:577.
14. Satsangi J, Silverberg MS, Vermeire S, et al. The Montreal classification of inflammatory bowel disease: controversies, consensus, and implications. Gut. 2006;55(6):749–53.
15. Ruedi F, Thoeni, John PC. CT imaging of colitis. Radiology. 2006;240(9):623–38.
16. Wold PB, Fletcher JG, Johnson CD, Sandborn WJ. Assessment of small bowel Crohn disease: noninvasive peroral CT enterography compared with other imaging methods and endoscopy—feasibility study. Radiology. 2003; 229:275–81.
17. Stange EF, Travis SPL, Vermeire S, et al. European evidence-based consensus on the diagnosis and management of ulcerative colitis: definitions and diagnosis. J Crohn's Colitis. 2008;2:1–23.
18. Turner D, Levine A, Escher JC, et al. Management of pediatric ulcerative colitis: joint ECCO and ESPGHAN evidence-based consensus guidelines. J Pediatr Gastroenterol Nutr. 2012;55:340–61.
19. Civitelli F, Di Nardo G, Oliva S, et al. Ultrasonography of the colon in pediatric ulcerative colitis: a prospective, blind, comparative study with colonoscopy. J Pediatr. 2014;165(1):78–84.
20. James D, Lewis MD. M.S.C.E. use of the non-invasive components of the Mayo score to assess clinical response in ulcerative colitis. Inflamm Bowel Dis. 2008;14(12):1660–6.
21. Turner D, Griffiths AM, Mack D, et al. Assessing disease activity in ulcerative colitis: patients or their physicians? Inflamm Bowel Dis. 2010;16:651–6.
22. Paraskeva KD, Paspatis GA. Management of bleeding and perforation after colonoscopy. Expert Rev Gastroenterol Hepatol. 2014;8(8):963–72.
23. Paulsen SR, Huprich J, Fletcher JG, et al. CT Enterography as a diagnostic tool in evaluating small bowel disorders: review of clinical experience with over 700 case. Radiographics. 2006;26:641–62.
24. Michael P, Federle. CT of the small intestine Enterography and angiography. Supplement to applied radiology. 2007:55–62.
25. Alexander J, Towbin, Sullivan J, et al. CT and MR enterography in children and adolescents with inflammatory bowel disease. Radiographics. 2013; 33(7):1843–60.
26. Johnson KT, Hara AK, Johnson CD. Evaluation of colitis:usefulness of CT enterography technique. Emerg Radiol. 2009;16:277–82.
27. Andersen K, Vogt C, Blondin D, et al. Multi-detector CT-colonography in inflammatory bowel disease: prospective analysis of CT-findings to high-resolution video colonoscopy. Eur J Radiol. 2006;58:140–6.
28. Fletcher JG, Fidler JL, Bruining DH, et al. New concepts in intestinal imaging for inflammatory bowel diseases. Gastroenterology. 2011;140:1795–806.
29. Yang XY, Dong Z, Luo YJ, et al. Multi-slice computed tomography enteroclysis in evaluation of active ulcerative colitis. Chinese journal of medical imaging. 2014;22(10):760–3.

25

Relevance of vitamin D deficiency in patients with chronic autoimmune atrophic gastritis: a prospective study

Sara Massironi[1], Federica Cavalcoli[1,2*], Alessandra Zilli[1,2], Alessandro Del Gobbo[3], Clorinda Ciafardini[1], Susanna Bernasconi[1], Irene Felicetta[4], Dario Conte[1] and Maddalena Peracchi[1]

Abstract

Background: Chronic autoimmune atrophic gastritis (CAAG) is an autoimmune disease characterized by hypo/achlorhydria. A role of CAAG in the pathogenesis of nutritional deficiencies has been reported, therefore we hypothesized a possible association between CAAG and 25-OH-Vitamin D [25(OH)D] deficiency. Aim of the present study is to evaluate the prevalence of 25(OH)D deficiency in CAAG patients. Methods: 87 CAAG patients (71 females; mean age 63.5 ± 12.8 years) followed at our Centre from January 2012 to July 2015 were consecutively evaluated. 25(OH)D, vitamin B_{12}, parathormone, and calcium were measured in all the CAAG patients. The results were compared with a control group of 1232 healthy subjects.

Results: In the CAAG group the mean 25(OH)D levels were significantly lower than in the control group (18.8 vs. 27.0 ng/ml, $p < 0.0001$). 25(OH)D levels < 20 ng/ml was observed in 57 patients, while levels < 12.5 ng/ml in 27 patients. A significant correlation between vitamin B_{12} values at diagnosis and 25(OH)D levels was observed ($r_s = 0.25$, $p = 0.01$). Interestingly, the CAAG patients with moderate/severe gastric atrophy had lower 25(OH)D values as compared to those with mild atrophy (11.8 vs. 20 ng/ml; $p = 0.0047$). Moreover, the 25(OH)D levels were significantly lower in CAAG patients with gastric carcinoid as compared to those without gastric carcinoid (11.8 vs. 19.8 ng/ml; $p = 0,0041$).

Conclusion: Data from the present study showed a significant reduction of 25(OH)D levels in CAAG patients and a possible impairment of vitamin D absorption in CAAG may be postulated. Any implication to the genesis of gastric carcinoids remains to be elucidated.

Keywords: Chronic autoimmune atrophic gastritis, Vitamin D deficiency, Gastric carcinoid, Bone health, Osteoporosis

Background

Chronic autoimmune atrophic gastritis (CAAG) is an immune-mediated inflammatory condition involving the parietal cells in the gastric fundus and body [1, 2]. Parietal cells secrete intrinsic factor and hydrochloric acid, via the H+/K+ adenosine triphosphatase proton pump, and are the main determinant of gastric acidification. The chronic inflammation results in mucosal atrophy with a progressive destruction and ultimate complete loss of parietal cells [3], increase in gastric pH, hypergastrinemia and intrinsic factor deficiency [4].

Intrinsic factor is a co-factor essential for vitamin B12 absorption in the terminal ileum and its deficiency in CAAG leads to vitamin B12 deficiency [5, 6]. In this setting, also iron insufficiency and iron deficiency anemia have been recently observed, especially in premenopausal women [7, 8]. The relevance of physiological gastric acid secretion for iron absorption has been suggested by several authors. In fact, nutritional iron is usually bound to proteins and requires the gastric acidification for its solubilization and uptake [9]. Furthermore, an increased incidence of different vitamins and micronutrients deficiency (e.g. ascorbic acid C and folate) in CAAG was reported [10–12]. It has been postulated that hypochlorhydria and bacterial overgrowth

---

* Correspondence: cavalcoli.federica@gmail.com
[1]Gastroenterology and Endoscopy Unit, Fondazione IRCCS Ca' Granda Ospedale Maggiore Policlinico, Milan, Italy
[2]Department of Pathophysiology and Transplantation, Università degli Studi di Milano, Milan, Italy
Full list of author information is available at the end of the article

in CAAG patients may cause a decreased absorption or increased loss of nutrients in the stomach [11].

A higher incidence of osteopenia and osteoporosis in conditions determining gastric hypochlorhydria, such as gastric resection [13], proton pump inhibitors (PPIs) therapy and CAAG [14–17] has been suggested. However, the pathogenic mechanism leading to these alterations has not been clarified yet. A few studies have reported about a reduced absorption of calcium in patients affected by CAAG [18, 19], while a study by Eastell et al. did not find any significant differences in calcium absorption in CAAG patients as compared with controls [20]. Interestingly, two studies have recently reported an association between CAAG and vitamin D deficiency [21, 22] and a possible role of vitamin D deficiency in the increased risk of osteopenia/osteoporosis in these patients has been proposed.

Therefore, a possible role of CAAG in determining a vitamin D deficiency could be hypothesized, however, to date there is lack of studies investigating the relevance of vitamin D deficiency in CAAG patients.

Objective of present study was to prospectively establish the prevalence of 25-OH-Vitamin D (25(OH)D) deficiency in a cohort of patients with CAAG. Secondary aims were to evaluate possible association between 25(OH)D levels and histological findings as well as between 25(OH)D and vitamin B12 levels. To the best of our knowledge, this is the first study aimed at investigating the presence of vitamin D deficiency in CAAG patients.

Methods

From January 2012 to September 2015, 87 patients with histologically confirmed CAAG followed at our Gastroenterology and Endoscopy Unit, Fondazione IRCCS Ca´ Granda Ospedale Maggiore Policlinico of Milan, Italy (16 males and 71 females; mean age 64 ± 13 years) were consecutively evaluated.

Moreover, a control group of 1232 healthy subjects (276 males and 956 females, mean age 62.3 ± 13.2 years) referred to the "Fondazione IRCCS Ca´ Granda Ospedale Maggiore Policlinico of Milan as outpatients for routine laboratory tests was matched for age and gender with the patient group. The criteria for exclusion for both groups were: primary hyperparathyroidism, abnormal calcium values, ongoing vitamin D supplementation or other medication that can interfere with calcium metabolism, renal failure, pancreatic insufficiency, gastrointestinal disease causing malabsorption (e.g. coeliac disease and inflammatory bowel disease), severe hepatic failure, and concomitant malignancy.

All the subjects, after full explanation of the purpose and nature of all procedures used, gave their written informed consent to participate in the study, which was approved by the local Ethics Committee.

All the CAAG patients underwent initial assessment including upper gastrointestinal endoscopy with complete biopsy sample and blood tests with APCA, anti-intrinsic factor antibodies and fasting gastrin determination. The diagnosis of CAAG was established based on the histological confirmation of gastric body mucosal atrophy and/or enterochromaffin-like (ECL) cell hyperplasia, associated with fasting hypergastrinemia and/or presence of APCA or anti-intrinsic factor antibodies.

In case of 25(OH)D deficiency (defined when dealing with values < 20 ng/mL), patients were given cholecalciferol supplementation, with a loading dose of 300,000 U/month for the first 2 months and then 100,000 U every 4 months and interrupted in case of values exceeded 60 ng/ml.

Laboratory investigations

In all CAAG patients, the levels of total and ionized calcium (Ca^{2+}), albumin, phosphate (P), intact PTH, 25(OH)D, creatinine, vitamin B_{12}, gastrin and CgA were measured in venous samples obtained after overnight fasting; anticoagulant-free tubes were used for the serum samples and tubes containing EDTA (1 mg/mL of blood) or heparin were utilized for the plasma ones. Serum calcium, albumin, creatinine and urinary calcium and creatinine were measured by standard colorimetric techniques. Total calcium levels were corrected using serum albumin measurements. Plasma ionized calcium was measured using a potentiometric method (Radiometer ABL System 625, Copenhagen, Denmark) on heparinized blood samples within 30 min from blood collection (reference range: 1.15–1.29 mM). Serum intact PTH was measured by chemiluminescence (Elecsys Intact PTH assay, F. Hoffmann-La Roche, Basel, Switzerland) with a sensitivity of 4.0 pg/mL. 25(OH)D was measured by using a commercial available kit (LIAISON® 25-OH Vitamin D TOTAL Assay ref. 310,600, DiaSorin Inc., Stillwater, MN, USA).

Histological examination

Upper gastrointestinal endoscopy was performed by trained endoscopists using standard endoscopes (Olympus, Japan and Pentax, Japan). Extensive gastric biopsies (2 from the antrum, 2 from the corpus, and 2 from the fundus, larger curvature, in addition to any endoscopically evident mucosal lesion) were obtained in all the cases. Formalin-fixed-paraffin-embedded biopsies were stained with hematoxylin-eosin and Alcian blue–periodic acid-Schiff (PAS) histochemical staining in order to evaluate morphological features. Immunohistochemistry with antibodies anti-chromogranin A, gastrin and Ki-67, when required, was performed using the automatic system DAKO Omnis (Agilent, Santa Clara, California, USA) according to the manufacturer's instructions. All the samples were evaluated by an experienced pathologist.

The degree of gastritis was classified according to the Sydney classification system [23] which provides guidelines on how to incorporate etiology (i.e. H.pylori, autoimmune), topography (antrum, corpus) and morphological features (chronic inflammation, activity, atrophy and intestinal metaplasia) in pathologist reports of gastric biopsies. More in detail, gastric atrophy defined as loss of appropriate glands, has been classified in mild (reduction of appropriate glands from 1 to 30%), moderate (loss of glands from 31 to 60%) and severe (loss of glands > 60%) (Table 1) [23, 24].

The status of the enterochromaffin-like (ECL) cells was classified according to Solcia et al. [25] as: hyperplastic changes in case of ECL cells proliferation < 150 μm (diffuse, linear, micronodular, or adenomatoid hyperplasia); dysplastic lesions for ECL proliferation between 150 and 500 μm (microinvasive lesions, enlarged or fused micronodules, and nodular growth), and neoplasia for ECL proliferation > 500 μm (intramucosal or invasive carcinoids). Minute ECL cell nests characterized by small aggregates less than 50 μm in diameter were separated from true hyperplastic micronodules and were not considered as signs of hyperplasia [26].

Patients characteristics'

According to the Sydney classification [23], 37 patients had mild, 34 moderate and 16 severe chronic gastritis. The status of the entero-chromaffin-like (ECL) cells was classified according to Solcia et al. [25]. In our series, 24 patients had no cell hyperplasia, 23 had linear hyperplasia and 17 had micronodular hyperplasia, whereas 23 patients had type 1 gastric carcinoids (GC1), of variable size (range 0.2–3 cm), single in 10 cases and multiple in 13.

Representative microphotographs of our series are depicted in Fig. 1.

Anti-parietal cell antibodies (APCA) were present in 79 patients (91%). The associated reported autoimmune diseases were: primary hypothyroidism in 30 patients, vitiligo in four, Graves' disease in two, mixed connective tissue disease in two, multiple sclerosis, psoriasis, alopecia, PGA type 1, myasthenia gravis and scleroderma were reported in one patient each. Previous *Helicobacter pylori* (*H. pylori*) infection was reported in 20 CAAG patients, all of them having been treated with successful eradication. Active infection was present in two patients, who have been treated successfully.

Among the CAAG patients, dual-energy X-ray absorptiometry (DXA) to evaluate bone mineral density (BMD) (g/cm^2) was available for 39 out of 87 patients. Lumbar spine BMD was measured using the average value for L1 to L4. Femur BMD was measured at femoral neck. Low bone density and osteoporosis were diagnosed using the World Health Organization criteria (– 2.5 < T-score < – 1.0 and T-score ≤ – 2.5 respectively).

Statistical analysis

Continuous variables were reported as mean ± standard deviation (SD) or median and range; categorical variables were reported as count (percentage). All data were tested for distribution normality via the Kolmogoroff-Smirnoff test. The differences between groups were assessed with the Mann-Whitney and Kruskal-Wallis test as appropriate. Differences between percentages were evaluated by Fisher's exact test. The relationships between variables were determined by Spearman's coefficient. A p value < 0.05, two-sided, was considered statistically significant. The analyses were carried out by software Graph Pad Prism version 5.00 and Graph Pad State Mat version 2, for Windows (GraphPad Software, San Diego, California, USA).

Results

The CAAG group showed significantly lower 25(OH)D mean levels (18.8 ± 9.7 ng/ml) compared with the control group (27.0 ± 16.3 ng/ml) ($p < 0.0001$). 25(OH)D deficiency, defined as 25(OH)D levels lower than 20 ng/ml, was observed in 57 (66%) of the 87 CAAG patients and in 438 (36%) of the patients in the control group, (Fisher's exact test $p < 0.0001$) (Table 2).

25(OH)D levels lower than 12.5 ng/ml, was present in 27 of 87 patients (31%) in the CAAG group and in 160 of 1232 (13%) patients in the control group (Fisher's exact test $p < 0.0001$). The mean 25(OH)D values were not significantly different between female and male patients, neither among CAAG patients (female mean 19.2 vs. male 17.0 ng/ml, $p = 0.65$) nor among controls (female mean 26.9 vs. male 27.0 ng/ml, $p = 0.07$). A

Table 1 Atrophy in the gastric mucosa: histological classification and grading [26]

0. Absent (= score 0)				
1. Indefinite (no score is applicable)				
2. Present	Histological type	Location & key lesions		Grading
		Antrum	Corpus	
	2.1. Non-metaplastic	Gland disappearance (shrinking) Fibrosis of the lamina propria		2.1.1. Mild = G1 (1–30%) 2.1.2. Moderate = G2 (31–60%) 2.1.3. Severe = G3 (> 60%)
	2.2. Metaplastic	Metaplasia: – Intestinal	Metaplasia: – Pseudo-pyloric – Intestinal	2.2.1. Mild = G1 (1–30%) 2.2.2. Moderate = G2 (31–60%) 2.2.3. Severe = G3 (> 60%)

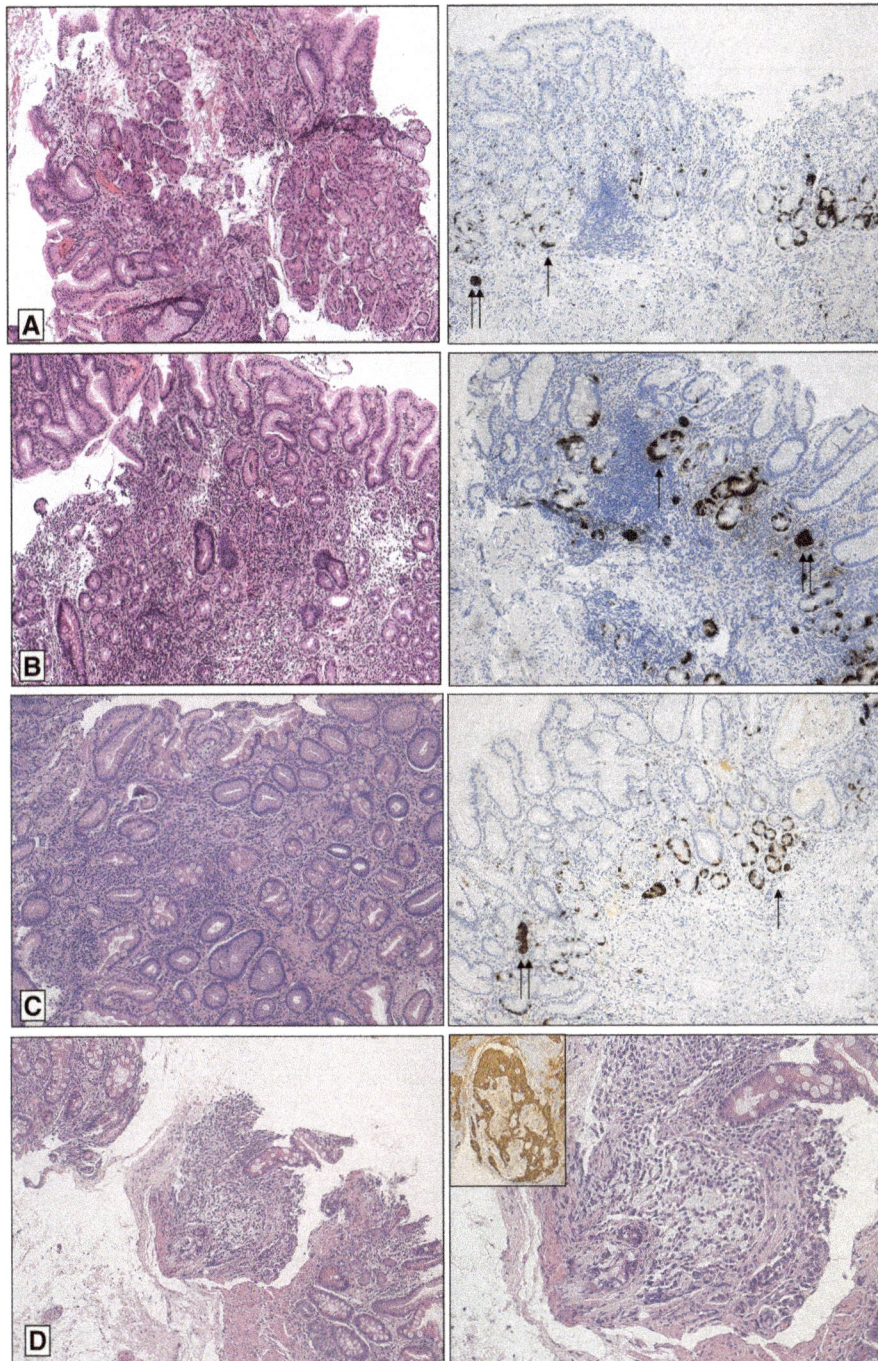

Fig. 1 Histological features of atrophic gastritis. **a** Mild atrophic chronic gastritis, showing focal loss of mucosal glands associated with mild chronic inflammation (EE 10x). Chromogranin A immunohistochemical stain shows linear (one arrow) and micronodular (two arrows) neuroendocrine cells hyperplasia. **b** Moderate atrophic chronic gastritis, showing moderate loss of mucosal glands associated with moderate chronic inflammation (EE 10x). Chromogranin A immunohistochemical stain shows linear (one arrow) and micronodular (two arrows) neuroendocrine cells hyperplasia. **c** Severe atrophic chronic gastritis, showing diffuse and severe loss of mucosal glands associated with mild chronic inflammation (EE 10x). Chromogranin A immunohistochemical stain shows linear (one arrow) and micronodular (two arrows) neuroendocrine cells hyperplasia. **d** Gastric carcinoid, characterized by nodular and solid growth pattern of monomorphous neuroendocrine cells (EE 10x left and 20x right), immunoreactive for Chromogranin A (insert)

Table 2 Demographic and biochemical data of CAAG patients and healthy controls

	CAAG patients ($n = 87$)	Healthy control ($n = 1232$)	p value
Female (%)	71 (82)	956 (76)	ns
Age (years) Mean ± SD	63.5 ± 12.8	62.3 ± 13.2	ns
25(OH)D ng/ml Mean ± SD	18.8 ± 9.7	27.0 ± 16.3	< 0.0001
25(OH)D < 20 ng/ml n (%)	57 (66%)	438 (36%)	< 0.0001
25(OH)D < 12.5 ng/ml n (%)	27 (31%)	160 (13%)	< 0.0001

CAAG chronic autoimmune atrophic gastritis, *25(OH)D* 25-OH-Vitamin D, *ns* not significant

statistical difference in the number of patients diagnosed in summer/spring vs winter/autumn was not observed ($p < 0.001$).

The demographic and biochemical data of CAAG patients with and without vitamin D deficiency are detailed in Table 3.

In CAAG patients a deficit of vitamin B12, defined as vitamin B12 levels below 190 ng/ml, was present in 28 cases (32%). In this setting, a significant correlation between vitamin B_{12} values at diagnosis and 25(OH)D levels was observed ($r_s = 0.25$, $p = 0.01$). In detail, mean 25(OH)D was lower in patients with vitamin B_{12} deficiency ($15.9 ± 9.9$ ng/ml) compared with patients without vitamin B_{12} deficiency ($20.2 ± 9.7$ ng/ml) ($p = 0.025$).

All the CAAG patients had normal serum calcium levels (mean $9.6 ± 1.8$ mg/dl) and ionized calcium levels ($1.2 ± 0.1$ mmol/l). Elevation in PTH levels, defined as PTH levels > 65 pg/ml was observed in 22 of the 87 CAAG patients (25%) (mean $74 ± 24.2$ pg/ml). In all

these cases, proper vitamin D supplementation led to PTH levels normalization, thus the diagnosis of secondary hyperparathyroidism due to vitamin D deficiency was made.

In our series, the CAAG patients with moderate to severe gastric atrophy at histology presented significantly lower 25(OH)D values than those with mild atrophy (11.8 vs. 20 ng/ml; $p = 0.0047$). Moreover, 25(OH)D levels were significantly lower in CAAG patients with gastric carcinoid as compared to the group of CAAG patients without ECL hyperplasia or having linear or micronodular ECL hyperplasia (11.80 vs. 19.75 ng/ml; $p = 0.0041$) (Fig. 2).

A significant inverse correlation ($r_s = -0.25$, $p = 0.032$) between 25(OH)D and BMI was observed in CAAG patients. A direct correlation was observed between 25(OH)D and circulating vitamin B_{12} ($r_s = -0.28$, $p = 0.009$), whereas there was not any significant correlation between 25(OH)D levels and gastrin levels ($p = 0.7$).

Table 3 Demographic and biochemical data of CAAG patients with and without vitamin D deficiency

Patients	25(OH)D deficiency ($n = 57$)	Normal 25(OH)D ($n = 30$)	p value
Female n (%)	47 (83)	24 (80)	ns
Age (years) Mean ± SD	63.4 ± 12.8	64.6 ± 12.9	ns
APCA positivity n (%)	50 (88)	29 (97)	ns
Atrophy n (%)			
• mild	24 (42)	13 (43)	ns
• moderate	20 (35)	14 (47)	
• severe	13 (23)	3 (10)	
ECL cell hyperplasia n (%)			
• normal	17 (30)	7 (23)	ns
• linear	12 (21)	11 (37)	
• micronodular	10 (17)	7 (23)	
• gastric carcinoid	18 (32)	5 (17)	

APCA Anti-parietal cell antibodies, *ECL* entero-chromaffin-like, *25(OH)D* 25-OH-Vitamin D

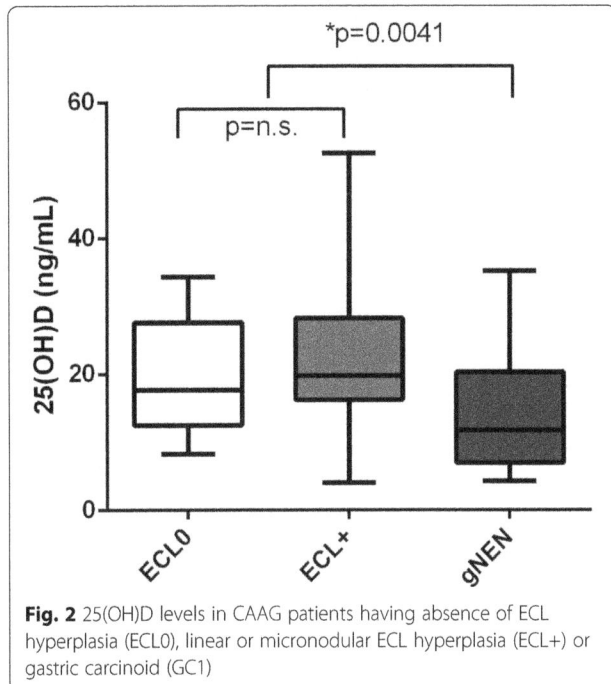

Fig. 2 25(OH)D levels in CAAG patients having absence of ECL hyperplasia (ECL0), linear or micronodular ECL hyperplasia (ECL+) or gastric carcinoid (GC1)

Among the 39 CAAG patients who underwent DXA, 17 patients had osteoporosis, 14 had low bone density/osteopenia, while in the remaining 5 patients the DXA scan was normal. 25(OH)D levels did not significantly differ among patients with osteoporosis/osteopenia and normal DXA.

Discussion

The present study has documented significantly lower mean 25(OH)D values in CAAG patients as compared with outpatient controls. Moreover, in CAAG patients a significantly higher rate of 25(OH)D deficiency, considering 25(OH)D values lower either than 20 ng/ml or 12.5 ng/ml, was observed. These results are similar to those observed by Antico et al. [22] that reported lower 25(OH)D values in CAAG patients when compared to patients with non-specific gastritis or healthy controls. The authors reported 25(OH)D mean levels in CAAG patients to be 9.8 ± 5.6 ng/mL versus 21.3 ± 12.2 ng/mL in controls. On the basis of their results, the authors speculated that vitamin D deficiency may play a role in the pathogenesis of the autoimmune processes [22]. In addition a previous study from our group [21] observed an higher rate of hyperparathyroidism secondary to vitamin D deficiency in CAAG patients. On the other hand, Eastell et al. [20] did not show a significant difference in 25(OH)D values among 21 CAAG patients and healthy controls [20], even though the low number of cases evaluated may have limited the results of their study.

To date the pathogenesis of hypovitaminosis D in CAAG patients has not been clarified. However, as for other micronutrients [11], a decreased absorption/increased destruction of vitamin D in the gastrointestinal mucosa due to the hypochlorhydria and bacterial overgrowth might be hypothesized. Interestingly, this is the first study showing significantly lower 25(OH)D values in CAAG with moderate to severe gastric atrophy as compared to those with mild atrophy ($p = 0.0047$). This finding strongly suggests a causal association between the degree of mucosal atrophy and 25(OH)D levels. It may be postulated that in patients with mild atrophy the residual production of gastric acid can preserve a sufficient rate of vitamin D absorption, which, however, becomes insufficient in more advanced stages of the disease.

The hypothesis of a progressive functional alteration in the gastric mucosa over time has been already proposed with regard to patients with CAAG so as to explain the progression from microcytic anemia to macrocytic anemia [9, 27]. Indeed, CAAG patients with iron deficiency anemia have been reported to be younger than patients presenting with pernicious anemia. This suggests iron deficiency to be an early manifestation of CAAG, while the depletion of vitamin B_{12} stores appears to take many years longer and to reveal in older patients, when a severe deficiency of the intrinsic factor has been established [9, 27]. Accordingly, in our study CAAG patients' presented a significant correlation between vitamin B_{12} values at diagnosis and 25(OH)D levels ($p = 0.009$), probably because these levels are both dependent on the residual gastric function and are reduced in the advanced stages of disease.

Interestingly, our study has showed significantly lower 25-OHvitD levels in patients with gastric neuroendocrine neoplasms (NENs) as compared to patients without gastric NENs. The pathogenic mechanism leading to this association has not been fully elucidated yet, however vitamin D has proved to be involved in cell growth, apoptosis, differentiation, cell adhesion, immune regulation, angiogenesis, and metastasis in epithelial tissues [28, 29] Therefore, the possible role of hypovitaminosis D in the development of gastric NENs may be postulated. In the last few years a number of studies have focused on the antineoplastic properties of vitamin D in different solid neoplasms [30–32] and recently a paper from our group showed a significant higher prevalence of vitamin D deficiency among NEN patients [33]. Moreover, in the same study we observed an improved clinical outcome for patients supplemented by vitamin D, reinforcing the hypothesis on an antiproliferative effect of vitamin D supplementation on NEN.

Gastric achlorhydria secondary to gastric surgery, long-term PPI intake or CAAG has been reported to increase the risk of bone health impairment [14]. A recent meta-analysis has shown that PPIs increase the rate of any site fractures of 16% and in particular the risk of hip (30%) and spine fractures (56%) [34]. However, to date the studies investigating the occurrence of osteoporosis in the setting of CAAG are rare and inconclusive [20]. In the present series, DXA scan results did not significantly differ between CAAG patients with vitamin D deficiency and those with normal levels. However, this can be owed to the small number of patients who underwent bone densitometry in the present study (39 out of 86). Therefore, the exact influence of vitamin D deficiency on osteopenia/osteoporosis in CAAG patients remains to be accurately evaluated. Some previous reports have suggested a reduction of bone density in the lumbar spine of patients with pernicious anemia, even though negative reports have also been published [35–37]. A recent study by Kim et al. has found a significant association between atrophic gastritis and osteoporosis in post-menopausal women aged 60 or older, after adjusting for age, body mass index, triglycerides, cholesterol, alcohol consumption, and smoking status [16]. Interestingly, a previous study had not found a significant association between bone mass density and atrophic gastritis [38], however, the participants in that study were relatively young. Therefore, it is possible that the onset of 25(OH)D deficiency in patients with CAAG is a long-developing process leading to significant alterations in older patients with a long-standing history of disease.

A decrease in calcium salts dissolution and absorption in non-acidic conditions has been previously suggested as the main pathological mechanism for bone impairment in patients with achlorhydria. Remarkably, the active transcellular absorption of ionized calcium in the duodenum and proximal small intestine represents the most important physiological pathway for calcium absorption and is highly dependent on vitamin D. Thus, it seems possible that the vitamin D deficiency in CAAG patients also explains calcium malabsorption and alterations in bone mineralization.

Possible limitations of our study are the relatively small number of patients evaluated and that 25(OH)D determination were obtained during outpatient's examination during all the year; however we did not observe a statistical difference in the number of patients diagnosed in summer/spring vs winter/autumn. Strengths of presents study were the use of strict diagnostic criteria for CAAG which enables to obtain a highly homogenous group of study and the centralization of all laboratory tests.

Conclusions

This study has clearly demonstrated that vitamin D deficiency is more frequent in patients affected by CAAG than in the general population and correlates with the grade of gastric atrophy. The pathogenic mechanism

underlying this association has not been fully elucidated, but it is probably due to a decreased absorption of vitamin D secondary to gastric hypo-achlorhydria. Further larger studies are necessary to evaluate the relevance of vitamin D deficiency in the occurrence of osteopenia and osteoporosis in CAAG patients.

Abbreviations

25(OH)D: 25-OH-Vitamin D; APCA: Anti-parietal cell antibodies; BMD: Bone mineral density; BMI: Body mass index; Ca^{2+}: Ionized calcium; CAAG: Chronic autoimmune atrophic gastritis; CgA: Chromogranin A; DXA: Dual-energy X-ray absorptiometry; ECL: Entero-chromaffin-like; GC1: Type 1 gastric carcinoids; NENs: Neuroendocrine neoplasms; P: Phosphate; PTH: Parathormone

Acknowledgements

Marc Hinxman-Allegri as an English native speaker revised the manuscript for language and style.

Funding

This research did not receive any specific grant from funding agencies in the public, commercial, or not-for-profit sectors.

Authors' contributions

SM planned the work; IF and CC performed the literature search; FC and AZ wrote the first draft of the manuscript; SM, SB and FC edited the subsequent versions of the manuscript; DC and MP critically revised the manuscript for relevant intellectual content. Finally, all authors read and approved the final manuscript.

Competing interests

The authors declare that there is no conflict of interest that could be perceived as prejudicing the impartiality of the research reported.

Author details

[1]Gastroenterology and Endoscopy Unit, Fondazione IRCCS Ca' Granda Ospedale Maggiore Policlinico, Milan, Italy. [2]Department of Pathophysiology and Transplantation, Università degli Studi di Milano, Milan, Italy. [3]Division of Pathology, Fondazione IRCCS Ca' Granda Ospedale Maggiore Policlinico, 20122 Milan, Italy. [4]Laboratory of Clinical Chemistry and Microbiology, Fondazione IRCCS Ca' Granda Ospedale Maggiore Policlinico, Milan, Italy.

References

1. Toh BH, van Driel IR, Gleeson PA. Pernicious anemia. N Engl J Med. 1997; 337:1441–8.
2. Toh BH. Diagnosis and classification of autoimmune gastritis. Autoimmun Rev. 2014;13:459–62.
3. Toh BH, Alderuccio F. Pernicious anaemia. Autoimmunity. 2004;37:357–61.

4. Solcia E, Capella C, Fiocca R, Cornaggia M, Rindi G, Villani L, et al. Exocrine and endocrine epithelial changes in type A and B chronic gastritis. In: Malfertheiner P, Ditschuneit H, editors. Helicobacter pylori, Gastritis and Peptic Ulcer. Berlin: Springer Berlin Heidelberg; 1990. p. 245–58.

5. Wintrobe M, Lee G, Boggs D, Bithell T, Foerster J, Athens J, et al. Megaloblastic and nonmegaloblastic macrocytic anemias. In: Wintrobe M, Lee G, Boggs D, Bithell T, Foerster J, editors. Clinical hematology. 8th ed. Philadelphia: Lea & Febiger; 1981. p. 559–604.

6. Kozyraki R, Cases O. Vitamin B12 absorption: mammalian physiology and acquired and inherited disorders. Biochimie. 2013;95:1002–7.

7. Gonçalves C, Oliveira ME, Palha AM, Ferrão A, Morais A, Lopes AI. Autoimmune gastritis presenting as iron deficiency anemia in childhood. World J Gastroenterol. 2014;20:15780–6.

8. Lagarde S, Jovenin N, Diebold MD, Jaussaud R, Cahn V, Bertin E, et al. Is there any relationship between pernicious anemia and iron deficiency? Gastroenterol Clin Biol. 2006;30:1245–9.

9. Hershko C, Ronson A, Souroujon M, Maschler I, Heyd J, Patz J. Variable hematologic presentation of autoimmune gastritis: age-related progression from iron deficiency to cobalamin depletion. Blood. 2006;107:1673–9.

10. Alt H, Chinn H, Farmer C. The blood plasma ascorbic acid in patients with achlorhydria. Am J Med Sci. 1939;197:222–32.

11. Ludden J, Flexner J, Wright I. Studies on ascorbic acid deficiency in gastric diseases: incidence, diagnosis, and treatment. Am J Dig Dis. 1941;8:249–52.

12. Cavalcoli F, Zilli A, Conte D, Massironi S. Micronutrient deficiencies in patients with chronic atrophic autoimmune gastritis: a review. World J Gastroenterol. 2017;23:563–72.

13. Vilarrasa N, San José P, García I, Gómez-Vaquero C, Miras PM, de Gordejuela AG, et al. Evaluation of bone mineral density loss in morbidly obese women after gastric bypass: 3-year follow-up. Obes Surg. 2011;21:465–72.

14. Sipponen P, Harkonen M. Hypochlorhydric stomach: a risk condition for calcium malabsorption and osteoporosis? Scand J Gastroenterol. 2010;45:133–8.

15. Goerss JB, Kim CH, Atkinson EJ, Eastell R, O'Fallon WM, Melton LJ. Risk of fractures in patients with pernicious anemia. J Bone Miner Res. 1992;7:573–9.

16. Kim HW, Kim YH, Han K, Nam GE, Kim GS, Han BD, et al. Atrophic gastritis: a related factor for osteoporosis in elderly women. PLoS One. 2014;9:e101852.

17. Aasarød KM, Mosti MP, Stunes AK, Reseland JE, Basso T, Syversen U, et al. Impaired skeletal health in patients with chronic atrophic gastritis. Scand J Gastroenterol. 2016;51:774–81.

18. Recker RR. Calcium absorption and achlorhydria. N Engl J Med. 1985;313:70–3.

19. Ivanovich P, Fellows H, Rich C. The absorption of calcium carbonate. Ann Intern Med. 1967;66:917–23.

20. Eastell R, Vieira NE, Yergey AL, Wahner HW, Silverstein MN, Kumar R, et al. Pernicious anaemia as a risk factor for osteoporosis. Clin Sci (Lond). 1992;82:681–5.

21. Massironi S, Cavalcoli F, Rossi RE, Conte D, Spampatti MP, Ciafardini C, et al. Chronic autoimmune atrophic gastritis associated with primary hyperparathyroidism: a transversal prospective study. Eur J Endocrinol. 2013;168:755–61.

22. Antico A, Tozzoli R, Giavarina D, Tonutti E, Bizzaro N. Hypovitaminosis D as predisposing factor for atrophic type a gastritis: a case-control study and review of the literature on the interaction of vitamin D with the immune system. Clin Rev Allergy Immunol. 2012;42:355–64.

23. Dixon MF, Genta RM, Yardley JH, Correa P. Classification and grading of gastritis. The updated Sydney system. International workshop on the histopathology of gastritis, Houston 1994. Am J Surg Pathol. 1996;20:1161–81.

24. Solcia E, Fiocca R, Villani L, Luinetti O, Capella C. Hyperplastic, dysplastic, and neoplastic enterochromaffin-like-cell proliferations of the gastric mucosa. Classification and histogenesis. Am J Surg Pathol. 1995;19:S1–7.

25. Marignani M, Delle Fave G, Mecarocci S, Bordi C, Angeletti S, D'Ambra G, et al. High prevalence of atrophic body gastritis in patients with unexplained microcytic and macrocytic anemia: a prospective screening study. Am J Gastroenterol. 1999;94:766–72.

26. Rugge M, Pennelli G, Pilozzi E, Fassan M, Ingravallo G, Russo VM, et al. Gastritis: the histology report. Dig Liver Dis. 2011;43(Suppl 4):S373–84.

27. Solcia E, Fiocca R, Villani L, Gianatti A, Cornaggia M, Chiaravalli A, et al. Morphology and pathogenesis of endocrine hyperplasias, precarcinoid lesions, and carcinoids arising in chronic atrophic gastritis. Scand J Gastroenterol Suppl. 1991;180:146–59.

28. Swami S, Raghavachari N, Muller UR, Bao YP, Feldman D. Vitamin D growth inhibition of breast cancer cells: gene expression patterns assessed by cDNA microarray. Breast Cancer Res Treat. 2003;80:49–62.

29. Whitfield GK, Jurutka PW, Haussler CA, Hsieh JC, Barthel TK, Jacobs ET, Dominguez CE, Thatcher ML, Haussler MR. Nuclear Vitamin D Receptor: Structure-Function, Molecular Control of Gene Transcription, and Novel Bioactions. in: Feldman D, Pike JW, Glorieux FH, editors. Vitamin D. vol. 1. Oxford: Elsevier Academic Press; 2005. pp. 219-261. https://doi.org/10.1016/B978-012252687-9/50016-4.

30. Leyssens C, Verlinden L, Verstuyf A. Antineoplastic effects of 1,25(OH)2D3 and its analogs in breast, prostate and colorectal cancer. Endocr Relat Cancer. 2013;20:R31–47.

31. Feldman D, Krishnan AV, Swami S, Giovannucci E, Feldman BJ. The role of vitamin D in reducing cancer risk and progression. Nat Rev Cancer. 2014;14:342–57.

32. Jacobs ET, Kohler LN, Kunihiro AG, Jurutka PW. Vitamin D and colorectal, breast, and prostate cancers: a review of the epidemiological evidence. J Cancer. 2016;7:232–40.

33. Massironi S, Zilli A, Bernasconi S, Fanetti I, Cavalcoli F, Ciafardini C, et al. Impact of vitamin D on the clinical outcome of gastro-Entero-pancreatic neuroendocrine neoplasms: report on a series from a single institute. Neuroendocrinology. 2017;105:403–11.

34. Yu EW, Bauer SR, Bain PA, Bauer DC. Proton pump inhibitors and risk of fractures: a meta-analysis of 11 international studies. Am J Med. 2011;124:519–26.

35. Bo-Linn GW, Davis GR, Buddrus DJ, Morawski SG, Santa Ana C, Fordtran JS. An evaluation of the importance of gastric acid secretion in the absorption of dietary calcium. J Clin Invest. 1984;73:640–7.

36. Knox TA, Kassarjian Z, Dawson-Hughes B, Golner BB, Dallal GE, Arora S, et al. Calcium absorption in elderly subjects on high- and low-fiber diets: effect of gastric acidity. Am J Clin Nutr. 1991;53:1480–6.

37. Adachi Y, Shiota E, Matsumata T, Iso Y, Yoh R, Kitano S. Bone mineral density in patients taking H2-receptor antagonist. Calcif Tissue Int. 1998;62:283–5.

38. Kakehasi AM, Carvalho AV, Maksud FA, Barbosa AJ. Serum levels of vitamin B12 are not related to low bone mineral density in postmenopausal Brazilian women. Rev Bras Reumatol. 2012;52:863–9.

26

Noninvasive biomarkers of gut barrier function identify two subtypes of patients suffering from diarrhoea predominant-IBS

Michele Linsalata, Giuseppe Riezzo, Benedetta D'Attoma, Caterina Clemente, Antonella Orlando and Francesco Russo* (ID)

Abstract

Background: Alterations of the small-intestinal permeability (s-IP) might play an essential role in both diarrhoea-predominant IBS (D-IBS) and celiac disease (CD) patients. Our aims were to analyse in D-IBS patients the symptom profile along with the levels of urinary sucrose (Su), lactulose (La), mannitol (Ma), and circulating biomarkers (zonulin, intestinal fatty acid binding protein - I-FABP, and diamine oxidase - DAO) of the gastrointestinal (GI) barrier function. The pro-inflammatory interleukins 6 and 8 (IL-6 and IL-8), the plasma values of lipopolysaccharide (LPS), and Toll-like receptor 4 (TLR-4) were also investigated. Besides, these biomarkers were compared with those in CD and healthy controls (HC). Finally, comparisons were performed between D-IBS patients with [D-IBS(+)] and without [D-IBS(−)] increased s-IP according to normal or altered La/Ma ratio.

Methods: The study included 39 D-IBS patients, 32 CD patients, and 20 HC. GI permeability was assayed by high-performance liquid chromatography determination in the urine of Su and La/Ma ratio. ELISA kits assayed circulating concentrations of zonulin, I-FABP, DAO, IL-6, IL-8, LPS, and TLR-4. The Mann–Whitney or the Kruskal–Wallis with Dunn's post-test was used to assess differences among the groups.

Results: As for the La/Ma ratio, %Su, and I-FABP levels, D-IBS patients were significantly different from CD, but not HC. IL-6 levels were significantly higher in CD than HC, whereas IL-8 levels were significantly higher in both D-IBS and CD patients than HC. By opposite, LPS, and TLR-4 concentrations did not differ significantly among the groups. When D-IBS patients were categorised according to normal or altered s-IP, D-IBS(+) patients had %La, %Su, I-FABP, and DAO levels significantly higher than D-IBS(−) ones. The inflammatory parameters and markers of bacterial translocation (namely, IL-6 and LPS) were significantly higher in D-IBS(+) patients than D-IBS(−) ones.

Conclusions: The present study suggests that two distinct D-IBS subtypes could be identified. The investigation of possible s-IP alterations (i.e., considering the La/Ma ratio) might be useful to assess better and categorise this heterogeneous D-IBS population.

Keywords: Celiac disease, Diarrhoea-predominant irritable bowel syndrome, Gut barrier, Interleukins, Intestinal permeability, Lipopolysaccharide

* Correspondence: francesco.russo@irccsdebellis.it
Laboratory of Nutritional Pathophysiology, National Institute of Gastroenterology, "S. de Bellis" Research Hospital, Via Turi 27, I-70013 Castellana Grotte, Bari, Italy

Background

Irritable bowel syndrome (IBS) is a prevalent functional disorder in Italy, with percentages in the urban area (13.7%) double that in the rural area (5.9%) [1]. Although IBS still represents an underdiagnosed condition, it is one of the most important reasons for care-seeking within gastroenterology. The current IBS diagnosis is mainly based on the symptom criteria, stool characteristics [2], and specific questionnaires [3]. Additionally, as reported by the Bristol Stool Form Scale, the stool pattern features allow the categorisation of IBS subtypes in diarrhoea-predominant IBS (D-IBS), constipation-predominant IBS (C-IBS), mixed-type, and not classified [4].

Of note, the classic gastrointestinal (GI) symptom profile of the D-IBS subtype often mimics that of patients who have celiac disease (CD) (e.g., abdominal pain, bloating and diarrhoea) [5]. CD is a widespread auto-immune disorder characterised by chronic inflammation of the proximal small intestine, resulting in villous atrophy and malabsorption in genetically susceptible individuals after the ingestion of gluten [6]. Although clear key differences exist in their aetiology and treatment, the last years data in the literature has suggested that alterations in the intestinal barrier, mainly in the upper gut, might play an essential role in the development and perpetuation for both diseases [7, 8]. If on the one hand, gluten toxicity is a well-known cause of alterations in the small intestinal permeability (s-IP) of CD patients [9], on the other new insights into the aetiology of IBS have pointed out a role for low-grade inflammation in s-IP alterations of patients suffering from D-IBS [10]. Altered gut permeability can permit the passage of the luminal contents into the underlying tissues and thus into the bloodstream, resulting in both the activation of the immune response and the induction of gut inflammation. This permeability alteration is now considered the basis for the pathogenesis of many diseases, including IBS and CD. Therefore, the assessment of s-IP and the related molecular mechanisms may become an interesting parameter to consider in clinical practice for studying and treating these diseases [11]. However, no study has previously been performed aimed at comparing s-IP changes in these two diseases by applying the same methodologies.

Initial studies considered the use of single probes, such as ^{51}Cr-EDTA, to assess the site of increased IP. This procedure, however, proved to be dependent on many non-mucosal factors, which not only reduced the sensitivity and specificity of the test but also posed a problem in the data interpretation. Moreover, the use of a radioactive substance such as ^{51}Cr-EDTA exposes patients to radiation, thus putting a limit in its application in some patients (e.g. paediatric subjects, women of childbearing age, healthy subjects and patients requiring multiple permeability analyses) [12].

Nowadays, current methods for evaluating upper gut (gastric and small bowel) permeability use probes, such as small sugar molecules of different sizes. Among them, the most used are sucrose (Su), lactulose (La), and mannitol (Ma) [13]. Su, a disaccharide hydrolysed by the enzyme sucrase in the duodenum, has been proposed as a marker of gastric permeability [14]. La crosses the small intestinal barrier by paracellular passage if it is compromised, and it is considered a marker of tight junction (TJ) integrity. The smaller probe, Ma, crosses the epithelial barrier by transcellular passage, giving information on the whole epithelial absorptive area [15]. Since their urinary recovery is affected by several non-mucosal factors (e.g., gastric emptying, intestinal transit, and renal clearance), using a ratio rather than the single urinary recovery percentages overcomes such variations. For this reason, the La/Ma ratio in urine is considered a reliable parameter to evaluate the impairment of s-IP [14].

The intestinal barrier may be considered as a dynamic system also responding to humoral signals, and zonulin is one of the physiological modulators that regulate s-IP by changing TJ protein-protein interaction. It has been studied as a peripheral marker of IP in some diseases, and potential intestinal stimuli, such as gluten, can increase its secretion [16]. Intestinal barrier integrity is essential for s-IP. In this context, the intestinal fatty acid binding protein (I-FABP), a small cytosolic protein of 14 kDa specific to mature small bowel enterocytes, has proven to be a sensitive marker of damage to the intestinal epithelium, and its detection in the serum is suggestive for a breakdown of the enterocyte membrane [17]. Likewise, diamine oxidase (DAO), an intracellular enzyme with a high level of activity in the upper layer of intestinal villi, is considered another marker for the integrity of intestinal epithelium, whose serum levels increase in the case of damage and loss of barrier function [18]. Overall, few studies [19] have been conducted to evaluate these putative biomarkers of gut integrity in patients suffering from D-IBS.

In order to improve our knowledge about s-IP and the integrity of the GI barrier as well as their implications for D-IBS pathophysiology, the aims of this study were to (a) analyse the symptom profile using a validated questionnaire such as the Gastrointestinal Symptom Rating Scale (GSRS) [20] in D-IBS patients and compare it with those recorded in CD patients and healthy controls (HC); (b) evaluate the levels of urinary (La, Ma, and Su) and circulating (zonulin, I-FABP, and DAO) biomarkers of function and integrity of the GI barrier along with the pro-inflammatory interleukins 6 and 8 (IL-6 and IL-8), the plasma values of lipopolysaccharide (LPS), and Toll-like receptor 4 (TLR-4) in D-IBS patients. Comparisons with the results obtained from CD patients and HC subjects were then performed; and (c) compare GI symptoms and the above-mentioned urinary and circulating markers in D-IBS patients with increased s-IP, as diagnosed by the La/Ma ratio, [D-IBS(+)], with those in D-IBS patients with normal s-IP, [D-IBS(–)].

Methods
Study participants
Patients suffering from diarrhoea-predominant IBS according to Rome III criteria, were recruited in this prospective case-control study from among the outpatients of the National Institute of Gastroenterology, "S. de Bellis" Research Hospital, Castellana Grotte, Italy.

The inclusion criteria were: (*a*) age more than 18 years; (*b*) a symptom profile resembling D-IBS with a stool pattern, as described according to Schmulson et al. [21]; (*c*) active symptoms for at least 2 weeks; (*d*) a minimum average of 3.0 on the seven-point Likert scale of the GSRS composite symptom score [20]; (*e*) a diet without any restrictions on eating and drinking (in particular, no previous period of gluten free diet (GFD) before examination); (*f*) as gluten-sensitive diarrhoea without CD is a clinical entity that has been observed in IBS patients positive for HLA-DQ2 or HLA-DQ8 [22], only the HLA-DQ2/HLADQ8-negative/negative D-IBS patients were considered for this study; (*g*) age, body mass index (BMI), anxiety or depression, smoking, alcohol intake and use of medication were accurately checked in order to obtain a group of D-IBS patients as homogeneous as possible.

All the patients underwent a physical examination, whole blood count, liver function tests, stool routine, faecal occult blood test, stool culture, stool examination for parasites, C-reactive protein, thyroid function test, gastroscopy, and colonoscopy in order to exclude patients with organic diseases. As concerns the female patients, to avoid any possible interference and contamination of the urine samples with blood, the urinary and blood samples were obtained within 10 days of the onset of the most recent menstrual cycle (follicular phase).

The diagnosis of CD was performed following the international guidelines and published data [23]. Serologic testing, with a combination of tissue transglutaminase (tTG) and anti-endomysium antibodies (EMA), was used. For recruitment in the study as CD patients, the diagnosis of CD had to be confirmed with a duodenal biopsy sample according to the modified Marsh–Oberhuber criteria (grades 3b–3c) [24].

Exclusion criteria included: post-infectious IBS, hepatic, renal or cardiovascular disease, constipation, metabolic and endocrine disorders, fever, intense physical activity, previous abdominal surgery, history of malignancy, secondary causes of intestinal atrophy, pregnancy, lactose intolerance or giardiasis. Besides, patients did not have to consume medication for the treatment of IBS for 2 weeks before evaluation, antibiotic therapy or probiotic agents, and other drugs known to cause abdominal pain.

The reasons for study discontinuation were recorded in the case report form and could include: death, adverse event (specified), ineligibility to continue the study, lost to follow-up, withdrew consent, and other (including the administrative closure of trial).

Healthy individuals were enrolled from among the administrative staff of our Institute as healthy controls (HC). They denied having metabolic, endocrine, or immunological diseases, dyspepsia, or other GI diseases and did not take any medication. Information on the health status of participants was obtained by an interview on the current diet, lifestyle, medical history, and a physical examination. As criteria for admission, EMA and tTG had to be negative. Besides, metabolic parameters (blood glucose, HbA1c, lipid profile, body weight, and blood pressure) had to be within the normal range of values. The absence of major psychiatric disorders, cancer, and pregnancy were also inclusion criteria. All the women, either patients or controls, were examined during the follicular phase of the menstrual cycle.

All the participants belonging to the three distinct groups (D-IBS, CD, and HC) were subjected to all the scheduled analyses. The CD patients were considered as positive controls. The HC subjects were enrolled as negative controls (study 1). After the D-IBS patients were separated into the D-IBS(+) and D-IBS(–) groups, according to whether s-IP was altered or not at the La/Ma ratio, the clinical characteristics and the urinary and circulating parameters of the two D-IBS subgroups, were evaluated (study 2).

All the subjects were compliant and were willing to participate in the study. Written informed consent was obtained from all the patients and healthy participants for blood testing and clinical data collection. This study was approved by the Institutional Ethics Committee of IRCCS Ospedale Oncologico di Bari - Istituto Tumori Giovanni Paolo II, Bari, Italy, DDG reg. 1227/2013, and it was part of registered research on http://www.clinical-trials.gov (reg. Number: NCT01574209).

Symptom assessment
Patients were evaluated with the GSRS, a validated questionnaire for GI symptoms [20]. GSRS utilizes a seven-level Likert scale (1–7), depending on intensity and frequency of GI symptoms experienced during the previous week. A higher score indicates mainly inconvenient symptoms. Combination scores among the questions can assess the following five domains: "*reflux syndrome*" (halitosis, heartburn, dysphagia and acid regurgitation: max. Score: 28), "*abdominal pain*" (pain referred as epigastric, colic, continuous or indefinite pain, gastric hunger pains and nausea: max. Score: 42), "*indigestion syndrome*" (postprandial fullness, early satiety,

borborygmi, bloating, eructation/belching and increased flatus, max. Score: 42), *"diarrhoea syndrome"* (increased frequency of evacuation, loose stools and urgent need to defecate, max. Score: 21), and *"constipation syndrome"* (reduced frequency of evacuation, hard stools and feeling of incomplete evacuation, max. Score: 21). In the case of D-IBS patients, *"abdominal pain"*, *"indigestion syndrome"*, and *"diarrhoea syndrome"* were taken into account. The stool consistency was investigated using the Bristol stool form chart [4].

Serological assay

All the analytical measurements were performed at the time of enrolment using blind-coded samples (no name or personal identifiers). Peripheral venous blood samples were obtained from participants in the study in the fasting state at least 12 h after the last meal.

After allowing to clot for at least 30 min, the samples were centrifuged at 1600 g for 15 min.

The serum samples were stored at – 80 °C until the assay and tested for immunoglobulin A (IgA) anti-EMA by the indirect immunofluorescence technique using sections of Monkey oesophagus as a substrate and anti-human IgA fluorescein as a conjugate (NOVA Lite Monkey Esophagus IFA it/slides; Inova Diagnostic Inc., San Diego, California, USA) following the instructions of the manufacturer. Slides were examined under a fluorescence microscope to identify the presence of autoantibody. Endomysial positive control, derived from human serum, and negative control, entirely negative for all autoantibodies, were included in every run.

The analysis of IgA anti-tTG was carried out using an enzyme immunoassay (EliACelikey IgA Well; Thermo Fisher Scientific, Waltham, Massachusetts, USA) and performed on the fully automated system (Phadia 250; Phadia GmbH, Freiburg, Germany). All samples were double analysed in a blinded manner, with the addition of positive and negative controls for each analysis run.

Serum levels of I-FABP in peripheral blood were evaluated by enzyme-link immunosorbent assay (ELISA) using a specific anti-human I-FABP antibody (Thermo Fisher Scientific, Waltham, Massachusetts, USA). DAO levels were determined by a commercially available ELISA Kit (Cloud-Clone Corp. Houston, USA). Zonulin was assayed using the specific ELISA kit (Immunodiagnostik AG, Bensheim, Germany).

Plasma levels of IL-6, IL-8, LPS, and TLR-4 were measured in duplicate using commercially available sandwich enzyme-linked immunosorbent assay kits (Human IL-6 ELISA and Human IL-8 ELISA, BD Biosciences, Milan, Italy; Lipopolysaccharide (LPS) ELISA kit Cloud-Clone Corp., Katy, TX, USA; Human Toll-Like Receptor 4 (TLR-4) ELISA kit Cloud-Clone Corp., Katy, TX, USA).

Sugar absorption tests

For the evaluation of GI permeability, all the participants fasted overnight. In order to check for the possible presence of endogenous sugars, a pretest urine was collected in our laboratory. Then subjects drank a sugar test solution containing 10 g of lactulose, 5 g of mannitol and 40 g of sucrose in a volume of 100 ml. Urine samples from control and patient subjects were collected up to 5 h after administration. A l-ml volume of 20% (w/v) chlorohexidine was added to each collection as a preservative regardless of the final total volumes. The total urine volumes from individuals were measured and recorded. After thoroughly mixing, a portion of 2 ml was taken and stored at – 80 °C until analysed.

The detection and measurement of the three sugar probes, Su, La, and Ma in urine were performed by chromatographic analysis as described previously by our group [25]. Briefly, high-performance anion exchange chromatography coupled with pulsed amperometric detection was performed on a Dionex Model ICS-5000 with a gold working electrode, and a 25 μl peek sample loop (Dionex Corp., Sunnyvale, California, USA).

The carbohydrate separation was performed using a Carbopac PA-10 pellicular anion-exchange resin connected to a Carbopac PA-10 guard column (Thermofisher Scientific, Waltham, Massachusetts, USA) at 30 ° C. The samples were eluted with 50 mmol/l NaOH at a flow rate of 1 ml/min. The percentage of ingested Su (%Su) together with those of La (%La) and Ma (%Ma) in urine were evaluated, and the La/Ma ratio was calculated for each sample.

Patients with a La/Ma ratio lower than 0.035 were considered as D-IBS(–); patients with a value equal to or higher than 0.035 were considered D-IBS(+). This cut-off value (mean + 2SD) derived from our previous study performed on a large group of healthy subjects [26].

Statistical analysis

All results are expressed as mean ± SEM unless otherwise specified. Data analysis concerned the comparisons of symptom profile, s-IP, markers of barrier function, and markers of inflammation among HC, D-IBS and CD patients (Study 1) and the comparison of the same variables when D-IBS patients were categorized as D-IBS(–) and D-IBS(+) (Study 2). Non-parametric tests were performed to avoid violation of the assumption of normal distribution. The Mann–Whitney or the Kruskal–Wallis with Dunn's post-test was used to assess differences among two or more the groups, respectively. Pearson's correlation coefficient measures the statistical relationship, or association, between two continuous variables. It is known as the best method of measuring the association between variables of interest because it is based on the method of covariance. The correlation coefficient r was calculated among the urinary and circulating IP biomarkers and the inflammatory parameters. All the differences were considered significant at a 5% level. A specific statistical package for exact nonparametric inference (2005 Stata Statistical Software Release 9; Stata Corp., College Station, Texas, USA) was used.

Results
Study 1. Comparisons among D-IBS patients, celiac disease patients, and healthy controls

Figure 1 shows the flow of participants through the study. Four hundred and three participants were included. Of these, 184 patients did not fulfil the inclusion criteria; 88 patients were excluded due to refusal to undergo endoscopy; 49 patients did not enter the study for other reasons. Thus, 82 patients were considered for

the study: 34 adult celiac patients with diarrhoea as the prevalent GI symptom and 48 D-IBS patients. One CD patients declined to participate, and one underwent major surgery. Three D-IBS patients refused to participate, four suffered from organic diseases, and two did not meet Rome III criteria when they were re-evaluated. The HC group comprised 28 subjects, but 8 of them did not complete the study. As a result, 20 HC subjects were analysed.

Table 1 describes the anthropometric characteristics and clinical data of the HC, D-IBS, and CD patients.

Anthropometric data were not significantly different among the groups. GSRS questionnaire items, such as single and combination items, were similar between D-IBS and CD patients. As expected, the GSRS scores recorded in both patients groups were significantly ($p < 0.05$) different from that in HC subjects.

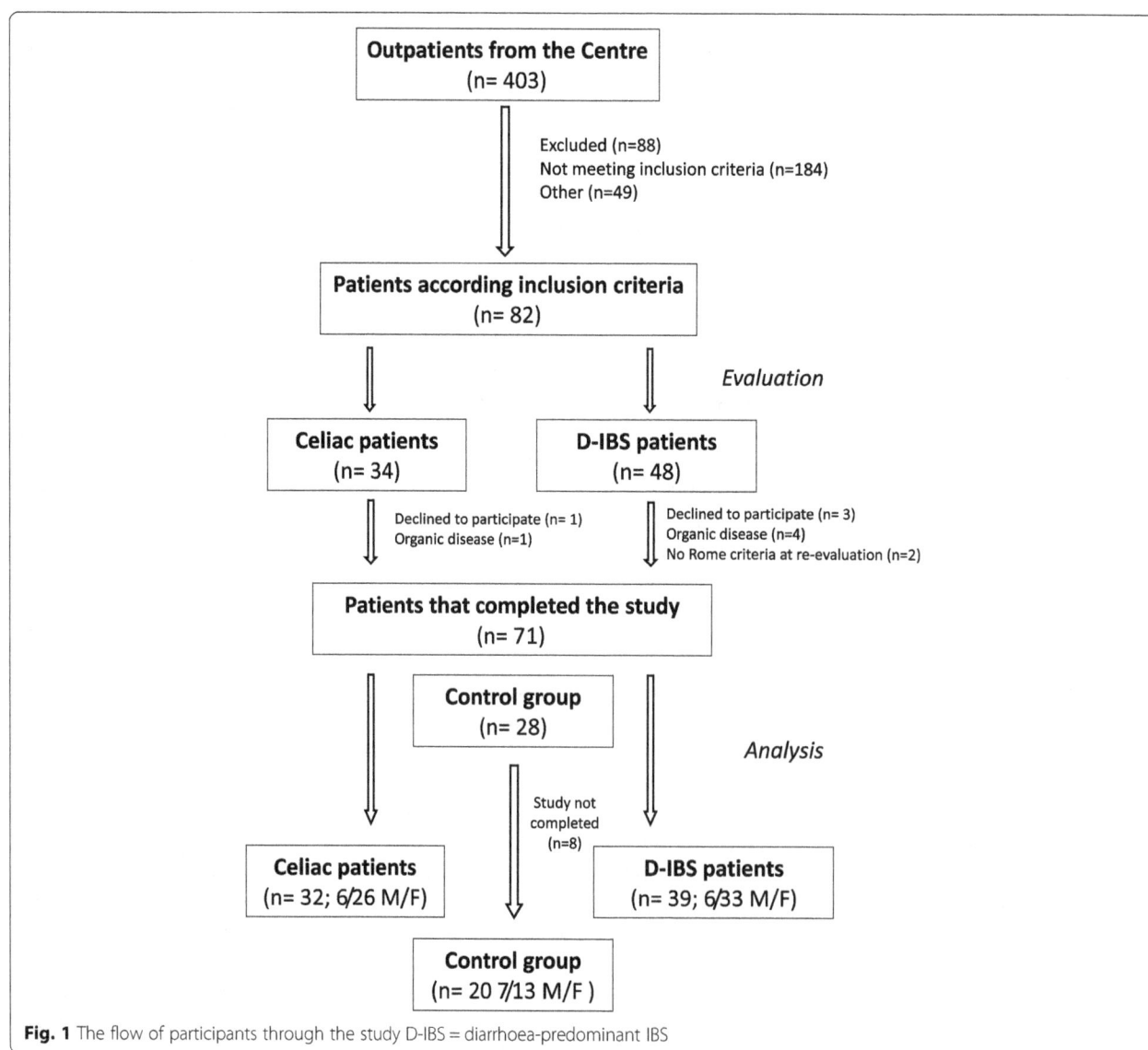

Fig. 1 The flow of participants through the study D-IBS = diarrhoea-predominant IBS

Table 1 Anthropometric and clinical data (GSRS items) of HC, D-IBS, and CD patients

	HC	D-IBS	CD
Anthropometric parameters			
Sex	7/13 (M/F)	6/33 (M/F)	6/26 (M/F)
Age (yrs.)	39.7 ± 7.2[a]	40.05 ± 12.2[a]	35.9 ± 3.71[a]
BMI	23.8 ± 2.9[a]	23.9 ± 3.3[a]	22.39 ± 3.65[a]
GSRS single items			
Nausea/vomiting	1.0 (1–1)[a]	1.0 (1–6)[b]	1.0 (1–6)[b]
Abdominal pain (colic pain)	1.0 (1–1)[a]	3.0 (1–7)[b]	2.0 (1–7)[b]
Gastric hunger pain	1.0 (1–1)[a]	2.0 (1–7)[b]	2.0 (1–7)[b]
Abdominal distension	1.0 (1–1)[a]	5.0 (1–7)[b]	5.0 (1–7)[b]
Burping	1.0 (1–1)[a]	2.0 (1–7)[b]	1.0 (1–7)[b]
Borborygmi	1.0 (1–1)[a]	3.0 (1–7)[b]	3.0 (1–7)[b]
Flatulence	1.0 (1–1)[a]	4.0 (1–7)[b]	4.0 (1–7)[b]
Increased passage of stools	1.0 (1–1)[a]	1.0 (1–7)[b]	2.0 (1–7)[b]
Bristol score	3.0 (3–4)[a]	4.0 (3–7)[b]	4.0 (2–7)[b]
Urgent bowel movement	1.0 (1–1)[a]	3.0 (1–7)[b]	3.0 (1–7)[b]
Feeling of incomplete defecation	1.0 (1–1)[a]	3.0 (1–7)[b]	2.5 (1–5)[b]
GSRS combination scores			
Abdominal pain	6.0 (6–6)[a]	14 (6–25)[b]	13.5 (6–29)[b]
Indigestion syndrome	6.0 (6–6)[a]	19.0 (7–38)[b]	20.0 (7–42)[b]
syndrome	3.0 (3–3)[a]	5.0 (3–21)[b]	6.5 (3–19)[b]

HC healthy controls, *D-IBS* diarrhoea-predominant IBS patients, *CD* celiac disease patients. Continuous data are expressed as Mean ± SD, and discrete data are expressed as Median and range. All data were analysed by Kruskal–Wallis test with Dunn's post-test. Different superscripts differ significantly ($p < 0.05$)

All the HC, D-IBS, and CD subjects underwent IP testing (Fig. 2). As for Ma (Fig. 2A), significant differences were present among the groups ($p = 0.0002$). D-IBS patients and HC subjects showed significantly higher %Ma compared to CD patients ($p < 0.05$ and $p < 0.01$, respectively) at the post hoc test. Significant differences were also present among the three groups ($p < 0.0001$) for %La. D-IBS patients and HC subjects showed significantly ($p < 0.001$) lower %La compared to CD patients at the post hoc test (Fig. 2B). Consequently, the La/Ma ratio differed significantly among the groups ($p < 0.0001$), and D-IBS patients and HC subjects had significantly ($p < 0.001$) lower ratio values than CD patients (Fig. 2C). Finally, %Su also differed significantly ($p = 0.0009$) among the groups, and both D-IBS and HC subjects had significantly ($p < 0.01$) lower values than CD patients (Fig. 2D).

Figure 3 shows the zonulin, I-FABP, and DAO levels in the serum of patients and controls. Zonulin levels differed significantly ($p = 0.021$) among the HC, D-IBS, and

CD groups. The latter group had significantly ($p < 0.05$) higher circulating levels than HC subjects but not D-IBS patients (Fig. 3A). I-FABP concentrations were significantly ($p < 0.0001$) different among the groups, and both D-IBS patients and HC subjects had significantly ($p < 0.001$) lower values than CD patients (Fig. 3B). On the contrary, the DAO levels were not significantly ($p = 0.087$) different among the groups (Fig. 3C).

Figure 4 reports the values of circulating IL-6 and IL-8 along with the circulating concentrations of LPS and TLR-4. As concerns cytokines, the values of IL-6 were significantly ($p = 0.024$) different among the three groups, and CD patients showed significantly ($p < 0.05$) higher levels than HC subjects at the post hoc test (Fig. 4A). IL-8 was also significantly ($p < 0.0001$) different among the groups and not only CD but also D-IBS patients had significantly ($p < 0.001$) higher concentrations than HC subjects (Fig. 4B). Lastly, both the plasma LPS and TLR-4 levels did not differ significantly among the groups ($p = 0.132$ and $p = 0.832$, respectively) (Fig. 4C and D).

Table 2 reports the Pearson correlation coefficients (r) between the urinary and circulating IP biomarkers and the inflammatory parameters in the whole population studied. Significant positive correlations ($p < 0.0001$) were present between I-FABP and IL-8, I-FABP and %La, I-FABP and La/Ma ratio. The La/Ma ratio positively and significantly ($p < 0.0001$) also correlated with IL-8. A significant negative correlation ($p < 0.001$) was present between %Ma and IL-8. Of note, %Su, a marker of gastroduodenal permeability, significantly ($p < 0.0001$) correlated with %La, La/Ma ratio, and I-FABP. No correlations between GSRS symptoms and urinary sugars as well as GSRS symptoms and each serum biomarker were recorded. The length of time since the IBS started and the symptoms and permeability markers did not correlate (data not shown).

Study 2. Differences between D-IBS patients with normal and altered s-IP

When the patients were categorised according to normal or altered s-IP, 28 out 32 CD patients (87.5%) and 18 out 39 D-IBS patients (46.2%) had a La/Ma ratio equal to or higher than 0.035 [D-IBS(+)]. All the controls and 21 out of 39 D-IBS patients (53.8%) had a La/Ma ratio lower than 0.035 [D-IBS(−)].

Table 3 describes the anthropometric and clinical data of D-IBS(+) and D-IBS(−) patients. As for the GSRS single and combination scores, the two groups showed no significant difference for both the GSRS single items and combination scores.

Figure 5 reports the urinary markers of GI barrier function in HC, D-IBS(−), D-IBS(+), and CD patients.

%Ma differed significantly ($p = 0.0004$) among the four groups, and both D-IBS(+) patients and HC subjects had

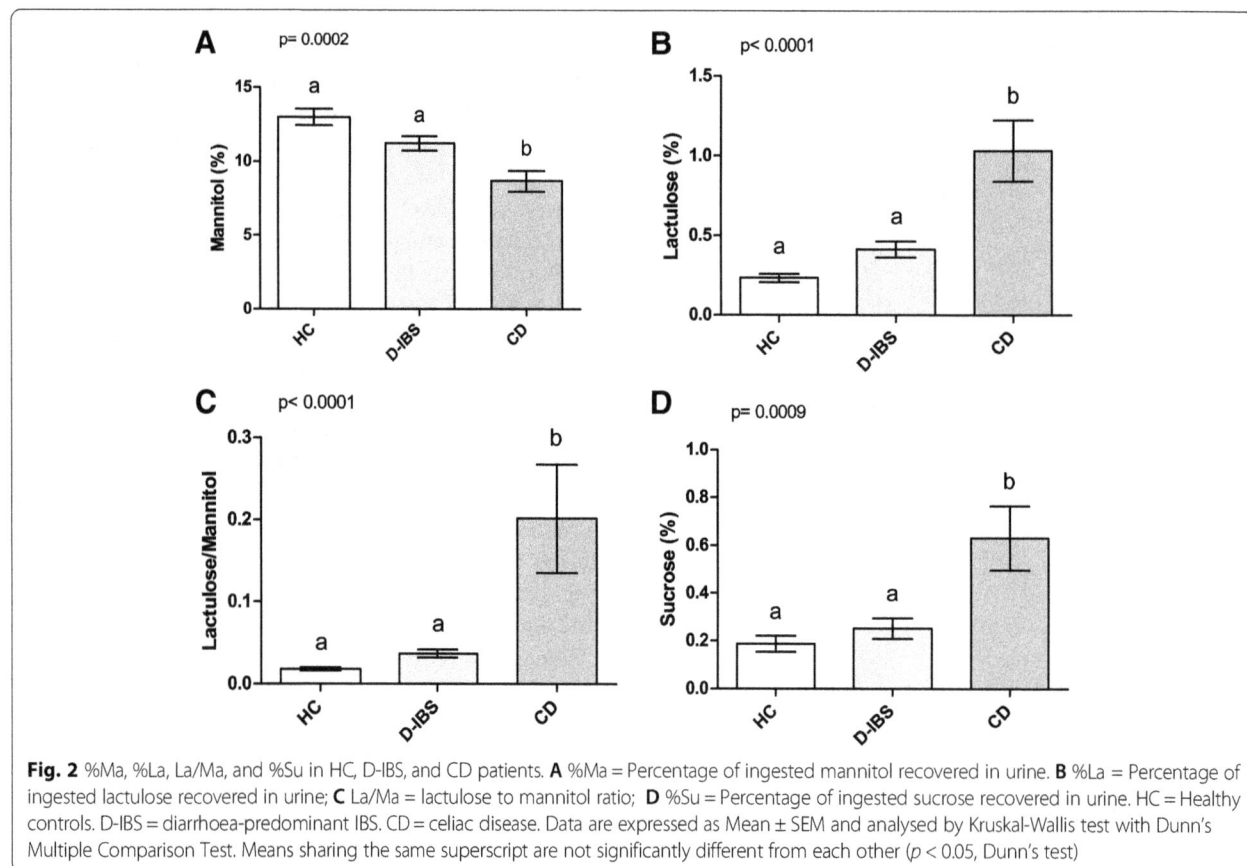

Fig. 2 %Ma, %La, La/Ma, and %Su in HC, D-IBS, and CD patients. **A** %Ma = Percentage of ingested mannitol recovered in urine. **B** %La = Percentage of ingested lactulose recovered in urine; **C** La/Ma = lactulose to mannitol ratio; **D** %Su = Percentage of ingested sucrose recovered in urine. HC = Healthy controls. D-IBS = diarrhoea-predominant IBS. CD = celiac disease. Data are expressed as Mean ± SEM and analysed by Kruskal-Wallis test with Dunn's Multiple Comparison Test. Means sharing the same superscript are not significantly different from each other ($p < 0.05$, Dunn's test)

significantly higher percentages of sugar excretion than CD patients ($p < 0.05$ and $p < 0.001$, respectively) (Fig. 5A). As concerns %La, significant ($p < 0.0001$) differences were present among the groups. At the post hoc test, both D-IBS(+) and CD patients had significantly ($p < 0.001$) higher %La than D-IBS(–) patients and HC subjects (Fig. 5B). This evidence indicates a failure in the paracellular permeability of the former two groups. Consequently, the La/Ma ratio differed significantly ($p < 0.0001$) among the groups, and both D-IBS(+) and CD patients had significantly ($p < 0.001$) higher ratio values than

D-IBS(–) patients and HC subjects (Fig. 5C). A significant difference was also found in %Su among the groups ($p < 0.0001$), and D-IBS(+) and CD patients had significantly ($p < 0.001$) higher concentrations compared to D-IBS(–) patients. Besides, %Su in CD patients was significantly higher than that in HC subjects ($p < 0.05$) (Fig. 5D). When the serum markers of barrier function were compared (Fig. 6), significant ($p = 0.0039$) differences in the zonulin levels were present among the groups, and the CD patients showed significantly ($p < 0.05$) higher levels than HC subjects at the post hoc test (Fig. 6A). The circulating

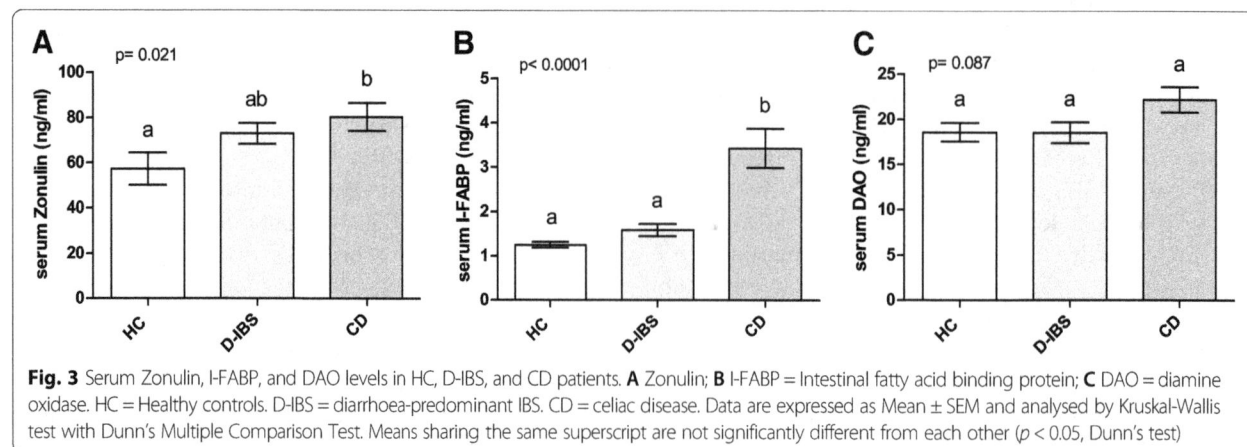

Fig. 3 Serum Zonulin, I-FABP, and DAO levels in HC, D-IBS, and CD patients. **A** Zonulin; **B** I-FABP = Intestinal fatty acid binding protein; **C** DAO = diamine oxidase. HC = Healthy controls. D-IBS = diarrhoea-predominant IBS. CD = celiac disease. Data are expressed as Mean ± SEM and analysed by Kruskal-Wallis test with Dunn's Multiple Comparison Test. Means sharing the same superscript are not significantly different from each other ($p < 0.05$, Dunn's test)

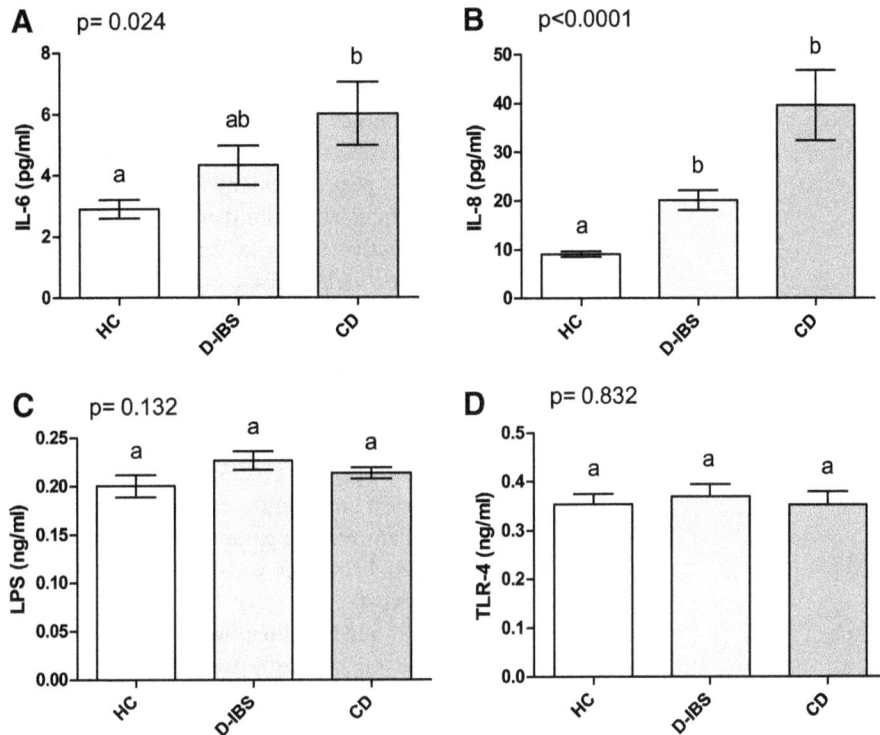

Fig. 4 Plasma concentrations of IL-6, IL-8, LPS, and TLR-4 in HC, D-IBS, and CD patients. **A** IL-6 = Interleukin-6; **B** IL-8 = Interleukin-8; **C** LPS = Lipopolysaccharide; **D** TLR-4 = Toll-like receptor 4. HC = Healthy controls. D-IBS = diarrhoea-predominant IBS. CD = celiac disease. Data are expressed as Mean ± SEM and analysed by Kruskal-Wallis test with Dunn's Multiple Comparison Test. Means sharing the same superscript are not significantly different from each other ($p < 0.05$, Dunn's test)

Table 2 The Pearson correlation coefficients (r) among the inflammatory parameters and the urinary and circulating intestinal permeability biomarkers in the whole population studied (n. 91 cases)

	%Ma	%La	La/Ma	%Su	Zonulin	IFAB-P	DAO	IL-6	IL-8	LPS	TLR-4
%Ma	1										
%La	−0.13	1									
La/Ma	−0.41****	0.93****	1								
%Su	0.09	0.67****	0.58****	1							
Zonulin	−0.22*	0.12	0.17	− 0.12	1						
IFAB-P	−0.26*	0.61****	0.67****	0.47****	0.10	1					
DAO	0.04	0.23*	0.27**	0.17	0.10	0.24*	1				
IL-6	0.05	0.32**	0.32**	0.18	0.24*	0.33**	0.23*	1			
IL-8	−0.36***	0.33**	0.42****	0.16	0.31**	0.45****	0.22*	0.31**	1		
LPS	0.05	0.15	0.14	0.06	0.15	0.07	−0.02	0.27*	0.18	1	
TLR-4	0.16	0.14	0.04	0.7	0.14	0.07	−0.15	0.09	0.07	0.26*	1

%La percentage of ingested lactulose recovered in the urine, *%Ma* percentage of the ingested mannitol recovered in urine, *La/Ma* lactulose to mannitol ratio, *%Su* percentage of ingested sucrose recovered in the urine, *I-FABP* Intestinal fatty acid binding protein, *DAO* diamine oxidase
*$p < 0.05$
**$p < 0.01$
***$p < 0.001$
****$p < 0.0001$

Table 3 Anthropometric and clinical data (GSRS items) of D-IBS patients according to normal D-IBS(–) or altered D-IBS(+) small intestinal permeability

	D-IBS(–)	D-IBS(+)	
Anthropometric parameters			
Sex	2/19 (M/F)	4/14 (M/F)	
Age (yrs.)	39.89 ± 11.25	40.19 ± 13.24	ns
BMI	24.48 ± 2.69	23.44 ± 3.76	ns
GSRS single items			p
Nausea/vomiting	2.0 (1–6)	1.0 (1–4)	ns
Abdominal pain (colic pain)	2.0 (1–6)	4.5 (1–7)	ns
Gastric hunger pain	5.0 (1–7)	2.0 (1–6)	ns
Abdominal distension	5.0 (1–7)	5.0 (1–7)	ns
Burping	1.0 (1–7)	3.0 (1–7)	ns
Borborygmi	3.0 (1–7)	2.5 (1–7)	ns
Flatulence	5.0 (1–7)	3.0 (1–6)	ns
Increased passage of stools	1.0 (1–3)	1.0 (1–7)	ns
Bristol score	5.0 (3–6)	4.0 (3–7)	ns
Urgent bowel movement	3.0 (1–7)	3.0 (1–7)	ns
Feeling of incomplete defecation	4.0 (1–7)	3.0 (1–7)	ns
GSRS combination scores			
Abdominal pain	13.0 (8–25)	14.0 (6–25)	ns
Indigestion syndrome	19.0 (12–36)	19.5 (7–39)	ns
Diarrhea syndrome	8.0 (3–21)	6.0 (3–13)	ns

D-IBS diarrhoea-predominant IBS, *D-IBS* patients with a lactulose to mannitol ratio lower than 0.035 were considered D-IBS(–); patients with a ratio value equal to or higher than 0.035 as D-IBS(+). Continuous data are expressed as Mean ± SD, and discrete data are expressed as Median and range. Data were analysed by Mann Whitney test

levels of I-FABP were significantly ($p < 0.0001$) different among the four groups, and both D-IBS(+) and CD patients showed significantly ($p < 0.01$) higher levels than D-IBS(–) and HC subjects (Fig. 6B). Finally, DAO concentrations differed significantly ($p = 0.0002$) among the four groups. At the post hoc test, both D-IBS(+) and CD patients showed significantly ($p < 0.001$) higher circulating levels compared to D-IBS(–) patients (Fig. 6C).

Figure 7 reports the circulating levels of IL-6, IL-8, LPS, and TLR-4 in HC, D-IBS(–), D-IBS(+), and CD patients. Significant differences ($p = 0.0007$) were found in the IL-6 levels among the groups. D-IBS(+) and CD patients had significantly ($p < 0.05$) higher concentrations than D-IBS(–) patients and HC subjects (Fig. 7A). As concerns IL-8, D-IBS(+) and CD patients had significantly ($p < 0.01$) higher circulating levels compared to HC but not D-IBS(–) patients (Fig. 7B). LPS concentrations were significantly ($p = 0.0043$) different among the groups (Fig. 7C). At the post hoc test, D-IBS(+) patients showed the highest LPS levels reaching a significant ($p < 0.01$) difference compared to both D-IBS(–) patients and

HC subjects. Finally, TLR-4 did not show significant differences among the groups ($p = 0.669$) (Fig. 7D).

Discussion

Although contrasting and often unclear, many pieces of evidence suggest that alterations of the intestinal barrier may play an essential role in the pathogenesis of IBS, particularly in its diarrhoea-predominant variant [27]. A defective epithelial barrier function, which can be measured as increased gut permeability, could facilitate passage of luminal antigens and lead to a mucosal immune response. The identification of increased s-IP in patients with D-IBS may become relevant from a therapeutic perspective [28].

In the present study, we firstly focused on the evaluation of the D-IBS symptom profile, the urinary and serum markers of the GI epithelium function and inflammatory parameters. Then, we compared the obtained findings with those from CD patients and healthy subjects.

In spite of their well-known different aetiology, D-IBS and CD patients were not different in their symptomatology as concerns bowel habits and abdominal symptoms. This finding may account for the limited ability of questionnaires in efficiently discriminating between patients, due to the frequent overlapping symptom profiles, as also described in other GI diseases [29]. Moreover, it suggests the need for new strategies for IBS classification and diagnosis, with the use of new bio-humoral markers that can help clinicians in its management. In this context, our cohort of D-IBS patients showed significantly lower levels of La/Ma ratio and I-FABP levels compared to CD patients. This finding may be imputable to the minor altered epithelium permeability as well as the less evident damage in the intestinal integrity in D-IBS patients compared to patients suffering from systemic autoimmune diseases (e.g., celiac disease, considered here as a putative positive control). Evident alterations in GI permeability characterise celiac disease, and as expected, the excretions of Su, La, and Ma as well as the La/Ma ratio were significantly different from those in the HC group. These data are in full agreement with the previously reported alterations in CD patients for gastric and s-IP, the latter characterised by both modifications of TJ and decreased mucosal absorptive surface [30]. In line with the results obtained with urinary markers, serum levels of I-FABP were higher in CD patients compared to both D-IBS patients and HC subjects. As a further demonstration of the close relationship between altered s-IP and mucosal damage, I-FABP strongly and positively correlated with either %La or La/Ma ratio. Finally, zonulin levels were also significantly higher in CD patients than in HC subjects, in full accordance with published data [31].

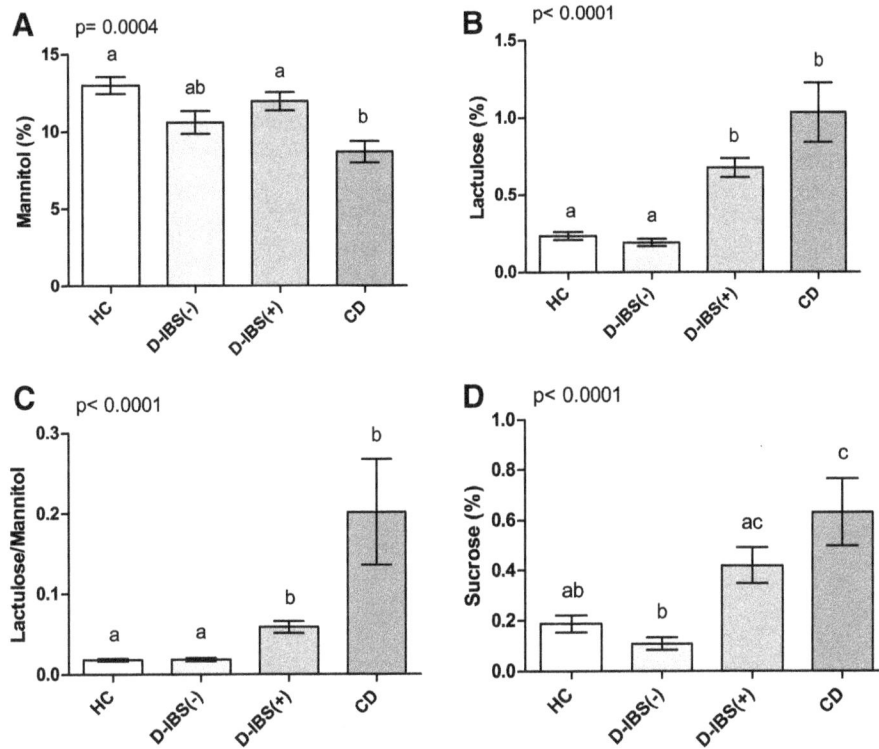

Fig. 5 Urinary markers of gastrointestinal barrier function in HC, D-IBS(−),D-IBS(+) patients, and CD patients HC = healthy controls. D-IBS = diarrhoea-predominant IBS. D-IBS patients with a Lactulose to Mannitol ratio lower than 0.035 were considered D-IBS(−). D-IBS patients with a ratio value equal to or higher than 0.035 were considered as D-IBS(+). CD = celiac disease. Urinary parameters of gastrointestinal permeability are expressed as percentages of ingested sugars recovered in urine: **A** mannitol (%Ma), **B** lactulose (%La), **C** the La/Ma ratio, and **D** sucrose (%Su). Data are expressed as Mean ± SEM and analysed by Kruskal-Wallis test with Dunn's Multiple Comparison Test. Means sharing the same superscript are not significantly different from each other (*p* < 0.05, Dunn's test)

As a whole group, D-IBS patients did not significantly differ from HC subjects for the secretion of the urinary markers of GI permeability. Unfortunately, there is no uniformity of data on this issue. Some papers already reported no alterations in the GI permeability of IBS patients [32–34], whereas other studies described impairment in the GI barrier function when D-IBS patients were evaluated [28, 35, 36]. These divergent findings could be due to either the different methods applied or the different criteria adopted for patient selection and diagnosis. Additionally, recent studies showed that epithelial barrier dysfunction is localised only to the

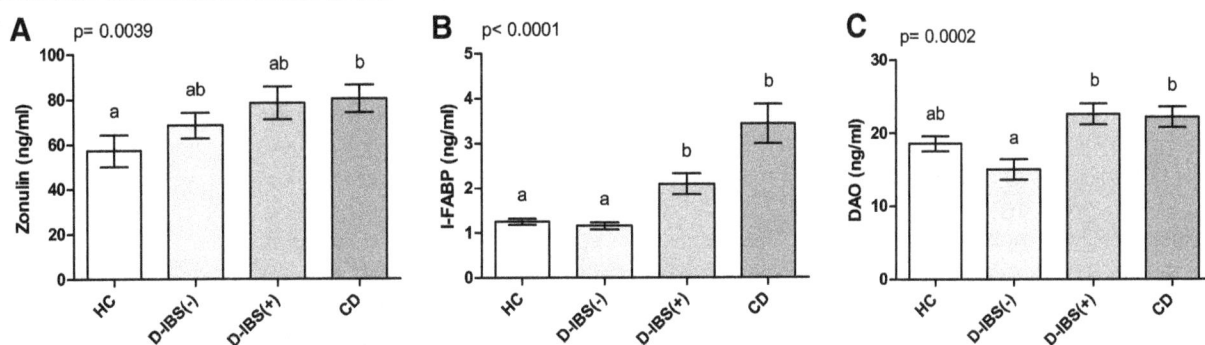

Fig. 6 Circulating markers of intestinal barrier function in HC, D-IBS(−), D-IBS(+) patients, and CD patients. HC = healthy controls. D-IBS = diarrhoea-predominant IBS. D-IBS patients with a Lactulose to Mannitol ratio lower than 0.035 were considered D-IBS(−). D-IBS patients with a ratio value equal to or higher than 0.035 were considered as D-IBS(+). CD = celiac disease. Circulating parameters of gastrointestinal permeability are expressed as: **A** Zonulin; **B** I-FABP = Intestinal fatty acid binding protein; **C** DAO = diamine oxidase. Data are expressed as Mean ± SEM and analysed by Kruskal-Wallis test with Dunn's Multiple Comparison Test. Means sharing the same superscript are not significantly different from each other (*p* < 0.05, Dunn's test)

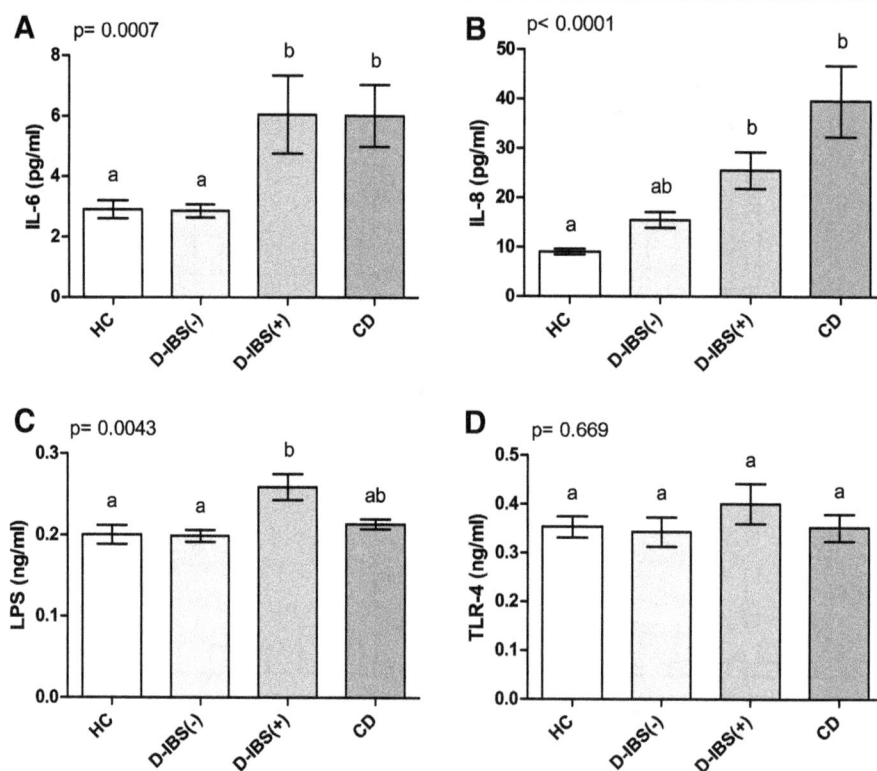

Fig. 7 Circulating levels of IL-6, IL-8, LPS, and TLR-4 in HC, D-IBS(−), D-IBS(+) patients, and CD patients. HC = healthy controls. D-IBS = diarrhoea-predominant IBS. D-IBS patients with a Lactulose to Mannitol ratio lower than 0.035 were considered D-IBS(−). D-IBS patients with a ratio value equal to or higher than 0.035 were considered as D-IBS(+). CD = celiac disease. **A** IL-6 = Interleukin-6; **B** IL-8 = Interleukin-8; **C** LPS = Lipopolysaccharide; **D** TLR-4 = Toll-like receptor 4. Data are expressed as Mean ± SEM and analysed by Kruskal-Wallis test with Dunn's Multiple Comparison Test. Means sharing the same superscript are not significantly different from each other (p < 0.05, Dunn's test)

small intestine in D-IBS patients, and no differences between IBS patients and controls in colonic permeability has been found [37]. However, the involvement of changes in colonic permeability in IBS is still under debate, since other studies reported increased colonic permeability [32].

Our results on the urinary markers of GI permeability were confirmed by those of zonulin and the serum integrity markers of the epithelium. Firstly, there were no significant differences between D-IBS patients and HC subjects in zonulin levels. These findings are congruent with a recent study by Ohlsson et al. [38]. In that study, subjects with a history of functional GI symptoms (IBS and also functional dyspepsia) had the same zonulin levels as those without symptoms. This result may not be unexpected if we consider that the pathophysiology of D-IBS is still under investigation and several agents might play a role in its aetiology. Although zonulin regulates TJ and IP permeability, a plethora of different proteins are known to participate in this regulation. So, in agreement with Ohlsson et al. [38], attention must be paid before considering only serum zonulin as a biomarker of s-IP. Secondly, as concerns I-FABP levels, following our results, the only

study available in the literature [33] showed no significant differences between HC and IBS patients, either before or after NSAID consumption, indicating the absence of damage to the intestinal epithelium in this functional GI disease. We also found no significant increase in the DAO serum levels of D-IBS patient compared to HC subjects, although this evidence is not in agreement with available data [19]. However, given the limited experience in the clinical use of serum DAO by our and other groups, it needs to be verified by further investigation. Of note, the analysis of the pro-inflammatory IL-8 and IL-6 showed higher levels in D-IBS patients compared to HC subjects, although statistical significance was present only for the former cytokine. This finding supports the notion of low-grade inflammation in this disease [10]. Besides, significant correlations between these pro-inflammatory cytokines and the circulating and urinary markers of GI permeability were found in the whole population studied. These pieces of evidence suggest the close relationship between the changes in barrier function and inflammatory processes. Under physiological conditions, the GI epithelium provides an effective barrier between the internal and external environment, protecting the body from potentially harmful luminal substances such as bacterial products, digestive enzymes, and antigens. The loss of integrity of the GI barrier is accompanied by an increase in epithelial permeability, reflecting a state in which luminal substances can permeate the barrier and enter the systemic circulation, where they may contribute to a systemic inflammatory response and organ dysfunction [12].

Another aim of the present work was to evaluate D-IBS patients according to the presence of normal or increased s-IP. Categorisation was performed to investigate whether this alteration could affect the symptom profile as well as biomarkers of gut barrier function and inflammation. In our study, 46% of D-IBS patients showed increased s-IP as diagnosed by the La/Ma ratio, in spite of the absence of significant differences in the symptom profile.

To date, differences in the symptomatology between D-IBS patients with normal or increased s-IP have not been investigated in-depth. In 2009, Zhou et al. [39] observed that 39% of the evaluated D-IBS patients had increased IP, which was associated with an increased severity index score of functional bowel disorder and with hypersensitivity to visceral and thermal nociceptive pain stimuli. More recently, Li et al. [37] demonstrated that 47% of D-IBS patients with increased s-IP tend to be more severely impaired with regard to psychological effects and quality of life. In particular, the authors found that D-IBS patients with increased s-IP were experiencing higher levels of psychological stress than those with normal s-IP. It has been hypothesised that stress can lead to a more permeable intestinal wall that increases the availability of water, sodium, and energy-rich substances necessary to meet the increased metabolic demand induced by the stressors. Besides, the stress-induced increases in IP raise the possibility of bacterial translocation, which in turn can stimulate an innate and adaptive immune response [37, 40].

In the present study, the alterations of the mucosal barrier in D-IBS(+) patients resembled those found in CD patients. As for the urinary markers of permeability, D-IBS(+) showed La/Ma ratio values not significantly different from those in CD patients, but three-fold higher than those in D-IBS(–) patients. The latter group, in turn, had a La/Ma ratio equal to that of HC subjects and significantly different from that of CD patients. Of note, the two D-IBS groups did not show significant differences in Ma excretion. As a consequence, the functional integrity of Ma recovery reflecting the transcellular pathway lets us hypothesise that our D-IBS patients did not suffer from villous atrophy. Besides, per inclusion criteria, D-IBS patients had to be negative for serologic markers of CD.

Additionally, the higher La excretion in D-IBS(+) patients compared to D-IBS(–) and HC subjects

suggests that impairment in the paracellular permeability characterises the small intestinal epithelium of D-IBS(+) patients. These data encourage us to further investigate the possible alterations in the TJ proteins, such as the Claudin and Occludin families [10]. Lastly, D-IBS(+) patients also had higher Su excretion than D-IBS(–) ones, with values closer to those in CD patients. This evidence allows us to hypothesise that D-IBS(+) patients might also suffer from an increase in gastro-duodenal permeability.

The urinary markers were in agreement with significantly higher levels of I-FABP and DAO observed in D-IBS(+) patients compared to D-IBS(–) ones, with the former showing values similar to those in CD patients. This evidence suggests the loss of integrity of the intestinal epithelium in D-IBS(+) patients. Enterocytes express I-FABP and DAO abundantly, and in the present study, significant correlations were found between these proteins and the La/Ma ratio in the overall population. Probably, some injury to the enterocytes could increase the release of I-FABP and DAO and compromise s-IP, even though it may not be solely responsible, as already observed in response to other physiological stressors [41].

The significant differences in these circulating proteins along with those of the La pathway proved that the D-IBS group was not a homogeneous class regarding s-IP and that two subtypes can be identified.

Moreover, the two D-IBS subtypes showed a different inflammatory status, as demonstrated by the higher IL-6, IL-8 and LPS levels in D-IBS(+) patients compared to D-IBS(–) patients. Based on these data, we can suppose that the altered GI barrier function observed in the former group may allow easier passage of bacteria and inflammatory agents through the mucous layer of the intestine. In turn, this cascade of events could also influence the course of the disease.

A major limitation of this case-control study was that the investigated parameters might not give an overview of whether bacterial translocation is mutually related to the observed alterations of s-IP in our D-IBS(+) patients. Thus, the analysis of IP in the large bowel (e.g., by analysing the urinary excretion of sucralose) as well as the investigation of the microbiota of these patients may improve the clinical relevance of the present findings. Another limitation was that the influence of hormones on gut permeability and differences between the genders concerning IBS and CD were not evaluated due to the small number of patients for gender subgroups. The role of sex steroids in the regulation of IP has not been fully elucidated, even if oestrogens can significantly modulate GI motility and visceral hypersensitivity [42]. CD is more frequent in women than men. Women suffer from nausea/vomiting and constipation, while greasy stools are more prevalent in men. Besides, depression, osteoporosis, fibromyalgia and unexplained hypochromic anaemia predominate in women [43]. Further investigation is needed to demonstrate how gender may influence s-IP as well as circulating biomarkers of GI barrier function.

Conclusion

Our current study is of particular interest, since it demonstrates the presence of significant differences in the profiles of biomarkers related to the intestinal barrier function among HC, D-IBS, and CD patients. Besides, present data support the concept that the intestinal barrier injury and low-grade inflammation could be involved in the pathophysiology of D-IBS, even if they represent a feature that is not always detectable and two distinct D-IBS subtypes could be identified. The investigation of possible s-IP alterations (i.e., considering the La/Ma ratio) might be useful to assess better and categorise this heterogeneous D-IBS population.

Abbreviations

%La: Percentage of ingested lactulose recovered in the urine; %Ma: Percentage of ingested mannitol recovered in the urine; %Su: Percentage of ingested sucrose recovered in the urine; BMI: Body mass index; CD: Celiac disease; C-IBS: Constipation-predominant IBS; DAO: Diamine oxidase; D-IBS: Diarrhoea-predominant IBS; ELISA: Enzyme-link immunosorbent assay; EMA: Anti-endomysium antibodies; GFD: Gluten free diet; GI: Gastrointestinal; GSRS: Gastrointestinal Symptom Rating Scale; HC: Healthy Controls; IBS: Irritable bowel syndrome; I-FABP: Intestinal fatty acid binding protein; IgA: Immunoglobulin A; IL-6: Interleukin-6; IL-8: Interleukin-8; La: Lactulose; LPS: Lipopolysaccharide; Ma: Mannitol; s-IP: Small intestinal permeability; Su: Sucrose; TJ: Tight junction; TLR-4: Toll-like receptor 4; tTG: Tissue transglutaminase

Acknowledgements

The authors thank Dr. Marianna Annese, HCA (IRCCS "Saverio de Bellis"), for her valuable technical assistance.

Funding

Italian Ministry of Health RC21-2015. The funding body had no role in the design of the study and collection, analysis and interpretation of data and in writing the manuscript.

Authors' contributions

ML and FR were responsible for data analysis and interpretation, wrote the manuscript and contributed to the intellectual content of the article; ML and CC performed the experiments; GR, BD, CC, and AO collected and interpreted the data and made intellectual contributions to the article. All authors participated in the study to a significant extent and read and approved the submitted manuscript.

Competing interests

The authors declare that they have no competing interests.

References

1. Usai P, Manca R, Lai MA, Russo L, Boi MF, Ibba I, Giolitto G, Cuomo R. Prevalence of irritable bowel syndrome in Italian rural and urban areas. Eur J Intern Med. 2010;21(4):324–6.
2. Drossman DA, Dumitrascu DL, Rome III. New standard for functional gastrointestinal disorders. J Gastrointestin Liver Dis. 2006;15(3):237–41.
3. Mearin F. Irritable bowel syndrome (IBS) subtypes: nothing resembles less an IBS than another IBS. Rev Esp Enferm Dig. 2016;108(2):57–8.
4. Blake MR, Raker JM, Whelan K. Validity and reliability of the Bristol stool form scale in healthy adults and patients with diarrhoea-predominant irritable bowel syndrome. Aliment Pharmacol Ther. 2016;44(7):693–703.
5. Shahbazkhani B, Forootan M, Merat S, Akbari MR, Nasserimoghadam S, Vahedi H, Malekzadeh R. Coeliac disease presenting with symptoms of irritable bowel syndrome. Aliment Pharmacol Ther. 2003;18(2):231–5.
6. Lebwohl B, Sanders DS, Green PHR. Coeliac disease. Lancet. 2018; 391(10115):70–81.
7. Heyman M, Abed J, Lebreton C, Cerf-Bensussan N. Intestinal permeability in coeliac disease: insight into mechanisms and relevance to pathogenesis. Gut. 2012;61(9):1355–64.
8. Gonzalez-Castro AM, Martinez C, Salvo-Romero E, Fortea M, Pardo-Camacho C, Perez-Berezo T, Alonso-Cotoner C, Santos J, Vicario M. Mucosal pathobiology and molecular signature of epithelial barrier dysfunction in the small intestine in irritable bowel syndrome. J Gastroenterol Hepatol. 2017;32(1):53–63.
9. Schumann M, Siegmund B, Schulzke JD, Fromm M. Celiac disease: role of the epithelial barrier. Cell Mol Gastroenterol Hepatol. 2017;3(2):150–62.
10. Piche T. Tight junctions and IBS--the link between epithelial permeability, low-grade inflammation, and symptom generation? Neurogastroenterol Motil. 2014;26(3):296–302.
11. Lopetuso LR, Scaldaferri F, Bruno G, Petito V, Franceschi F, Gasbarrini A. The therapeutic management of gut barrier leaking: the emerging role for mucosal barrier protectors. Eur Rev Med Pharmacol Sci. 2015;19(6):1068–76.
12. van Wijck K, Bessems BA, van Eijk HM, Buurman WA, Dejong CH, Lenaerts K. Polyethylene glycol versus dual sugar assay for gastrointestinal permeability analysis: is it time to choose? Clin Exp Gastroenterol. 2012;5:139–50.
13. Bischoff S, Bischoff SC, Barbara G, Buurman W, Ockhuizen T, Schulzke JD, Serino M, Tilg H, Watson A, Wells JM. Intestinal permeability - a new target for disease prevention and therapy. BMC Gastroenterol. 2014;14:189.
14. van Wijck K, Verlinden TJ, van Eijk HM, Dekker J, Buurman WA, Dejong CH, Lenaerts K. Novel multi-sugar assay for site-specific gastrointestinal permeability analysis: a randomized controlled crossover trial. Clin Nutr. 2013;32(2):245–51.
15. Aguirre Valadez JM, Rivera-Espinosa L, Mendez-Guerrero O, Chavez-Pacheco JL, Garcia Juarez I, Torre A. Intestinal permeability in a patient with liver cirrhosis. Ther Clin Risk Manag. 2016;12:1729–48.
16. Sturgeon C, Fasano A. Zonulin, a regulator of epithelial and endothelial barrier functions, and its involvement in chronic inflammatory diseases. Tissue Barriers. 2016;4(4):e1251384.
17. Pelsers MM, Hermens WT, Glatz JF. Fatty acid-binding proteins as plasma markers of tissue injury. Clin Chim Acta. 2005;352(1–2):15–35.
18. Honzawa Y, Nakase H, Matsuura M, Chiba T. Clinical significance of serum diamine oxidase activity in inflammatory bowel disease: importance of evaluation of small intestinal permeability. Inflamm Bowel Dis. 2011;17(2):E23–5.
19. Xu XJ, Zhang YL, Liu L, Pan L, Yao SK. Increased expression of nerve growth factor correlates with visceral hypersensitivity and impaired gut barrier function in diarrhoea-predominant irritable bowel syndrome: a preliminary explorative study. Aliment Pharmacol Ther. 2017;45(1):100–14.
20. Svedlund J, Sjodin I, Dotevall G. GSRS--a clinical rating scale for gastrointestinal symptoms in patients with irritable bowel syndrome and peptic ulcer disease. Dig Dis Sci. 1988;33(2):129–34.
21. Schmulson M, Lee OY, Chang L, Naliboff B, Mayer EA. Symptom differences in moderate to severe IBS patients based on predominant bowel habit. Am J Gastroenterol. 1999;94(10):2929–35.

Noninvasive biomarkers of gut barrier function identify two subtypes of patients suffering from diarrhoea...

237

22. Verdu EF, Armstrong D, Murray JA. Between celiac disease and irritable bowel syndrome: the "no man's land" of gluten sensitivity. Am J Gastroenterol. 2009;104(6):1587–94.

23. El-Salhy M, Hatlebakk JG, Gilja OH, Hausken T. The relation between celiac disease, nonceliac gluten sensitivity and irritable bowel syndrome. Nutr J. 2015;14:92.

24. Antonioli DA. Celiac disease: a progress report. Mod Pathol. 2003;16(4):342–6.

25. Russo F, Linsalata M, Clemente C, D'Attoma B, Orlando A, Campanella G, Giotta F, Riezzo G. The effects of fluorouracil, epirubicin, and cyclophosphamide (FEC60) on the intestinal barrier function and gut peptides in breast cancer patients: an observational study. BMC Cancer. 2013;13:56.

26. Linsalata M, D'Attoma B, Orlando A, Guerra V, Russo F. Comparison of an enzymatic assay with liquid chromatography-pulsed amperometric detection for the determination of lactulose and mannitol in the urine of healthy subjects and patients with active celiac disease. Clin Chem Lab Med. 2014;52(4):e61–4.

27. Martinez C, Gonzalez-Castro A, Vicario M, Santos J. Cellular and molecular basis of intestinal barrier dysfunction in the irritable bowel syndrome. Gut Liver. 2012;6(3):305–15.

28. Mujagic Z, Ludidi S, Keszthelyi D, Hesselink MA, Kruimel JW, Lenaerts K, Hanssen NM, Conchillo JM, Jonkers DM, Masclee AA. Small intestinal permeability is increased in diarrhoea predominant IBS, while alterations in gastroduodenal permeability in all IBS subtypes are largely attributable to confounders. Aliment Pharmacol Ther. 2014;40(3):288–97.

29. Russo F, Chimienti G, Clemente C, Riezzo G, D'Attoma B, Martulli M. Gastric activity and gut peptides in patients with functional dyspepsia: postprandial distress syndrome versus epigastric pain syndrome. J Clin Gastroenterol. 2017;51(2):136–44.

30. Vogelsang H, Schwarzenhofer M, Oberhuber G. Changes in gastrointestinal permeability in celiac disease. Dig Dis. 1998;16(6):333–6.

31. Vorobjova T, Raikkerus H, Kadaja L, Talja I, Uibo O, Heilman K, Uibo R. Circulating Zonulin correlates with density of enteroviruses and Tolerogenic dendritic cells in the small bowel mucosa of celiac disease patients. Dig Dis Sci. 2017;62(2):358–71.

32. Del Valle-Pinero AY, Van Deventer HE, Fourie NH, Martino AC, Patel NS, Remaley AT, Henderson WA. Gastrointestinal permeability in patients with irritable bowel syndrome assessed using a four probe permeability solution. Clin Chim Acta. 2013;418:97–101.

33. Kerckhoffs AP, Akkermans LM, de Smet MB, Besselink MG, Hietbrink F, Bartelink IH, Busschers WB, Samsom M, Renooij W. Intestinal permeability in irritable bowel syndrome patients: effects of NSAIDs. Dig Dis Sci. 2010;55(3):716–23.

34. Gecse K, Roka R, Sera T, Rosztoczy A, Annahazi A, Izbeki F, Nagy F, Molnar T, Szepes Z, Pavics L, et al. Leaky gut in patients with diarrhea-predominant irritable bowel syndrome and inactive ulcerative colitis. Digestion. 2012; 85(1):40–6.

35. Rao AS, Camilleri M, Eckert DJ, Busciglio I, Burton DD, Ryks M, Wong BS, Lamsam J, Singh R, Zinsmeister AR. Urine sugars for in vivo gut permeability: validation and comparisons in irritable bowel syndrome-diarrhea and controls. Am J Physiol Gastrointest Liver Physiol. 2011;301(5):G919–28.

36. Dunlop SP, Hebden J, Campbell E, Naesdal J, Olbe L, Perkins AC, Spiller RC. Abnormal intestinal permeability in subgroups of diarrhea-predominant irritable bowel syndromes. Am J Gastroenterol. 2006;101(6):1288–94.

37. Li L, Xiong L, Yao J, Zhuang X, Zhang S, Yu Q, Xiao Y, Cui Y, Chen M. Increased small intestinal permeability and RNA expression profiles of mucosa from terminal ileum in patients with diarrhoea-predominant irritable bowel syndrome. Dig Liver Dis. 2016;48(8):880–7.

38. Ohlsson B, Orho-Melander M, Nilsson PM. Higher levels of serum Zonulin may rather be associated with increased risk of obesity and hyperlipidemia, than with gastrointestinal symptoms or disease manifestations. Int J Mol Sci. 2017;18(3):582.

39. Zhou Q, Zhang B, Verne GN. Intestinal membrane permeability and hypersensitivity in the irritable bowel syndrome. Pain. 2009;146(1–2):41–6.

40. de Punder K, Pruimboom L. Stress induces endotoxemia and low-grade inflammation by increasing barrier permeability. Front Immunol. 2015;6:223.

41. March DS, Marchbank T, Playford RJ, Jones AW, Thatcher R, Davison G. Intestinal fatty acid-binding protein and gut permeability responses to exercise. Eur J Appl Physiol. 2017;117(5):931–41.

42. Mulak A, Tache Y. Sex difference in irritable bowel syndrome: do gonadal hormones play a role? Gastroenterol Pol. 2010;17(2):89–97.

43. Rubio-Tapia A, Jansson-Knodell CL, Rahim MW, See JA, Murray JA. Influence of gender on the clinical presentation and associated diseases in adults with celiac disease. Gac Med Mex. 2016;152(Suppl 2):38–46.

Permissions

List of Contributors

Daniel Stram and Neal Tambe
Department of Preventive Medicine, Keck School of Medicine of University of Southern California, Los Angeles, California, USA

Jane C. Figueiredo
Department of Preventive Medicine, Keck School of Medicine of University of Southern California, Los Angeles, California, USA
Samuel Oschin Comprehensive Cancer Institute, Cedars-Sinai Medical Center, Los Angeles, California, USA

Christopher Haiman and Veronica Wendy Setiawan
Department of Preventive Medicine, Keck School of Medicine of University of Southern California, Los Angeles, California, USA
Norris Comprehensive Cancer Center, Keck School of Medicine of University of Southern California, Los Angeles, California, USA

Wendy Cozen
Department of Preventive Medicine, Keck School of Medicine of University of Southern California, Los Angeles, California, USA
Norris Comprehensive Cancer Center, Keck School of Medicine of University of Southern California, Los Angeles, California, USA
Department of Pathology, Keck School of Medicine, University of Southern California, Los Angeles, California, USA

Jacqueline Porcel
Norris Comprehensive Cancer Center, Keck School of Medicine of University of Southern California, Los Angeles, California, USA

James Buxbaum
Department of Medicine, Keck School of Medicine, University of Southern California, Los Angeles, California, USA

Lynne Wilkens and Loic Le Marchand
Epidemiology Program, University of Hawaii Cancer Center, Honolulu, Hawaii, USA

Sonia Alonso, Adriana-René Guerra, Lourdes Carreira, Juan-Ángel Ferrer, María-Luisa Gutiérrez and Conrado M. Fernandez-Rodriguez
Unit of Gastroenterology, Hospital Universitario Fundación Alcorcón, Av. Budapest-1, 28922 Alcorcon, Madrid, Spain

Nai-Hsuan Chien
Cathay General Hospital, Taipei, Taiwan
School of Medicine, Fu Jen Catholic University, New Taipei, Taiwan
Sijhih Cathay General Hospital, New Taipei, Taiwan

Chi-Yang Chang and Jaw-Town Lin
School of Medicine, Fu Jen Catholic University, New Taipei, Taiwan
Division of Gastroenterology, Fu-Jen Catholic University Hospital, New Taipei, Taiwan
Division of Gastroenterology, E-Da Hospital/I-Shou University, Kaohsiung, Taiwan

Yao-Chun Hsu
School of Medicine, Fu Jen Catholic University, New Taipei, Taiwan
Division of Gastroenterology, Fu-Jen Catholic University Hospital, New Taipei, Taiwan
Division of Gastroenterology, E-Da Hospital/I-Shou University, Kaohsiung, Taiwan
No.510, Zhongzheng Rd., Xinzhuang Dist, New Taipei City 24205, Taiwan

Yen-Tsung Huang
Institute of Statistical Science, Academia Sinica, Taipei, Taiwan

Chun-Ying Wu
Division of Gastroenterology, Taichung Veterans General Hospital, Taichung, Taiwan
Faculty of Medicine, School of Medicine, National Yang-Ming University, Taipei, Taiwan

Ming-Shiang Wu
Department of Internal Medicine, National Taiwan University Hospital, Taipei, Taiwan

Jia-Horng Kao
Department of Internal Medicine, National Taiwan University Hospital, Taipei, Taiwan
Graduate Institute of Clinical Medicine, National Taiwan University, Taipei, Taiwan

Lein-Ray Mo
Department of Internal Medicine, Tainan Municipal Hospital, Tainan, Taiwan

Chi-Ming Tai and Chih-Wen Lin
Division of Gastroenterology, E-Da Hospital/I-Shou University, Kaohsiung, Taiwan

Tzeng-Huey Yang
Department of Internal Medicine, Lotung Poh-Ai Hospital, Yilan Country, Taiwan

Lianjun Di, Huichao Wu, Rong Zhu, Youfeng Li, Rui Xie, Hongping Li, Haibo Wang, Hua Zhang, Hong Xiao, Kui Zhao and Bigung Tuo
Department of Gastroenterology, Affiliated Hospital, Zunyi Medical College, Zunyi 563003, China
Digestive Endoscopy Center, Affiliated Hospital, Zunyi Medical Colleage, Zunyi, China

Xinglong Wu and Hong Zhen
Department of Pathology, Affiliated Hospital, Zunyi Medical College, Zunyi, China

Hui Chen
Department of Anesthesiology, Affiliated Hospital, Zunyi Medical College, Zunyi, China

Xuefeng Yang and Ming Xie
Department of Gastrointestinal Surgery, Affiliated Hospital, Zunyi Medical College, Zunyi, China

Nadeem Kalak and Edith Holsboer-Trachsler
Psychiatric Clinics of the University of Basel, Centre for Affective, Stress and Sleep Disorders, University of Basel, Wilhelm Klein-Strasse 27, Ch-4012 Basel, Switzerland

Serge Brand
Psychiatric Clinics of the University of Basel, Centre for Affective, Stress and Sleep Disorders, University of Basel, Wilhelm Klein-Strasse 27, Ch-4012 Basel, Switzerland
Department of Sport, Exercise and Health, Sport Science Section, University of Basel, Basel, Switzerland
Substance Abuse Prevention Research Center; Sleep Disorders Research Center, Psychiatry Department, Kermanshah University of Medical Sciences, Kermanshah, Iran

Laura Mählmann
Psychiatric Clinics of the University of Basel, Centre for Affective, Stress and Sleep Disorders, University of Basel, Wilhelm Klein-Strasse 27, Ch-4012 Basel, Switzerland
United Nations University - Maastricht Economic and Social Research Institute on Innovation and Technology (UNU-MERIT), Maastricht University, Maastricht, The Netherlands

Raoul I. Furlano and Corinne Legeret
Pediatric Gastroenterology and Nutrition, University Children's Hospital Basel, Basel, Switzerland

Markus Gerber
Department of Sport, Exercise and Health, Sport Science Section, University of Basel, Basel, Switzerland

Sarah K. Schäfer and Nicolas Becker
Department of Psychology, Saarland University, Saarbrücken, Germany

Kathrin Julia Weidner
University Mannheim, I. Medical Clinic-Cardiology, Pneumology and Angiology Mannheim, Mannheim, Germany

Jorge Hoppner
University Heidelberg, Clinic for Diagnostic and Interventional Radiology Heidelberg, Heidelberg, Germany

Dana Friedrich, Caroline S. Stokes and Frank Lammert
Saarland University, Department of Medicine II – Gastroenterology und Endocrinology, Homburg, Germany

Volker Köllner
Department of Psychosomatic Medicine, Rehabilitation Clinic Seehof, Lichterfelder Allee 55, 14513 Teltow, Germany
Psychosomatic Rehabilitation Research Group, Department of Psychosomatic Medicine, Center for Internal Medicine and Dermatology Charité – Universitätsmedizin Berlin, Berlin, Germany

Qi Cheng and Xiaoyan Shao
State Key Laboratory of Pharmaceutical Biotechnology, Jiangsu Key Laboratory of Molecular Medicine and School of Medicine, Nanjing University, Nanjing, Jiangsu Province, China

Xianwen Yuan
State Key Laboratory of Pharmaceutical Biotechnology, Jiangsu Key Laboratory of Molecular Medicine and School of Medicine, Nanjing University, Nanjing, Jiangsu Province, China
Department of Hepatobiliary Surgery, the Affiliated Drum Tower Hospital of Nanjing University Medical School, Nanjing 210008, Jiangsu Province, China

Bin Xue
State Key Laboratory of Pharmaceutical Biotechnology, Jiangsu Key Laboratory of Molecular Medicine and School of Medicine, Nanjing University, Nanjing, Jiangsu Province, China
State Key Laboratory of Natural Medicines, China Pharmaceutical University, Nanjing, Jiangsu Province, China

Liver Disease Collaborative Research Platform of Medical School of Nanjing University, 22Hankou Road, Gulou District, Nanjing 210093, Jiangsu Province, China

Xiaolei Shi, Yitao Ding and Xitai Sun
Department of Hepatobiliary Surgery, the Affiliated Drum Tower Hospital of Nanjing University Medical School, Nanjing 210008, Jiangsu Province, China

Jun Chen
Department of Pathology, the Affiliated Drum Tower Hospital of Nanjing University Medical School, Nanjing, Jiangsu Province, China

Yinjuan Zhao
Collaborative Innovation Center of Sustainable Forestry in Southern China, College of Forestry, Nanjing Forestry University, Nanjing, China

Pengzi Zhang and Yan Bi
Department of Endocrinology, the Affiliated Drum Tower Hospital of Nanjing University Medical School, Nanjing, Jiangsu Province, China

Jacob J. Hughey
Department of Biomedical Informatics, Vanderbilt University School of Medicine, Nashville, TN, USA

Bonnie K. Ray
Talkspace, New York, NY, USA

Anne R. Lee
Celiac Disease Center, Columbia University Medical Center, New York, NY, USA

Kristin N. Voorhees
BeyondCeliac, Ambler, PA, USA

Ciaran P. Kelly
Division of Gastroenterology, Beth Israel Deaconess Medical Center, Boston, MA, USA

Detlef Schuppan
Division of Gastroenterology, Beth Israel Deaconess Medical Center, Boston, MA, USA
Institute of Translational Immunology, University Medical Center, Mainz, Germany

Liu Hui
Department of Clinical Immunology, Dalian Medical University, Dalian 116044, People's Republic of China

Daiki Hirano, Shiro Oka, Kyoku Sumimoto, Yuki Ninomiya, Yuzuru Tamaru, Kenjiro Shigita, Yuji Urabe and Kazuaki Chayama
Department of Gastroenterology and Metabolism, Hiroshima University Hospital, 1-2-3 Kasumi, Minami-ku, Hiroshima 734-8551, Japan

Shinji Tanaka and Nana Hayashi
Department of Endoscopy, Hiroshima University Hospital, Hiroshima, Japan

Koji Arihiro
Department of Anatomical Pathology, Hiroshima University Hospital, Hiroshima, Japan

Yasuhiko Kitadai
Department of the Faculty of Human Culture and Science, Prefectural University of Hiroshima, Hiroshima, Japan

Fumio Shimamoto
The Faculty of Humanities and Human Sciences, Hiroshima Shudo University Hiroshima, Hiroshima, Japan

Amit Goel, Ankur Singh and Avani Sasi
Department of Gastroenterology, Sanjay Gandhi Postgraduate Institute of Medical Sciences, Lucknow 226014, India

Aditya Narayan Sarangi and Rakesh Aggarwal
Department of Gastroenterology, Sanjay Gandhi Postgraduate Institute of Medical Sciences, Lucknow 226014, India
Biomedical Informatics Center, Sanjay Gandhi Postgraduate Institute of Medical Sciences, Lucknow, India

Hanifah Oswari, Fatima Safira Alatas, Badriul Hegar, William Cheng and Arnesya Pramadyani
Department of Child Health, Gastrohepatology Division, Cipto Mangunkusumo Hospital, Faculty of Medicine, Universitas Indonesia, Jakarta, Indonesia

Marc Alexander Benninga
Department of Pediatric Gastroenterology and Nutrition, Emma Children's, Hospital, Academic Medical Centre, Amsterdam, The Netherlands

Shaman Rajindrajith
Department of Paediatrics, University of Kelaniya, Ragama 11010, Sri Lanka

Wei Lu, Yan-Bing Wang and Zhan-Qing Zhang
Department of Hepatology, Shanghai Public Health Clinical Center, Fudan University, Caolang Road 2901, Shanghai 201508, China

Xiao-Nan Zhang
Research Unit, Shanghai Public Health Clinical Center, Fudan University, Caolang Road 2901, Shanghai 201508, China

Qi-Cheng Weng
Shanghai Representative Office, Fujirebio Inc., Shanghai, China

Yan-Ling Feng
Department of Clinical Pathology, Shanghai Public Health Clinical Center, Fudan University, Shanghai, China

A. Drori, D. Rotnemer-Golinkin, L. Zolotarev and Y. Ilan
Gastroenterology and Liver Units, Department of Medicine, Hadassah-Hebrew University Medical Center, -91120 Jerusalem, IL, Israel

S. Avni O. Danay and D. Levanon
Migal, Galilee Research Institute, Kiryat Shmona, Israel

A. Drori and J. Tam
Obesity and Metabolism Laboratory, The Institute for Drug Research, School of Pharmacy, Faculty of Medicine, The Hebrew University of Jerusalem, Jerusalem, Israel

Chia-Chen Lin and Shih-Huan Su
School of Medicine, College of Medicine, Chang-Gung University, 5, Fu-Xin street, Quain San, TaoYuan 330, Taiwan

Yi-Cheng Chen, Chun-Yen Lin and I-Shyan Sheen
School of Medicine, College of Medicine, Chang-Gung University, 5, Fu-Xin street, Quain San, TaoYuan 330, Taiwan
Division of Hepatology, Department of Hepato Gastroenterology, Chang-Gung Memorial Hospital, Linkou Medical Center, TaoYuan, Taiwan

Wen-Juei Jeng, Chien-Hao Huang, Wei Teng and Wei-Ting Chen
Division of Hepatology, Department of Hepato Gastroenterology, Chang-Gung Memorial Hospital, Linkou Medical Center, TaoYuan, Taiwan

Shoji Yamada, Toshiaki Nakaoka and Masaki Kimura
Division of Pharmacotherapeutics, Faculty of Pharmacy, Keio University, 1-5-30 Shiba-Kohen, Minato-ku, Tokyo 105-8512, Japan

Yoshimasa Saito and Hidetsugu Saito
Division of Pharmacotherapeutics, Faculty of Pharmacy, Keio University, 1-5-30 Shiba-Kohen, Minato-ku, Tokyo 105-8512, Japan
Division of Gastroenterology and Hepatology, Department of Internal Medicine, Keio University, Shinjuku-ku, Tokyo 160-8582, Japan

Nobuhiko Kamada
Division of Gastroenterology, Department of Internal Medicine, The University of Michigan Medical School, Ann Arbor, MI 48109, USA

Takeru Amiya, Nobuhiro Nakamoto and Takanori Kanai
Division of Gastroenterology and Hepatology, Department of Internal Medicine, Keio University, Shinjuku-ku, Tokyo 160-8582, Japan

Chieko Ejima
Research Institute, EA Pharma Co. Ltd, Kawasaki, Kanagawa 210-8681, Japan

Wenfei Li, Hongjie Chen, Shuai Wu and Jie Peng
Department of Infectious Diseases, Nanfang Hospital of Southern Medical University, Guangzhou 510515, China

Jian Yang, Bin Yan, Lihong Yang and Jie Zheng
Clinical Research Center, the First Affiliated Hospital, Xi'an Jiaotong University, Xi'an 710061, People's Republic of China

Huimin Li, Yajuan Fan and Xiancang Ma
Department of Psychiatry, the First Affiliated Hospital, Xi'an Jiaotong University, No.277 Yanta West Road, Yanta District, Xi'an 710061, People's Republic of China

Feng Zhu
Center for Translational Medicine, the First Affiliated Hospital, Xi'an Jiaotong University, Xi'an 710061, People's Republic of China

Jesús-Miguel Herrero, Pablo Vega, María Salve and Joaquín Cubiella
Department of Gastroenterology, Complexo Hospitalario Universitario de Ourense, Ourense, Spain
Instituto de Investigación Biomédica Galicia Sur, Centro de Investigación Biomédica en Red de Enfermedades Hepáticas y Digestivas (CIBERehd), , Ourense, Spain

Luis Bujanda
Donostia Hospital, Biodonostia Institute, University of the Basque Country UPV/EHU, CIBERehd, San Sebastian, Spain

Nadia Pallotta, Giuseppina Vincoli, Danilo Badiali, Piero Vernia and Enrico Stefano Corazziari
Dipartimento di Medicina Interna e Specialità Mediche, Università "Sapienza", Policlinico "Umberto I", V.le del Policlinico, 155, 00161 Rome, Italy

Patrizio Pezzotti
Dipartimento di Malattie Infettive, Istituto Superiore di Sanità, Rome, Italy

Maurizio Giovannone and Alessandro Gigliozzi
UOC di Gastroenterologia, Ospedale San Camillo De Lellis, Rieti, Italy

Xinchun Liu, Qiuyang Chen, Junli Wu, Wentao Gao, Kuirong Jiang, Yi Miao and Jishu Wei
Pancreas Center, The First Affiliated Hospital of Nanjing Medical University, 300 Guangzhou Road, Nanjing, Jiangsu Province, China
Pancreas Institute, Nanjing Medical University, Nanjing, China

Yue Fu
Pancreas Center, The First Affiliated Hospital of Nanjing Medical University, 300 Guangzhou Road, Nanjing, Jiangsu Province, China
Department of Gastrointestinal Surgery, The Affiliated Changzhou No.2 People's Hospital of Nanjing Medical University, Changzhou, China

Qiang Li, Leilei Pei and Hong Yan
Department of Epidemiology and Health Statistics, School of Public Health, Xi'an Jiaotong University Health Science Center, Xi'an, China

Song Leng
Department of Epidemiology and Health Statistics, School of Public Health, Xi'an Jiaotong University Health Science Center, Xi'an, China
Health Management Center, The Second Hospital of Dalian Medical University, Dalian, China

Rui Liang
Health Management Center, The Second Hospital of Dalian Medical University, Dalian, China

Ai Zhao
School of Public Health, Peking University Health Science Center, Beijing, China

Wei Zheng
Division of Endocrinology and Metabolism, Department of obstetrics, Beijing Obstetrics and Gynecology Hospital, Capital Medical University, Beijing, China

Norio Akuta, Yusuke Kawamura, Yasuji Arase, Satoshi Saitoh, Shunichiro Fujiyama, Hitomi Sezaki, Tetsuya Hosaka, Masahiro Kobayashi, , Yoshiyuki Suzuki, Fumitaka Suzuki, Kenji Ikeda and Hiromitsu Kumada
Department of Hepatology, Toranomon Hospital and Okinaka Memorial Institute for Medical Research, 2-2-2 Toranomon, Minato-ku, Tokyo 105-0001, Japan

Mariko Kobayashi
Liver Research Laboratory, Toranomon Hospital, Tokyo, Japan

Yingmei Jia, Chang Li, Zhi Dong, Kun Huang, Yanji Luo, Xuehua Li, Canhui Sun, Shi-Ting Feng and Zi-Ping Li
Department of Radiology, The First Affiliated Hospital, Sun Yat-Sen University, 58th, The Second Zhongshan Road, Guangzhou 510080, Guangdong, China

Xiaoyan Yang
Department of Radiology, Shenzhen Traditional Chinese Medicine Hospital, Shenzhen 518000, China

Sara Massironi, Clorinda Ciafardini, Susanna Bernasconi, Dario Conte and Maddalena Peracchi
Gastroenterology and Endoscopy Unit, Fondazione IRCCS Ca' Granda Ospedale Maggiore Policlinico, Milan, Italy

Federica Cavalcoli and Alessandra Zilli
Gastroenterology and Endoscopy Unit, Fondazione IRCCS Ca' Granda Ospedale Maggiore Policlinico, Milan, Italy
Department of Pathophysiology and Transplantation, Università degli Studi di Milano, Milan, Italy

Alessandro Del Gobbo
Division of Pathology, Fondazione IRCCS Ca' Granda Ospedale Maggiore Policlinico, 20122 Milan, Italy

Irene Felicetta
Laboratory of Clinical Chemistry and Microbiology, Fondazione IRCCS Ca' Granda Ospedale Maggiore Policlinico, Milan, Italy

Michele Linsalata, Giuseppe Riezzo, Benedetta D'Attoma, Caterina Clemente, Antonella Orlando and Francesco Russo
Laboratory of Nutritional Pathophysiology, National Institute of Gastroenterology, "S. de Bellis" Research Hospital, Via Turi 27, I-70013 Castellana Grotte, Bari, Italy

Index

www.ingramcontent.com/pod-product-compliance
Lightning Source LLC
Chambersburg PA
CBHW080508200326
41458CB00012B/4126